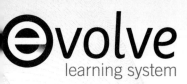
evolve
learning system

To access your Student Resources, visit:

http://evolve.elsevier.com/Jenkins/Hollinshead/

Register today and gain access to:

- **Answers to chapter Review Questions and Exercises from the book**

- **WebLinks**
  An exciting source that lets you link to hundreds of websites carefully chosen to supplement the content of the textbook by chapter

- **Labeling exercises**
  Exercises that reinforce what you have learned from the book

ELSEVIER

Hollinshead's

Functional Anatomy of the Limbs and Back

Hollinshead's Functional Anatomy of the Limbs and Back

NINTH EDITION

DAVID B. JENKINS, PhD
Chair, Department of Growth, Development and Structure
Head, Section of Anatomy
School of Dental Medicine
Southern Illinois University
Alton, Illinois

SAUNDERS

SAUNDERS
ELSEVIER

11830 Westline Industrial Drive
St. Louis, Missouri 63146

HOLLINSHEAD'S FUNCTIONAL ANATOMY OF THE LIMBS AND BACK, NINTH EDITION 978-1-4160-4980-7

Notice

Knowledge and best practice in this field are constantly changing. As new research and experience broaden our knowledge, changes in practice, treatment and drug therapy may become necessary or appropriate. Readers are advised to check the most current information provided (i) on procedures featured or (ii) by the manufacturer of each product to be administered, to verify the recommended dose or formula, the method and duration of administration, and contraindications. It is the responsibility of the practitioner, relying on their own experience and knowledge of the patient, to make diagnoses, to determine dosages and the best treatment for each individual patient, and to take all appropriate safety precautions. To the fullest extent of the law, neither the Publisher nor the Author assumes any liability for any injury and/or damage to persons or property arising out of or related to any use of the material contained in this book.

The Publisher

Library of Congress Cataloging-in-Publication Data

Jenkins, David B.
   Hollinshead's functional anatomy of the limbs and back / David B. Jenkins. — 9th ed.
      p. ; cm.
   Includes bibliographical references and index.
   ISBN 978-1-4160-4980-7 (pbk. : alk. paper)
   1. Extremities (Anatomy) 2. Back—Anatomy. I. Title. II. Title: Functional anatomy of the limbs and back.
   [DNLM: 1. Musculoskeletal System—anatomy & histology. 2. Movement. 3. Musculoskeletal Physiology. WE 101 J52h 2009]
   QM548.J46 2009
   611'.98—dc22

                                        2008034348

Vice President and Publisher: Linda Duncan
Executive Editor: Kathy Falk
Senior Developmental Editor: Christie M. Hart
Publishing Services Manager: Catherine Jackson
Senior Project Manager: Gena Magouirk-Singh
Design Direction: Jessica Williams

Printed in Canada.

Last digit is the print number: 9 8 7 6 5 4 3 2 1

*To the most important people in my life—my wife, Rita, and our family—
Kathie and Daren, Ben and Paige, Tim and Michelle, and grandsons,
Brad, Adam, Josh and Zach—for their love, support, and understanding.*

PREFACE

Dr. W. Henry Hollinshead, while heading the Section of Anatomy at the Mayo Clinic, realized a deficiency in available anatomical texts and wrote the first edition of what was then called *Functional Anatomy of the Limbs and Back*. His basic premise for creating the book was "to provide a readable account of that portion of anatomy which is of particular interest to those interested in the functions of muscle and movements of the body," a text which could be utilized by the "beginning non-medical student of muscular movement" and as a "ready reference or review for the more advanced student or the medical graduate especially interested in this field." With the death of Dr. Hollinshead before work on the sixth edition was started, the book's title was changed to *Hollinshead's Functional Anatomy of the Limbs and Back* in honor of a friend, mentor, colleague, and superb anatomist who contributed so much to the discipline. As the text has evolved through its numerous subsequent editions, the main coverage has remained true to the title, and it has been expanded to provide a more complete coverage of the body to create a better resource for those who use the book.

With the ninth edition, additional modifications will be evident. The text has been edited and modified, and the terminology has been updated to conform to the internationally accepted *Terminologia Anatomica: International Anatomical Terminology* developed by the Federative Committee on Anatomical Terminology. New "Analyses of Activities and Associated Movements" have been added. These discussions demonstrate the correlation between anatomy and function and illustrate how they relate to everyday activities. At the end of each chapter, separate sections with review questions and exercises have been expanded. These are included to assist readers in evaluating their understanding of the material and to provide examples of questions and practical exercises that can be used as a basis for developing additional questions for testing comprehension. Since anatomy is such a visual discipline, considerable emphasis has been placed upon evaluation and revision of the artwork. Over 60 new illustrations have been created to replace some of the original figures. Of the artwork that remains from the previous edition, significant changes have been made in the labeling, content, and color.

I hope you find the ninth edition of *Hollinshead's Functional Anatomy of the Limbs and Back* to be an informative, user-friendly, and useful resource in your studies and career. Anatomy is a fascinating discipline, particularly when you apply the information functionally and clinically.

David B. Jenkins, PhD

ACKNOWLEDGMENTS

I extend my sincere thanks to Christie Hart, Kathy Falk, Gena Magouirk-Singh, and all at Elsevier who contributed to the preparation of this edition. To Jodie Bernard, Lima Colati, and the art team at LASERWORDS, thank you for the illustrations you modified and created and your patience through numerous revisions. Thanks also to Rita Jenkins for her capable help in text preparation.

CONTENTS

SECTION 1   **THE ORGANIZATION OF THE BODY**

CHAPTER 1   **Anatomical Terminology, *1***
    Introduction to Terminology, *1*
    Regions and Parts of the Body, *2*
    Anatomical Position and Terms of Direction and Relationship, *2*
    Planes of the Body, *3*
    Terms of Movement, *4*
    Center and Line of Gravity, *4*

CHAPTER 2   **Tissues of the Body, *8***
    Epithelial Tissue, *8*
    Connective Tissue, *9*
    Muscle Tissue, *14*
    Nervous Tissue, *16*

CHAPTER 3   **Organs and Organ Systems, *19***
    Skeletal System, *19*
    Muscular System, *26*
    Nervous System, *38*
    Circulatory System, *50*
    Digestive System, *53*
    Respiratory System, *53*
    Urogenital System, *53*
    Endocrine System, *53*
    Skin, *54*

SECTION 2   **THE UPPER LIMB**

CHAPTER 4   **General Survey of the Upper Limb, *57***
    Development, *57*
    Skeleton, *58*
    Muscles, *58*
    Nerves, *60*
    Arteries, *60*
    Veins, *61*
    Bursae, *62*

CHAPTER 5   **The Shoulder, *64***
    General Considerations, *64*
    Movements of the Scapula and Arm, *65*
    Bones and Joints of the Shoulder, *66*
    Fascia and Superficial Nerves and Vessels, *72*
    Axilla, *73*
    Muscles, *79*
    Movements of the Shoulder, *90*
    Bursae and Shoulder Lesions, *97*
    Nerve Injuries: Brachial Plexus, *98*
    Analyses of Activities and Associated Movements, 102

CHAPTER 6   **The Arm, *107***
    General Considerations, *107*
    Bones and Joints, *108*
    Fascia and Superficial Nerves and Vessels, *112*
    Muscles, *114*
    Nerves and Vessels, *117*
    Movements at the Elbow Joint, *121*
    Analyses of Activities and Associated Movements, 123

CHAPTER 7   Forearm and Hand: General
             Survey, *126*
                 General Considerations, *126*
                 Movements, *127*
                 Nerves and Arteries, *128*
                 Bones and Joints, *128*
                 Fascia and Superficial Nerves
                     and Vessels, *130*

CHAPTER 8   Flexor Forearm, *133*
                 Bones, *133*
                 Muscles, *134*
                 Nerves and Vessels, *139*

CHAPTER 9   Extensor Forearm, *147*
                 Muscles, *147*
                 Nerves and Vessels, *152*

CHAPTER 10   Radioulnar and Wrist
             Movements, *159*
                 Movements at the Radioulnar
                     Joints, *159*
                 Movements at the Wrist
                     Joint, *160*
                 *Analyses of Activities and
                     Associated Movements, 164*

CHAPTER 11   The Hand, *167*
                 General Considerations, *167*
                 Bones and Joints, *167*
                 The Palmar Fascia, *173*
                 The Flexor Synovial Sheaths,
                     Tendons, and Lumbrical
                     Muscles, *174*
                 Fascial Spaces of the Palm, *177*
                 Muscles, *177*
                 Nerves and Vessels, *182*
                 Dorsum of the Hand, *188*
                 Nerve Injuries, *190*

CHAPTER 12   Movements of the Digits, *195*
                 Flexion of the Fingers, *195*
                 Extension of the Fingers, *196*
                 Abduction and Adduction
                     of the Digits, *197*
                 Movements of the Little
                     Finger, *197*

                 Movements of the Thumb, *197*
                 Types of Grips Involved in
                     Grasping, *199*
                 *Analyses of Activities and
                     Associated Movements, 201*

SECTION 3   **THE BACK**
CHAPTER 13   The Back, *204*
                 General Considerations, *204*
                 Vertebral Column, *204*
                 Vertebrae, *206*
                 Joints of the Vertebral
                     Column, *210*
                 Movements and Stability, *216*
                 Musculature of the Back, *219*
                 The Meninges and the Spinal
                     Cord, *229*
                 *Analyses of Activities and
                     Associated Movements, 235*

SECTION 4   **THE LOWER LIMB**
CHAPTER 14   General Survey of the Lower
             Limb, *238*
                 General Considerations, *238*
                 Development, *238*
                 Skeleton, *239*
                 Muscles, *241*
                 Nerves, *241*
                 Arteries, *241*
                 Veins, *243*

CHAPTER 15   The Bony Pelvis, Femur, and Hip
             Joint, *245*
                 Bones and Joints of the Bony
                     Pelvis, *245*
                 Femur and Hip Joint, *249*
                 Movements, *253*

CHAPTER 16   The Thigh and Knee, *255*
                 General Considerations, *255*
                 Bones and Joints, *256*
                 Fascia and Superficial Nerves
                     and Vessels of the Thigh, *261*
                 Lumbar Plexus, *261*
                 Muscles, *263*
                 Anteromedial Nerves
                     and Vessels, *272*

CHAPTER 17   Gluteal Region and Posterior
                   Thigh, 279
                       Sacral Plexus, 279
                       Fascia and Superficial Nerves
                          and Vessels of the Gluteal
                          Region, 281
                       Muscles, 281
                       Nerves and Vessels, 289
                       Movements of the Bony
                          Pelvis, 292

CHAPTER 18   Movements of the Thigh
                   and Leg, 294
                       Movements at the Hip
                          Joint, 294
                       Movements at the Knee
                          Joint, 299
                       Maintenance of Stability at
                          the Hip and Knee Joints, 302
                       *Analyses of Activities and
                          Associated Movements, 303*

CHAPTER 19   The Leg, 307
                       General Considerations, 307
                       Bones, 308
                       Fascia and Superficial Nerves
                          and Vessels, 310
                       Muscles, 312
                       Nerves and Vessels, 320
                       Movements of the Foot, 323
                       *Analyses of Activities and
                          Associated Movements, 329*

CHAPTER 20   The Foot, 332
                       General Considerations, 332
                       Bones and Joints, 332
                       Superficial Nerves and
                          Vessels, 340
                       Fascia and the Plantar
                          Aponeurosis, 340
                       Plantar Muscles, 341
                       Plantar Nerves and Vessels, 347
                       Dorsum of the Foot, 349
                       Movements of the Toes, 351
                       The Ankle and Foot in
                          Supporting Weight, 351
                       Gait, 353

SECTION 5   THE HEAD, NECK,
                   AND TRUNK
CHAPTER 21   The Head and Neck, 356
                       Skull, 356
                       Meninges and Brain, 360
                       Facial Muscles, 364
                       Orbit, 366
                       Muscles of Mastication and the
                          Temporomandibular Joint, 367
                       Muscles of the Tongue, 370
                       Muscles of the Neck, 372
                       Pharynx, Larynx, Trachea,
                          and Esophagus, 377
                       Nerves and Vessels, 378
                       Surface Anatomy, 386

CHAPTER 22   The Thorax, 389
                       Thoracic Wall, 389
                       Pleural and Pericardial Sacs, 393
                       Thoracic Viscera, 395
                       Vessels, 398
                       Nerves, 398
                       Surface Anatomy, 399

CHAPTER 23   The Abdomen and Pelvis, 401
                       Abdominal Wall, 401
                       Pelvic Floor and Perineum, 405
                       Abdominal Viscera, 407
                       Pelvic Viscera, 411
                       Vessels, 411
                       Nerves, 413
                       Surface Anatomy, 413

Suggested Readings/References, 415
Glossary, 417
Index, 421

Hollinshead's

Functional Anatomy of the Limbs and Back

SECTION 1

The Organization
of the Body

1 ANATOMICAL TERMINOLOGY

CHAPTER CONTENTS

Introduction to Terminology

Regions and Parts of the Body

Anatomical Position and Terms of Direction
and Relationship

Planes of the Body

Terms of Movement

Center and Line of Gravity

INTRODUCTION TO TERMINOLOGY

Learning and understanding the terminology of any discipline are key components to mastery of the information. In the anatomical sciences, much of the terminology originated from Latin and Greek roots. Over the years, several published official guidelines have modified these terms to better fit the modern languages in which they were being used and to standardize the terms. The most recent guidelines, *Terminologia Anatomica: International Anatomical Terminology* (Federative Committee on Anatomical Terminology, 1998), were approved by the International Federation of Associations of Anatomists to provide an internationally accepted terminology for anatomy. Many commonly used, well-established terms have been modified or replaced to provide more clarity and to minimize the confusion associated with some of the older terms. For example, the terms *common peroneal nerve* and *peroneus longus muscle*, two structures within the leg, have been changed to *common fibular nerve* and *fibularis longus muscle*, respectively. Although *peroneal* and *peroneus* are derived from the Greek term *perone*, meaning "fibula," for those not familiar with the derivation, *fibular* and *fibularis* localize the terms to the leg

1

through an association with a bone of the leg, the fibula.

Not all terms, even with the new terminology, enable immediate recognition, but a medical dictionary can be consulted to obtain information on the original meaning of the term. In studying anatomy, it is most beneficial to understand the terminology rather than to simply memorize it. This makes the material easier to learn, because the terminology has meaning.

Eponyms (terms incorporating the proper name of an individual) have commonly been used in anatomy. Although a list of eponyms has been included in the new terminology, use of eponyms is discouraged.

This edition of *Hollinshead's Functional Anatomy of the Limbs and Back* contains the terminology presented in *Terminologia Anatomica*. When appropriate, older terms have been included parenthetically with the new term so that the reader is not at a disadvantage when using older textbooks or when communicating with instructors and clinicians who use other terminology.

REGIONS AND PARTS OF THE BODY

The major subdivisions of the body are the head, neck, trunk, and limbs. Although the terms for these subdivisions are commonly used in anatomy, the subdivisions also have Latin names that are used in many terms related to these areas. The Latin term for **head** is *caput*, and *capitis* means "of the head." The Latin term for **neck** is *collum; cervix* also means "neck," especially its anterior part, and *nucha* refers to its posterior part. Therefore, *colli* means "of the neck," and the terms *cervical* and *nuchal* or *nuchae* are also used in referring to structures in the neck.

The word **trunk** is obviously the same as the Latin *truncus*, but there is no particular reason to use the latter word. The Latin names for the subdivisions of the trunk, however, need to be understood. The Latin word for chest is *thorax*, and this word is often used in this form, in its possessive form, *thoracis* (which means "of the chest"), and in its adjectival form, *thoracic*. The term *abdomen* refers to the part of the trunk with muscular walls that lies below the thorax. It is most easily translated as the word "belly", but because this is considered inelegant and there is no acceptable translation, the words *abdomen* and *abdominal* are used. ("Stomach", commonly used and understood to mean the abdomen, means no such thing. The stomach is one of many organs in the abdominal cavity.) The lowest part of the trunk is the *pelvis* (meaning "basin"), and the Latin term is always used for this area. *Pelvic* is the adjective pertaining to the pelvis.

The Latin word for **limb** is *membra* (member), but this has no common usage. *Appendage* is a term long used by zoologists to describe limbs in general and sometimes appears in human anatomy in the adjectival form *appendicular*. The limbs are typically designated as the *upper and lower limbs*. Names of smaller subdivisions of the limbs are discussed in later chapters.

ANATOMICAL POSITION AND TERMS OF DIRECTION AND RELATIONSHIP

Certain general terms describe surfaces of the body, planes through the body, and relative positions of one structure to another. The surfaces of the trunk are described as the *anterior (ventral)*, or front, surface; the *posterior (dorsal)*, or back, surface; and the *lateral* surfaces, or sides. The *cranium* is the skull, and *cephalon* is the Greek word for *head;* therefore, both *cranial* and *cephalic* mean "toward the head." Similarly, *caudal* means "toward the tail" or, in humans, toward where the tail would be had it persisted from embryonic life.

These terms are all understandable regardless of the position of the body. However, in order to understand other terms, the orientation of the body must first be established. For instance, *superior,* meaning "up" or "upward," implies a relation to gravity and might differ entirely in meaning according to whether the person is erect, lying on the back, or standing on the head. For this reason, such terms of relative position should always be used in relation to a fixed position of the body, termed the anatomical position. The **anatomical position** (Fig. 1-1) is an erect position with the heels together and the feet

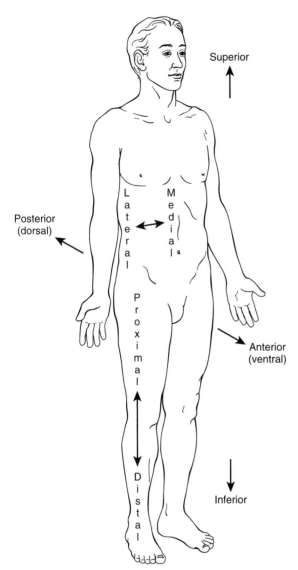

Figure 1-1 The anatomical position and terms of position.

Superior — toward the head

Inferior — toward the feet

Anterior (ventral) — toward the front of the body

Posterior (dorsal) — toward the back of the body

Medial — closer to the median plane of the body or midline of a structure

Lateral — farther from the median plane of the body or midline of a structure

Proximal — closer to the trunk or point of origin

Distal — farther from the trunk or point of origin

Superficial — closer to the surface

Deep — farther from the surface

For the limbs, some confusion might exist in regard to whether the terms *medial* and *lateral* refer to the body as a whole or to the limb itself. The little finger is medial to the other fingers in regard to the midline of the hand, but it is lateral, as is the thumb, in regard to the midline of the body. In this case, it is best to use *medial* and *lateral* only when referring to the limb as a whole and to its relation to the body in the anatomical position. If relative mediolateral relationships of structures within the limb are to be described, the terms *radial* and *ulnar* or *tibial* and *fibular* would be more meaningful. These terms refer to the paired bones of the limbs. In the upper limb, the radius is on the thumb side and the ulna on the little finger side (see Fig. 4-1), and in the lower limb, the tibia is on the side of the big toe and the fibula is on the side of the little toe (see Fig. 14-2). The sides of the limbs are therefore named according to the positions of these bones.

PLANES OF THE BODY

Considering the body in the anatomical position, several planes can be defined (Fig. 1-2). The **median plane** passes vertically through the body, dividing it into right and left halves; the median plane is occasionally referred to as a *median sagittal* or *midsagittal plane*. A **sagittal plane** parallels the median plane, dividing the body into unequal right and left parts. A **frontal (coronal) plane** divides the body into an anterior and a posterior portion, running approximately parallel with the coronal suture of the skull. A **transverse (horizontal) plane** divides the body or limbs into upper and lower parts; it is oriented at a right angle to the long axis of the body or limb.

pointing somewhat outward (laterally), the arms by the sides, and the palms facing forward or anteriorly. With reference to the anatomical position, *superior* always means "toward the head" and is used interchangeably with *cephalic* or *cranial*. Similarly, *inferior* means "toward the feet" and is usually synonymous with *caudal*. These and other terms are defined as follows (see Fig. 1-1):

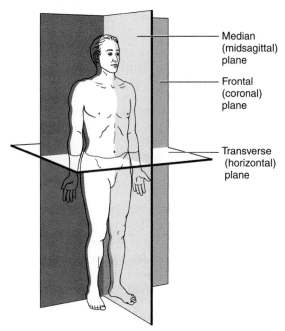

Median (midsagittal) plane

Frontal (coronal) plane

Transverse (horizontal) plane

Figure 1-2 Planes of the body.

TERMS OF MOVEMENT

The movement of **flexion,** which means "bending," decreases the angle between two parts and brings the original anterior surfaces closer together (Figs. 1-3 and 1-4). In flexion of the forearm at the elbow, the forearm initially moves anteriorly in a sagittal plane (see Fig. 1-3, *B*). In flexion of the leg at the knee (see Fig. 1-4, *B*), the leg moves posteriorly (approximating the original anterior surfaces). **Extension,** the opposite of flexion, usually straightens out a bent part. If movement is continued, it is often termed **hyperextension. Abduction** means "moving apart," or away from the midline, and **adduction,** the reverse, means "moving together," or toward the midline; both of these terms are particularly useful in describing movements of the limbs (see Figs. 1-3 and 1-4). **Protraction** means moving a part forward or anteriorly; **retraction** means moving it backward or posteriorly. **Elevation** means lifting a part (moving it superiorly), while **depression** means lowering it (moving it inferiorly). **Rotation** is the twisting of a part around its longitudinal axis. **Lateral (external) rotation** occurs if the anterior surface of the part is turned laterally, and **medial (internal) rotation** occurs if it is turned medially. **Circumduction** is a combination of successive movements of flexion, abduction, extension, and adduction in such a way that the distal end of the part being moved, moves in a circle. More detailed descriptions of movements as they relate to specific regions are provided in later chapters.

CENTER AND LINE OF GRAVITY

Reference is made in this book to the center of gravity and the line of gravity, particularly in discussions of the stability and movements of the back and lower limbs. In brief, the **center of gravity,** or center of mass of the body, is considered the imaginary point around which the weight of all parts of the body is in balance. The location of this point depends on many factors, including the proportions of body parts, the distribution of fat and muscle mass in the body, posture, structural deformities, and external forces (such as in carrying a suitcase, in which extra weight is placed on one side of the body). In the "average" body, the center of gravity is *a point on the midline, just anterior to the level of the second sacral vertebra.* The **line of gravity** is a vertical line that passes through the center of gravity (Fig. 1-5).

In the erect human body, the line of gravity normally passes through the junctions of the various regions of the vertebral column: the skull with the cervical vertebrae, the cervical vertebrae with the thoracic vertebrae, the thoracic vertebrae with the lumbar vertebrae, and the lumbar vertebrae with the sacrum. At the hip, the line passes posterior to the joint but lies anterior to the knee and ankle joints. Muscles and ligaments help maintain the position of the body in relation to the line of gravity. Only minimal muscle activity at the vertebral column is necessary if the weight is balanced properly. Because of the position of the line of gravity at the hip and knee, weight supported by the lower limb helps keep these joints in extension, which limits muscle activity necessary to maintain the vertical support of the limb. The ligaments at these joints can provide much of the support needed in quiet standing. At the ankle, however, with the line of gravity passing anterior to the joint, there is a tendency of the joint to *dorsiflex*—that is, for the body to bend forward at the ankle joint. Muscle activity at this joint (particularly

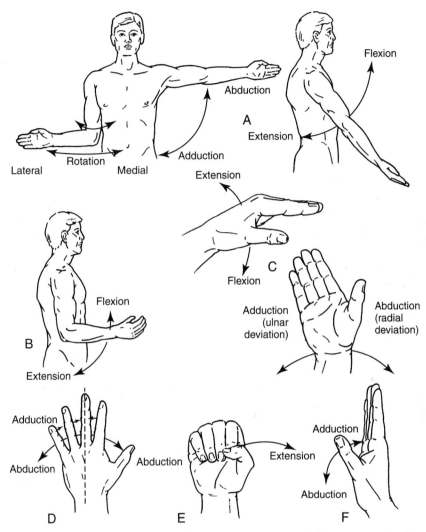

Figure 1-3 Movements of the upper limb. **A,** Movements at the glenohumeral joint. **B,** Movements at the elbow joint. **C,** Movements at the wrist joint. **D to F,** Movements of the digits. **D,** The *dashed line* indicates the midline axis of the hand, around which abduction and adduction of the four fingers are defined. **E,** All digits are in flexion, and the *arrow* indicates the direction of movement for extension of the thumb; note that this movement is in a different plane than is extension-flexion of each of the other digits. **F,** Abduction of the thumb moves the thumb away from the plane of the palm, and adduction moves it toward the plane of the palm.

of the calf muscles) is necessary to maintain the body in an erect and balanced position.

Any change in the distribution of weight (e.g., bending over, reaching out to pull a book from a shelf, or standing on one leg) results in a change in the center of gravity and also in the line of gravity. More muscles must then be used to maintain balance.

The feet provide a **base of support** for the erect body. This area of the ground is occupied by the feet and the space between them. To maintain balance, the line of gravity must fall within this area. The area can be increased by widening the stance or by adding another point of support, such as a cane. As the line of gravity moves toward the perimeter of the base of support, muscle activity increases. Once the line falls outside of the base of support, an erect position cannot be maintained without external support (e.g., a hand rail, a wall, or the support provided by another person).

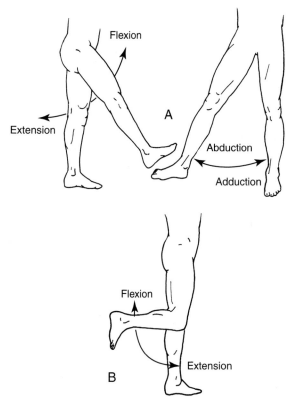

Figure 1-4 Movements of the lower limb. **A,** Movements at the hip joint. **B,** Movements at the knee joint.

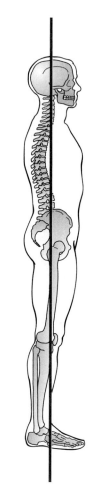

Figure 1-5 Line of gravity.

REVIEW QUESTIONS

1 Describe the anatomical position.

2 Define the following terms:
   a distal
   b lateral
   c anterior
   d superficial

3 Which structure has a more proximal position, the big toe or the patella (knee cap)? Which is positioned more medially, the big toe or the little toe?

4 Which plane divides the body into anterior and posterior parts? Which plane divides the body into right and left halves?

5 Which movement refers to moving toward the midline? Which refers to moving away from the midline?

6 Carrying a bucket of water on one side of the body would have what effect on the center and line of gravity? What is the effect if the bucket is positioned in front of the body and lifted with both upper limbs? What actions would be necessary to compensate for the weight of the bucket?

EXERCISES

1 Demonstrate the following movements:
   a flexion of the forearm at the elbow
   b extension of the thigh at the hip joint
   c abduction of the fingers
   d adduction (ulnar deviation) of the hand at the wrist
   e circumduction of the upper limb

2 Stand in an erect position with the feet about 1 foot apart. Lean anteriorly, posteriorly, and laterally, noting the increasing muscle activity as each movement progresses and the point where balance is lost. Try the same movements with the support of a cane (or an umbrella or a stick) and with the feet 2 feet apart. How do these changes (additional support and wider stance) affect the amount of movement possible before balance is lost?

2 TISSUES OF THE BODY

CHAPTER CONTENTS

Epithelial Tissue

Connective Tissue

Muscle Tissue

Nervous Tissue

The human body, like most of the better-organized forms of animal life, consists of various types of specialized cells and a varying amount of intercellular substance. Much of the actual weight of the body is water, both inside and outside the cells. The cells represent the living portion of the organism, whereas the intercellular substance, regardless of its nature, represents nonliving material that owes its existence to the activities of the cells.

Most types of cells tend to occur in groups in which the component parts are somewhat similar in appearance and in function. Such organized groups of cells are known as **tissues.** The tissues of the body, in turn, are not independent of one another. Tissues are combined to form more complex anatomical and functional units known as **organs** or **organ systems.**

According to their general appearance and functions, the various tissues of the body are usually classified into four major types: *epithelial tissue, connective tissue, muscular tissue,* and *nervous tissue.*

EPITHELIAL TISSUE

Epithelial tissue occurs most commonly in sheets and is adapted especially for covering other tissues (Fig. 2-1). It serves the general functions of protection, absorption, and secretion. An epithelium is characterized by cells that are closely packed, with a minimum of intercellular material between them. The cells have various shapes: flat ones, called *squamous* cells (*squama* means "scale," such as that of a fish); *cuboidal* cells, shaped somewhat like children's blocks; and tall *columnar* cells. There are many subvarieties in shape, general appearance, and function.

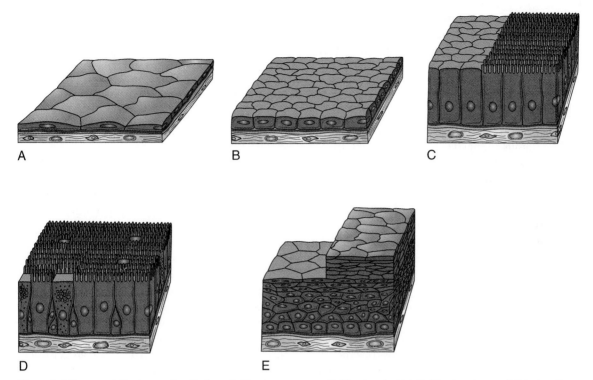

Figure 2-1 Representative types of epithelium. **A,** Simple squamous. **B,** Simple cuboidal. **C,** Simple columnar (ciliated on the right). **D,** Pseudostratified ciliated columnar. **E,** Stratified squamous (keratinized on the right).

An epithelium may take the form of a single-layered sheet of cells *(simple)*, a multilayered sheet *(stratified)*, or essentially tubular outgrowths (glands) from such sheets. A *pseudostratified* epithelium is one that seems to be stratified but really is composed of only one layer of cells. All of the cells are positioned in the base of the epithelium, but not all of them reach the surface of the epithelium.

One type of epithelium covers the external surface of the body as the outer layer of the skin (epidermis). It is a stratified or multilayered epithelium with dead outer cells *(keratinized layer)*. This stratified epithelium protects the more delicate deeper lying cells and helps seal off intercellular spaces from contact with the outside. Another type of epithelium, adapted for absorption and secretion, lines the digestive tract. Outgrowths from this epithelium form the digestive glands, including the characteristic cells of such large organs as the liver and pancreas. Other types of epithelium line the tubules of the kidneys, the ureters, and the urinary bladder and continue

along the urethra (the tube leading from the bladder) to unite with the epithelium of the skin. Therefore, epithelium occurs primarily either on the outside of the body or as a lining of the cavities of the body that communicate with the exterior.

Two specialized types of epithelium are also found lining closed cavities within the body. **Mesothelium** is a single-layered, squamous epithelium. It lines the four great cavities of the trunk: the two pleural cavities surrounding the lungs, the pericardial cavity surrounding the heart, and the peritoneal cavity surrounding the abdominal viscera. **Endothelium,** essentially similar to mesothelium in appearance, forms the inner linings of the heart, of all the blood vessels, and of the lymphatic vessels.

CONNECTIVE TISSUE

Connective tissue, in sharp contrast to epithelial tissue, has cells that are more widely dispersed and separated from each other by nonliving intercellular material. The presence and character of this inter-cellular material gives connective tissue its specific characteristics. (The category of connective tissue includes blood, but blood is not discussed here.)

Fibrous Connective Tissue

The most pervasive type of connective tissue in the body is **fibrous connective tissue** (Fig. 2-2). In this tissue, the spaces between the cells are occupied by numerous fibers that make the tissues tough and capable of withstanding distortions and strains. The fibers between the cells may be of several types. They may occur in the form of a loosely woven net, with large quantities of fluid in the intervening spaces within the net, or as an apparently solid structure, such as a tendon, with closely packed fibers and very little interfibrillar space.

The most common type of fiber found in connective tissue is the **collagen fiber.** These fibers are essentially nonelastic. When they occur in places in which some deformation must be possible, they are arranged in wavy bundles that allow movement until the slack of these bundles is taken up. **Elastic fibers** are the other important type of intercellular fibers. These fibers actually are elastic, as their name implies. They may be stretched, and when the tension on them is relaxed, they shorten again. They are frequently mixed with more numerous collagen fibers, but in certain locations, great bundles of almost pure elastic tissue are found.

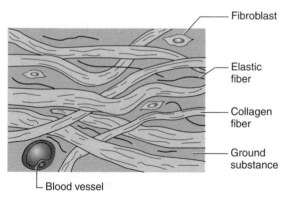

Figure 2-2 Connective tissue, illustrating collagen and elastic fibers embedded within the ground substance.

At intervals, in the spaces between connective tissue fibers, connective tissue cells occur. Some of these are responsible for the formation and repair of the connective tissue fibers; they are known as *fibroblasts.* Other cells possess the property of ingesting formed material. In this function, they may be aided by cells from the blood, some of which pass freely into the fibrous connective tissues as a part of the reaction of inflammation.

Collagen tissue, with or without elastic fibers, is the most widespread of all tissues. Taking various forms, they permeate and surround practically all the tissues of the body, serving as a binding agent for these tissues. If all the tissues of the body were removed so as to leave only the fibrous connective tissues, the essential organization of the body would still be represented and recognizable through the arrangement of this fibrous tissue.

The connective tissue underlying the epithelium (epidermis) of the skin is called the *dermis.* The dermis consists of a *papillary layer* of loose connective tissue immediately adjacent to the epidermis. The deeper lying part of the dermis, the *reticular layer,* is made up of dense irregular connective tissue. Most of fibers within the dermis are collagen fibers, but there are also elastic fibers to lend resiliency to the skin. The dermis of animals is the source of leather.

Deep to the skin, elastic and collagen fibers are more loosely woven (loose connective tissue) to form a subcutaneous layer, the *superficial fascia,* which allows movement of the skin over the deeper structures (see the following section). To a varying extent in different parts of the body and in different individuals, this subcutaneous connective tissue contains modified tissue cells that are filled with fat. If these fat cells are sufficiently numerous, the tissue is known as *adipose tissue* or *fat.*

Varying amounts of loose connective tissue, often containing fat, occur elsewhere throughout the body. This type of tissue forms padding between various organs, around blood vessels, and so forth. Special accumulations of connective tissue form the outer wall of blood vessels and surround and permeate nerves to bind their nerve fibers together. Epithelia are regularly supported by connective tissue. Muscles are surrounded and their cells are held together by connective tissue. Bone also contains large quantities of connective tissue fibers, and fibrous tissue permeates practically all the organs of the body.

FUNCTIONAL/CLINICAL NOTE 2-1

Because of its prevalence, fibrous connective tissue is almost always involved in any injury to the body. It normally plays an important part in the healing process. New connective tissue fibers form in the injured area and reunite the parts that were separated by the injury. Connective tissue formed in an attempt to repair an injury is known as **scar tissue.** If the injury is severe or of long duration, more scar tissue than necessary is formed to repair the defect. As this newly formed tissue grows older, the fibers shorten and become more densely packed together. They may form a hard mass of considerable size, which may—on a finger, for instance—interfere with movement of the part. Moreover, if the scar tissue is attached to a movable part—for example, a tendon in the finger that normally glides freely back and forth—it may interfere with movement by binding the part too closely to its less movable surroundings. As the scar tissue contracts and becomes denser, it may pull upon the tendon, which, in turn, forces the part to maintain a flexed and useless position. Therefore, scar tissue, although necessary for healing, also has its drawbacks. One of the common functions of a physical therapist or occupational therapist is to minimize the unwanted effects of scar formation after operation, accident, or disease, through the use of such methods as heat, massage, and exercise.

Fascia

When the normal connective tissues of the body are arranged in the form of enveloping sheaths, each layer is usually known as a **fascia** (meaning "bandage" or "band" and indicating a layer binding together other structures). The subcutaneous tissue is called the **superficial fascia.** Fascia deep to this superficial layer is termed **deep fascia.** Deep fascia can be especially well developed: for example, in the limbs, it forms heavy membranes surrounding the entire limb. Individual muscles are also surrounded by thin fascia called *perimysium* and are separated from each other by looser connective tissue. This is especially well developed where two adjacent muscles cross each other rather than running parallel. The fluid between the fibers of the tissue acts as a lubricant to allow free movement of one muscle upon the other. From the fascia surrounding a muscle, connective tissue septa pass into the muscle and subdivide it into bundles. These septa, in turn, divide until delicate connective tissue fibers surround each muscle fiber within a muscle.

In some locations between muscles, or between muscles or tendon and bone, or even beneath the skin over bony prominences, connective tissue spaces coalesce to form pocket-like accumulations of fluid. These structures are known as **bursae** (see Chapter 3).

Tendons and Ligaments

The connective tissue fibers of a fascia, although arranged in approximately the same plane to form membranes, run in various directions within this plane so that they appear interwoven, usually with no main direction of fibers predominating. In tendons and ligaments, in contrast, connective tissue fibers are arranged roughly parallel to one another and are closely packed to form definite cords or bands, specially adapted to resist movement in one direction.

Tendons are formed by heavy collagen bundles and delicate cross-fibers. A tendon is defined as such a bundle that attaches muscle to bone or, occasionally, to some other structure. A broad, flattened tendon is known as an **aponeurosis.** The tendons of most muscles are more narrow bands or, frequently, as is true of many of the tendons of the limbs, rounded cords. The fibers of the tendons are attached firmly to the muscle cells at one end; at the other end, they enter the bone and blend both with the connective tissue surrounding the bone (periosteum) and with the fibers within the bone itself.

Although most of the collagen fibers composing a tendon run in the same direction, they are not strictly parallel. Instead, they intertwine to form small bundles that, in turn, intertwine to form the larger parallel bundles that give tendons their distinctive appearance. Near the tendon's attachment to the bone, the larger tendon bundles also intertwine with each other. The end result is that the pull of any part of the muscle, instead of being limited to a tendon bundle originating in that part, is widely spread through the tendon.

Ligaments represent another type of dense connective tissue, frequently similar to tendons in appearance but uniting bone to bone rather than muscle to bone. Most ligaments are composed of dense collagenous tissue, but a few are almost pure elastic tissue.

Cartilage

A type of connective tissue that at first sight appears to have little in common with fibrous connective tissue is **cartilage.** Like fibrous connective tissue, however, cartilage consists largely of intercellular material that contains scattered cells. Although it is frequently not apparent, the groundwork of intercellular material of cartilage is a feltlike mass of fibrous tissue. This fibrous tissue is, in turn, impregnated by a matrix that renders it harder, tougher, and more homogeneous than ordinary fibrous tissue. The fibers within cartilage are usually collagenous in nature, but in cases in which brittleness would be a disadvantage, as in the cartilages of the external ear and the tip of the nose, the cartilages contain elastic fibers.

Cartilage serves as a supporting framework for softer tissues because it is more resistant to deformation than is fibrous connective tissue but less resistant, and therefore more resilient, than is bone. The embryonic and fetal skeletons consist almost entirely of cartilage, but in the adult skeleton, most of this cartilage has been replaced by bone, and cartilage is found in relatively few locations. The thyroid cartilage (Adam's apple) in the neck and the cartilaginous rings that support the trachea (windpipe) represent a supportive type of cartilage that is sufficiently strong to keep the airway to the lungs open and yet is less brittle than similar-sized bones would be. Because the most common type of cartilage, called **hyaline cartilage** due to its glassy appearance, has a much smoother surface than does bone, this type of cartilage is well suited for covering the ends of bones at joints that are freely movable. Hyaline cartilage typically forms the bearing surfaces between two adjacent bones as they move one upon the other. In other locations, where cartilage must support great crushing force, the collagen fibers within the cartilage are exceedingly heavy and prominent, and the cartilage is then known as **fibrocartilage.** Examples of fibrocartilage are the intervertebral discs, heavy pads forming a part of the vertebral column that must withstand the weight of the body while still allowing some movement between bones.

Bone

Bone is the hardest of the connective tissues and forms most of the skeleton of the adult human body. Like cartilage, bone consists of a fibrous connective tissue embedded in a more solid matrix. The matrix of bone contains a large amount of minerals, primarily in the form of tiny crystals of a complex compound of calcium and phosphorus, which are responsible for the hardness of bone.

FUNCTIONAL/CLINICAL NOTE 2-2

In young children, in whom the deposition of calcium has not been completed, the fibrous tissue of bone overbalances the mineral content, and the bone has toughness without adequate hardness. Therefore, the bones of young children are relatively easily deformed by weight bearing, and when young bones are broken, they tend to break irregularly, splintering like a greenstick. The disproportion between crystalline minerals and fibers leads to this splintering, which is termed a **greenstick fracture** because of its appearance. In young adults, the balance between calcium deposit and fibrous content of the bone is usually well maintained so that the bone possesses both maximum hardness and resistance to stress. In older adults, the ratio changes. The bone remains hard but is less resilient; this loss of resiliency, combined with a decrease in bone tissue volume, results in bones' being more susceptible to fractures.

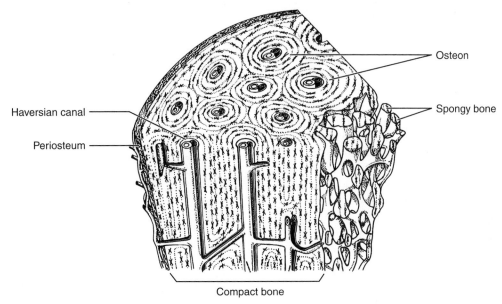

Osteon

Spongy bone

Haversian canal

Periosteum

Compact bone

Figure 2-3 Typical structure of bone. Although the major part of the medullary (marrow) cavity is not illustrated, it would include the spaces between the bony processes of the spongy bone in this figure.

Bone occurs in two typical forms: compact and spongy. **Compact bone** forms the outer surface of all bones. **Spongy** (trabeculated or cancellous) **bone** is surrounded by compact bone. Compact bone varies in hardness and thickness but is distinguished by the fact that it is laid down in concentric layers and appears solid. Spongy bone actually appears spongy in texture. It is composed of very thin plates of bone that meet other plates at various angles, and the spaces between these plates, or *trabeculae* (*trabecula* means "beam"), are relatively large. In a typical long bone, such as one in the limbs (Fig. 2-3; see Fig. 3-1), compact bone forms the entire outer layer of the bone. Spongy bone lines the inside of the compact bone, surrounding the medullary (marrow) cavity, and is also found within each end of the bone.

In a segment from a typical long bone of a limb (see Fig. 2-3), the bone is arranged mostly in layers around a series of branching tubes that contain the blood vessels. Each cylindrical unit, which contains a canal and its blood vessels, the concentric layers of bone tissue that surround it, and the bone cells in those layers, is known as an *osteon* or *haversian system*.

The canal of the osteon is more specifically called the *haversian canal*. The concentric layers of bone around a haversian canal contain the bone cells, or *osteocytes*. The layers belonging to one osteon are bound to those of adjacent ones by layers resembling parts of osteons, the *interstitial lamellae*.

The blood vessels entering the bone are so distributed through the haversian canals that none of the cells that lie between the layers of bone is far removed from a blood vessel. The living cells within the bone, although separated by the layers of bone matrix, communicate with one another and, finally, with the haversian canal, by means of tiny threadlike processes. Through these communications, substances from the blood, especially calcium salts, may be passed out into the bone, or calcium from the bone may be passed back into the blood stream. Even the bone of an adult, in which both the growths in length and diameter have ceased, is not an inert, unresponsive mass of tissue. Rather, the living cells in and about the bone are capable of bringing about modifications within this tissue; therefore, bones constantly adapt themselves to changes in the body as a whole.

Modification of the calcium deposit within the bone is especially striking in connection with tumors of the parathyroid glands. In persons with such tumors, calcium may be so withdrawn from the bones that even turning over in bed may cause fracture of a rib or a limb. Similarly, modifications of the entire bony structure may occur when a fractured bone is improperly set or when the forces exerted upon a bone, in the form of weight bearing and muscle pull, are markedly changed. In normal spongy bone, for instance, the trabeculae are arranged to support the stresses normally placed upon that bone. If the direction of these stresses is changed, much of the bone may undergo reorganization. This results in an entire rearrangement of the trabeculae with disappearance of those no longer useful and formation of new trabeculae to withstand the new forces acting upon the bone.

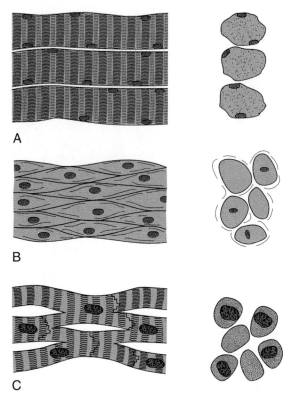

Figure 2-4 The three types of muscle tissue in longitudinal section *(left)* and cross-section *(right)*. **A,** Skeletal muscle. **B,** Smooth muscle. **C,** Cardiac muscle.

MUSCLE TISSUE

Muscle is a specialized type of tissue adapted for shortening or contraction, and it therefore consists of rather long cells. There are three distinct types of muscle in the human body: smooth muscle, cardiac muscle, and skeletal muscle.

Smooth Muscle

Smooth muscle (Fig. 2-4, *B*) typically occurs in sheets surrounding hollow viscera, such as the walls of the digestive tract and the walls of blood vessels. The individual smooth muscle cell is elongated with tapering ends and contains delicate muscle fibrils within its cytoplasm. Smooth muscle cells are usually firmly interlocked, and contraction occurs regionally rather than involving individual cells. Smooth muscle forms one of the two types of involuntary muscle. Involuntary smooth muscle is responsible for the movement of material along the digestive tract, for the contractive ability of such other hollow viscera as the urinary bladder and uterus, for the control of the very small arteries whose diameter is in turn so important in affecting the blood pressure, and for various other activities, including even the formation of "goose bumps" or "goose flesh" by small smooth muscle bundles connected with hair follicles.

Cardiac Muscle

Cardiac muscle (see Fig. 2-4, *C*) is confined to the heart and the bases of the great vessels immediately adjacent to the heart. Physiologically, this muscle resembles smooth muscle in that it also is involuntary. Anatomically, it appears to be somewhat intermediate between smooth muscle and skeletal muscle, because its cells, like those of skeletal muscle, have a striated appearance when viewed under the microscope. Cardiac muscle, however, differs sharply from skeletal

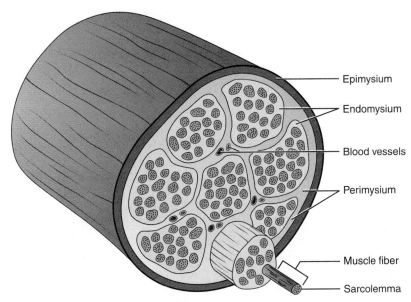

— Epimysium

— Endomysium

— Blood vessels

— Perimysium

— Muscle fiber

— Sarcolemma

Figure 2-5 Cross-section of a skeletal muscle.

muscle in one regard: its cells branch and are closely united to each other so that contraction starting within one localized region of cardiac muscle spreads widely over the heart through the close contact of the cardiac muscle cells with one another. Essentially, the cardiac muscle of the atria of the heart contracts as a unit, and that of the ventricles also contracts as a unit. Although various muscles or muscle layers in the heart are described, these consist of only partially separable sheets of fibers. As a whole, they form interconnecting layers by means of which an impulse for contraction may travel over the entire cardiac muscle of the atria or of the ventricles.

Skeletal Muscle

Skeletal muscle (see Fig. 2-4, *A*) constitutes by far the greatest mass of muscle in the body and is the tissue that in domestic animals is usually recognized as meat. The individual cells of skeletal muscle, which are very threadlike, are also termed *muscle fibers* (Fig. 2-5). Only a small fraction of a millimeter in diameter, they extend as much as 2 inches (about 5 cm) or more in length. The cell membrane of the fiber is called the *sarcolemma*. Immediately outside the sarcolemma is a very delicate layer of connective tissue,

the *endomysium*. The endomysium binds the muscle fiber loosely to other muscle fibers and, of more importance, binds the end of the fiber to the end of another fiber or to the tendon. Bundles of muscle fibers are surrounded by the *perimysium,* and a connective tissue layer called the *epimysium* surrounds the entire muscle. These three layers are interconnected and contribute to the structure of the tendon of the muscle.

Each skeletal muscle cell or fiber contains (1) numerous nuclei that are usually close to the sarcolemma and (2) closely packed, longitudinally arranged myofibrils that appear as alternating light and dark areas. The light and dark areas of each myofibril are approximately adjacent to the similar areas of other myofibrils, causing a striated appearance in these closely packed areas. This type of muscle differs from cardiac muscle in that the fibers run approximately parallel to one another, do not branch, and have no anastomoses with adjacent fibers. Each cell in skeletal muscle is associated with a nerve ending that deeply indents the sarcolemma. Under normal conditions, the muscle fiber contracts only as a result of impulses received through this nerve ending.

Myofibrils are the contractile elements of muscle fibers. They are present not only in skeletal muscle but also in smooth and cardiac muscle. Each myofibril, in turn, contains still smaller filamentous structures, visible only with the electron microscope, called *myofilaments.* Two types of myofilaments are described: thick ones that are composed primarily of the protein *myosin* and thin ones composed chiefly of another protein, *actin.*

Contraction of Muscle

Contraction of cardiac muscle cells and of many smooth muscle cells spreads from one cell to the next, although the contraction of one skeletal muscle fiber has no effect on adjacent muscle fibers. Cardiac muscle needs no nerve impulse to initiate its contraction, while skeletal muscle cannot contract (except by direct stimulation, as through an electrode) without a nerve impulse. The response of smooth muscle is somewhat in between. Some smooth muscle—for instance, that of much of the digestive tract—can contract in the absence of nerve impulses; other smooth muscle, such as that of blood vessels, is dependent on nerve impulses for contraction.

There are two aspects to the contraction of muscle: the mechanics of shortening and the biochemical basis of this shortening. In the uncontracted or resting skeletal muscle, the thick (myosin) myofilaments, which form the dark band of the fiber as a whole, are only partially overlapped by the thin (actin) myofilaments. These project beyond the ends of the thick filaments into the light band in the muscle fiber and are the only filamentous occupants of that band. During contraction, the light band shortens and finally disappears. This results from a sliding of the thin filaments toward each other, between the thick filaments, until they meet and are completely overlapped by the latter.

In contrast to this relatively simple mode of change in length, the biochemical changes responsible for and associated with contraction are very complicated and are only briefly summarized here. In the case of skeletal muscle, the nerve impulse initiates contraction by releasing acetylcholine at the nerve endings on the muscle. Acetylcholine changes the permeability of the sarcolemma to allow an influx of sodium ions. The resulting depolarization causes a high-velocity impulse to travel along the length of the muscle fiber. The impulse then causes release of calcium ions, which enables interaction of actin and myosin filaments to produce contraction.

The immediate source of energy for contraction is adenosine triphosphate (ATP). Glucose, derived from glycogen stored in the muscles and in the liver, is the chief original source of energy for muscle contraction. When sufficient oxygen is available, the glucose is oxidized to carbon dioxide (CO_2) and water, and the energy released is used in part to form additional ATP (some, of course, is wasted in heat). When the respiratory and vascular systems cannot supply sufficient oxygen, as during vigorous exercise, the glucose is converted to lactic acid, but the lesser energy liberated by that reaction also helps form additional ATP. Because lactic acid is essentially a poison to the muscle and oxygen is necessary to remove it, the muscle is said to have accumulated an "oxygen debt." The resting muscle, now receiving sufficient oxygen, uses that oxygen in part to re-form glucose and glycogen from lactic acid and in part to oxidize the lactic acid to CO_2 and water.

NERVOUS TISSUE

Nervous tissue is specialized for conduction. The essential part of nervous tissue is the nerve cell, or **neuron** (Fig. 2-6), which has a somewhat rounded cell body distorted by processes that extend outward from this cell body. Every neuron has at least one process, and most neurons have many processes. One process of the neuron, the *axon,* is threadlike and rarely branches until it is close to its ending. Most neurons have other processes, known as *dendrites,* that are relatively short and branch abundantly, like the branches of a tree. The axon is the fiber that takes the nerve impulses away from the cell body. Dendrites, which are not as specialized in structure as are axons, conduct nerve impulses toward the cell body. As a rule, the dendrites of a cell are limited in their distribution to the immediate region of the cell body, but the axon may be short or long. The axons of some cells extend only to closely adjacent cells and may be only a fraction of a millimeter in length. In contrast, there are cells in the brain that have axons measuring up to 20 inches (about 500 mm) or more in length, and the neurons that supply the muscles of the foot

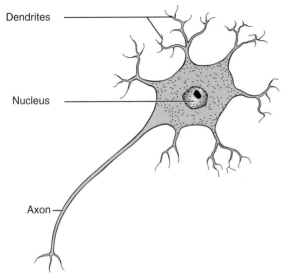

Dendrites

Nucleus

Axon

Figure 2-6 Diagram of a neuron.

have axons that extend the whole length of the lower limb and may be a yard or more (approximately 9000 mm) long, in spite of the fact that the axon may be approximately 10 μm (0.01 mm) or less in diameter.

Most cell bodies of neurons lie within the central nervous system, forming a part of the brain or spinal cord. In these locations, the bodies of the neurons and their fibers are held in place by a special connective tissue, specific to the nervous system, known as the **neuroglia.** Other neurons routinely lie outside the central nervous system, forming groups of cell bodies known as **ganglia.** The term *ganglion*, which means "swelling," may be applied to any swelling but is more often limited to a swelling produced by an accumulation of nerve cell bodies outside the central nervous system.

The bodies of neurons vary greatly in size and shape, but the largest ones rarely exceed 100 μm (0.1 mm) in diameter. Their shapes depend primarily on the number of processes to which they give rise. Because the process represents a nonnucleated extension of the cytoplasm of the cell body (the nucleus being located in this cell body), nerve fibers cannot survive after they have been detached from their connections with the cell bodies. Therefore, when a nerve fiber is cut in two, the part lying distal to the cut dies because it no longer has a connection with

the nucleated part of the cell. Nerve fibers that have been interrupted outside the central nervous system can, under the proper circumstances, grow back and form connections that replace the old degenerated ones. However, when nerve fibers within the central nervous system are interrupted, there is no functional restitution of the degenerated fibers. Once neurons are formed, they are incapable of replacing themselves.

Nerve impulses typically travel through the cell body and out along the axon. These nerve impulses are initiated by an ionic change in the cytoplasm of the cell, which is essentially similar to that initiating contraction of muscle. An adequate stimulus allows the influx of sodium ions into the cytoplasm, producing a reversal of polarity so that the inside of the cell very briefly becomes positive in regard to the outside. The electrical change, in turn, triggers a similar change in polarity in the immediately adjacent part of the cell, so that the impulse travels through the cell or along the fiber. Through this electrical change, the speed and progress of the nerve impulse can be followed. The speed of the impulse varies according to the diameter of the fiber along which it is traveling, being faster in large axons and slower in small ones. Nevertheless, it is very fast in all types of nerve fibers: approximately 120 m/second in the faster fibers.

Nerve fibers are capable of conducting a nerve impulse in either direction, but nerve impulses proceeding in the wrong direction are kept from being propagated farther by the **synapse,** or junction between two neurons. The synapse, usually formed by the close apposition of the terminal branches of the axon of one cell to the dendrites or cell body of another cell, allows the nerve impulse to pass across it only in one direction. This is because conduction across the synapse involves chemical rather than electrical transmission, and neither dendrites nor the cell body can release the chemical substance; it can be released only by axons. The chemical substances (neurotransmitters) released by axons vary, but the best known are acetylcholine and noradrenaline (norepinephrine). Transmission across the synapse (and from axons to an effector organ, such as muscle) is brought about when the electrical nerve impulse reaches the axonal ending, where it causes the release of the chemical transmitter.

Neurons and nerve fibers usually conduct only in one direction. **Motor (efferent) cells and fibers** conduct impulses away from the central nervous system and to some effector organ such as a gland or muscle, and **sensory (afferent) cells and fibers** conduct impulses to the central nervous system from the skin, muscles, joints, viscera, and so forth. Within the central nervous system, many neurons have such numerous connections that it is difficult to classify them as motor or sensory. Instead, the cells are usually described as sending their fibers primarily up the central nervous system—that is, toward the brain—or down the central nervous system or making relatively local connections. Therefore, within the central nervous system, there are ascending fibers, descending fibers, and intercalary or connecting fibers and neurons.

REVIEW QUESTIONS

1 What is the difference between a tissue and an organ?

2 What are the four basic tissues?

3 Where would a mesothelium be found?

4 What type of tissue forms a scar?

5 Describe the following:
   a fascia
   b bursa
   c tendon
   d aponeurosis
   e ligament

6 What is the difference between compact and spongy bone?

7 What are the three types of muscle tissue? Compare and contrast their structural characteristics.

8 What is a ganglion?

9 In what direction does an impulse associated with a motor or efferent fiber travel? In what direction does a sensory or afferent impulse travel?

EXERCISES

1 Make a simple sketch illustrating the features of the following:
   a simple squamous epithelium
   b simple columnar epithelium
   c pseudostratified ciliated columnar epithelium

2 Draw a neuron and label its parts.

3 ORGANS AND ORGAN SYSTEMS

CHAPTER CONTENTS

Skeletal System

Muscular System

Nervous System

Circulatory System

Digestive System

Respiratory System

Urogenital System

Endocrine System

Skin

An **organ** is a combination of several different tissues that work together to perform a given function, whereas **organ systems** are groups of organs of somewhat similar makeup and with somewhat similar functions. The stomach, for instance, an organ of the digestive system, is composed of epithelial tissue, connective tissue, and smooth muscle, with smaller amounts of vascular and nervous tissues. All of these tissues are necessary for the proper functioning of the stomach. In turn, the digestive organs as a whole are built on the same fundamental plan as the stomach, and each of the various organs contributes something toward the total digestive process.

In the same way that a single muscle can be considered an organ because it contains several different tissues, all the skeletal muscles together constitute the muscular system. The various individual bones (organs) together form the major portion of the skeletal system, and this is the pattern for other organ systems. In this chapter, only the general features of the various organs and organ systems are considered.

SKELETAL SYSTEM

The skeleton of the body consists largely of bones, with cartilage of one type or another located at strategic points. Bone, however, is usually preceded by a cartilaginous model. This is known as *endochondral bone formation* and includes the type of growth that occurs, for example, at the ends of long bones such as the femur. Some bones, however, such as the flat bones of the skull, are derived from mesenchymal tissue in what is termed *intramembranous bone formation.* This type of bone formation also occurs on the surface of the shaft of long bones.

In enchondral bone formation, while the cartilage is still growing, a blood vessel erodes the cartilage and grows into it near the midportion of the bone. The blood vessel brings with it bone-forming cells that begin to lay down bone. As the cartilage is eroded, bone is also laid down on the inside and outside, so that a hollow bone replaces the solid cartilage in the middle of the structure. In order to grow in diameter, this bone must be remodeled, with bone being removed on the inside and added on the outside. Therefore, growth of a bone from its first appearance as cartilage to its fully developed form involves a simultaneous destruction of previously formed cartilage or bone and addition of new bone. All of this must occur while the bone is providing support for surrounding tissues. This process is approximately comparable to enlarging the exterior of a house by advancing its outer walls while at the same time enlarging and changing the number of rooms and keeping the roof intact.

Bones

Bones can be classified according to their shape as *long* (e.g., femur), *short* (e.g., carpal bones), *flat* (e.g., parietal bone in the skull), *irregular* (e.g., vertebrae), and *sesamoid* (e.g., sesamoid bones in the foot) *bones.* Sesamoid bones are a special type, usually developed in connection with tendons. Most of these bones are tiny nodules, as implied by their name, which refers to a sesame seed, although the patella, which is quite large, is also a sesamoid bone.

A typical, mature long bone, such as most of those of the limbs, consists of a *diaphysis,* or shaft, and two *epiphyses,* one at each end of the bone (Fig. 3-1). The tapered junction between an epiphysis and the diaphysis is termed the *metaphysis.* The diaphysis of the bone is formed of cortical (compact) bone that surrounds a large *medullary* or *marrow cavity.* The red blood cells and many of the white blood cells are formed within the medullary cavity during a period of fetal life. During adult life, the marrow of many of the bones of the body ceases its function of producing blood cells. This function is then primarily restricted to the flat bones. The long bones may resume this

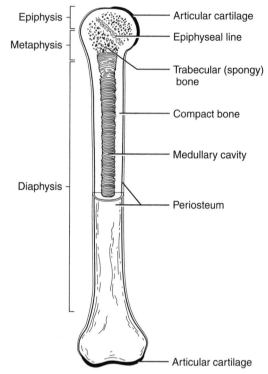

Figure 3-1 Features of a typical long bone.

function if there is an excessive demand for newly formed blood elements. In the bones not actively forming blood cells, the connective tissue of the marrow develops numerous fat cells, causing a yellowish-white appearance. Marrow active in the formation of red blood cells is known as *red marrow.* The marrow cavity is supplied by a *nutrient artery* that pierces the body of the bone to pass into and branch within the cavity. This artery is also the chief supply of the bone tissue itself, for many of its branches enter the bone to run in haversian canals.

The ends of long bones are provided with a thin outer shell of compact bone but are largely filled by spongy bone. There the marrow cavity is subdivided by the bony trabeculae.

The diaphysis and epiphyses of adult long bones are firmly united at the metaphyses. In childhood and early adolescence, however, there is a cartilaginous plate, the *epiphyseal plate,* between the diaphysis and each epiphysis. The epiphyseal plates are responsible for the growth in length of the diaphysis.

As the epiphyseal plate grows, the part of it nearest the diaphysis is being constantly transformed into bone. As long as the epiphyseal plates are growing and are not being replaced by bone faster than new cartilage is formed, growth in a long bone continues. When the destruction of the epiphyseal plate and its replacement by bone proceed faster than the cartilage can grow, the cartilage soon disappears, and no further growth in length of the bone is possible. For a time after the epiphyseal plate has disappeared, its former position in the bone is often fairly apparent as the *epiphyseal line.*

The importance of the epiphyseal plates in growth in length of the long bones is dramatically illustrated by a condition, *achondroplasia,* in which for unknown reasons the epiphyseal plates cease their growth early in life. Because growth in diameter of a bone does not depend on the presence of cartilage but occurs as a result of deposition of successive layers of new bone on the periphery, the bones of the limbs continue to grow in diameter even though they have ceased to grow in length. In consequence, the limbs remain short, not much longer than those of an infant, although they attain a diameter approaching that in an adult. The trunk and head also usually reach normal size. The adult so affected has extremely short limbs attached to a more normal-sized trunk and is known as an *achondroplastic dwarf.*

Bone Growth and Formation

A number of factors may affect the growth of the epiphyseal plates and their transformation into bone. An important mechanical one is pressure, which must be much greater than that exerted by the weight of the body before it has any effect. It once was common for a limb paralyzed by poliomyelitis to grow more slowly than did the normal limb. One of the factors in this slower growth may have been the pressure exerted when the bone grew and paralyzed muscles failed to grow likewise. It is possible to insert staples across an epiphyseal plate so that they hold the diaphysis and epiphysis of a bone together, and as the growing cartilage builds up pressure, growth ceases. This stapling technique has been used to retard or halt growth of a normal limb so that there will not be too great a difference in length between the otherwise normal limb and a paralyzed one. Another method of accomplishing the same result is to remove one or more epiphyseal plates.

Hormones that affect growth of the body as a whole, particularly thyroxine secreted by the thyroid gland in the neck, and the growth hormone of the pituitary gland (hypophysis) lying in the skull just below the brain, also affect growth of bone. Too little secretion of either hormone leads to *dwarfism.*

In contrast to hyposecretion, hypersecretion of the growth hormone leads to growth that may go on far beyond the age at which the epiphyseal plates normally disappear. Such an overgrowth may produce marked *gigantism.* Sex hormones also affect epiphyseal plates but in a different manner than the growth hormone. They hasten the replacement of cartilage by bone and lead to total disappearance of the cartilage. Earlier sexual maturity is the cause of the earlier cessation of growth in girls than in boys.

The ages at which epiphyseal plates disappear and growth in length at that end stops have been carefully recorded. They vary greatly for different bones and even for the two ends of a single bone. There are also variations among individuals, but epiphyseal fusion tends to follow a general pattern in which there is usually a range of only a year or two among individuals of the same sex. Girls, however, typically have epiphyseal fusion as much as 3 years before boys.

Other bones that are first formed in cartilage— the ribs, most of the bones of the wrist and ankle, and many bones of the skull—do not have epiphyseal plates. In these cases, once the growing cartilage has been destroyed, the growth, like that of the diameter of long bones, occurs by addition of bone to the outside surfaces.

Although most bones are first formed in cartilage, some of the flat bones of the skull never go through a cartilaginous stage, and as mentioned previously, are formed in the process of *intramembranous bone formation.* The membranes connecting the bones of the roof of the skull have not, at birth, been completely transformed into bone, and the bones of the skull of an infant can overlap somewhat during childbirth.

Bones are covered by a dense fibrous connective tissue membrane called the *periosteum* (meaning "around the bone"). This tough membrane is usually united firmly to the bony tissue through some of its fibers, which penetrate the bone to mingle with the collagenous tissues. The tendons of muscles insert into the periosteum, blend with it, and send many of their fibers into the bone.

In addition to its fibrous, relatively vascular outer layer, periosteum has a more delicate and more cellular inner layer, lying against the outer surface of the compact bone. The cells (osteoblasts) of this inner layer are capable of forming bone, and in the fetus and child, these cells lay down new bone on the outside of the old bone, producing growth in the diameter of the bone. Other bone-forming cells lie on the inner surface of the cortical bone, lining the medullary cavity, to form the *endosteum.* There are also cells (osteoclasts) in the endosteum that are capable of destroying bone to allow enlargement of the medullary cavity and to prevent the bone from becoming too thick as more bone is added to the outer surface.

Although the cells within the cortical bone are living, it is the potential bone-forming cells of the endosteum and periosteum that are especially capable of new bone formation in the adult. When a fracture occurs, these bone-forming cells begin to lay down bone across the break. They usually overdo the process of repair and form an enlargement, or *callus,* where the fracture occurred.

Bone Strength

Although cortical bone varies much in strength, both its tensile strength (resistance to being pulled apart) and its compressive strength (resistance to being crumbled) exceed those of granite and of white oak, although they do not approach those of medium steel. Bone is reported to have a tensile strength along its long axis of 13,200 to about 17,700 lb/in.[2] (91 to about 122 MPa) and a compressive one of 18,000 to 24,700 lb/in.[2] (124 to 170 MPa). The corresponding statistics for granite are a tensile strength of 1500 lb/in.[2] (10 MPa) and a compressive strength of 15,000 lb/in.[2] (103 MPa); for white oak along the grain, a tensile strength of 12,500 lb/in.[2] (86 MPa) and a compressive strength of 7000 lb/in.[2] (48 MPa) and for medium steel, a tensile strength of 65,000 lb/in.[2] (448 MPa) and a compressive strength of 60,000 lb/in.[2] (414 MPa).

Joints

A joint (articulation) is defined as a union between two or more bones. Joints are typically classified into three major groups according to the method of union between the bones: fibrous joints, cartilaginous joints, and synovial joints. There are also subcategories of each group (Fig. 3-2).

Fibrous joints

In **fibrous joints**, the bones are united by connective tissue fibers. Many of these joints are immovable because of the shapes of the articulating surfaces and because of the shortness of the collagenous fibers that bind them together. The subcategories of fibrous joints include suture, syndesmosis, and gomphosis.

A **suture** is the type of joint occurring between most of the bones of the skull (see Fig. 21-1). At a suture, the bones often have serrated edges that interlock and are held firmly together by a small amount of fibrous tissue.

In a **syndesmosis**, the two bones entering into this fibrous joint may be some distance from each other but are connected by a ligament or interosseous membrane. An example is the laminae of adjacent vertebrae (see Fig. 13-6), which are connected by ligaments made of elastic tissue (called the *ligamenta flava*); these ligaments allow considerable movement between the laminae. Another example of a syndesmosis is the connection of the shafts of the tibia and fibula by an interosseous membrane.

A **gomphosis** is a fibrous joint in which a tooth is held in place in the mandible or maxilla.

Cartilaginous Joints

The bones entering into a cartilaginous joint are united by hyaline cartilage or fibrocartilage; therefore, little or no movement is possible between the bones. Two subcategories are usually described: synchondrosis and symphysis.

A **synchondrosis** (primary cartilaginous joint) is the junction between two parts of a bone and consists of hyaline cartilage. This is a temporary, immovable joint formed by the epiphyseal plate that unites the shaft and ends of the bone. When bone growth ceases and the epiphyseal plate is replaced by bone, this

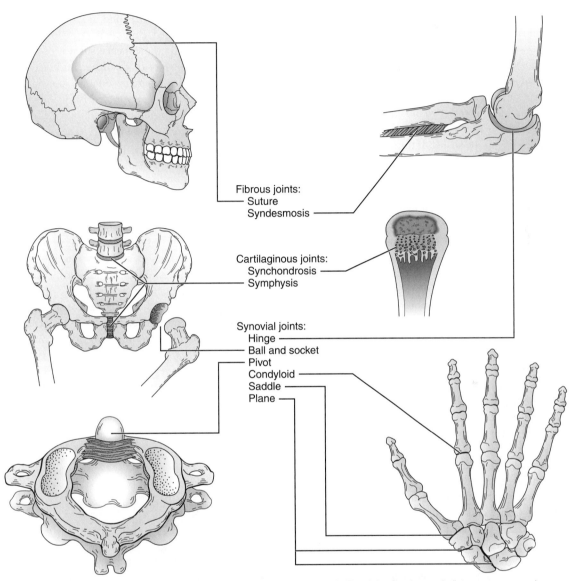

Figure 3-2 Examples of joints. *Top left,* Suture (between bones of the skull). *Top right,* Syndesmosis (interosseous membrane between the radius and ulna of the forearm) and hinge (elbow joint). *Middle left,* Symphysis (joint between vertebral bodies [intervertebral disc] and at the symphysis pubis) and ball-and-socket (hip joint). *Middle right,* Synchondrosis (epiphyseal plate of a growing long bone). *Bottom left,* Pivot (between the atlas and the dens process of the axis). *Bottom right,* Condyloid (metacarpophalangeal joint of a finger), saddle (carpometacarpal joint of the thumb), and plane (between carpal bones).

joint is obliterated. Synchondroses are also found in some bones located in the base of the cranial cavity.

In most cartilaginous joints of the adult, union is by fibrocartilage instead of hyaline cartilage, and a small amount of movement is possible. Such a joint is called a **symphysis** (secondary cartilaginous joint).

Examples of this type of cartilaginous joint are the unions between the bodies of the vertebrae, in which heavy fibrocartilaginous discs, the intervertebral discs (see Fig. 13-6), unite the bones and allow the limited movement between any two vertebrae that is necessary for movements of the back. Another example of a symphysis is the pubic symphysis between the two hip (pelvic) bones.

Synovial joints

Synovial joints, in which there is a cavity between the articular surfaces, are movable joints. Synovial joints may be simple (between two bones) or composite (between several bones). They are more completely classified according to the shapes of the articulating surfaces (see Fig. 3-2). These shapes in turn determine the type of movement allowed at the joint. Synovial joints can be further categorized by the movement occurring at the joint: A uniaxial synovial joint allows movements occurring in one plane or axis; a biaxial joint allows movements in two planes or axes; and a triaxial joint allows movements in three planes or axes.

In general, where two surfaces come together to form a synovial joint, they are reciprocally curved. The two curves are usually not identical. However, a certain amount of discrepancy allows better lubrication of the joint.

A **hinge (ginglymus) joint** is uniaxial. It allows primarily back-and-forth movement, similar to that which occurs at the hinge of a door. Examples of this type of joint are found at the elbow or the knee, where flexion and extension occur.

In a **pivot (trochoid) joint,** one element forming the joint resembles a peg and is held against the second element so that rotation is the primary movement allowed (uniaxial). An example of this type of joint is that within the neck between the first cervical vertebra (atlas) and the dens process of the second cervical vertebra (axis).

At a **plane joint,** the two articulating surfaces are almost flat and allow only a gliding movement. These joints are found between some of the carpal bones of the wrist. Movement is usually uniaxial; however, some joints may move in more than one plane or axis.

In a **condyloid (ellipsoid) joint** the surface of one bone entering the joint is typically convex in shape, whereas that of the other bone is concave. This type of articulation occurs at the bases of the fingers (metacarpophalangeal joints). Because the articular areas are often oval in shape, little or no rotation is possible and the joint is considered to be biaxial, enabling movement in two planes.

A **saddle (sellar) joint** is one in which both surfaces are saddle-shaped, concave in one direction and convex in the other; the concave surface of one fits onto the convex surface of the other, and vice versa. This structural arrangement enables considerable movement. An example of this type is the joint at the base of the thumb (carpometacarpal joint). This type of joint is considered to be a biaxial joint.

Ball-and-socket (spheroid) joints are triaxial joints, permitting movement in multiple planes or axes. At such a joint, one of the articular surfaces is rounded and the other is concave, as at the glenohumeral (shoulder) or hip joint. Unless movement is restricted by ligaments or muscles, this joint allows the greatest freedom of movement: flexion, extension, abduction, adduction, and even rotation around the long axis of the bone (circumduction).

A typical synovial joint, regardless of the shape of the articulating surfaces, has a constant structure (Fig. 3-3). The portions of the bones that are in contact with and move on each other constitute the *articulating surfaces.* These surfaces are typically covered with cartilage. This cartilage, usually of the hyaline type, offers a much smoother surface than can be obtained from the bone itself. These surfaces

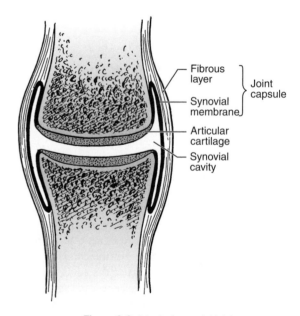

Figure 3-3 A typical synovial joint.

may be subject to considerable pressure, even in non–weight-bearing joints. For instance, when flexion of the extended forearm is attempted, the line of pull of the flexor muscles is almost parallel to the bones. Therefore, much of the muscle's force is exerted on the elbow joint, forcing the articular surfaces against each other. Because of the lack of complete congruency, this pressure is concentrated into an area less than that of the apposed articular surfaces. If there is a weight in the hand, the muscles must contract still more strongly in order to flex the forearm, therefore exerting more pressure on the joint.

In weight-bearing joints, the pressure on the joint may be greatly increased by the pull of supporting muscles. If all the weight of a 200-lb (91-kg) man is supported on one limb, the hip joint is subject not only to that weight minus the weight of one limb but also to the pull of the muscles necessary to maintain the weight on one limb. One limb should be about 15% of the body weight, or 30 lb (14 kg), leaving 170 lb (77 kg) to be supported. Using the formula for calculating the force necessary to balance the body on one limb (see the "Levers and Muscular Action" section), it can be calculated that this amounts to 425 lb. The hip joint is subjected to a pressure of 425 lb plus 170 lb, or a total of 595 lb. This is during quiet standing. Imagine the total stress on the joint when the person is running instead of standing still.

The ends of the bones entering into a synovial joint are enclosed by the **joint (articular) capsule,** which connects from one bone to the other. The outer layer of the joint capsule is the *fibrous layer (membrane),* which is composed typically of collagenous tissue. This layer completely surrounds the joint and blends with the periosteum of the bones entering into the joint. In many joints, this layer attaches some distance from the articular surfaces. The inner layer of the joint capsule is the *synovial membrane.* The synovial membrane is more vascular than the fibrous layer, is quite thin, and consists of an outer layer of connective tissue and a single layer of cells on its inner surface. The synovial membrane lines the inner surface of the fibrous layer but is also reflected along the bones to the edges of the articular cartilages. Therefore, a synovial cavity is lined by the synovial membrane except over the articular cartilages. The synovial membrane produces a viscous substance, the

synovia or *synovial fluid,* that somewhat resembles the white of an egg (*synovium* means "like an egg"). The synovial fluid is the lubricant of the joint and also the source of nourishment to the articular cartilage.

The fibrous layers of synovial joints are thickened in certain locations by **ligaments.** These bands consist of dense fibrous connective tissue that is almost always collagenous. The constituent bundles run largely in the same direction (see Fig. 15-7). Most ligaments blend with the joint capsule on their deep surfaces and are really local thickenings of the capsule. In the case of a hinge joint, the anterior and posterior parts of the capsule are usually thin and protected by the muscles passing in front of and behind the joint, and the sides are reinforced by well-developed ligaments. In this way, the ligaments do not interfere with the moves of flexion and extension at the joint.

Ligaments play an important part in the physiology of the joints. Although the type of movement allowed at a joint usually depends primarily on the shape of the articular surfaces, ligaments sometimes guide the movement and regularly assist muscles in limiting the amount of movement. They are an important source of strength to the joint and are typically much stronger than is necessary to resist the forces that ordinarily act on them.

FUNCTIONAL/CLINICAL NOTE 3-1

If unusual forces act on the ligaments over a long period, the ligaments gradually stretch and allow the bones to slide out of their normal positions. An excellent example of this is acquired *flatfoot,* in which carrying the weight constantly on the inner border of the foot leads to stretching of the supporting ligaments and flattening of the arch. A certain amount of dislocation (termed *subluxation*) between bones may occur as a result of lax or stretched ligaments. For complete *dislocation* to occur, ligaments must be torn. A *sprain* is a tearing of ligaments without dislocation.

Any swelling of the capsules and ligaments of joints, whether produced by strain or sprain, infection, or arthritis, is painful because the

Continued

capsules and ligaments are provided with nerve endings, some of which belong to pain fibers (sensory nerve fibers that conduct impulses associated with the sensation of pain). The articular cartilage itself has no nerve fibers in it. *It is a general rule that a joint is innervated mainly by the nerves supplying the muscles that produce movement at that joint.*

The swelling and stiffness typical of a joint that has been immobilized for a long time, as by a splint or cast, are caused, at least in part, by faulty circulation to the joint. When possible, joints distal to the immobilized one should be regularly exercised in order to increase the circulation.

MUSCULAR SYSTEM

Muscles are composed primarily of skeletal muscle fibers but also contain a certain amount of connective tissue and abundant blood vessels and nerves. A typical muscle moves bone on bone and is attached to each of the two bones across a movable joint. For purposes of description, it is preferable to have terms by which one attachment of the muscle may be distinguished from the other attachment. The terms adopted for this purpose are *origin* and *insertion.* The **origin** of a muscle is considered to be the attachment that is, under usual circumstances, the less movable end of the muscle. Similarly, the **insertion** of a muscle is the attachment to the more movable part. Difficulties sometimes arise in deciding which of the skeletal attachments of a muscle is more likely to move when the muscle shortens, but as a whole, it is usually easy to distinguish between origin and insertion. In regard to the limbs, it is clear that in general, a more distal part of the limb may be moved more easily than a more proximal part. Therefore, the origins of limb muscles are usually at their proximal ends, and their insertions are at their distal ends.

The definitions of *origin* and *insertion* do not imply that the origin of a muscle may not be moved by contraction of that muscle. As a muscle shortens, its ends move closer together, but if particular circumstances cause the insertion of the muscle to be at the moment more fixed than is the origin, the origin of the muscle is then moved by contraction of the muscle. For instance, muscles that pass across the glenohumeral (shoulder) joint and move the arm generally have their origin on the shoulder or the back and their insertion on the arm. If the body is suspended by the arms, as in doing a pull-up, contraction of the shoulder muscles moves the body as a whole, because the limbs are then the fixed points. This reverses the typical description of origin and insertion and their relation to fixed versus movable attachment points.

An alternative terminology for attachment points, especially for muscles associated with the limbs, is to describe them as **proximal** or **distal attachments.** This terminology simply categorizes the attachments of a muscle according to their relative location with regard to the limb and body. (Where appropriate in the tables in this text, this terminology is used in addition to the terms *origin* and *insertion.*) Regardless of the terminology used, knowing the attachment points of a muscle provides a basis for understanding the various actions it is capable of performing.

Muscles are regularly attached to bone by dense fibrous connective tissue. At one end, this tissue attaches to the ends of the muscle fibers, and at the other end, it blends with the periosteum of the bone and with the fibrous connective tissue within the bone itself. If these connective tissue fibers are short, the muscle fibers may appear to arise almost directly from the bone, described as a *fleshy origin* of the muscle.

Many muscles arise by longer connective tissue bundles that are aggregated to form a **tendon,** and most muscles insert by tendons. A tendon has several advantages over muscle fibers. In crossing a bone or joint, for instance, a muscle closely applied to bone may be subjected to considerable wear and tear in this location, which may then lead to the injury or death of the muscle fibers. On the contrary, a tendon is composed of nonliving fibers and is much tougher than are living muscle cells. Tendons are much more suited to withstand strain. Another advantage of a tendinous insertion is that it allows a bulky muscle to insert on a very small area of bone, because tendon is much stronger than muscle and small tendons can withstand the pull of large muscle bellies. For instance, most of the muscles of the forearm attach in the hand. Obviously, if these muscles continued as muscle tissue into the hand, the hand would have to be much larger to accommodate them. The muscles are therefore replaced by tendons as they near the wrist, and the reduced bulk of these tendons contributes considerably to the flexibility of the hand.

As stated previously, tendons are much stronger than the muscles that act on them. A very large muscle can act through a small tendon or even a small part of a small tendon. The maximal tensile strength of muscle (its resistance to a pull) has been reported to be about 77 lb/in.^{2} (0.5 MPa), while tendons have been found to have a tensile strength of 8600 to 18,000 lb/in.^{2} (59 to 124 MPa).

FUNCTIONAL/CLINICAL NOTE 3-2

Although there is a great difference in the strength of different tendons, they are all much stronger than muscle. This strength accounts for the fact that normal tendons that are ruptured by sudden force never break in their middles but instead pull away from one end. If this occurs at the bony attachment, a piece of bone may be torn away from the tendon. If it is at the other end, the tear comes at the musculotendinous attachment. Certain tendons around the glenohumeral joint sometimes rupture in or near their middles, but this is a result of repeated damage to the tendon with its eventual weakening.

Bursae and Synovial Sheaths

Bursae were described briefly in Chapter 2 but merit a more detailed description here. A **bursa** is a flattened connective tissue sac that is lined by a synovial membrane (Fig. 3-4). It contains a small amount of fluid that eliminates friction on the opposing inner surfaces, allowing them to slide freely against each other. Bursae can lie between a muscle and bone, a tendon and bone, skin and bone, or another combination of structures, and they facilitate free movement of these structures on each other. Bursae lying adjacent to joints may communicate with the articular cavity of the joint.

FUNCTIONAL/CLINICAL NOTE 3-3

Bursitis, or inflammation of a bursa, can be caused by injury, chronic pressure, or infection. Inflammation causes additional fluid to be produced within the bursa, causing swelling. Application of pressure to the area or movement of structures between which the bursa lies can cause pain.

A **synovial sheath** (synovial tendon sheath) may be regarded as a bursa that completely surrounds a tendon. It has two walls. The *inner wall* (visceral layer) is closely attached to the tendon and forms a smooth, glistening outer surface on the tendon; the *outer wall* (parietal layer) of the sheath forms a closed sac, uniting with the inner layer at the edges of the sheath (see Fig. 3-4). Where the two sides of the sheath come together, a *mesotendon* is formed. It unites the inner and outer walls and serves as a point of entrance and exit for tiny blood vessels. The cavity of the synovial tendon sheath, between its inner and outer walls, contains a thin layer of fluid (similar to that occurring in joints) that acts as a lubricant to allow frictionless movement of the tendon. Synovial sheaths are especially numerous at the wrist and ankle, where the tendons pass close to bone and are held down by heavy ligaments.

Mechanics of Muscular Action and Arrangement of Muscle Fibers

The strength of a muscle and the range of movement that it can produce at a joint vary with several factors. The strength ultimately depends on the number and size of the constituent muscle fibers. However, the mechanical factors—the arrangements of fibers within muscles and the varying leverage afforded by the attachments of muscles across the joints—make it impossible to compare the effective movements and strengths of different muscles solely on the basis of their sizes. Individual muscle fibers, regardless of what muscle they are in, apparently can contract maximally to the same percentage of their length, about 50%. Each muscle crossing a joint, however,

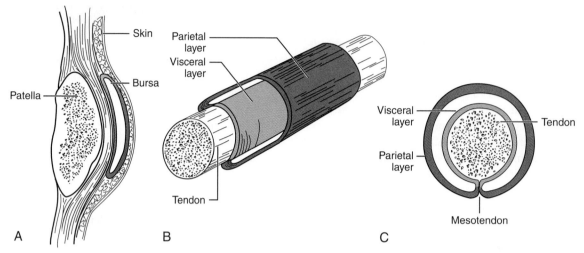

Figure 3-4 Bursa and synovial sheath. **A,** Drawing depicting a section through the patella and subcutaneous prepatellar bursa at the knee joint. **B,** Cut-away view of a synovial sheath surrounding a tendon. The visceral layer of the sheath lies on the surface of the tendon. **C,** Cross-section view of the tendon and sheath. The mesotendon enables vessels to gain access to the tendon. The size of the space between the visceral and parietal layers has been exaggerated for clarity; normally the two layers are closely apposed with only a thin layer of fluid between them.

may contract by a different amount. The extent to which a muscle as a whole can contract is the distance over which it normally shortens as the part to which it is attached moves through its complete range of movement, from the extreme in one direction to the extreme in the other. Each muscle is accurately adapted to the amount of movement it can perform, and this adaptation depends on both the length of the muscle fibers and their arrangement in the muscle.

There are various arrangements of the fibers within muscles (Fig. 3-5). In muscles in which the fibers are arranged essentially parallel to the long axis of the muscle, most of the fibers run the length of the muscle, and the amount of shortening the muscle can undergo is approximately 50% of its length. A long muscle with parallel fibers (see Fig. 3-5, *A-C*) therefore produces a great range of movement. **Strap muscles** (e.g., the sartorius muscle of the thigh) and **fusiform muscles** (e.g., the biceps brachii muscle of the arm) are muscles in which the fibers have a parallel organization. The rectus abdominis in the abdominal wall is a strap-type muscle, but it is interrupted along its length by tendinous intersections into which its fibers attach. Its fibers are therefore

shorter and do not run the length of the muscle. In the fusiform type, the muscle belly is rounded with tapering ends, and the fibers curve between their origins and insertions. Other groups of muscles in which the fibers have a parallel arrangement include **flat, triangular,** and **quadrate muscles.**

In some muscles, the fibers insert at an angle into a tendon that passes through the muscle, somewhat as the barbs of a feather attach to its quill. In this case, the length of the muscle fibers is always less than the total length of the muscle. These are called **pennate muscles.** The distance over which the muscle can contract bears no fixed relation to the length of the muscle. Instead, it is proportional to the length of its muscle fibers. This characteristic varies from muscle to muscle, depending on the angle at which the fibers approach their insertion, the width of the muscle, and whether the muscle belly is flat or rounded.

There are several types of pennate muscles (see Fig. 3-5, *D-F*). In a **unipennate** (semipennate) **muscle,** the fibers are attached to only one side of a tendon (e.g., the flexor pollicis longus of the forearm). In a **bipennate muscle,** the fibers attach to two sides of a tendon that runs through the muscle.

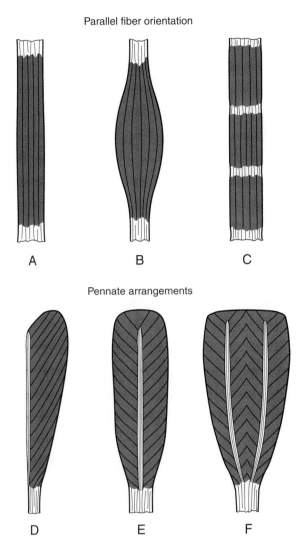

Parallel fiber orientation

A   B   C

Pennate arrangements

D   E   F

Figure 3-5 Muscle fiber arrangements. **A** to **C,** Muscles with parallel fiber orientation: strap **(A)**, fusiform **(B)**, and parallel with tendinous intersections **(C)**. **D** to **F,** Muscles with pennate arrangements: unipennate **(D)**, bipennate **(E)**, and multipennate **(F)**.

the strength of contraction depends on the size and number of contracting fibers. The maximal strength of contraction of a muscle is therefore determined by the total cross-sectional size of all its muscle fibers. In the parallel type, this is also the cross-sectional area of the muscle, but in all other types it is different. Obviously, for a given muscle length, there are more muscle fibers in a unipennate muscle than in a parallel one of the same width and even more in a bipennate one. It is impossible to compare two muscles of different types on the basis of their sizes alone. Moreover, of two muscles of the same size in which the fibers are not parallel, the one with the longer fibers has fewer of them, so that although it has the greater range of contraction, it also has less strength.

Levers and Muscular Action

A similar inverse relationship between range and strength of movement, one being sacrificed to a greater or lesser extent for the other, appears when two muscles of similar size and shape differ appreciably in the distance of their insertion from the joint over which they act. Mechanical levers are used in many daily activities to increase strength (using a claw hammer to pull a nail) or to increase the range and rapidity of movement (swinging a golf club). Similarly, the musculoskeletal system is largely a series of levers.

The following are the four components of a *lever system:*

The *lever* itself, typically a rigid bar: in the case of the body, a bone or bones

A *fulcrum,* the axis or point at which movement of the lever takes place: the joint

An *effort* or *force:* the muscle acting on the lever

The *resistance* (load or weight) that the force must overcome to move the lever: the weight of the body part being moved; e.g., the forearm and hand and any additional weight, such as a hammer, being held by the hand

Levers are categorized into three classes, depending on the relationship among the fulcrum, the point at which the force is applied (*effort point,* which in the body is the insertion of the muscle), and the resistance.

The rectus femoris of the thigh is an example of a bipennate muscle. In the **multipennate muscle**—for example, the deltoid muscle in the shoulder region—there are many tendons within the muscle to which the fibers attach.

Although the distance over which a muscle can contract depends on the length of its muscle fibers,

In a **first-class lever,** the fulcrum (F) lies between the effort point (E) and the resistance (R); for example, a seesaw or an oar with the support of the seesaw or the oar holder representing the fulcrum:

In a **second-class lever,** the resistance lies between the fulcrum and the effort point; for example, a wheelbarrow with the wheel being the fulcrum:

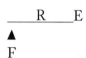

In a **third-class lever,** the effort point lies between the fulcrum and the resistance; for example, an automatic storm door closer with the hinges being the fulcrum:

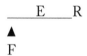

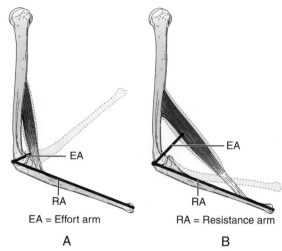

EA = Effort arm   RA = Resistance arm

A   B

Figure 3-6 Third-class levers illustrating the effect of the place of attachment of a muscle on the range of movement. Both muscles are shown shortening the same amount with contraction, but the one attached closer to the joint **(A)** moves the lever much more (the difference between the solid and broken outlines of the bones) than does the one farther from the joint **(B).**

All or almost all the levers in the body belong to either the first or third class. Figure 3-6 depicts two third-class levers; in both cases, the insertions of the muscles, the effort points lie between the joint (fulcrum) and the resistance or weight. All the muscles arising from the bone of the arm and passing in front of the elbow joint to either bone of the forearm use these bones as third-class levers.

Figure 3-6 indicates how a difference in the point of the attachment of the muscle affects the range of action, and a simple calculation shows how it also affects the strength the muscle needs to overcome a given resistance. In a lever system, a perpendicular line from the line of force (a line passing through the length of the muscle) to the fulcrum is called the *effort arm* (or *effort moment arm*), and a line from the resistance to the fulcrum is called the *resistance arm* (or *resistance moment arm*). In Figure 3-6, the effort arm is a measurement of a line that extends from the fulcrum (the joint) perpendicularly to a line that passes through the long axis of the muscle belly. Therefore, the value

of the effort arm for Figure 3-6, *A* is less than that of Figure 3-6, *B* because the muscle belly of the latter is further from the joint. The resistance arm is the distance from the joint to the tip of the bone being moved, which is the same in both parts of the figure. For the lever to be in balance, the effort (E) multiplied by the length of the effort arm (EA) must equal the resistance (R) multiplied by the length of the resistance arm (RA), or E × EA must equal R × RA. In Figure 3-6, *A*, the effort arm is initially about 0.2 in. and the resistance arm is about 1.5 in.; in Figure 3-6, *B*, the effort arm is initially about 0.5 in., and the resistance arm is, again, about 1.5 in. Assuming a weight or resistance of 10 lb, the equations would read as follows:

$$E \times EA \quad = \quad R \times RA$$

Figure 3-6, *A* : E × 0.2 in. = 10 lb × 1.5 in.
Figure 3-6, *B* : E × 0.5 in. = 10 lb × 1.5 in.

When these equations are solved, the required efforts (E) for Figures 3-6, *A* and 3-6, *B* are 75 lb and 30 lb, respectively. Therefore the muscle in Figure 3-6, *A* would have to contract with 2.5 times the strength of the muscle in Figure 3-6, *B* in order to produce any movement. Through its closer attachment to the joint, the muscle in Figure 3-6, *A* has sacrificed strength in favor of range of movement and speed, inasmuch as range and speed parallel each other. The muscle in Figure 3-6, *B,* however, has gained effective strength at the expense of range and speed of movement.

The resistance arm has been found to be about 2.5 times greater than the effort arm. Therefore, in the calculation of the stress on the hip joint when standing on one limb (p. 25), the equation is as follows:

$$E \times 1 = 170 \times 2.5, \text{ or } E = 425$$

The muscles shown in Figure 3-6 are flexors. A muscle arising from the posterior surface of the upper bone and inserting into the proximal end of the lower bone would be an extensor, and the lower bone would then function as a lever of the first class, the joint being between the insertion of the muscle and the resistance. There is a muscle of the arm, the triceps, that has these attachments. Obviously such a muscle, because it inserts so close to the joint, produces rapid movement over a wide range. However, a similar muscle inserting farther from the joint, an insertion that could be afforded by a longer posterior projection of the lower bone, would have greater effective strength but produce a smaller range of movement. Therefore, regardless of the type of lever,

effective strength of a muscle and range and rapidity of movement vary inversely with each other.

Types of Contraction

In the previous discussion, shortening of a muscle as a result of its contraction has been assumed. In a smooth movement, such *shortening* may or may not demand any great variation in the strength of contraction but is called a **concentric contraction** nevertheless. If a movement that can be carried out by gravity, such as bending the knees, is to be controlled, muscles that oppose this movement must first contract and then gradually lengthen. This lengthening reaction is known as an **eccentric contraction.** Concentric and eccentric contraction are sometimes grouped together and known as **isotonic contraction.** In general, an isotonic contraction results in movement at the joint with either muscle shortening or lengthening. Muscle, however, may contract and perform work in other ways. If opposing muscles across a joint act with equal strength, there is no movement of the part, and neither set of muscles shortens in spite of their contraction. Because they retain the same length, this is called an **isometric contraction.**

Determination of the Actions of Muscles

The action of a muscle, meaning how it moves a part of the body, was originally determined from observations of the origin, insertion, and placement of the muscle. In time, these observations were supplemented by electrical stimulation of many of the muscles to obtain information on what muscles can do when they contract alone. Careful studies of patients with various paralyses have further defined the possible contribution of unparalyzed muscles to movements that they do not necessarily normally carry out. Palpation of superficial muscles during various movements has revealed in part which muscles normally do participate in a given movement.

With the technique of *electromyography,* or recording the electrical impulses generated by muscular contraction, it is possible to determine very precisely which muscles, superficial and deep, contract during a given movement. Electromyography

---

FUNCTIONAL/CLINICAL NOTE 3-4

Another important aspect of levers in relation to muscular contraction is the effect of the length of the lever on speed. For instance, if the arm with extended forearm is abducted at the shoulder to an angle of 45 degrees, the elbow and the hand, although moving together, travel at different speeds, because the tips of the fingers are approximately twice as far from the side as is the elbow. The use of multiple levers can increase this effect. Compare, for instance, throwing a baseball while limiting the movement to the shoulder and the usual throwing movement in which the lower limb, the trunk, and the upper limb act together to multiply the speed at which the ball leaves the hand.

can also provide information on the sequence in which each of several participating muscles contracts and can help in estimating the strength of contraction of each muscle.

Through electromyography, more accurate information concerning the actions of many muscles has been obtained, although the knowledge of others is still incomplete and research is continuing. Although the method is precise, the results must be interpreted very carefully in order to understand not only which muscles are contracting but also how they are participating in the movement or why they are contracting.

In analyzing the participation of various muscles in a movement, it has been customary to categorize them as prime movers, as synergists, and as antagonists. A **prime mover,** or *agonist,* is a muscle that carries out an action. When the chief action or actions of a muscle are described, it is the prime mover that is being defined. A **synergist** (*synergy* means "working together") is a muscle that contracts at the same time as the prime mover, whereas an **antagonist** has an action that is, in varying degrees, directly opposed to that of the prime mover. Depending on the movements being considered, the same muscle may at one time be classified as a prime mover, at another as an antagonist, and perhaps at another as a synergist.

Although synergists are muscles that contract at the same time as the prime mover in order to facilitate or potentiate the effect of the prime mover, the term is a loose one. In a broad sense, it can include the second of any two muscles that regularly contract together, regardless of the function of the second muscle, and the term is sometimes used to describe the second of two muscles that carry out the same action. A more useful definition of a synergist is to regard it as a fixating or stabilizing muscle, one that contracts at the same time as the prime mover in order to prevent some unwanted movement that would otherwise take place.

It may be difficult to determine in the restricted sense whether a contracting muscle is serving as a second prime mover or as a synergist (although it can also be obvious), and examples of the latter function have long been known. For instance, clenching the fingers should also flex the wrist because the tendons of the fingers cross the front of the wrist, but if the wrist does flex, the fingers cannot make a tight fist because of the limited range of contraction of the finger flexors. (Grip a pencil with a clenched fist, and use the other hand to push the clenched hand with the pencil into flexion at the wrist. The tight grasp is lost.) In clenching the fingers, muscles that cross the back of the wrist contract synergistically to bend the wrist a little posteriorly (extension) and make the muscles moving the fingers more effective. Similarly, some muscles around the shoulder regularly contract synergistically with other muscles. The purpose is not to move the arm but to prevent displacement at the glenohumeral joint through the action of the prime mover.

Antagonists also require further definition. The word is useful in designating a muscle that has approximately the opposite action of the prime mover, but only in this sense can it be called an *antagonist.* In the normal individual, an antagonist does not fight against the prime mover. Instead, it either relaxes completely or cooperates with it, preventing some unwanted effect and actually acting as a synergist. In other instances, such as in lowering the outstretched arm or in bending over, gravity substitutes for the prime mover while the antagonist, by its lengthening reaction or eccentric contraction, controls the movement. Thus, in general, once a movement is learned, antagonists contract only when they can in some way aid the movement.

Nerve Supply

The nerve supply of a muscle is limited to the one or several nerves specifically destined for that muscle, while the blood supply is usually derived from all the blood vessels in the neighborhood. Learning the blood supply to a muscle is simply combining general knowledge concerning the location of that muscle and knowledge of the blood vessels in that area. However, a general knowledge of the locations of various nerves is of little significance in predicting which of these nerves will supply the muscle. Of several nerves in the neighborhood of a muscle, as a rule, only one supplies it. Therefore, nerve supplies of muscles must be learned.

Every muscle receives at least one but sometimes two or more nerve branches. These are regularly derived from more than one spinal nerve, so that most muscles have a multisegmental innervation. (In other words, they are supplied with fibers from two or more spinal nerves.) The activity of the muscle depends on the nerve or nerves reaching it. If the nerve supply to a muscle is destroyed, the muscle is paralyzed and remains so until a nerve supply is reestablished. As a nerve enters a muscle, it divides to be distributed within it. The branching is, for the most part, the separation of smaller bundles of nerve fibers. Eventually, however, individual nerve fibers branch, and every muscle fiber receives a nerve supply.

A typical nerve to a muscle does not consist entirely of motor fibers (i.e., fibers that cause the contraction of the muscle); it also contains a large number of sensory fibers. About 40% to 60% of the nerve fibers entering a muscle are sensory in character. Some of these are *pain fibers,* responsible for the conduction of impulses associated with the sensation of pain, as evidenced by the feeling of soreness in a muscle from overexertion or strain or the pain arising from tears of the muscles or tendons. These pain fibers are probably associated with the connective tissue and blood vessels of the muscle, rather than with the muscle fibers themselves, and are relatively few in number. Most of the sensory fibers are of the type known as *proprioceptive fibers.* These fibers are concerned with registering the stretch or contraction of a muscle and the tension within a tendon and with carrying impulses concerning the activity of the muscles and the pull on their tendons to the central nervous system.

The majority of the sensory or afferent impulses from muscle do not reach the level of consciousness but do play an extremely important part in the subconscious regulation of muscular contraction. Practically all movements require the coordination of a number of individual muscles, and each of these muscles must contract at exactly the proper moment and with exactly the proper force if the movement is to be a smooth one.

FUNCTIONAL/CLINICAL NOTE 3-5

The afferent fibers from muscles and tendons, together with similar fibers from around the joints, play a determining role in this coordination. Their importance is clearly highlighted in such diseases as *tabes dorsalis* (tabetic neurosyphilis), in which the larger fibers from muscles and joints are among the first to be affected. Such apparently simple everyday actions as buttoning a dress or coat, or even walking (really very complicated actions from the standpoint of the muscular coordination required) become difficult for a patient afflicted with tabes. The lack of both conscious and subconscious information as to what the muscles are doing and what the position of the fingers or limbs is at any particular moment results in clumsy and poorly coordinated movements that must be guided primarily by the eyes. Therefore, a patient with tabes, although suffering no paralysis or weakness of skeletal musculature, walks with a peculiar gait. The individual is unable to estimate how high the foot has been lifted from the ground. In order to keep from stumbling, the person may lift it too high. As the foot is put down, the person cannot estimate the movement required, and the foot is dropped or flung to the ground. The patient with tabes is able to walk better in the light because he or she can watch the feet and guide them somewhat consciously. In the dark, walking is much more difficult or even impossible. The learning of movements, both in infancy and in adulthood, and the acquisition of greater skill in movements are dependent primarily on the proprioceptive sensory fibers. These fibers from muscles, tendons, and joints are of great importance for the proper functioning of the muscles.

Muscle spindles

Nerve endings in tendons, in muscles, and around joints are of several different types. Some of those related to joints are particularly important in the conscious awareness of position and movement.

In muscle, the chief sensory structure is the **muscle spindle,** a group of 2 to 10 small muscle fibers. One sensory nerve fiber winds intricately around the center of the muscle spindle and is called an *annulospiral*

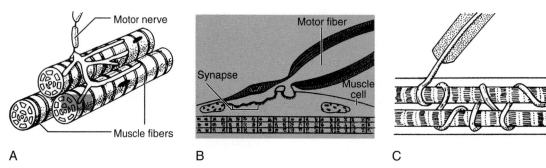

Figure 3-7 Motor and sensory (proprioceptive) nerve endings in skeletal muscle. **A,** Illustration of a small motor unit in which one nerve fiber innervates three muscle fibers. **B,** Enlargement of the shaded area shown in *A:* a motor end plate showing the synapse between a motor nerve fiber and a muscle fiber is seen here. **C,** Sensory ending at a muscle spindle.

or *primary ending* (Fig. 3-7, *C*). Other nerve fibers form what are called *flower spray* or *secondary endings* closer to the two extremities of the muscle fibers of the spindle. In addition, the tendons of muscles typically contain afferent end organs *(Golgi tendon organs)* close to the attachment of tendon and muscle fibers. None of the afferent fibers from these endings gives rise to impulses that reach consciousness.

Muscle spindles respond to stretching of their annulospiral regions. Therefore, they are commonly stimulated by stretching of the muscle as a whole. The annulospiral afferent fibers from the muscle spindles of a muscle make direct contact with the motor nerve cells in the central nervous system that supply that muscle, and contraction of the muscle in response to this stretch then ensues and relaxes the tension on the annulospiral region. The response of muscle to stretch is one of the basic reflexes (p. 42). This particular reflex is fundamental in resisting gravity and therefore in maintaining posture. It is the predominant reflex activity resulting from muscle stretch. Flower spray endings in muscle also respond to stretch but end differently in the central nervous system. Their activation facilitates flexion, regardless of the muscle stimulated. Finally, the tendon organs also respond to stretch, but because they do not lie within the muscle, this stretch can be imposed by either stretch of muscle and tendon or contraction of the muscle. Their sensitivity to stretch is far less than that of the annulospiral ending, and their action, which is inhibiting contraction of the muscle concerned, becomes prominent only when the stretch is excessive. It is a protective effect, tending to prevent undue strain on muscle and tendon.

The muscle fibers of the muscle spindle, like all skeletal muscle fibers, receive motor nerve fibers. These are distinctly smaller than the motor fibers to the rest of the muscle and arise from a different set of cell bodies in the central nervous system. They, and the neurons of which they are a part, are called *gamma fibers* and neurons; the neurons and fibers to the bulk of the muscle are designated as *alpha fibers*. The gamma neurons, in contrast to the alpha neurons, receive no impulses from the muscle spindles but do receive impulses from higher centers in the central nervous system. Their activity produces contraction of the two ends of muscle fibers of the spindle, therefore stretching the annulospiral region and sensitizing the spindle to stretch the muscle as a whole.

FUNCTIONAL/CLINICAL NOTE 3-6

Disturbance of the normal control over the gamma innervation in various disease conditions apparently accounts for the occurrence of the abnormal states of contraction of muscle known as *spasticity* and *rigidity*.

Motor nerve fibers

The motor nerve fibers to the muscles all end on muscle fibers and indent the cell membrane in such a way that they appear to be actually in the fiber (see Fig. 3-7, *A* and *B*). The specialized ending and the modified portion of muscle fiber in which it lies are called a **motor end plate.** The number of motor fibers entering a muscle is always disparate with the approximate number of muscle fibers within that muscle. For instance, in a certain muscle, the muscle fibers may outnumber the entering motor nerve fibers by about 100 to 1; in other words, there are about 100 muscle fibers for every motor fiber in the nerve or nerves entering the muscle. Normally, every muscle fiber within a muscle is capable of contraction, and no skeletal muscle fiber can contract unless it is supplied with a functional nerve ending. Therefore, each nerve fiber must branch repeatedly after it enters the muscle. Although the ratio between muscle fibers and nerve fibers varies greatly from one muscle to another, an average nerve fiber in the example given must give off about 100 branches or sub-branches in order to supply its quota of muscle fibers. Each of these terminal branches then ends on a single muscle fiber.

According to the "all-or-none law" of physiology in regard to muscle, if a given muscle fiber contracts, it contracts with all the force of which it is capable at that particular moment. Stated differently, a stimulated muscle fiber contracts with all its strength or does not contract at all. Although the all-or-none law is true concerning the contraction of individual muscle fibers, it is obvious that it does not apply to a muscle as a whole. For instance, the same muscles used to grasp and pick up a heavy steel ball could also be used to grasp and pick up a delicate eggshell. If the strength exerted to grasp the shell is the same as that used to lift the steel ball, the shell would be destroyed. It is evident with this example that voluntary movements are graded and that only the desired strength and speed are exerted during muscle activity. As far as any one muscle fiber is concerned, such gradation is impossible. Similarly, it is impossible to send an impulse of contraction to only one muscle fiber of the many innervated by a single nerve fiber. A nerve impulse, once started along a nerve fiber, is propagated along all the branches of that fiber. There is no known mechanism by which a nerve impulse can be routed along only certain branches of a single fiber.

It follows from this discussion that regulation of the strength of a movement depends on activation of groups of muscle fibers. If a delicate movement is desired, possibly only 10% of the nerve fibers to a muscle may be used to activate 10% of the muscle fibers in that muscle. If the strongest possible movement is required, impulses are sent along all the nerve fibers to the muscle, and all of the muscle fibers are activated. In any muscle, it is possible to get a smooth gradation of contraction, from a minimal one that produces no movement to a maximal one that produces the strongest movement possible.

Because all the muscle fibers that are innervated by a single nerve cell and its branching nerve fiber contract at the same time, the neuron and the group of muscle fibers it innervates constitute a **motor unit** (see Fig. 3-7, *A*). The size of the motor unit is determined by the number of muscle fibers composing it and varies from muscle to muscle. Because the motor unit represents the smallest number of fibers in a muscle that can contract at one time and the smallest increment by which strength of contraction can be increased, it might be expected that its size would vary with the type of movement demanded of the muscle. Therefore, some of the muscles around the hip and thigh, concerned in general with very coarse movements, have motor units variously reported as ranging from approximately 150 to possibly 1,600 muscle fibers. Those governing the rather delicate movements of the thumb have much smaller motor units. The muscles governing movements of the eye, which must be very precise, have the smallest motor units of all, averaging perhaps no more than three muscle fibers per nerve fiber. Some muscles, therefore, have a built-in delicacy of movement that others do not have and that no amount of training could establish.

Just as all the muscle fibers within a muscle do not have to contract together, the various larger portions of a muscle do not necessarily contract together. For instance, the pectoralis major muscle on the thorax is arranged so that some of its fibers aid in elevation of the arm and others aid in depressing the raised arm. Obviously, if both upper and lower fibers acted together, they would tend to cancel the action of each other. They are used together in some movements, and this use of the muscle as a whole results simply in pulling the arm toward the side or across the front of the chest. Either some of the upper fibers or some of the lower fibers, however, may be used alone. For example, if the upper limb is to be raised forward, the upper part of the pectoralis major, but not the lower part, is used with other muscles to accomplish this action. The lower fibers of the pectoralis major then assist in bringing the limb back to the side of the body. This selection of the proper portion of a muscle to carry out a given action is obviously brought about by selective activation of the nerve fibers going to that part of the muscle.

Integration of Muscular Action

The sending of impulses along only the nerve fibers that end in parts of muscles useful in carrying out a desired movement is automatic, effected by cellular arrangements within the brain. Although it is possible with special training to learn to contract a single motor unit, most individuals cannot at will contract only part of a muscle except by carrying out a movement that has been learned through experience to involve contraction of the desired part. Obviously, then, this selection lies largely below the conscious level. A given movement is produced not by deciding what muscles should be used but rather by deciding simply that a given movement is desired. Learning is involved here, but the important point is that the motor centers, especially the voluntary movement center in the cerebral cortex, are organized both anatomically, on the basis of muscles, and physiologically, on the basis of movements. Artificial stimulation of the motor cerebral cortex regularly produces integrated movements, and only in appropriate cases does it produce isolated contraction of an individual muscle. Similarly, movements are consciously and subconsciously learned, whereas integrated movements are produced when the motor centers are consciously stimulated. Depending on the movement and on the strength necessary to carry it out, one or several muscles, or only appropriate parts of one or several muscles, may be involved.

Many movements require, of course, very precise coordination in the timing and strength of contraction of various muscles and their synergists. Learning a movement often requires that a person first learn not to use the antagonists to that muscle, which interfere with it and make movement clumsy and difficult. Greater skill is then acquired by learning to use more precisely only the muscles that produce the desired effect.

Although everyone, in general, uses the same muscles in the same way, electromyography has shown that there may be differences among individuals. Of two muscles that produce the same movement, for instance, one may initiate the movement in one person, but the other one may do so in another person.

Consequences of Muscle Contraction

Mechanisms of muscle action have already been discussed, as have the physicochemical changes involved in the contraction of muscle fibers. Under conditions of insufficient oxygen, metabolites from the oxygenation of glucose, particularly lactic acid, accumulate in the muscle. This accumulation of metabolites is thought to be a cause of soreness after excessive exercise. Both massage and heat increase the blood circulation within the muscle and aid in the destruction or the removal of the metabolites and in the consequent relief from soreness.

Muscles, like engines, are not completely efficient in their use of energy, and some of the energy is dissipated in the form of heat. This production of heat as a result of muscular contraction is obvious and needs little comment. Exercise may lead to such increased body heat that the production and evaporation of sweat and the dilation of the blood vessels in the skin occur in order to dissipate this heat. Similarly, when a person is too cold, the skeletal muscles are called on to produce more heat, and *shivering* is the response of the muscles to this demand.

Neuromuscular Ending

Discussion of functional aspects of muscular contraction would be incomplete without some further reference to the neuromuscular endings or motor end plates. Anatomically, the neuromuscular end plate or junction represents the point of contact between two different tissues: nerve fibers and muscle fibers. Physiologically, it represents the mechanism by which the nerve impulse is transmitted to the muscle fiber and creates the muscle impulse that results in contraction. Because this transmission takes place through a humoral mechanism, and because transmission of the nerve impulse and spread of contraction along the muscle fiber are electrical phenomena, the neuromuscular ending presents features that are found neither in the nerve fiber nor in the muscle fiber. It is, instead, essentially similar to the synapse, or junction, between two nerve cells.

This similarity is emphasized by the presence of acetylcholine, which is the transmitter involved at the neuromuscular junction and is also the active agent at many synapses. Because the acetylcholine stored at the nerve endings cannot be replaced as rapidly as it can be released, the repetitive stimulation of the nerve fiber can result in such depletion of the acetylcholine that transmission between nerve and muscle becomes largely ineffective or ceases entirely. This is often referred to as *fatigue of the neuromuscular junction*. Continuous stimulation of a nerve to a muscle results at first in a *tetanic* (constantly maintained) *contraction* of the muscle, because the nerve impulses reach the individual muscle fibers so fast that none of the fibers relax. If such stimulation is of long duration, the muscle begins to relax in spite of stimulation and eventually becomes completely relaxed because of fatigue at the neuromuscular ending. This fatigue then prevents further contraction of the muscle until recovery has taken place. It can be shown, however, that the muscle fibers themselves are still capable of contraction (inasmuch as they can be stimulated directly with an electric current) and that the nerve fibers can still conduct impulses. Complete tiring of the muscle really involves an inability of the nerve impulses to pass the neuromuscular junction.

Under ordinary circumstances, fatigue at the motor end plate is minimized through a rotation of contraction among the muscle fibers that carry out a given movement or maintain a certain posture. If all a person's strength is exerted in carrying out a certain movement, the person tires very quickly, and the movement soon becomes progressively weaker. The same movement, however, may be repeated for a much longer time if less effort is involved. If the desired strength of a movement requires only 5% of the total number of muscle fibers capable of carrying out that movement, then obviously any one motor unit could be used on an average of only once in every 20 contractions, which allows a considerable rest period before the same unit must be used again.

In addition to its susceptibility to fatigue, the neuromuscular junction is also susceptible to certain chemical agents. Among the best known of these is *curare,* long used by certain South American Indians as a poison to paralyze game and now of clinical importance. Curare blocks the neuromuscular junction, paralyzing skeletal muscles. In contrast to anesthetics, which affect primarily the nervous system rather than the neuromuscular junction, the carefully controlled clinical use of curare produces relaxation of the skeletal muscle without undue effect on the nervous system.

Effects of Training and Exercise on Muscle

FUNCTIONAL/CLINICAL NOTE 3-7

The supervision of therapeutic exercise plays an important part in the activities of the physical therapist and occupational therapist, and the physical educator must supervise normal motions. These clinicians should know what can and what cannot be accomplished through exercise. No amount of exercise will increase the number of muscle fibers in a muscle. Increase in size and strength of a muscle results from increase in the size (hypertrophy) of the muscle fibers already present. Because there are a maximal size and a maximal strength that muscle fibers can reach, the useful effects of exercise in increasing the strength of a muscle are limited. There is no way of restoring a muscle to normal if many fibers have completely degenerated and been replaced by fibrous tissue. All that can be done is to ensure the most effective action of the remaining muscle fibers and to hope that this action is functionally adequate.

The training of muscle really involves training the nervous system, because the activities of muscle depend entirely on the nervous system. If, in trying to produce a movement, the antagonists are also used, training must include relaxation of the antagonists, as well as the most efficient use of the prime movers. Also, because patterns of movement are learned, reeducation in a movement may allow a new pattern of muscular contraction to be set up in the central nervous system. In this way, the weakness of a given muscle or muscle group is at least partially compensated for by the use of other muscles, perhaps not habitually used in the weakened movement, but having functions overlapping with those of the weakened group.

An important factor in muscular imbalance is the fact that muscle fibers tend to adjust their lengths (under the control of the nervous system) so that they are exactly long enough, but no longer than is necessary, to bring about the range of movement ordinarily required of them. In order to retain their original lengths, they need to be stretched and made to contract over the total distance that they normally do. Therefore, if a part is so bent that the muscle or muscles crossing it need to contract over only half the distance ordinarily necessary, these muscles contract enough to take up the slack. The longer the part is kept in such a position, the more "set" the muscle fibers become in this short, partially contracted condition, and the more difficult it is later to stretch them back to their original lengths.

This shortening, or *contracture,* of muscle can occur either through a part being kept in a flexed position by splints or as a result of weakness of an opposing muscle group. In paralyses caused by peripheral nerve injuries, it often occurs that the unparalyzed muscles draw the part toward themselves, and if the regenerative process is lengthy, they can become fixed in this shortened position before the paralyzed muscles can recover. This shortening can be prevented by passively carrying the affected part through its complete range of movement to subject the unparalyzed muscles to a normal amount of stretch.

Another type of contracture that has nothing directly to do with muscle results from the deposition of collagen in joints, ligaments, and tendons, as in a completely paralyzed (flail) limb. Here also, the physical therapist, by taking the part through its complete range of normal movement, can stretch the newly formed tissue and prevent deformity.

Closely related to the problem of reeducation in cases of loss of muscular power is the possibility of substitute movements, sometimes known as "trick" movements. These depend primarily on taking advantage of some mechanical disposition of muscles and tendons at joints so that a movement that is otherwise impossible can be carried out. For instance, in paralysis of the extensors of the wrist and fingers, the wrist can frequently be extended adequately by clenching the fingers tightly, and some extension of the fingers can be obtained by sharply flexing the wrist. Both of these flexion movements mechanically put tension on the extensor tendons. Such substitute movements are very important, and the therapist must become familiar with many of these in order to aid the patient in overcoming physical disabilities.

NERVOUS SYSTEM

The essential elements of the nervous system are neurons and their processes: that is, cells that are especially differentiated for the conduction of impulses. These important cells are described briefly in Chapter 2. However, it is the arrangement of these cells, and their functional connections, that is important in understanding the nervous system. Although an adequate discussion of either the anatomy or the physiology of the nervous system is beyond the scope of this book, certain fundamentals of the organization and function of this system are necessary to understand the function of muscles and of the body in general.

Anatomically, the nervous system is divisible into two major parts: the central nervous system and the peripheral nervous system. The **central nervous system** is composed of the *brain* and *spinal cord.* The **peripheral nervous system** is made up of the *cranial* and *spinal nerves* and of the *autonomic nervous system.* Such a division is useful for descriptive purposes, but it must be clearly understood that all parts of the nervous system are dependent on one another. The peripheral nervous system arises in part within the central nervous system, and it both receives impulses from and sends impulses into the central nervous system. The central nervous system, in contrast, obtains all its information from and is able to exert its effects only through the peripheral nervous system. Various details of the distribution of the peripheral nervous system are described throughout this book. Some further basic features of the anatomy of the spinal cord and brain are described in Section 3 ("The Back") and Section 5 ("The Head, Neck, and Trunk").

Origin

The central nervous system arises as a thickening of the epithelium on the dorsal surface of the embryo. This thickening sinks into the underlying tissue to form a groove. The lips of the groove then roll together to form the **neural tube,** which separates from the overlying epithelium. As this separation occurs, epithelium at the junction of the neural groove and the overlying epithelium separates from both, to lie alongside the neural tube. This, the **neural crest,** forms the sensory ganglia of the spinal nerves and some cranial nerves, as well as the ganglia of the autonomic nervous system.

Only the cells adjacent to the lumen of the spinal cord and brain retain their epithelial shape. The others, after a period of proliferation, differentiate either into connective tissue unique to the central nervous system or into neuroblasts. A neuroblast becomes a neuron by giving rise to sprouts that grow out as dendrites and axons. Axons in the central nervous system grow for varying distances within that system or, if they are to emerge as motor fibers, leave it as components of a root of the nerve (anterior root for a spinal nerve). Each axon then must continue to grow until it reaches the muscle or other structure in which it is to end. The neuroblasts of the sensory ganglia likewise give rise to sprouts, but only two are formed. One grows centrally into the central nervous system, and the other grows peripherally to form a sensory ending.

Synapse

The essential feature of the organization of neurons is their functional connection to one another by their processes. Unless they end peripherally on muscle or glands, axons of neurons end primarily in connection with the dendrites or cell bodies of other neurons. Through these connections, the cells of the central nervous system are arranged in innumerable interconnecting "circuits" or nerve pathways. If there were no designation as to the routing of a nerve impulse, it might wander haphazardly from one "circuit" to another. It might also spread simultaneously in many directions so as to eventually involve the entire nervous system in aimless and uncoordinated activity.

However, once an impulse is initiated in a neuron, there is no variation as to the pathway within that cell: The impulse must follow out the axon and travel along all its branches. When, however, the impulse arrives at the terminations of the axon, other conditions prevail. There exists between one axon and the next neuron a slight gap (minute anatomically, but very important physiologically) that the nerve impulse must cross if it is to affect the next neuron. This tiny gap is known as the **synapse,** and because of the character of the synapse, coordinated activity of the nervous system is possible.

At the synapse, a determination is made as to whether an impulse will cross to the next neuron or be obliterated. Some synapses are much more resistant to the passage of a nerve impulse than are others. If resistance at the synapses is generally broken down, as occurs in strychnine poisoning, then nerve impulses spread through the nervous system without order, and totally uncoordinated activity results. The response of the synapse to the timing and the number of nerve impulses reaching it plays a decisive role in the activity of the nervous system. Knowledge of the important functional connections existing among neurons, and under what conditions certain synapses become usable, enable an outline of some of the more simple features of neural activity, especially in relation to sensation and to activity of skeletal muscles.

Spinal Cord

The spinal cord, the lower and least complicated portion of the central nervous system, is continuous with the brain. Its diameter is about the size of a finger and in an average adult is about 17 or 18 inches long. It is protected by the vertebral (spinal) column and is connected to skeletal muscles, skin, and other structures by the spinal nerves. In cross-section, the fresh spinal cord can be seen to contain a center of pinkish-gray material (shaped approximately like a butterfly or a distorted letter H) known as the *gray matter* (Fig. 3-8). The peripheral glistening white area is known as the *white matter*. Both gray and white matter extend throughout the length of the spinal cord and continue upward into the brain. The horns seen in cross-sections of the cord are actually parts

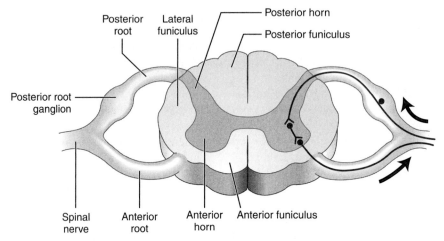

Figure 3-8 A spinal cord segment. The gray matter of the cord is surrounded by white matter (funiculi). On the right, a simple spinal reflex arc is illustrated. This particular arc is diagrammed as involving only three elements: a sensory neuron, which brings an impulse originating in the sensory receptor into the nervous system; an intercalated neuron located in the anterior horn that transmits this impulse to the motor neuron; and the lower motor neuron, which transmits the impulse to the effector organ, the skeletal muscle. Other connections of the sensory fiber are not shown, nor are the many other fibers that end in connection with the lower motor neuron, the final common path to the muscle. *Arrows* indicate the direction flow of the nerve impulse.

of continuous gray columns, and the words *horns* and *columns* are used somewhat interchangeably in referring to the gray matter. The gray matter of the spinal cord consists primarily of cell bodies of neurons but also contains the fibers leaving these cell bodies and the fibers entering the gray matter to end on them.

The posterior or dorsal projections of the gray matter on either side are known as the **posterior, or dorsal, horns.** They are concerned especially with receiving impulses coming in through the spinal nerves and with routing such impulses upward to the brain. The anterior or ventral projections of the gray matter are the **anterior, or ventral, horns.** Many of the cells of these horns give rise to fibers that leave the spinal cord as the anterior (ventral, motor) roots of the spinal nerves, to end eventually on skeletal muscles. Associated with the motor fibers to skeletal muscles as they emerge to form the anterior roots of the nerves are motor fibers controlling the activity of smooth muscles and glands. These are the sympathetic (and, to a more limited extent, parasympathetic) fibers, which arise from cells situated laterally in the posterior parts of the anterior horns of some, but not all, parts of the spinal cord. There are also many cells in both horns that receive impulses from higher centers

or from incoming nerve fibers and distribute them to other cells of the cord.

The white matter is composed of nerve fibers. The spinal cord is partially divided into right and left halves by a posterior septum and an anterior fissure. The projecting anterior and posterior horns of the gray matter tend, in turn, to divide the white matter of one side into three great bundles, the **funiculi,** or **white columns:** a *posterior,* a *lateral,* and an *anterior* funiculus. Each of the funiculi is, in turn, composed of several variously definitive, but often overlapping, smaller bundles of fibers. These smaller fiber bundles *(fasciculi)* are also known as the *tracts of the spinal cord.* These tracts represent groupings of fibers of a similar function and are discussed briefly in Section 3 ("The Back"). For purposes of this discussion, it need be noted only that they include groups of nerve fibers that connect different parts of the spinal cord, ascend to various parts of the brain, or descend from the brain to the cord. Fibers in the *lateral* and *anterior funiculi* consist of all three types and are derived almost entirely from cells that lie in the central nervous system. Those of the *posterior funiculus* are mostly ascending fibers and are the central processes of neurons that form the posterior root ganglia and send their peripheral processes, as sensory fibers, into the spinal nerves.

Afferent fibers

Afferent fibers entering the spinal cord arise from cell bodies that are located in the posterior roots of the spinal nerves, where they form the posterior root ganglia (see Fig. 3-8). The peripheral processes from these ganglion cells end in connection with many tissues in the body and are variously concerned with impulses of touch, pressure, temperature, or pain or with impulses from other structures, including muscles, joints, and tendons. As the central processes of these neurons enter the spinal cord, each fiber branches. Some branches end in the gray matter of the spinal cord at the level at which the nerve fiber enters the cord. Others run upward or downward within the white matter of the cord for varying distances. Through these branches of a single entering nerve fiber, it is possible for an incoming sensory impulse to travel in several directions within the spinal cord at one time. Many of the branches of the sensory fiber end on cells of the posterior horn, through which their impulses are propagated both within the cord and, by way of the long ascending tracts, upward to various parts of the brain. Some end also on the large cells in the anterior horn that control skeletal muscle.

Motor neurons

The long descending tracts of the cord originate from neurons in many parts of the brain. The majority of their fibers end either on the anterior horn cells supplying skeletal muscle or on cells that in turn send fibers to these anterior horn cells. Therefore, most of these tracts are known as **motor tracts**, and the groups of cells from which they originate in the brain constitute **motor centers**. The pathway by which the motor centers of the brain influence skeletal muscle always involves at least two neurons: one in the brain and one in the anterior horn of the spinal cord. Because both are motor neurons, they are distinguished as follows: the cell in the anterior horn is the *lower motor neuron*, and the cell in the brain is the *upper motor neuron*.

The large **lower motor neurons** of the anterior horn not only receive connections from all the motor tracts of the cord that affect skeletal muscle but also are influenced by incoming sensory fibers of various types. Therefore, nerve impulses from many different sources converge on the lower motor neuron. *The lower motor neurons and their fibers constitute the only connection between the spinal cord and skeletal muscles.* It does not matter whether the muscle cell is to be affected by a nerve impulse originally derived from stimulation of the skin, from stretching of a muscle or movement of a joint, or from any of those numerous parts of the brain having to do with the action of skeletal muscle; the lower motor neuron of the anterior horn, with its fiber (axon) ending on the muscle, constitutes the only pathway to this muscle. This cell and its axon were therefore called the *final common path* by Sir Charles Scott Sherrington (1857–1952), a famous neurophysiologist.

Destruction of the lower motor neuron, the final common path, means that no impulses, whatever their original sources, can reach the skeletal muscle. Therefore, such destruction leads to complete paralysis of the muscle concerned. If the paralysis of the muscle is the result of a peripheral nerve injury (damage to the axons of the lower motor neurons), the body attempts to repair the nerve injury. The complete lack of activity in the paralyzed muscle, however, leads to atrophy and degeneration of the muscle fibers. Thus, while the nerve repair is awaited, the therapist attempts to halt the atrophy as much as possible by stimulating the circulation to the muscle and, perhaps, stimulating contraction of the muscle fibers through an electric current.

FUNCTIONAL/CLINICAL NOTE 3-8

If all the lower motor neurons to a given muscle are destroyed, that muscle always remains paralyzed because new neurons cannot be formed to replace those destroyed. Lower motor neurons may also be so damaged that they cease to function for a while, which also results in paralysis of the muscle; however, the neurons may later recover, with consequent recovery of function on the part of the muscle. It is impossible to distinguish between paralysis caused by total destruction of the

Continued

neurons supplying the muscle and paralysis caused by their temporary injury. Hope of recovery after muscular paralysis should not be abandoned until it seems obvious that the neurons innervating the muscles have actually been destroyed.

Reflex arc

The least complicated of the controls over the lower motor neuron is that of incoming sensory fibers at the spinal level. These fibers, their connections with the lower motor neuron, and this neuron itself can be regarded as forming an anatomical and functional unit called a simple **spinal reflex arc** (see Fig. 3-8). A particular characteristic of a reflex (a reflex being the activity resulting from the functioning of a reflex arc) is that the response after the application of a given stimulus is stereotyped; that is, the nerve connections are so relatively simple that there is little choice as to the routing of the nerve impulse, and, therefore, little opportunity for deviation from one particularly appropriate action. All human activities are built upon reflex arcs of varying complexity. The simple spinal reflexes constitute the basis of all muscular activity, even though, in normal life, spinal reflexes are much affected, modified, and sometimes rendered almost unrecognizable by impulses from numerous other reflex arcs and from conscious centers.

A pure spinal reflex, free from inhibiting or inciting influences from higher centers, can occur only when the spinal cord is cut in two so as to isolate a lower portion of the cord. In an animal or a human with the cord so cut, the muscles supplied from this lower segment of the cord are paralyzed, for they can no longer respond to the efforts of the individual to move them. They are not paralyzed, however, in the sense that they cannot contract, for indeed a great deal of activity is maintained in them through the activity of the reflex arc. If the muscles supplied from an isolated segment of the cord are palpated, they are relaxed even less than in the normal individual. The limbs may be maintained in abnormal postures by this excessive contraction and may offer considerable resistance to passive movement by the clinician. This is because various sensory impulses arising both from the skin and from the muscles, tendons, and joints are being constantly poured into the spinal cord, in which they act on the lower motor neuron. This lower motor neuron, being now freed of all impulses from centers in the brain, responds more actively than normal to the incoming impulses at its own level. If all sensory impulses coming into the cord are abolished, the activity of the muscles then ceases. If, on the other hand, sensory impulses are increased by stimulation, then the activity of a certain muscle or muscle group is likewise increased and may produce a definite movement or reflex action. In physiological terms, a simple spinal reflex involves stimulation of receptors, transmission (of the nerve impulses set up) along the sensory fibers of the spinal nerve to the cord, and relay of these impulses to the motor neurons, with subsequent transmission to an effector organ.

In an animal with a severed spinal cord, a simple type of spinal reflex may be elicited by pricking the skin of the foot. Regardless of how many times this is done, if proper attention is paid to the conditions of the experiment, the result are always the same: The animal withdraws the foot as if to escape from the source of the pain—an obviously useful movement.

Another simple spinal reflex is the muscle stretch reflex. If a muscle is stretched, nerve endings within that muscle are stimulated, and this stimulation, being transmitted to the central nervous system, brings about the activity of the lower motor neuron and contraction of the muscle. A very familiar example of this stretch reflex is the *patellar reflex,* or *knee jerk.* Tapping the tendon below the patella (knee cap) results in a contraction of the extensor muscle of the knee, causing a sudden kick. Although this reflex as elicited may seem purposeless, it is actually the basis of the support of the body weight. Stretching of the large muscle (quadriceps femoris) on the front of the thigh (and stretching of the tendon) usually means that the knee is being bent and is therefore giving way beneath its load. Further contraction of the extensor of the knee is a logical response to control of this movement, to prevent tumbling to the ground.

Not all spinal reflexes are as simple as those just mentioned. For instance, experimental results have demonstrated that if the foot of a dog with a severed spinal cord were pricked with a pin, the dog would withdraw that foot (despite the fact that because the pain impulse cannot reach the brain, the dog feels nothing). This reaction is a simple spinal withdrawal reflex. At the same time that the dog withdraws the pricked foot, the extensor muscles of the other limbs would increase their contraction in order to support the shift in weight of the body. Spinal reflexes, whether simple or complicated, are coordinated reactions that seem to be carefully planned to bring about an appropriate response to a given stimulus. They differ from more complicated reactions in the nervous system through their relative simplicity and the inevitability of their results. An intact dog, when pricked on the foot, will usually lift that foot, but they may also turn to bite what is pricking them or attempt to run away; therefore, there is a choice among several courses of action. The injured dog (with a severed spinal cord), on the other hand, would simply continue to lift the pricked paw, making no effort either to bite what pricks it or to run away. In fact, such a dog does not know the foot is being injured or lifted because severing of the cord prevents sensory impulses of any type from reaching the brain.

FUNCTIONAL/CLINICAL NOTE 3-9

As evidenced by the preceding examples, some of the more important spinal reflexes involving skeletal muscle are concerned with the protection of the body from harmful influences or with the maintenance of posture. Because harmful stimuli usually cause pain, reflexes initiated by pain are of common occurrence. For example, people "double up" with abdominal pain because this pain causes increased tension in the abdominal muscles, which contract in order to protect the abdominal contents from outside pressure. The contraction of the muscles, consequently, increases intra-abdominal pressure, which is relieved by flexing the trunk and therefore approximating the origins and insertions of the muscles concerned. The physician, in examining the abdomen, notes the occurrence and the location of muscle spasm as one clue to where the pain originates.

In a similar way, meningitis, or inflammation of the coverings of the brain and spinal cord may result in the head and back's being arched backward by the contraction of the back muscles. This posture somewhat relieves the tension of the coverings over the convexity of the brain. Another example of the protective reflex action of muscle is found in the fixation of a painful joint. All the muscles around such a joint may go into spasm to prevent that joint from being further moved.

Because flexion, representing a withdrawal movement, is a basic reflex response to pain, the flexor muscles frequently contract more than do the extensors around a painful joint, thus maintaining the joint in flexion in spite of the fact that the extensors (usually the antigravity muscles) are typically the stronger muscles. In very painful rheumatoid arthritis, for instance, the limb is characteristically maintained in flexion spasm.

Supraspinal Influences

The activity of the lower motor neuron is obviously maintained in part by spinal reflexes. In the intact (noninjured) individual, however, this cell is also under the control of the various descending motor pathways from the brain. Therefore, its final action is a summation of all of the various excitatory and inhibitory impulses reaching it. The physician examines spinal reflexes because these can be affected not only by damage to the components of the spinal reflex arc but also by damage to various higher centers or pathways. A change from normal in a reflex may give important information concerning the functional activities of these higher centers or their descending tracts.

The motor pathways descending into the cord are responsible for all the voluntary and much of the automatic or higher reflex control over the lower motor neuron. A typical result of an upper motor neuron lesion is paralysis of voluntary movement, as in a stroke in which a whole side of the body is paralyzed. The same injury that prevents impulses for voluntary movement from reaching the lower motor neurons also cuts off a variable number of other impulses, especially inhibitory ones, so that the lower motor neuron is simultaneously deprived of its ability to carry out voluntary movements and yet excited more than normally by various reflex arcs converging on it. Many peripheral stimuli may produce a contraction of the affected muscles. Upper motor neuron paralysis, therefore, is typically a spastic paralysis in which the muscles cannot be used voluntarily, and at the same time, their contraction and their resistance to passive movement are increased markedly above normal. This type of paralysis is in sharp contrast to lower motor neuron paralysis, in which, again, the muscles are not subject to voluntary influence but are in addition completely relaxed or flaccid, because destruction of the lower motor neurons prevents any nerve impulses from reaching the muscles.

Other motor centers in the brain are concerned not with initiating a voluntary movement but with coordinating the action of the numerous lower motor neurons involved so that a movement is carried out smoothly and accurately. Disease of some of these centers results in abnormal distribution of impulses to the lower motor neuron. Depending on the center involved, a number of situations may occur. There may be almost constant contraction of all muscles, known as *rigidity* because the part is then hard to move. There may be trembling whenever a part is moved, and it may be moved inaccurately and weakly. There may also be trembling at rest and, perhaps, uncontrollable movement of a part, such as flinging a limb around in a purposeless manner. All these situations provide evidence of the intricacy of control needed to ensure proper function of the lower motor neurons and, through them, the muscles.

Nerves

The nerves arising from the brain and spinal cord are bundles of axons of neurons that connect the central nervous system to the rest of the body. The voluntary motor fibers of a nerve arise from lower motor neurons and extend to the skeletal muscle, however remote that muscle may be from the central nervous system. The cell bodies of sensory fibers of a nerve are located in ganglia (collections of cell bodies of neurons outside the central nervous system). The ganglia are very close to the central nervous system and are protected by the skull and vertebral column, which also protect the central nervous system. A sensory neuron in a ganglion has two processes that arise together but soon separate. One is usually very long and runs peripherally in the nerve to reach skin, muscle, or other tissue with a sensory innervation. The other enters the central nervous system and then branches to end on cells located there.

The nerves containing fibers traveling to and from the central nervous system can be classified into two groups: spinal and cranial nerves. *Spinal nerves*, which attach to the spinal cord, are associated with the vertebral column at their formation (see also Chapter 13). *Cranial nerves*, which attach to the brain, make their exits through the skull. (Cranial nerves are considered in Chapter 21.) All the smaller nerves found in the body are branches of either the spinal or the cranial nerves.

Spinal nerves

There are 31 pairs of spinal nerves. To differentiate between the various spinal nerves, they are all named and numbered according to the segment of the spinal cord to which they are related. The eight pairs that leave the vertebral column in the neck are called **cervical nerves** and are distinguished from each other by number—the first cervical nerve is the highest, the eighth the lowest. Similarly, there are 12 pairs of **thoracic nerves,** or nerves associated with the thorax; five pairs of **lumbar nerves,** which leave the mobile part of the vertebral column below the ribs; five pairs of **sacral nerves,** associated with the sacrum; and one pair of **coccygeal nerves,** which leave the lowest part of the vertebral column. In identifying the nerves, an abbreviated terminology is often used. The third cervical nerve, for instance, is labeled C3 (also written C-3), the letter *C* standing for *cervical;* similarly, T1 through T12 (also written T-1 and so forth) identifies thoracic nerves; L1 through L5, lumbar nerves; S1 through S5, sacral nerves; and Co, the coccygeal nerves.

Each spinal nerve is attached to the spinal cord (see Fig. 3-8) by a **posterior root** (also called a *dorsal root*), which is sensory, and an **anterior root** (also called a *ventral root*), which is motor. On the posterior root there is a swelling, the **posterior root ganglion,** produced by the accumulation of the cell bodies of the sensory fibers. The ganglion lies on the posterior root at the point where the nerve is about to leave the shelter of the vertebral column. Just distal to the ganglion, as the nerve emerges from between the adjacent vertebrae, the posterior and anterior roots join, and their fibers become mixed together. As a result of this mixing, almost all the branches of a spinal nerve contain both sensory and motor fibers. Although injury to or surgical section (cutting) of the posterior and anterior roots separately causes injury only to sensory or motor fibers, injury to the spinal nerves after their roots have joined involves both types of fibers.

After the mixed (sensory and motor) spinal nerve leaves the vertebral column, it divides into two branches, a **posterior (dorsal) ramus** that turns posteriorly to supply muscle and skin of the back, and an **anterior (ventral) ramus** that runs laterally and anteriorly (see Fig. 13-13). The anterior rami supply the muscles and skin of all parts of the body except the back. Except in the thoracic region, where they run between the ribs and are separated by these, the anterior rami run close together and exchange branches with each other. Such an exchange is known as a **nerve plexus** (e.g., see Fig. 5-7). Instead of containing fibers of only one spinal nerve, as the anterior rami entering the plexus obviously do, the nerves leaving the plexus usually contain fibers from more than one spinal nerve.

Because the nerves supplying the limbs form plexuses, it is difficult to determine the exact distribution of spinal nerves to the muscles and skin of the limbs. The peripheral nerves, containing fibers from several spinal nerves, can be traced by dissection. The clinician, however, must distinguish between segmental (spinal) nerve distribution and peripheral nerve distribution and must be familiar with both. **Segmental innervation** is the distribution of all motor and sensory nerve fibers from one spinal cord segment (in other words, of the pair of spinal nerves of that segment). For example, the segmental innervation of spinal cord segment C8 (the eighth segment in the cervical region of the cord) would include all skeletal muscles to which it provides motor fibers, sensory input to muscle tissue, and the area of skin innervated

exclusively by C8. Because fibers of C8 enter and mix with other fibers in the brachial plexus of the upper limb, the fibers can be included in several nerve branches of the plexus. Each peripheral nerve has a specific distribution. All motor and sensory innervation provided by each named nerve would be considered its **peripheral innervation.**

The innervation of skin can be described in terms of the segmental nerve innervation or the peripheral nerve innervation. Cutaneous peripheral nerve innervation can be reasonably determined accurately by dissection, although, because of overlap between adjacent nerves, the area of sensory loss after section of any one nerve is never as large as might be expected. The distribution of sensory fibers from one segment of the spinal cord to the skin is known as a **dermatome** (Fig. 3-9). Because there is overlap between adjacent spinal nerves, the most common method of determining dermatomes has been to record the area in which sensation remains when an intact spinal nerve is bordered above and below by nerves that have been interrupted. On the trunk—because the nerves are not branches of a nerve plexus—dermatomes and peripheral nerve distribution are identical, but on the limbs, the dermatomes bear no apparent relation to the distribution of the various peripheral nerves.

A comparison of segmental (as represented by a dermatome of the segment) and peripheral innervation of the skin of the upper limb is shown in Figure 3-10. The dermatome of C8 includes part of the medial side of the forearm. The peripheral nerve innervation to this area is provided by the medial cutaneous nerve of the forearm. This indicates that this nerve contains nerve fibers from C8. It is also apparent from the figure, in a comparison of the dermatome with the peripheral nerve, that the area innervated by the medial cutaneous nerve of the forearm also includes part of the dermatome of T1. Therefore, the medial cutaneous nerve of the forearm also includes fibers from the T1 segment of the spinal cord.

Knowledge of the approximate segmental innervation of the skeletal muscles is also useful (e.g., see Tables 5-7 and 6-4). Although there is disagreement on details, probably resulting both from incomplete knowledge and from variations among persons, a general rule is that most muscles are innervated

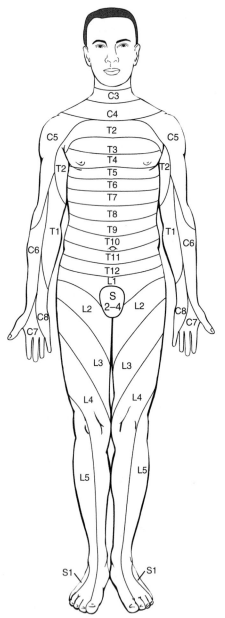

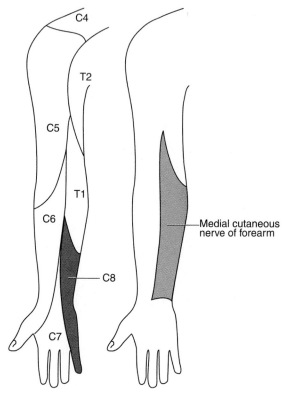

Figure 3-10 Cutaneous innervation of the upper limb. *Left,* Dermatomes, representing segmental innervation to the skin. *Right,* The cutaneous innervation provided by the medial cutaneous nerve of the forearm (providing an example of the distribution of a peripheral nerve). Comparison of the illustrations reveals that the medial cutaneous nerve of the forearm contains fibers from spinal cord segments C8 and T1. This illustrates that a peripheral nerve may contain nerve fibers from more than one spinal cord segment.

by two or more spinal nerves and that any one spinal nerve to the limbs helps to supply a large number of muscles.

Autonomic Nervous System

The autonomic nervous system is the portion of the motor nervous system that controls the activities of *smooth muscle, cardiac muscle,* and *certain glands.* It has, therefore, no direct effect on skeletal muscles, but its activities do influence the activities of the body as a whole. The autonomic nervous system is classified as a part of the peripheral nervous system because a large part of it lies outside the central nervous system.

Figure 3-9 Dermatomes of the anterior aspect of the body. Charts vary significantly because of differences in interpretation, anatomical variations between individuals, and methods of collecting data. Extent of dermatomes is approximate as a result of overlap of dermatomal areas.

There are, however, important centers and pathways within the brain and spinal cord that influence the activity of the autonomic system. These are referred to as *autonomic centers* and *pathways*. The autonomic nervous system is like the rest of the peripheral nervous system in that its activities are dependent on the activities of the central nervous system.

The autonomic nervous system can be classified into two parts: the **sympathetic nervous system** and the **parasympathetic nervous system.** Although there are anatomical and functional differences between the two systems, they also share some general characteristics. Both systems control involuntary structures, and two neurons are used to conduct impulses from the central nervous system to the structure to be innervated. (The latter is in contrast to the innervation of skeletal muscle, in which one neuron transmits the impulses from the central nervous system to the muscle.)

The first neuron, the **preganglionic neuron,** is located in the central nervous system. Its axon exits the central nervous system and passes out to the periphery to synapse with a second neuron, the **postganglionic neuron.** Collections of postganglionic neurons form a ganglion. These ganglia are always located in a position outside the central nervous system. The axon of the postganglionic neuron exits the ganglion and passes to the structure to which it provides innervation. Typically, one preganglionic fiber synapses with more than one postganglionic neuron. The sympathetic system typically has a larger number of postganglionic neurons associated with each preganglionic fiber than does the parasympathetic system.

Location and outflow of preganglionic neurons

All preganglionic neurons are located in either the brain or spinal cord. As noted previously, these fibers exit the central nervous system to synapse on postganglionic neurons. Some preganglionic fibers become associated with selected cranial nerves; others exit in the anterior roots of spinal nerves of the twelve thoracic, upper lumbar, and second to fourth sacral segments of the spinal cord (see Chapter 13 for more information on spinal cord segments). Therefore, the autonomic outflow of preganglionic fibers from the central nervous system occurs in three groups: *cranial, thoracolumbar,* and *sacral outflows.*

A **cranial outflow** is associated with certain cranial nerves and is separated from the **thoracolumbar outflow** by the cervical nerves, in which there is no preganglionic outflow. The thoracolumbar outflow then forms a second group and is in turn separated from the third or **sacral outflow** by the lower lumbar and one or more upper sacral nerves, which also have no preganglionic outflow.

The *thoracolumbar outflow* and its distribution make up the *sympathetic nervous system.* Figure 3-11 illustrates the essential structure of this system. The cranial and sacral outflows *(craniosacral outflow)* of the autonomic nervous system closely resemble each other in their anatomy and physiology, and they and their further distribution are grouped together as the *parasympathetic nervous system.*

Postganglionic neurons

The ganglia containing the postganglionic neurons of the sympathetic nervous system form paired **sympathetic trunks** or **chains** lying on the sides or front of the vertebral column. The trunks extend from the neck region (around the level of the second cervical vertebra) to the end of the vertebral column, where the two trunks join at the coccyx. The ganglia in the sympathetic trunk are sometimes termed the *paravertebral ganglia* to distinguish them from a second group of sympathetic ganglia that are located around the aorta and origins of the great vessels going to the abdominal viscera. Those ganglia are called the *prevertebral ganglia* because they are positioned in front of the vertebral column. The prevertebral ganglia, with their fibers entering and leaving them, form the celiac, or solar, plexus and other plexuses on the anterior surface of the aorta (see Fig. 23-8).

The **ganglia of the parasympathetic nervous system** are small and scattered, being located in or very close to the organ that they innervate. Except for a few parasympathetic ganglia in the head, most of the parasympathetic ganglia are too small to be seen during dissection.

Postganglionic fibers from both the sympathetic and parasympathetic ganglia usually run with other nerves or along blood vessels to the organs that they innervate. For instance, the postganglionic sympathetic fibers to the limbs join the spinal nerves close to the spinal cord and are distributed by these nerves

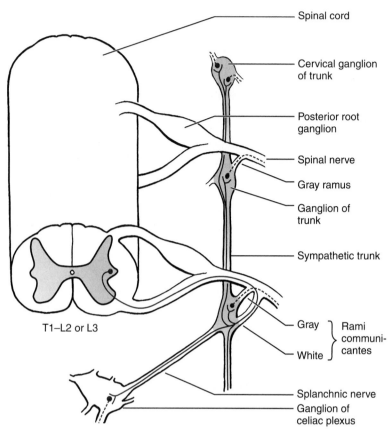

Spinal cord

Cervical ganglion of trunk

Posterior root ganglion

Spinal nerve

Gray ramus

Ganglion of trunk

Sympathetic trunk

Gray ⎤ Rami
White ⎦ communi-cantes

Splanchnic nerve

Ganglion of celiac plexus

T1–L2 or L3

Figure 3-11 Course of sympathetic fibers. The segment shown at the cross-section of the spinal cord is representative of the sympathetic outflow from T1 to L2 or L3. A single preganglionic fiber (*solid line*) is used to illustrate the possible courses that preganglionic fibers can take. They travel through the anterior root of a spinal nerve and leave the nerve to reach the sympathetic trunk. At the trunk, they have one of several courses: they may synapse with the ganglion cells in the first ganglion they reach; they may run up or down the trunk to synapse in ganglia above or below the level at which they enter the trunk; or they may leave the trunk without synapsing, to end in ganglia of the celiac or other ganglia around the aorta. Postganglionic fibers (*broken lines*) arise from cells of the trunk ganglia and return to the spinal nerves to be distributed with them, arise from the ganglia of the celiac and related plexuses to be distributed along the blood vessels to the viscera, or leave as a direct branch of a cervical ganglion to structures in the head and neck. (The association of the cervical ganglia to spinal nerves is the same as that for other ganglia of the trunk, but it is not illustrated.) Of note: There are preganglionic fibers that go to the medulla of the suprarenal gland to synapse directly on cells there.

along with other fibers to the various parts of the limb. The postganglionic sympathetic fibers to the head and to the abdominal viscera reach these parts mainly by following blood vessels.

Both sympathetic and parasympathetic fibers frequently go to the same organ; therefore, many involuntary structures have a double innervation. Typically, when both systems innervate an organ, they have opposite effects on it. For instance, the sympathetic innervation to the pupil of the eye dilates the pupil;

the parasympathetic innervation constricts the pupil. Not all organs, however, are supplied by both sets of fibers. The smooth muscle of the blood vessels in the limbs, for instance, is innervated only through sympathetic fibers (because parasympathetic fibers do not enter the extremities). The two systems do not actively oppose each other in the organs that have a double innervation. Instead, they cooperate in much the same manner that prime movers and antagonists of skeletal muscles do.

Sympathetic nerve fibers

As previously mentioned, the sympathetic system receives its preganglionic fibers from the thoracolumbar outflow. More specifically, these fibers arise from the lateral horn (intermediolateral nucleus) of the gray matter in spinal cord segments **T1 to L2 or L3.** The preganglionic fibers travel in the spinal nerves of those levels (see Fig. 3-11) and reach the sympathetic trunk by passing through the gray rami communicantes (gray rami are present only at the level of outflow of sympathetic preganglionic fibers). Once in the trunk, they have several possible courses. Some fibers synapse with postganglionic neurons at that level, and postganglionic fibers enter the spinal nerve by way of a white ramus. Those fibers then travel with the spinal nerve to reach the periphery. Other preganglionic fibers ascend or descend in the trunk to synapse at a higher or lower level; postganglionic fibers then exit in spinal nerves above and below the level of outflow from the central nervous system. By way of these various routes, sympathetic fibers can be provided to the periphery through all of the spinal nerves.

Sympathetic fibers are also needed within the cavities (thoracic, abdominal, and pelvic) and in the head region. After entering the sympathetic trunk, some preganglionic fibers exit from the trunk in the thorax without synapsing by way of the **splanchnic nerves.** The fibers travel to the abdomen, where most synapse in the ganglia around the aorta. The postganglionic fibers are then distributed within the abdomen and pelvis. (In addition, some fibers go directly to the suprarenal gland to synapse with cells in the medulla of the gland.)

From the cervical part of the trunk (see Chapter 21) some postganglionic fibers are given off from the ganglia and travel downward into the thorax to innervate the lungs and heart. Others are distributed, usually by way of blood vessels, to the head.

Parasympathetic nerve fibers

The craniosacral outflow of the parasympathetic system consists of preganglionic fibers from nuclei in the brain that are associated with four **cranial nerves—oculomotor (cranial nerve III), facial (VII), glossopharyngeal (IX), and vagus (X)**—and of fibers from spinal cord segments **S2, S3, and S4.** The sacral fibers exit the spinal cord with the corresponding spinal nerves but leave these nerves immediately to remain within the pelvis. (As mentioned earlier, no parasympathetic fibers are contained within spinal nerves in the periphery.)

All of the preganglionic parasympathetic fibers must synapse with postganglionic neurons that are located outside of the central nervous system. For the majority of the parasympathetic fibers in the cranial nerves, the synapses occur in specific ganglia located within the head. Fibers in the *oculomotor nerve* (cranial nerve III) have synapses in the **ciliary ganglion** within the orbit. Those in the *facial nerve* (cranial nerve VII) have synapses in either the **submandibular ganglion** (located deep to the mandible) or **pterygopalatine ganglion** (situated deep within the head), and those of the *glossopharyngeal nerve* (cranial nerve IX) have synapses in the **otic ganglion** (also located in a deep position in the head). The postganglionic fibers of these three nerves are distributed within the head region. The fibers of the *vagus nerve* travel to the thorax and abdomen and synapse in ganglia located in these areas. The postganglionic fibers innervate the organs within the thorax and most of those in the abdomen. Sacral fibers synapse within the pelvis and their postganglionic fibers innervate pelvic organs and the terminal part of the digestive tract.

Functions of the autonomic nervous system

The functions of the two parts of the autonomic nervous system can be broadly compared. The sympathetic nervous system is concerned with preparing the body for emergency actions and functions, especially in times of fright or anger. The parasympathetic nervous system is concerned with maintaining the everyday activities of the body and minimizing some of the strains put on its parts.

Sympathetic stimulation tends to stop the digestive functions and constricts the blood vessels to the digestive tract and to the skin, so that more blood can be available to go to the limb muscles where it may be needed. It *increases the cardiac output* so that the blood circulates faster, and it *dilates the air passages in the lungs* so that the blood may be fully aerated. These things being done, the body is better prepared to react to danger by either fleeing or fighting, whichever seems appropriate. On the other hand, the *parasympathetic nervous system promotes the orderly activity of the digestive tract, slows the heart, and aids in emptying the rectum and bladder.*

Because the *autonomic system is defined as a motor system,* the sensory fibers that accompany it to visceral structures are not, strictly speaking, a part of this system. Although it is not unusual to hear references to "sympathetic sensory fibers," such fibers are better called *visceral sensory fibers.* They are concerned especially with pain and with reflex activity initiated in the viscera. In their anatomy, they are similar to other sensory fibers, inasmuch as their cell bodies lie in the sensory ganglia (not in autonomic ganglia) and their processes extend to the sensory endings. In order to reach the viscera, however, they travel with autonomic fibers going to the same location. Therefore, most autonomic nerves and plexuses are really a mixture of autonomic and sensory fibers.

CIRCULATORY SYSTEM

The circulatory system can be divided into two parts: a blood vascular system and a lymph vascular system. The **blood vascular system** consists of the *heart and blood vessels;* the **lymph vascular system** is made up of the *lymphatic vessels, tissues, and organs.*

Blood Vascular System

The heart (see Chapter 22) is a muscular pump that propels the blood. The tubes along which the blood is pumped as it leaves the heart are known as **arteries.** Because the blood enters the arteries under pressure, the arteries must have strong walls to withstand this pressure. The walls are also somewhat elastic, being composed of varying mixtures of elastic tissue and smooth muscle. This elasticity in turn helps force the blood along, and when elasticity is lost through *arteriosclerosis* (hardening of the arteries), the heart must beat harder in order to move the same amount of blood.

As the arteries branch and become smaller, they eventually give rise to very small branches known as **arterioles.** The chief component of the arteriolar wall is smooth muscle, and the contraction of this smooth muscle under the control of the sympathetic nervous system determines the ease with which the blood can pass through these smaller vessels. The *blood pressure* depends on the amount of blood pumped into the arteries by the heart and on the size of the vascular bed into which this blood can pass. If the arterioles are constricted, the size of the vascular bed is decreased, and blood flows more slowly from the arteries, so that on the next beat, the heart must contract more forcibly in order to push its contained blood through the arterial bed. If the arterioles are contracted, the blood pressure rises. If they are relaxed, the peripheral resistance and, therefore, the blood pressure are lowered. The arterioles also control the distribution of blood through various parts of the body. If the arterioles of one part of the body or one organ contract more than usual, then that part receives less blood than normal, and some other part then receives more than normal.

The arterioles open into **capillaries,** tiny vessels whose walls consist only of endothelium. This endothelium, which is one cell layer thick, is the same lining found throughout the entire vascular system. The walls of the capillaries, however, have no elastic fibers or smooth muscle. Through these very thin walls, exchange between materials in the blood and materials in the fluid outside the vascular system can take place. The capillaries are responsible for supplying the cells of the surrounding tissue with their required food, oxygen, and hormones and for removing from the fluid around these cells the carbon dioxide and other metabolic products that should be eliminated. The capillaries are in turn continuous with the **venules,** which join together to form **veins** and eventually return the blood to the heart. The vascular system forms a closed circuit, the blood circulating from the heart through the arteries, capillaries, and veins and then back to the heart.

Lymphatic Vascular System

The lymphatic system consists of lymphatic vessels, lymphatic fluid (lymph), and lymphatic tissues and organs. The lymphatic vessels constitute the lymphatic vascular system. The role of these vessels is to remove the excess extracellular fluid left within the tissues by the blood vascular system and return the collected lymph back to the venous blood. In contrast to the blood vascular system, the lymphatic system begins in blind capillaries among the cells. These capillaries unite to form larger vessels and eventually one major and several minor chief lymphatic vessels, which empty their contents into the blood stream by way of the great veins in the base of the neck. Most lymphatic vessels (and the veins of the limbs but not the veins of many other parts of the body) have valves that allow the lymph to flow in one direction, toward the heart, but resist a backward flow.

Associated with lymphatic vessels are structures known as **lymph nodes.** These are, in general, bean-shaped structures varying in size from that of a pin-head to that of a lima bean. The nodes are interposed along the pathways of the lymphatic vessels and act essentially as filters for the lymph. Lymph passes through one or more of these lymph nodes before it is returned to the blood stream.

FUNCTIONAL/CLINICAL NOTE 3-10

The lymphatic system frequently acts as the pathway for migration of infections and cancer, and the lymph nodes act as filters along the lymphatic pathway, tending to catch and hold for a time such bacteria or cancer cells that may reach them. The physician may look for red streaks up the arm or for hard swollen lymph nodes in the armpit or elsewhere as a sign of infection. The pathologist may examine lymph nodes for cancer cells or for other pathological processes that may involve the nodes.

The surgeon likewise is extremely conscious of the importance of the lymph nodes. In removing a cancerous structure, an attempt is made to also remove the lymph nodes to which the cancer is most likely to have spread. With such a procedure, the hope is that all of the cancer cells within the body are removed and the disease is cured by being eliminated. If the cancer has not yet spread beyond the nodes that can be removed, cure should result. For example, the axillary lymph nodes (in the armpit), which receive most of the lymphatic drainage of the breast, must often be removed during a *mastectomy* (surgical removal of the breast). If the cancer has spread into the underlying muscle tissue, that tissue, too, may be removed.

All of the lymphatic drainage of the body is eventually carried by one of two lymphatic vessels to the venous system (Fig. 3-12). The **thoracic duct,** on the left side of the body, joins the venous system at or near the junction of the left internal jugular and left subclavian veins. The thoracic duct receives the lymphatic drainage from the lower limbs, pelvis, abdomen, left upper limb, and left side of the thorax, neck, and head. On the right, the smaller **right lymphatic duct** joins the venous system at or near the junction of the right internal jugular and right subclavian veins. It receives the remainder of the lymphatic drainage of the body, which is from the right upper limb and right side of the thorax, neck, and head.

Blood

The blood is composed of *plasma,* in which the red and white blood cells are suspended. Blood is the sole means by which most of the tissues of the body can obtain the elements they need for life and through which they can dispose of harmful products of metabolism. The *red blood cells (erythrocytes)* transport oxygen, picking it up as they circulate through the capillaries of the lung and, in turn, giving it up as they circulate in the capillaries of the body tissues in general. The *white blood cells (leukocytes)* serve primarily to repel invasions of the body by noxious agents or cells that are foreign to that body (for instance, tissues introduced by skin, kidney, or heart transplants). Although most of the white blood cells are carried passively in the blood, they are living cells and are capable of movement. Moreover, they can leave the blood stream by passing through the junctions between the capillary endothelial cells and therefore may congregate in any tissue in which they are needed.

FUNCTIONAL/CLINICAL NOTE 3-11

Large numbers of white blood cells leave the blood stream this way to enter an area of infection and to act to overcome this infection both by engulfing the bacteria concerned and by the production of chemical substances that interfere with the growth or further life

Continued

of the bacteria. In any localized area of severe infection, white blood cells form a prominent element of the pus produced by the infection. In regard to transplants, the white blood cells that are responsible for their rejection respond to immunological differences between host and transplant tissues. Therefore, skin grafted from one location to another in the same person, or a graft from an identical twin, provokes no immunological reaction. In grafts between persons of little or no blood relationship, however, the major problem is usually how best to minimize the immunological reaction. This is done typically by the infusion into the blood stream of various chemical substances.

The blood is normally protected from contact with other tissues by the endothelial walls that line the blood vessels. If the blood vessels are damaged, blood may spread among the tissue cells or perhaps be lost from the body through an external opening. In either case, there is a tendency for the blood to check its own flow by clotting. *Clotting* involves certain chemical

reactions in the plasma, and in the case of small vessels, it results in the formation of a fibrous plug at the break in the wall of the vessel. The addition of heat hastens the chemical reaction that leads to clotting. However, heat causes the smaller blood vessels to dilate, whereas cold causes them to contract. Therefore, there is room for argument as to the efficacy of hot packs versus cold packs for the control of minor hemorrhages.

Even a slight injury to the endothelial lining results in the formation of a clot at the point of injury. If the injury is extensive, a large clot may be formed. If this clot later breaks away from the vessel wall, it is carried along by the blood stream until it reaches a vessel of a diameter too small for it to continue. It then occludes this vessel, with varying results. There is little effect if other vessels supply the same tissue as the obstructed vessel. If there is no other blood supply, death of that tissue, and perhaps even death of the individual, results.

There is normally a constant interchange of the fluids found in the blood capillaries, in the tissue spaces (living cells have to be surrounded by fluid), and in the lymphatic capillaries. If there is obstruction of either the venous or the lymphatic drainage of a part, fluid is likely to accumulate in the tissues

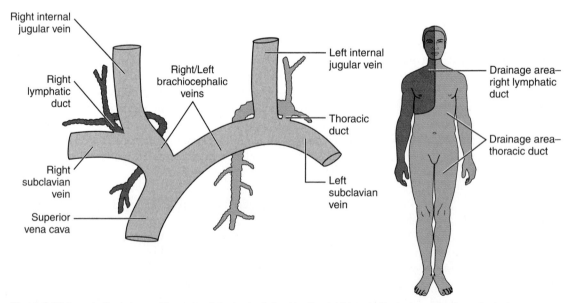

Figure 3-12 Lymphatic drainage. The areas of the body drained by the right lymphatic duct and the thoracic duct are illustrated. The right lymphatic duct and the thoracic duct return lymph to the venous system by joining the system at or near the junction of the internal jugular and subclavian veins on the right and left sides, respectively.

faster than it can be removed, leading to *edema,* or swelling of the tissues by the fluid. Another cause of local edema is infection.

DIGESTIVE SYSTEM

The digestive system includes the *mouth (or oral cavity), pharynx, esophagus, stomach, and intestines, with their associated glands.* The **oral cavity** is provided with three pairs of large salivary glands, whose secretion both moistens the food and starts the process of digestion. All three are closely associated with the mandible (lower jaw). The gland between the mandible and the ear that is involved in mumps is the *parotid gland.* The oral cavity opens into the **pharynx,** as does the nasal cavity, but the digestive and respiratory systems separate at the level of the larynx where the esophagus begins. The **esophagus** passes through the lower part of the neck and the entire thorax to reach the abdomen and ends in the **stomach.** The rest of the digestive tract consists of the **duodenum, jejunum,** and **ileum;** the **ascending, transverse, descending,** and **sigmoid colon;** the **rectum;** and the **anal canal.** The gross anatomy of these parts, beginning with the stomach, is described with the other abdominal viscera in Chapter 23.

Both the pharynx and the upper part of the esophagus are provided with skeletal muscle, but once swallowing is started, further propulsion through the essentially tubular digestive tract is carried out by smooth muscle. The digestive tract is lined with a highly glandular mucosa, which adds digestive enzymes and other substances to the ingested material and then absorbs the products of digestion and much of the water. The activity of the digestive tract is largely independent of nerves, but it is partly under the control of the autonomic nervous system.

RESPIRATORY SYSTEM

The respiratory system begins with the nose, in which the air passages are bilateral. The **nasal cavity** is provided with projections (conchae) from the walls that bring the air into close contact with the nasal mucosa. The nasal mucosa aids in warming and humidifying the air as it passes toward the lungs. Because both the nasal and oral cavities empty into the **pharynx,** the oral cavity can also be used for respiration, and it is used this way when the nasal passages cannot accommodate the sufficient airflow. The pharynx is held open by its attachments to the skeleton of the head and neck, allowing a free flow of air to the **larynx.** The **trachea** begins at the lower end of the larynx and is supported by a series of C-shaped cartilages that keep this part of the air passage open. In the upper part of the thorax, the trachea divides into two large **bronchi,** one for each lung. Within the lung, the bronchi divide and subdivide to end in tiny, very thin-walled air sacs called **alveoli.** The alveoli are surrounded by networks of blood capillaries. The air in the alveoli is therefore in close association with the blood within the capillaries, and interchange between the gaseous contents of blood and air takes place freely.

UROGENITAL SYSTEM

The urogenital system consists of the *kidneys, ureters, urinary bladder,* and *urethra* (which together constitute the urinary system) and the sex glands, or *gonads,* and their associated reproductive organs. The paired **kidneys** (see Fig. 23-6) lie within the abdomen. They filter the blood to remove impurities, which are then excreted in the urine. The urine formed in the kidneys is transported by the peristaltic action of the **ureters** to the **urinary bladder,** where it accumulates. The tube leading from the bladder to the exterior is the **urethra.** In the male, the urethra is also a part of the genital system.

Much of the urogenital system lies in the pelvis. The difference in position of the gonads, the **testes** in the male and the **ovaries** in the female, accounts for the greater incidence of inguinal hernia in males. Although the ovaries remains in the pelvis, the testes migrate into the *scrotum,* each carrying its duct and blood vessels (constituting the *spermatic cord*) with it. The testis and cord create a larger defect in the lower abdominal wall than does the small ligament that passes through the wall in the female body.

ENDOCRINE SYSTEM

The endocrine, or ductless, glands are a scattered rather than united system, unlike those already discussed. They are in the head, neck, and trunk and are dissimilar to one another in practically all details of their anatomy and physiology except that, unlike most glands, they have no ducts. Because they secrete hormones, which are discharged into the blood stream, endocrine glands are highly vascularized.

Hormones—chemical agents that in very tiny quantities affect the activity of cells and tissues—may be released by tissues that are not truly endocrine in structure. For instance, the cellular lining of the duodenum (first part of the intestine) releases a hormone into the blood stream that causes the gallbladder to contract. The majority of hormones that have been identified, however, are produced by the endocrine glands. The structures that are usually listed as endocrine glands are the *pituitary gland, thyroid gland, parathyroid glands, suprarenal glands,* certain parts of the *pancreas,* and certain parts of the *ovaries and testes.*

The **pituitary gland (hypophysis)** is located at the base of the skull immediately below the brain, to which it is attached (see Fig. 21-5). It is actually two different glands, although they are closely bound together. One part, the *adenohypophysis* (anterior lobe), produces hormones that regulate secretions of other glands and tissues. The other part, the *neurohypophysis* (posterior lobe), is concerned primarily with regulating the amount of water excreted by the kidneys.

The **thyroid gland** lies in the neck, largely on the sides of the trachea. Its two large lobes are connected anteriorly across the midline (see Fig. 21-12). The hormones it produces are involved with the regulation of metabolism and growth and development.

The **parathyroid glands,** typically four in number, are about the size of very small peas and usually lie on the posterior surface of the thyroid gland. They govern the level of calcium in the blood.

The paired **suprarenal (adrenal) glands** receive their name from the fact that they lie on the upper ends of the kidneys (rene). Each is really two glands. An inner part, the *medulla,* releases into the blood stream hormones called *epinephrine* (adrenaline) and *norepinephrine* (noradrenaline), which produce the same general effect that stimulation of the sympathetic nervous system does. For instance, these hormones increase the strength of the heartbeat and, at the same time, cause many arterioles to contract, so that the blood pressure rises. Epinephrine is released particularly when a person is frightened or angry.

The outer portion of the gland, the *cortex,* produces hormones that have numerous functions that include regulating electrolytes and metabolism.

Most of the cells of the pancreas produce digestive enzymes that reach the intestine through a duct. However, scattered throughout the pancreatic tissue are small groups of different cells, called the **pancreatic islets** (islets of Langerhans), which are endocrine glands. Some of the cells within the islets produce insulin, which is involved primarily with the level of blood sugar (glucose) and its storage as glycogen. An insufficient secretion of insulin produces the common form of *diabetes,* in which the high level of glucose in the blood leads to its appearance in the urine. Another hormone produced in the pancreatic islets is glucagon, which helps increase the glucose level in the blood.

In addition to the sex cells that they form, both the **testis** and the **ovary** also contain cell groups that release the sex hormones (hormones affecting sexual characteristics may also come from other places, such as the suprarenal cortex). In general, these sex hormones, of which there are a large number in post-pubertal girls and women, govern the growth and activity of the other parts of the reproductive system. The shifting balances of sex hormones are responsible for the menstrual cycle, which ceases when the ovaries atrophy. They are also responsible for the development of the secondary sex characteristics, such as the distribution of hair and the development of the female breast.

SKIN

The skin is composed of an outer layer of stratified squamous epithelium, the **epidermis,** and a deeper layer of connective tissue, the **dermis.** It varies in pigmentation and texture from person to person. It also varies in the same person according to differing circumstances. The skin may provide indications of good health or illness, or it may reflect the emotions, as in sweating from nervousness or blushing from embarrassment. It also gives evidence of the circulation to a part: it becomes flushed when the arterioles and capillaries are dilated (as they are by heat), and it becomes blanched, or even blue, when exposed to cold or when there is some other interference with the arterial supply. Because the nails are translucent, they also reflect these changes in blood supply.

The skin has many functions. A primary one is to seal off the body fluids, which living cells need to survive, from the surrounding air or water. Therefore, one of the problems in burns is the loss of body fluids that may result. The skin also protects against infection, and it offers first line of resistance to physical forces such as friction.

The skin of the posterior parts of the body is usually thicker than that of the anterior, less exposed parts, but the reverse is true of the palm and sole. On the palm and sole, the epidermis is particularly thick, and if subjected to more than the usual friction, it thickens still more to form calluses. The dermis is also thick and tightly bound down to deeper structures.

Nails, hair, and glands, developed from the epidermis, also have protective functions. Nails protect against mechanical trauma, hair protects against cold, and sweat glands protect against heat. These thermoregulatory properties, largely confined in humans to dissipation of heat through radiation, increase by the evaporation of sweat. Its various glands, which include the breast and the sebaceous glands connected with hairs, make it also a secretory organ.

The skin is also a particularly important sense organ containing, especially in the dermis immediately adjacent to the epidermis, nerve endings that respond to *touch, pressure, heat, cold,* and *painful stimuli.* These sensations are mediated through sensory fibers of the cranial and spinal nerves. Testing cutaneous sensation is a routine part of examining the nervous system.

REVIEW QUESTIONS

1 Give an example of each of the following synovial joints:
   a ball-and-socket
   b condyloid
   c hinge

2 Define the terms *origin* and *insertion* of a muscle. How do these terms compare with the terms *proximal attachment* and *distal attachment?*

3 Describe the arrangement of the fulcrum, effort point, and resistance in a third-class lever. Give an example of a joint that is a third-class lever.

4 What is a motor unit? Is the size of every motor unit the same? If not, how does the size affect muscle activity?

5 If the motor nerve to a muscle is completely severed, what happens to the muscle?

6 The nervous system can be subdivided into what two major parts? What are the components of these parts?

7 Preganglionic fibers of the sympathetic system originate in which areas of the central nervous system? Where do the preganglionic fibers of this system synapse?

8 What is a dermatome?

9 Explain the difference between segmental nerve and peripheral nerve innervation.

10 Where does the thoracic duct join the venous system? From what areas of the body does the thoracic duct receive lymphatic fluid?

EXERCISES

1 Draw the structure of a synovial joint. Include in the illustration the joint capsule, synovial membrane, joint cavity, and locations of the articular cartilage. How does this type of joint differ from fibrous and cartilaginous joints?

2 Draw a cross-section of the spinal cord. Include on the drawing the gray matter, anterior and posterior roots, posterior root ganglia, spinal nerves, and anterior and posterior rami. On the drawing, trace the course of a motor fiber that would innervate a striated muscle and a sensory fiber from the skin and trace the pathway of a simple reflex arc.

SECTION 2

The Upper Limb

4 GENERAL SURVEY OF THE UPPER LIMB

CHAPTER CONTENTS

Development

Skeleton

Muscles

Nerves

Arteries

Veins

Bursae

The upper limb can be divided into the **shoulder region;** the **arm,** or **brachium** (above the elbow); the **forearm,** or **antebrachium;** the **wrist,** or **carpus;** and the **hand.** The hand ends in five projections that can be termed the **digits** (numbered one through five from lateral to medial) or, more commonly, **four fingers and a thumb** *(pollex).* The four fingers can be more specifically termed the *index, middle (digitus medius), ring (digitus anularis),* and *little (digitus minimus) fingers.*

As the human upper limb has been freed from a weight-bearing function, it has been possible to sacrifice the greater stability necessary for weight bearing and to gain the mobility (stability and mobility are inversely related) that has added so much to human development. This mobility is especially marked in the hand and digits, but it extends, to a lesser degree, throughout the entire upper limb.

DEVELOPMENT

The upper limb first appears as a swelling on the side of the embryo. As it rapidly grows outward, it projects first laterally and then ventrally and slightly caudally. The distal end becomes a flattened plate for the hand, flexures indicating the elbow and wrist appear,

57

and ridges on the hand plate differentiate into digits. This growth, and a medial rotation of the growing limb, distorts the relations between the surfaces of the limbs and those of the trunk. The original relations can be restored in the adult, however, by simply raising the limb to the sides in a horizontal position with the palm facing anteriorly. In this position, the back of the hand, forearm, and arm face posteriorly. The thumb or radial side is directed cranially. The palm and the flexor side of the forearm and arm form the anterior or ventral surfaces, and the little finger is directed caudally.

The limb bud consists initially of a core of mesenchyme (embryonic connective tissue) within a thin sheet of epithelium. The latter forms only the outer layer of the skin, whereas the mesenchyme of the bud forms the remaining tissues except for the blood vessels and the nerves, which grow into the bud. The base of the bud is relatively broad, extending from about the fifth cervical segment to the first thoracic segment, and nerves from these segments grow into the developing limb. Condensations of mesenchyme (which are eventually transformed into cartilage and then bone) indicate the positions of the skeleton. Condensations around the primitive skeletal elements gradually differentiate into muscle groups (e.g., extensor on the posterior side, flexor on the anterior side) and then into individual muscles. Some of those at the base of the limb grow back into the trunk, to attach to the ribs, sternum, or vertebral column.

SKELETON

A convenient subdivision of the skeleton is into an **axial skeleton** (skull, ribs, sternum, and vertebral column) and an **appendicular skeleton** (the skeleton of the limbs, or appendages). For both the upper and lower limbs, the skeleton is divisible into a girdle and the skeleton of the free limb. The girdle of the upper limb is called the **pectoral** or **shoulder girdle.** It consists of the **clavicle** and the **scapula** (Fig. 4-1). The clavicle serves as a strut to keep the upper limb away from the body wall and provides the only bony "attachment" of the upper limb to the rest of the skeleton. The clavicle articulates by synovial joints with the **sternum** medially and with the scapula laterally

(see Fig. 5-1). The scapula is largely held in place by muscles.

The scapula has a shallow cavity that receives the upper rounded end, or head, of the **humerus,** the single bone of the arm. The glenohumeral (shoulder) joint is a shallow ball-and-socket joint that is freely movable in most directions. The forearm contains two bones: the **radius** on the thumb side and the **ulna** on the little-finger side. The ulna is articulated with the lower end of the humerus in a way that enables only movements of flexion and extension between the two bones. The radius participates in flexion and extension but also can rotate on its long axis, allowing the palm of the hand to be turned downward (in pronation) and upward (in supination) when the forearm is horizontal.

Although the ulna forms the chief articulation at the elbow, the distal expanded end of the radius is the chief forearm component at the wrist joint. At the wrist, eight small bones, or **carpals,** are arranged in two rows. Movements such as flexion and extension occur here, aided by movements between the carpals, especially between the proximal and distal rows of these elements.

The long bones of the palm of the hand are the **metacarpals**. For the most part, they are limited in their movements, but the first (or thumb metacarpal) is freely movable to allow opposition of the thumb (touching it to the tips of the fingers or to the palm). The fifth and fourth metacarpals are more movable than the second and third (which are essentially immovable), allowing a firmer grasp with the ulnar (little finger) side of the hand. The digits are composed of **phalanges;** the thumb has only two phalanges, and the four fingers each have three. The phalanges articulate with each other by hinge joints.

MUSCLES

Some of the muscles acting on the pectoral girdle and the free limb lie, for the most part, on the anterior (pectoral region) or lateral thoracic wall and are considered muscles of the thorax. Other muscles of the limb have spread over the back to attain an origin from the vertebral column. Therefore, in position, they are muscles of the back, although their primary

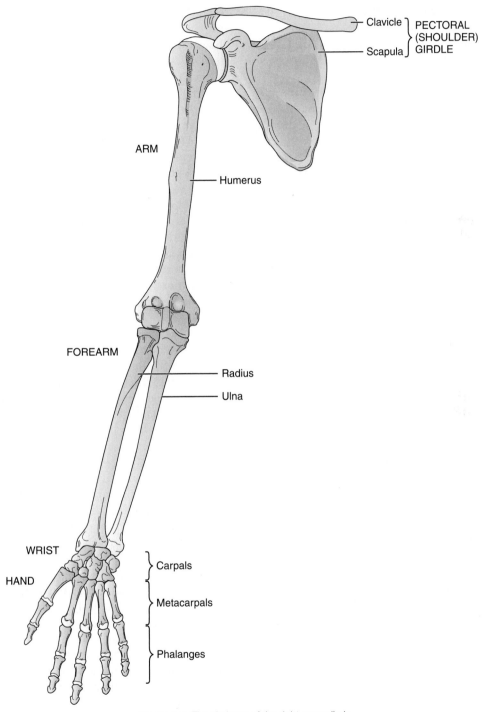

Figure 4-1 The skeleton of the right upper limb.

actions are on the girdle or the arm. Still other muscles of the shoulder arise from the girdle and insert on the humerus; these are listed as muscles of the upper limb proper. These muscles, as a whole, move the scapula or the arm on the scapula.

The muscles in the arm form fleshy masses on the anterior and posterior surfaces of the humerus and act primarily across the elbow joint, where they are flexors or extensors of this joint. They can also rotate (supinate) the radius. Some of these muscles arise from the girdle and can act either solely at the glenohumeral joint or at both the glenohumeral and elbow joints.

The muscles in the forearm, divided conveniently into **flexor** (anteromedial) and **extensor** (posterolateral) **muscle masses,** act primarily at the wrist or on the digits, but some of them have an accessory or chief action at the elbow. Among the forearm muscles are those that pronate or supinate the forearm.

Many of the muscles forming parts of the flexor and extensor masses in the forearm are connected with the fingers or thumb and have their chief action on the digits and a secondary action at the wrist joint. These longer muscles are continued into the hand by relatively narrow tendons, many of which can be easily palpated or seen at the wrist. Other muscles of the digits, situated in the hand itself, act on only the digits. Some of these shorter muscles form two prominent groups on the palmar surface, the **thenar** (thumb) and **hypothenar** (little finger) groups. Others lie deeper.

NERVES

The nerves of the upper limb are derived principally from the **anterior rami of the lower four cervical spinal nerves (C5 to C8)** and the **first thoracic spinal nerve (T1).** At their origins, these nerves are spread over an area considerably wider than the space available for their entrance at the base of the arm and, for the most part, are at a higher level than is the origin of the free limb. As they run into the arm, they give branches to some of the shoulder muscles and then pass between the clavicle and first rib to enter the axilla. In so doing, they converge and then branch in a complex pattern to form the **brachial plexus** (see Fig. 5-7). Essentially, the nerves come together in such a manner as to form three main cords arranged about the axillary artery (see next section). From these cords, branches are given off to the upper limb, including the shoulder region.

There are four main nerves continuing down into the limb: the musculocutaneous, median, ulnar, and radial (Fig. 4-2). Of these, the **musculocutaneous nerve,** derived from an anterior part of the brachial plexus, supplies anterior muscles of the arm. The **median** and the **ulnar nerves,** also derived from the anterior part of the plexus, supply anterior muscles of the forearm and hand. The **radial nerve,** the only posterior branch that runs down the limb, supplies the posterior muscles of the arm and forearm (there are no true posterior muscles in the hand). These nerves also help supply sensory innervation to the skin of the limb. Their distributions are best considered later, but that of the musculocutaneous nerve is shown diagrammatically in Figure 6-12; that of the median nerve, in Figure 8-6; that of the ulnar nerve, in Figure 8-7; and that of the radial nerve, in Figure 9-6. (Also shown in Fig. 9-6 is the **axillary nerve,** a branch of the brachial plexus that is distributed mainly within the shoulder region.)

ARTERIES

The chief artery to the upper limb is the **subclavian artery,** which is derived directly (on the left) or indirectly (on the right) from the aorta. In the base of the neck, the subclavian artery gives rise to branches that help supply shoulder muscles. As it crosses the first rib, it continues as the **axillary artery,** which gives off branches (some of which are not shown in Fig. 4-2) to muscles of the shoulder and to the wall of the thorax. The axillary artery then continues into the arm, where its name changes to the **brachial artery.** Branches of the brachial artery supply the arm, and in the upper part of the forearm, the brachial artery ends by dividing into **radial** and **ulnar arteries,** which run down the front of the forearm. There is no large posterior artery in the forearm, but the ulnar artery gives off a branch that runs deeply on the posterior aspect. Both ulnar and radial arteries go mainly to the palm of the hand.

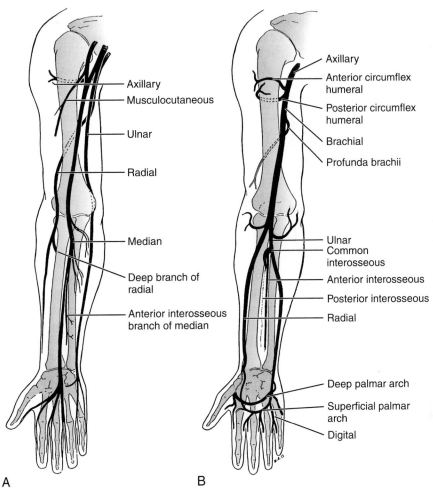

Figure 4-2 **A,** The principal nerves of the upper limb. The deep branch of the radial nerve is distributed on the back of the forearm to extensor muscles and continues as the posterior interosseous nerve. **B,** The chief arteries of the upper limb.

VEINS

The veins of the upper limb consist of both superficial and deep veins. The superficial veins (Fig. 4-3) are located in the subcutaneous tissue. In the hand, superficial drainage is predominantly onto the posterior surface, where two major veins are formed: the cephalic (laterally) and the basilic (medially). The **cephalic vein** courses proximally on the anterior surface of the forearm and arm, lies in a groove between the deltoid and pectoralis major muscles in the shoulder region, and then passes deeply to join the axillary vein. The **basilic vein** gains access to the anterior surface of the forearm just distal to

the elbow, continues onto the anteromedial aspect of the arm, and then passes deeply to continue as the **axillary vein.** At the elbow, the **median cubital vein** forms a communication between the cephalic and basilic veins.

The deep veins generally accompany the arteries and are usually paired. The veins of the hand drain laterally into the **radial vein** and medially into the **ulnar vein.** These receive tributaries in the forearm and join at the elbow to form two **brachial veins** that continue into the arm. The brachial veins join the axillary vein. As the axillary vein crosses the first rib, it continues as the **subclavian vein.**

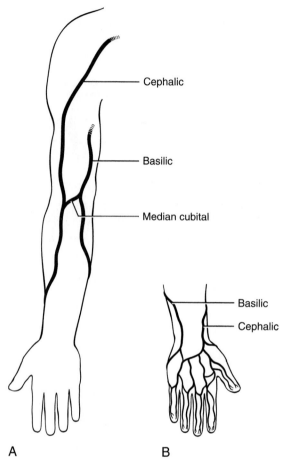

Cephalic

Basilic

Median cubital

Basilic

Cephalic

A

B

Figure 4-3 **A,** Main superficial veins of the anterior aspect of the upper limb. **B,** Superficial veins of the posterior aspect of the hand.

BURSAE

Subcutaneous bursae similar to other bursae are found in a few locations on the upper limb. The more constant of these are the *subacromial bursa,* over the acromion (shoulder tip) of the scapula; the *subcutaneous olecranon bursa,* between the olecranon process (back of the elbow) and skin; and dorsally placed bursae, lying over the knuckles or the proximal joints of the fingers. These bursae have essentially the same functions as bursae elsewhere in the body; in these particular cases, they enable the skin to slide freely over a projecting bony surface.

REVIEW QUESTIONS

1 The pectoral (shoulder) girdle is formed by which bones?

2 Which anterior rami contribute to the brachial plexus?

3 What group of muscles does the musculocutaneous nerve supply? Which groups does the radial nerve innervate?

4 After the subclavian artery crosses the first rib, it continues as the _____ artery.

5 Which vein, the cephalic or basilic, lies on the lateral side of the forearm? Which vein provides a communication between the cephalic and basilic veins?

EXERCISES

1 Demonstrate the two movements that are possible between the humerus and ulna.

2 Demonstrate the following:
   a extent of the arm
   b location and course of the median cubital vein
   c position of the radius
   d position of the thenar group of muscles
   e location of the metacarpals

5 THE SHOULDER

CHAPTER CONTENTS

General Considerations

Movements of the Scapula and Arm

Bones and Joints of the Shoulder

Fascia and Superficial Nerves and Vessels

Axilla

Muscles

Movements of the Shoulder

Bursae and Shoulder Lesions

Nerve Injuries: Brachial Plexus

Analyses of Activities and Associated Movements

GENERAL CONSIDERATIONS

The shoulder region in human anatomy includes, in a broad sense, not only the rounded contour between the arm and the body but also the pectoral region, the region of the back around the scapula (shoulder blade), and the axilla (armpit). The shoulder muscles cover the upper part of the chest and spread posteriorly so that they almost completely cover the true back muscles. Therefore, study of the shoulder must include much of the trunk and the upper part of the arm.

Muscles of the shoulder attach to the pectoral (shoulder) girdle, the skeleton of the anterior thoracic wall, and the vertebral column. The anterior thoracic wall is made up of the sternum and ribs (Fig. 5-1). Positioned in the anterior midline, the **sternum** consists of the *manubrium,* the *body of the sternum,* and the *xiphoid process.* Of the twelve pairs of **ribs,** only the upper seven pairs articulate directly with the sternum. Posteriorly, all ribs articulate with the thoracic vertebrae.

The pectoral (shoulder) girdle consists of the scapula and clavicle (see Figs. 4-l and 5-1). The **scapula,** largely suspended by muscles, is rather freely movable. The **clavicle** articulates on its lateral end with the scapula and moves primarily with it. Medially, it articulates with the sternum. The proximal end of the **humerus** articulates with the scapula to form the glenohumeral (shoulder) joint.

Muscles arising from the pectoral girdle (**intrinsic muscles** of the limb, so called because they both arise and insert on bones of the limb) insert on the humerus and act at the glenohumeral joint. Some of the muscles with origins from the axial skeleton

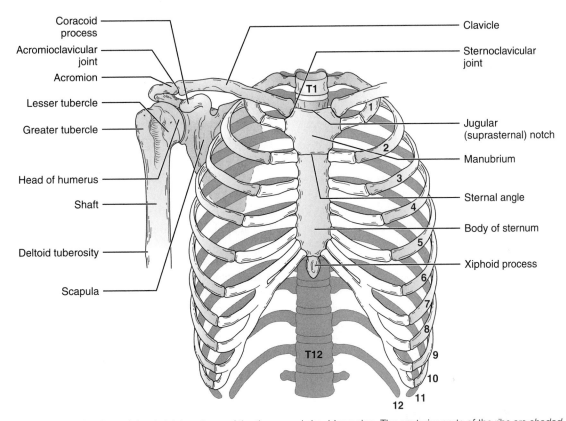

Figure 5-1 Anterior view, of the skeletal anatomy of the thorax and shoulder region. The posterior parts of the ribs are *shaded.*

(**extrinsic muscles,** so called because they are not confined to the limb) also attach to the humerus and act primarily at the glenohumeral joint. Other extrinsic muscles attach to the scapula and clavicle and move these bones.

Most of the nerves to the muscles of the shoulder are derived from the upper part of the **brachial plexus.** The blood supply of these muscles is chiefly from branches of the **subclavian** and **axillary arteries.**

MOVEMENTS OF THE SCAPULA AND ARM

The **movements of the scapula** (Fig. 5-2, *A-C*) are defined as *elevation* (raising the scapula toward the head), *depression* (lowering it), *protraction* (moving it forward), and *retraction* ("straightening" the shoulders). Rotation of the scapula also occurs and may be either upward or downward. In *upward rotation,*

the inferior angle is moved laterally and anteriorly around the thoracic wall, and the lateral angle and glenoid cavity (which articulates with the humerus) are tilted upward. In *downward rotation,* the inferior angle is moved toward the vertebral column and the lateral angle is lowered.

FUNCTIONAL/CLINICAL NOTE 5-1

These movements of the scapula accompany movements of the arm; for instance, when the arm reaches anteriorly, the scapula slips forward on the thoracic wall in protraction. When the arm is raised above the head, the accompanying upward rotation of the scapula also tilts the lateral angle upward. A combination of these movements occurs in reaching both forward

Continued

and upward, as in retrieving a book from a high shelf. As the scapula moves upward, downward, anteriorly, and posteriorly, the lateral end of the clavicle follows it, pivoting at the sternal end.

Movements of the arm at the glenohumeral joint (see Fig. 5-2, *D* and *E*) are particularly free and include flexion, extension, abduction, adduction, circumduction, medial rotation, and lateral rotation. *Flexion* of the arm (also called *flexion of the arm at the glenohumeral joint* or *flexion of the glenohumeral joint*) is an anterior movement of the arm. *Extension,* the reverse of this, is a posterior movement of the arm. *Abduction* is the action of raising the arm laterally away from the body; *adduction,* the opposite of this, is the action of bringing the arm toward the side (closer to the body). *Circumduction* is a combination of all four of these movements, so that the hand moves in a circle. *Medial rotation* (also called *internal rotation*) is a rotation of the arm about its long axis, so that the usual anterior surface is turned inward toward the body. *Lateral rotation* (also called *external rotation*) is the opposite of this.

FUNCTIONAL/CLINICAL NOTE 5-2

When the arm and forearm are at the side of the body (anatomical position), the apparent effects of rotation of the arm are increased by the somewhat similar movements of pronation and supination occurring in the forearm. Therefore, if the amount of rotation of the arm itself is to be observed, the forearm should be held in flexion while this movement is being tested. This allows dissociation between rotation of the arm and pronation-supination, which occur within the forearm.

All movements of the arm at the shoulder can be described by the terms used in the preceding section, although usually movements of the arm are combinations of two or more movements. In touching the opposite tip of the shoulder, for example, the arm, forearm, and hand are brought anteriorly across the thoracic wall. In this action, the arm is flexed and adducted (at the shoulder) and usually is also medially rotated. In scratching the lower part of the back, the arm is extended, medially rotated, and then alternately abducted and adducted.

BONES AND JOINTS OF THE SHOULDER
Bones

Scapula

The **scapula** is a triangular bone with three *borders* (*superior, medial,* and *lateral*) and three *angles* (*superior, inferior,* and *lateral*) (Fig. 5-3). The lateral angle is the expanded end on which the smooth *glenoid cavity,* the surface that articulates with the head of the humerus, is located. Attached around the edge of the glenoid cavity in the living person or cadaver specimen is a narrow rim of fibrocartilage, the *glenoid labrum,* which slightly widens and deepens the cavity. The hooked *coracoid process* projects forward from the scapula, close to the glenoid cavity. The costal (meaning "related to the ribs") surface of the scapula is relatively smooth, whereas the posterior or dorsal surface is divided into two parts by the projecting *spine.* The area of the posterior surface above the spine is the *supraspinous fossa;* the area below the spine is the *infraspinous fossa.* The costal surface is called the *subscapular fossa.* The supraspinatus, infraspinatus, and subscapularis muscles occupy these fossae, respectively. The spine of the scapula continues as a free projection, the *acromion,* which forms the point of the shoulder and articulates with the clavicle. The acromion is connected to the coracoid process by the coracoacromial ligament; the acromion and ligament form an arch above the glenohumeral joint. The scapula is largely suspended by muscles; its only articulations are with the humerus and clavicle.

Clavicle

The **clavicle** is a long bone that is approximately cylindrical and has a slightly S-shaped curve. Its sternal (medial) end is somewhat expanded and fits poorly into the notch on the manubrium of the sternum. Its acromial end is expanded and flattened and articulates

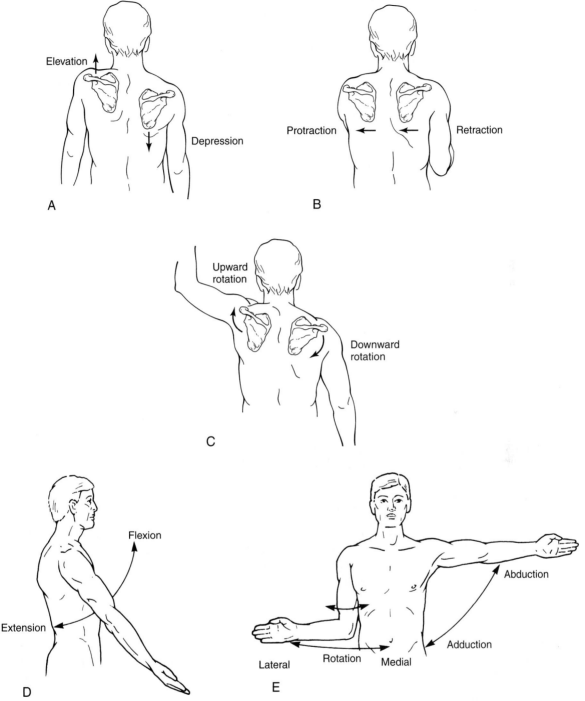

Figure 5-2 Movements of the scapula (**A** to **C**) and arm (**D** and **E**). **A,** Elevation of the left scapula (as in shrugging the shoulders) and depression of the right. **B,** Protraction of the left scapula (moved away from the midline as in reaching forward), and retraction of the right scapula, as in moving the arm posteriorly. **C,** Upward rotation of the left scapula, as in reaching laterally upward (abduction of the arm); the inferior angle moves away from the midline and the glenoid cavity is tilted upward. Also illustrated is downward rotation of the right scapula; the inferior angle of the scapula moves medially toward the midline and the glenoid cavity tilts downward. **D,** Flexion and extension of the arm at the glenohumeral joint are illustrated. **E,** Lateral/medial rotation and abduction/adduction of the arm are illustrated. In demonstrating rotation, the forearm is flexed to eliminate pronation/supination of the forearm.

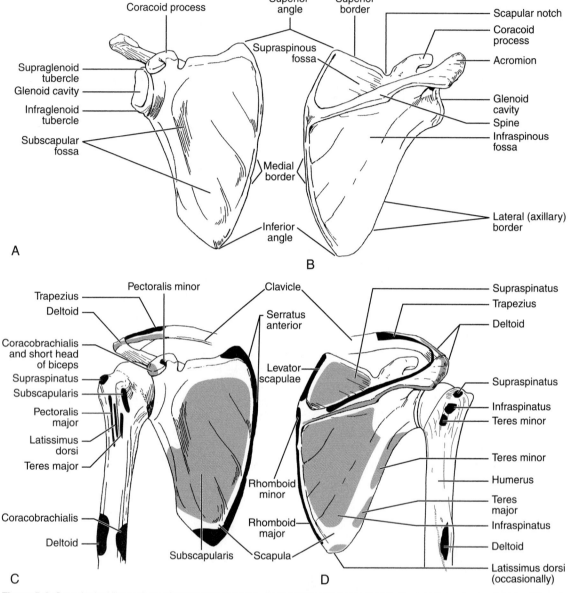

Figure 5-3 Osteological illustrations of the shoulder region. Anterior **(A)** and posterior **(B)** views of the scapula. Anterior **(C)** and posterior **(D)** views of the scapula and parts of the clavicle and humerus, showing origins of muscles *(color)* and insertions of muscles *(black)*.

with the acromion of the scapula. Because the clavicle acts primarily to keep the limb free or away from the body, it must be attached firmly at both ends. However, because it must allow movement of the scapula, it must also possess joints at both ends.

Joints

Sternoclavicular joint

The **sternoclavicular joint** contains two synovial cavities that are separated by an *articular disc* (Fig. 5-4). Although the adjacent surfaces of the clavicle and sternum do not fit well together, this articular disc allows the joint to move more freely, somewhat like a ball-and-socket joint. Up-and-down, anterior-and-posterior, and rotatory movements are all possible at the sternoclavicular joint. In up-and-down movement (the freest), the clavicle moves on the disc as on a hinge, whereas in the other movements, the disc moves with the clavicle. The joint also includes a small portion of the first rib as it attaches to the sternum.

The sternoclavicular joint slants in such a way that medial thrust on the clavicle tends to displace its sternal end upward and medially. Downward movement of the shoulder tends to bring the clavicle against the first rib and, if continued, to raise the sternal head of the clavicle from its bed, using the first rib as a fulcrum. Several ligaments resist these movements of dislocation. The *anterior and posterior sternoclavicular ligaments* reinforce the capsule (the posterior being the stronger) and are directed downward and slightly medially from clavicle to sternum. These ligaments help prevent both upward displacement and lateral displacement, which tend to occur if the arm is pulled. A similar function is served by the *costoclavicular ligament,* which runs downward and medially between the clavicle and the first rib, and by the articular disc. The ligament is attached inferiorly to the first rib and superiorly to the clavicle, so that any upward and medial movement of the sternal head of the clavicle produces tension on the disc. It tears away from the rib, however, if the posterosuperior part of the capsule, which offers most of the resistance against upward dislocation, is cut.

Lateral displacement is prevented not only by the sternoclavicular and costoclavicular ligaments, as already noted, but also, to some extent, by the *interclavicular ligament,* which extends from one clavicle to the other across both joints and also has some attachment to the sternum. *Sensory innervation to the sternoclavicular joint is provided by branches from the medial (anterior) supraclavicular nerve off the cervical plexus and the nerve to the subclavius muscle.*

Acromioclavicular joint

The **acromioclavicular joint** is small and its gliding surfaces are so sloped as to favor overriding of the acromion by the clavicle. An articular disc is usually present between the articular surfaces of the bones but may be incomplete. The joint capsule itself has little strength, and the scapula could be easily displaced medially beneath the clavicle if it were not for the *coracoclavicular ligament* (Fig. 5-5). This strong ligament is divided into two parts; the more medial and posterior part is the *conoid ligament,* and the more lateral and anterior is the *trapezoid ligament.* Both parts of this ligament prevent medial displacement of the scapula. The conoid passes upward and slightly posteriorly from the coracoid process to the clavicle and also resists forward movement of the scapula without corresponding movements of

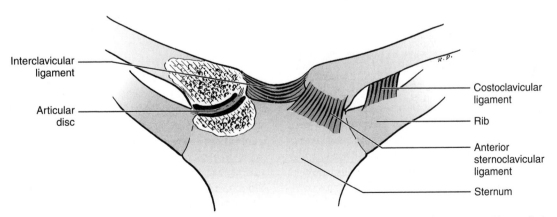

Interclavicular ligament

Articular disc

Costoclavicular ligament

Rib

Anterior sternoclavicular ligament

Sternum

Figure 5-4 The sternoclavicular joint and associated ligaments. The left joint is depicted as sectioned in a frontal (coronal) plane to expose the articular disc.

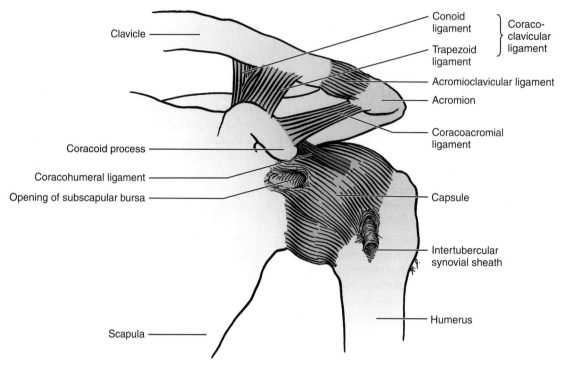

Clavicle

Conoid ligament

Trapezoid ligament

} Coraco-clavicular ligament

Acromioclavicular ligament

Acromion

Coracoacromial ligament

Coracoid process

Coracohumeral ligament

Opening of subscapular bursa

Capsule

Intertubercular synovial sheath

Humerus

Scapula

Figure 5-5 Ligaments of the glenohumeral joint and distal end of the clavicle.

the clavicle. The trapezoid resists independent backward movement of the scapula. In forcible dislocation at this joint ("shoulder separation"), the coracoclavicular ligament is usually torn, as are the muscles (trapezius and deltoid) attaching across the joint, and the scapula and upper limb are displaced inferiorly. *The acromioclavicular joint is usually innervated by branches of the suprascapular, pectoral, and axillary nerves.*

FUNCTIONAL/CLINICAL NOTE 5-3

The importance of the synovial joints at both ends of the clavicle is easily demonstrated by noting how the scapula and clavicle move together as the shoulders are raised or lowered or thrust forward or backward. In all these movements, the clavicle has to move rather freely at the sternoclavicular joint. The small gliding movement allowed at the acromioclavicular joint is necessary because

the lateral angle of the scapula follows the clavicle, defining an arc of which the clavicle is the radius. The medial border of the scapula follows the different curve of the thoracic wall, to which it is closely held by muscles. Therefore, constant adjustment at both ends of the clavicle is necessary for the scapula to move smoothly. These movements of the scapula, in turn, greatly increase the mobility of the glenohumeral joint because they result in alterations of the position of the glenoid cavity on which the head of the humerus moves.

Glenohumeral (shoulder) joint

To understand the glenohumeral joint and the muscles acting across it, the upper end of the **humerus** must be studied (see Figs. 5-1 and

6-1). The humerus is the long bone of the arm and consists of a *shaft (body)* and two expanded ends. The smooth articular part of the proximal end of the humerus is the *head.* A marked prominence of the anterior surface of the proximal end is the *lesser tubercle,* which is clearly separated from the more lateral *greater tubercle* by the *intertubercular groove.* Below the tubercles, this groove is bordered by *crests* that extend downward from each tubercle. The *anatomical neck* of the humerus is at the point of junction of the head with the shaft and lies in part between the head and the tubercles. The *surgical neck,* so called because of the frequent occurrence of fractures here, lies below both the head and tubercles and is a narrow, not clearly demarcated portion of the upper part of the shaft. Near the middle of the shaft (on its anterolateral surface) is the *deltoid tuberosity,* a prominence on which the deltoid inserts. (The remainder of the humerus and its participation in the elbow joint is described in Chapter 6.)

The **glenohumeral joint** is formed by the articular surfaces of the glenoid cavity, and the head of the humerus (see Fig. 5-5). It is surrounded by a thin joint capsule that has relatively little strength except above by a thickening known as the *coracohumeral ligament.* Internally, there are two or three very slightly thickened bands, the *glenohumeral ligaments,* on its anterior wall. The joint capsule of the glenohumeral joint is attached proximally to the glenoid labrum, which attaches it to the edge of the glenoid cavity. The capsule is very often deficient anteriorly close to the labrum, where the synovial cavity of the joint may communicate with a *subscapular bursa* lying on the anterior surface of the scapula. Distally, the capsule is attached to the anatomical neck of the humerus, but between the tubercles, it extends downward as a thin-walled tube, the *intertubercular synovial sheath,* that surrounds the tendon of the long head of the biceps brachii muscle. Through this sheath, the tendon enters the glenohumeral joint and runs through its cavity to an origin on the upper edge of the glenoid cavity. *Innervation to the glenohumeral joint is usually provided by the axillary, suprascapular, and lateral pectoral nerves.* These nerves supply muscles that act at this joint.

FUNCTIONAL/CLINICAL NOTE 5-4

The glenoid labrum may be torn partially from the edge of the glenoid cavity when there has been repeated dislocation of the shoulder, but it is also frequently torn in older persons who have never had dislocations. Although the coracohumeral ligament can support the weight of the arm hanging by the side, additional weight evokes muscular action. Even slight abduction of the arm releases the ligament, rendering it useless during almost all movements. The chief strength of the glenohumeral joint lies in certain muscles and tendons that are closely applied to the capsule anteriorly, above, and posteriorly. These together are called the *rotator cuff,* or *musculotendinous cuff,* of the shoulder.

The relatively free movements of the ball-and-socket or spheroid joint of the shoulder are limited by the short muscles around the glenohumeral joint, as well as by the tubercles and the overhanging acromion process. On the other hand, the apparent range of movement at the shoulder is greatly increased by movements of the scapula, as is the strength of the movements of the arm.

Surface Anatomy

Studying the surface anatomy of an area is a means of enabling "visualization" of structures beneath the skin. It is useful in conducting physical examinations and provides an opportunity to review anatomical structures and their relationships. Many of the bony landmarks in the shoulder region can be easily palpated. Knowledge of their location aids in locating the muscles, discussed later in this chapter. In examining the bones of the shoulder region, it is apparent that the pectoral girdle (clavicle and scapula) and proximal end of the humerus form the major framework of the area. Because many of the muscles acting at the glenohumeral joint are considered extrinsic muscles to that joint, other skeletal elements, including the sternum, ribs, and vertebral column, can also be examined to obtain a more complete understanding of the entire area.

A familiar landmark in the region is the **clavicle** at the base of the neck (see Fig. 5-1). The midline depression between the ends of the two clavicles (at the sternoclavicular joints) and the prominent muscles of the neck (sternocleidomastoids) that attach here is the *jugular (suprasternal) notch.* The clavicle can be traced laterally to its junction with the *acromion* of the scapula at the acromioclavicular joint. Inferior to the distal end of the clavicle is a depression, the *clavipectoral,* or *deltopectoral, triangle,* which is bordered by the clavicle, pectoralis major muscle, and deltoid muscle.

On the dorsal surface of the **scapula,** it is possible to palpate the *scapular spine.* The spine extends from the acromion to the medial border and separates the *supraspinous fossa* (above) and *infraspinous fossa* (below). Following the *medial border* of the scapula inferiorly enables palpation of the *inferior angle.* The freedom of movement of the scapula can be examined by placing a finger on the inferior angle and moving the arm through various motions, including full abduction. Only part of the *lateral border* can be felt because it is partially obscured by overlying muscles (teres major and minor). Anteriorly, the *coracoid process* can be examined by deep palpation in the clavipectoral (deltopectoral) triangle.

The proximal end of the **humerus** is evident deep to the deltoid muscle. Moving the humerus in medial and lateral rotation (with the forearm flexed at the elbow) enables palpation (or at least approximate identification) of the *greater and lesser tubercles.* The *shaft* of the humerus can easily be palpated laterally at the middle of the arm.

The skeleton of the thorax is partly covered anteriorly and almost entirely covered posteriorly by shoulder muscles. Many of the **ribs,** however, can be felt or are visually evident both anteriorly and laterally, and in the anterior midline, the **sternum** can easily be palpated. The uppermost rib that can be palpated attaching to the sternum is the second rib, because the first rib is covered by the clavicle. The point of attachment of the second rib to the sternum is regularly marked by the sternal angle, which can be felt by running a finger lightly down the upper portion of the sternum. The *sternal angle* is formed by the junction of the *manubrium* and *body* of the sternum, which lie in slightly different planes. The *xiphoid process* lies in the *infrasternal angle;* the angle is formed by the cartilage of some of the lower ribs of each side as they ascend to attach to the sternum.

On the back, the posterior tips, or *spinous processes* (see Fig. 13-3), of many of the **vertebrae** can be palpated or are visually evident in the midline, their prominence being increased by flexion (forward bending) of the trunk. Most of the cervical vertebrae lie so deeply buried in the muscles of the neck that they cannot be felt distinctly, and usually the first distinct spinous process is that of the seventh cervical vertebra. This usually forms a marked projection at the base of the neck, and the vertebra is sometimes known as the *vertebra prominens.* On occasion, the sixth cervical vertebra can be felt above the seventh, and sometimes, the spinous process of the first thoracic vertebra is more prominent than that of the seventh cervical vertebra. The spinous processes of the 12 thoracic vertebrae are, in general, long and pointed and overlap each other. Those of the five lumbar vertebrae are broad and blunt (see Figs. 13-1 and 13-3). Below the lumbar spinous processes, the **sacrum** can be palpated in the midline, and laterally, the attachment of the **hip bones** to the sacrum and the *crest of the ilium* can be felt.

On the posterior aspect of the *skull,* there are also markings that are of importance for the study of the limb muscles. These are the *external occipital protuberance,* which is the prominent posterior projection of the skull in the midline, and the *mastoid processes,* the bony enlargements behind the ears.

FASCIA AND SUPERFICIAL NERVES AND VESSELS

Fascia

The subcutaneous tissue, or **superficial fascia,** in the pectoral region contains a variable amount of fat and also encloses the glandular tissue of the breast, a gland of the skin that has expanded into the subcutaneous tissue. Elsewhere around the shoulder, superficial fascia is not as well developed and is fused with deep fascia.

The **deep fascia** of the shoulder splits to surround each structure it encounters and then unites again into a single layer on the other side of that structure. It is attached to various bony prominences and in certain regions—for instance, the supraspinous and infraspinous fossae—enables attachment to some of the fibers of the underlying muscles. The fascia on the deep surface of the pectoralis major muscle contains the larger nerves and vessels to the muscle. A special layer of fascia surrounding the pectoralis minor muscle, under cover of the pectoralis major, and extending up to the clavicle is the **clavipectoral fascia.**

Nerves

The skin over the shoulder is supplied by a number of nerves. Anteriorly and laterally, the **supraclavicular nerves,** which are branches of the cervical plexus (mostly nerve fibers from spinal cord segments C3 and C4), pass downward over the clavicle to supply the skin over the upper part of the thorax and the top of the shoulder. The skin of the pectoral region is supplied by branches of **intercostal nerves** (anterior rami of thoracic nerves). The skin over the shoulder muscles on the back is supplied partly also by branches of intercostal nerves, partly by the posterior rami of cervical, thoracic, and lumbar spinal nerves. Skin over the lateral side of the proximal part of the arm is supplied by a cutaneous branch of the **axillary nerve.** The skin of the floor of the axilla and the medial side of the upper part of the arm is supplied by a branch **(intercostobrachial nerve)** from the second or the second and third intercostal nerves and by a small branch from the medial cord of the brachial plexus.

Vessels

The only superficial vessel of any size in the shoulder region is the upper end of the **cephalic vein.** The cephalic vein lies between the deltoid and pectoralis major muscles and passes deeply between the two in the infraclavicular fossa. It then joins the axillary vein.

AXILLA

The axilla varies in shape and size, depending on the position of the arm. With the arm slightly abducted, it can be regarded as a space in the form of a somewhat misshapen, truncated pyramid, the **base**

of which is formed by the *skin* and *fascia* extending from the arm to the thoracic wall. The **anterior wall** of this space is formed by the *pectoralis major and minor* muscles, and the **medial wall** is formed by the *serratus anterior* muscle on the lateral thoracic wall (Fig. 5-6). The **posterior wall** is formed by shoulder muscles, the *latissimus dorsi* and *teres major* below and the *subscapularis* above. The narrow **lateral wall** of the axilla is the *intertubercular groove of the humerus.* The coracobrachialis muscle lies just medial to this groove. The misshapen **apex** of this pyramid lies *between the first rib*, the *clavicle*, and the *upper edge of the subscapularis* muscle, and through this apex pass the great nerves and vessels of the upper limb.

Brachial Plexus

Most of the nerves to muscles of the shoulder and those to muscles of the arm and forearm are derived from the **brachial plexus.** The plexus lies primarily deep within the lower part of the neck and extends between the clavicle and first rib into the axilla. On the lateral wall of the axilla, several components of the lower end of the brachial plexus can be rolled between a finger and the humerus.

The brachial plexus is formed by the *anterior rami of the fifth, sixth, seventh, and eighth cervical nerves* (C5, C6, C7, C8) and the *first thoracic nerve* (T1) (Fig. 5-7). (The posterior rami of these spinal nerves turn sharply posteriorly around the vertebral column to supply skin and muscles of the back.) To these five anterior rami there may be added small communications from the anterior rami of C4 or T2.[*] The anterior rami of C5 and C6 (with any contribution that there is from C4) join to form an **upper trunk.** C7 continues as a **middle trunk,** and C8 and T1 unite to form a **lower trunk.** Each of these three trunks then divides into an **anterior** and a **posterior division.** The posterior divisions of all three trunks unite to form the **posterior cord;** the anterior divisions of upper and middle trunks unite to form the **lateral cord;** and the anterior division of the lower trunk is continued as the **medial cord.** These cords are named

---

[*]Spinal nerves are often designated by letters and numerals, with the letter representing the region of the spinal cord (spinal cord segment) to which the nerve belongs and the numeral representing its place in the series; see p. 44.

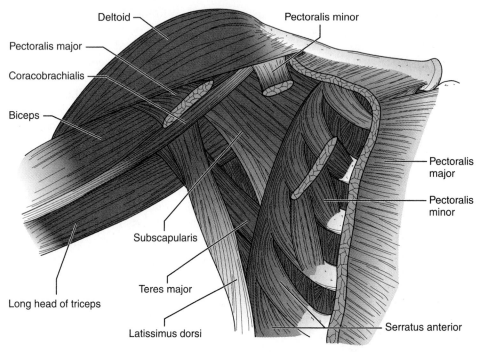

Deltoid

Pectoralis minor

Pectoralis major

Coracobrachialis

Biceps

Pectoralis major

Pectoralis minor

Subscapularis

Teres major

Long head of triceps

Latissimus dorsi

Serratus anterior

Figure 5-6 The axillary region. The pectoral muscles are omitted to reveal the deeper lying muscles.

according to their relations to the axillary artery, so that the lateral cord lies lateral to the artery (Fig. 5-8). The medial and posterior cords maintain a medial and posterior relation, respectively, to the axillary artery throughout the distal part of their course; however, as they emerge from deep to the clavicle, the posterior cord is at first lateral to the artery and the medial cord lies behind the artery.

The plexus is clearly divided into two basic parts: an anterior (flexor) and a posterior (extensor) portion. This division of the plexus corresponds to the division of the musculature of the limb into flexor and extensor groups. The medial and lateral cords of the brachial plexus form the anterior portion of the plexus. Through their branches, they supply the muscles of the pectoral region and all the muscles on the anterior aspects of the arm, forearm, and hand. Thus, they supply all the muscles originally arising on the anterior or flexor surface of the limb. The posterior cord represents the posterior element of the brachial plexus; it supplies most of the muscles of the shoulder proper and all the posterior muscles

in the arm and forearm: that is, muscles originally associated with the posterior or extensor surface of the embryonic limb.

The **lateral cord,** carrying fibers primarily from C5, C6, and C7, gives off the *lateral pectoral nerve* to the pectoralis major muscle at the level of the clavicle. A larger branch, the *musculocutaneous nerve*, penetrates and innervates the coracobrachialis muscle and the other anterior muscles of the arm. The remainder of the lateral cord serves as a *contribution to the median nerve*, passing anterior to the axillary artery to join a branch of the medial cord.

The **medial cord,** carrying fibers from C8 and T1, first gives off the *medial pectoral nerve* to the pectoralis minor and major muscles and then gives off two cutaneous branches: a tiny upper one, the *medial cutaneous nerve of the arm*, which supplies skin on the medial side of the arm, and a larger one, the *medial cutaneous nerve of the forearm*, which runs inferiorly to supply skin of the forearm. The medial cord then ends by dividing into the *ulnar nerve*, which passes distally in the arm (slightly posterior to the artery),

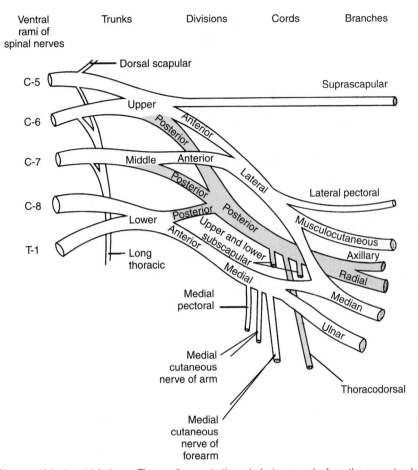

Ventral rami of spinal nerves	Trunks	Divisions	Cords	Branches

Dorsal scapular

Suprascapular

C-5

Upper

Posterior   Anterior

C-6

Anterior

Middle

C-7

Posterior   Lateral

Lateral pectoral

C-8

Posterior   Posterior

Lower

Upper and lower subscapular

Musculocutaneous

Anterior

Axillary

T-1

Long thoracic

Medial

Radial

Medial pectoral

Median

Ulnar

Medial cutaneous nerve of arm

Thoracodorsal

Medial cutaneous nerve of forearm

Figure 5-7 Diagram of the brachial plexus. The small nerve to the subclavius muscle, from the upper trunk, is omitted.

and a *contribution to the median nerve,* which crosses anterior to the axillary artery to join the contribution from the lateral cord. The median nerve is formed anterolateral to the axillary artery, and its two roots form a loop across the surface of this vessel.

The **posterior cord** lies on the surface of the subscapularis muscle deep to the axillary artery. It contains fibers from most of the anterior rami forming the brachial plexus but usually relatively few fibers from C8 and sometimes none from T1. The posterior cord gives off an *upper subscapular nerve* to the subscapularis muscle, the *thoracodorsal nerve* to the latissimus dorsi muscle, and a *lower subscapular nerve* to the subscapularis and teres major muscles, and then it divides into axillary and radial nerves. The *axillary nerve* immediately passes posteriorly around the

surgical neck of the humerus and supplies the teres minor and deltoid muscles. The larger *radial nerve* gives off small motor and cutaneous branches in the axilla and then disappears posteriorly, deep to the triceps muscle (the muscle of the back of the arm).

In addition to the branches from the three cords, other branches arise from the more proximal parts of the brachial plexus (i.e., closer to the origin of the plexus). The tiny *nerve to the subclavius* (not shown in Fig. 5-7) and the larger *suprascapular nerve* (to the supraspinatus and infraspinatus) arise from the upper trunk of the brachial plexus. The *dorsal scapular nerve* to the rhomboids arises from C5 before this joins the upper trunk, and the *long thoracic nerve* to the serratus anterior arises from the anterior rami of C5, C6, and C7, especially C6 (see Fig. 5-7).

Furthermore, the anterior rami, before their union, contribute *nerves to muscles of the neck,* and C5 also regularly sends *fibers into the phrenic nerve* which innervates the diaphragm.

FUNCTIONAL/CLINICAL NOTE 5-5

Because of its position between the first rib and clavicle, its relationship to structures within the neck (such as the anterior scalene muscle), and its proximity to the humerus in the axilla and arm, the brachial plexus is subject to injuries resulting from stretching and compression. A familiar example of temporary impairment of the function of the fibers of the brachial plexus is that involved in the upper limb "going to sleep" when a person lies in bed with the upper limb above the head. In that scenario, the brachial plexus is stretched over the clavicle and the head of the humerus. Although the discomfort ordinarily resulting from such abuse to the brachial plexus is mild with no accompanying permanent sensory or motor effects, exaggerated positions of the arm under some conditions may lead to more permanent damage. The brachial plexus may be injured by undue stresses exerted on it while an individual is under anesthesia or by abnormal postures of the arm maintained by the faulty application of casts or splints. Constant pressure in the axilla, as from a splint or a crutch, may also produce injury to the brachial plexus.

Chronic injury to the brachial plexus and the subclavian and/or axillary arteries at the base of the neck as they pass into the axilla has been attributed to a number of causes. The syndromes can be grouped generally as *neurovascular compression* or *entrapment syndromes,* implying the possible involvement of neural, vascular, or both components within the area. The syndromes described here can more specifically be grouped within the category of *thoracic outlet* (or *inlet*) *syndrome* (i.e., the symptoms resulting from injury at the upper border of the thorax).

In *cervical rib syndrome,* an abnormal (cervical) rib may be associated with the seventh cervical vertebra. The brachial plexus and associated vessels must pass across this extra rib rather than crossing the lower lying normal first rib and, in this relationship, may become stretched. This situation can be aggravated by the upper limb's being pulled inferiorly, as in carrying a bucket of water.

Scalenus anticus syndrome is the result of compression by a particularly broad and tendinous or spastic anterior scalene muscle that lies anterior to the brachial plexus and subclavian artery.

In *costoclavicular syndrome,* the plexus can be pinched between the clavicle and first rib, whereas in *pectoralis minor syndrome,* the plexus and vessels can be compressed between the pectoralis minor muscle and underlying ribs.

Most of these syndromes have one thing in common: Symptoms are brought on or increased by habitually carrying the shoulder lower than normal, so that the plexus is subjected to abnormal stretch and pressure. The primary neural component involved is the lower trunk of the brachial plexus. In many cases, patients have reported relief or cure by appropriate physical therapy, which involves a toning up of the elevators of the scapula so that the patient carries the shoulder higher. This avoids the surgical treatment that is otherwise necessary.

Vessels

The **axillary artery** is the direct continuation of the subclavian artery and continues into the arm as the brachial artery (Fig. 5-9). The axillary artery extends between the first rib and the lower border of the teres major muscle. It gives off branches to the thoracic wall and its covering muscles, to the shoulder, and to the uppermost part of the arm. It has six named branches. The first, the *supreme thoracic artery,* is a small artery to the upper thoracic wall. The *thoracoacromial artery* supplies primarily the pectoral muscles, the anterior part of the deltoid, and the joints at both ends of the clavicle. The *lateral thoracic artery* supplies both the

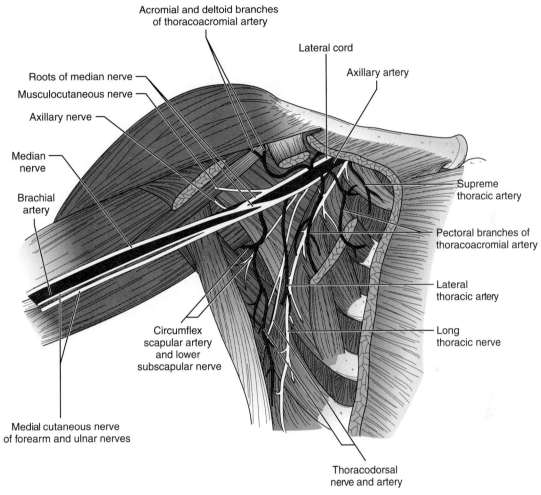

Acromial and deltoid branches
of thoracoacromial artery

Roots of median nerve

Musculocutaneous nerve

Axillary nerve

Median
nerve

Brachial
artery

Lateral cord

Axillary artery

Supreme
thoracic artery

Pectoral branches of
thoracoacromial artery

Lateral
thoracic artery

Long
thoracic nerve

Circumflex
scapular artery
and lower
subscapular nerve

Medial cutaneous nerve
of forearm and ulnar nerves

Thoracodorsal
nerve and artery

Figure 5-8 Nerves and arteries of the axilla.

thoracic wall and the pectoral muscles, especially the pectoralis minor. The *subscapular artery* is the largest branch of the axillary, and through its *circumflex scapular* branch, it supplies muscles on the posterior surface of the scapula (Fig. 5-10). Its continuation downward on the thoracic wall is the *thoracodorsal artery* (see Fig. 5-9). The last two branches of the axillary are the *anterior* and *posterior circumflex humeral arteries*; the posterior circumflex humeral is larger and encircles the surgical neck of the humerus with the axillary nerve (see Fig. 5-10).

The veins in the axilla are somewhat variable. A large superficial vein, the **basilic vein,** becomes the **axillary vein** as it crosses the lower border of the teres major to enter the axilla. The axillary vein is joined by **two brachial veins,** the **cephalic vein,** and various deep branches corresponding approximately to arterial branches of this region.

Most of the complex nerves and vessels described are surrounded by a tube of fascia, termed the **axillary sheath,** that is brought down from the neck. The additional space in the axilla is occupied by parts of muscles (the coracobrachialis and the short head of the biceps, both located laterally) and by connective tissue and fat in which numerous lymph nodes are embedded.

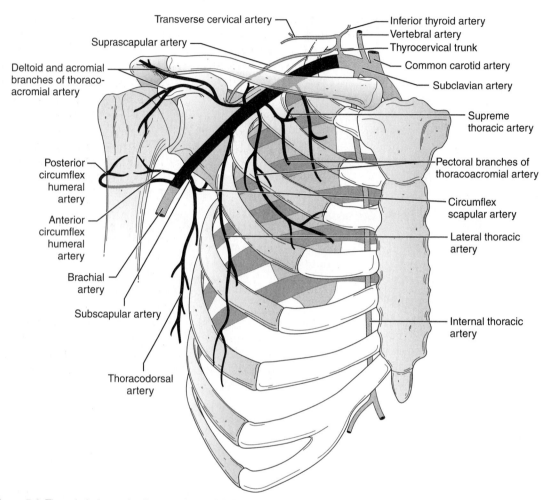

Figure 5-9 The subclavian and axillary arteries and their branches. The axillary artery and its branches are shaded in red. The origin of the suprascapular and transverse cervical arteries varies; each may arise directly from the subclavian artery. The branches of the transverse cervical may arise separately, one from the subclavian artery and the other from the thyrocervical trunk.

FUNCTIONAL/CLINICAL NOTE 5-6

Lymphatic drainage from the upper limb, shoulder, and most of the anterolateral thoracic wall, including the breast, ends in the axillary nodes. In removal of a cancerous breast (mastectomy), it may be necessary to remove these nodes. The subsequent swelling (edema) of the limb, resulting from interruption of lymphatic drainage, and the fact that much of the pectoralis major muscle may be removed in the course of the operation, may make physical therapy necessary.

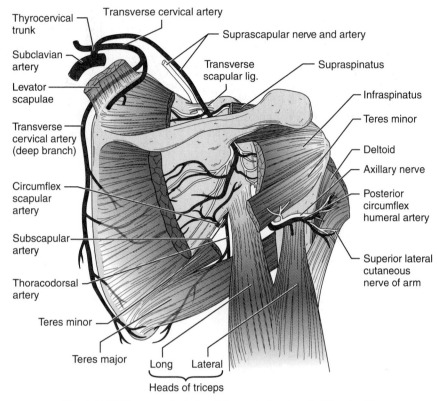

Figure 5-10 Nerves and arteries of the posterior aspect of the shoulder.

Surface Anatomy

Some of the vessels and nerves of the shoulder can be observed or palpated. The only nerves that can be palpated are those forming the lower part of the **brachial** plexus. These are not individually recognizable but can be rolled against the humerus by the thumb. The fact that nerves form at least a part of this mass (the axillary artery is also a part of it) can be recognized by the unpleasant sensation produced by slight pressure on the nerves. The **cephalic vein** is frequently visible through the skin as it runs up the anterolateral side of the arm, and it may be visible between the deltoid and pectoralis major muscles. It joins the axillary vein deep to the clavipectoral (deltopectoral) triangle. Unnamed superficial veins can frequently be seen through the skin of the pectoral region, especially in women, in whom these veins are larger because they participate in the drainage of the breast.

The pulse of the **subclavian artery** can be felt behind the clavicle in the depression at the base of the neck. The **axillary artery,** which gives rise to all the other important arteries to the shoulder, can be palpated in the axilla against the humerus.

MUSCLES

Muscles of the Pectoral Region

The muscles of this region are the pectoralis major and pectoralis minor, but other muscles are closely associated with this area. The two pectoralis major muscles are the large muscles covering most of the upper part of the thorax; each muscle forms the

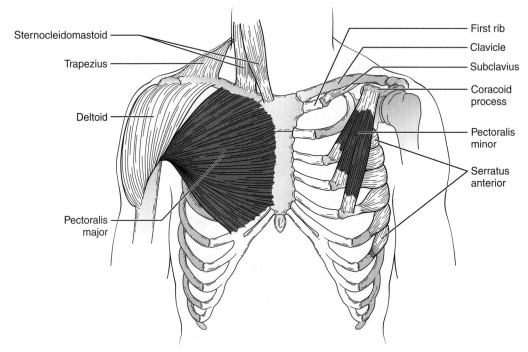

Figure 5-11 The pectoralis major and minor muscles *(color)* and related muscles.

anterior wall of the axilla as it extends across to attach to the humerus (Fig. 5-11). At its attachment to the clavicle, the muscle is covered by the thin platysma ("flat") muscle lying mostly in the fascia of the neck but extending downward over the clavicle (see Fig. 21-7). Attached to the upper border of the clavicle above the clavicular origin of the pectoralis major is the sternocleidomastoid, a prominent muscle of the neck. The pectoralis major lies medial to the anterior portion of the deltoid muscle, the large muscle below the point of the shoulder. Usually there is a distinct groove between these two muscles, occupied by the cephalic vein, which serves as a landmark for the boundary line between them. The pectoralis minor may or may not be evident at the lower lateral edge of the major. The external oblique muscle and its aponeurosis (see Fig. 23-1) and the serratus anterior muscle (see Fig. 5-11) can be identified laterally and inferiorly. As the pectoralis major proceeds to its insertion, it passes deep to the anterior fibers of the deltoid but superficial to the origin of two muscles of

the arm (the coracobrachialis and the short head of the biceps brachii; see Fig. 6-6).

Pectoralis major

The *origin* of the fan-shaped **pectoralis major** is from the medial two thirds of the clavicle, the length of the sternum, the upper six costal cartilages, and a small slip from the aponeurosis of the external oblique muscle (the most superficial of the lateral abdominal muscles). From this wide origin, the muscle bundles converge to a tendon of *insertion* that is attached to the crest of the greater tubercle, or lateral lip of the intertubercular groove. The tendon of insertion is bilaminar. The tendon from the fibers of the clavicular portion of the muscle blends with the tendon from the upper part of the sternocostal portion to form an anterior lamina. The fibers of the lower sternocostal and the abdominal parts pass upward deep to the insertion of the upper portion to form the posterior layer of the pectoralis tendon, the lowest fibers being inserted highest on the humerus.

The pectoralis major receives *innervation* from the medial and lateral pectoral nerves. The medial pectoral nerve, innervating the inferior part of the muscle, arises from the medial cord of the brachial plexus (hence the name *medial*) and runs around the lateral border of the pectoralis minor (the muscle deep to the pectoralis major) or pierces that muscle to enter the lateral part of the pectoralis major. It brings into the muscle nerve fibers from spinal cord segments C8 and T1. (Segmental levels for innervation of the muscles are summarized in Table 5-7 later in the chapter.) The lateral pectoral nerve arises from the lateral cord of the plexus and contains fibers derived from spinal cord segments C5 through C7. It runs anteriorly into the superior part of the pectoralis major with pectoral branches of the thoracoacromial artery (the first major branch of the axillary artery), passing superior to the pectoralis minor and perforating the fascia (clavipectoral) stretching from this muscle to the clavicle. In addition to the branches that the thoracoacromial artery sends into the pectoralis major, other branches emerge superior to the insertion end of the muscle to run toward the tip of the shoulder and also with the cephalic vein between the deltoid and pectoralis major muscles, supplying both. Deep to the pectoralis major, a twig of the thoracoacromial artery runs toward the sternoclavicular joint. On the thoracic wall, approximately along the lateral border of the pectoralis minor muscle, are the lateral thoracic vessels. (The artery arises also from the axillary, usually below the origin of the thoracoacromial artery but sometimes with that vessel.)

The *action* of the muscle as a whole is to adduct the arm and bring it anteriorly and medially across the chest. The clavicular fibers, working alone, add a movement of flexion, such as that involved in touching the lobe of the opposite ear. The lower fibers of the sternocostal portion depress the arm and may depress the shoulder. The sternocostal portion of the muscle, acting alone, extends the arm at the glenohumeral joint, if the arm is already flexed, but cannot hyperextend it (carry it backward beyond its normal position at the side). Also, because the muscle as a whole crosses anterior to the humerus to insert lateral to the intertubercular groove, it will, in contraction, produce medial rotation of the humerus.

FUNCTIONAL/CLINICAL NOTE 5-7

The pectoralis major is, on occasion, congenitally absent, and all or most of it is removed in radical mastectomy (removal of the breast and surrounding diseased tissue). The approximately normal movement of the arm across the thorax in the absence of the pectoralis major indicates the extent to which other muscles, especially the anterior portion of the deltoid and the coracobrachialis, can substitute for the functions of the missing muscle.

Pectoralis minor

The **pectoralis minor** is small and rather triangular and lies deep to the pectoralis major (see Fig. 5-11). Its *origin* is from about the third to the fifth ribs, with some variation in origin possible. It crosses the front of the axilla, where it is in close contact with the vessels and nerves in the area. The *insertion* of the muscle is on the coracoid process of the scapula behind its tip. The pectoralis minor receives *innervation* from the medial pectoral nerve and is usually pierced by the portion of this nerve that continues to the pectoralis major. The *action* of the pectoralis minor is to depress the shoulder, and, because it acts close to the lateral angle, it aids in downward rotation of the scapula (Table 5-1).

The pectoralis minor is supplied by branches of the various arteries appearing on the thoracic wall, notably the thoracoacromial and lateral thoracic arteries from the axillary.

The pectoralis minor is surrounded by a thin fascial sheath, the **clavipectoral fascia,** which has anterior and posterior layers that come together at the upper and lower edges of the muscle. Inferior and lateral to the pectoralis minor, the clavipectoral fascia is continuous with the fascia covering the superficial muscle (serratus anterior) of the anterolateral thoracic wall. Above and laterally, it joins fascia that forms the floor of the axilla. From the upper and medial border of the pectoralis minor, the clavipectoral fascia extends to the clavicle, being especially tough laterally. It is pierced by the lateral pectoral nerve and the large vessels to the pectoralis major. As the fascia

Table 5-1	PECTORAL MUSCLES			
Muscle	**Origin (Proximal Attachment)**	**Insertion (Distal Attachment)**	**Action**	**Innervation**
Pectoralis major	Medial two thirds of clavicle; sternum; costal cartilages 1–6	Lateral lip of intertubercular groove (crest of greater tubercle) of humerus	Adduction and medial rotation of arm; flexion (clavicular fibers) and extension (sternocostal fibers) of arm	Medial and lateral pectoral nerves
Pectoralis minor	Ribs 3–5	Coracoid process of scapula	Depression of shoulder; downward rotation of scapula	Medial pectoral nerve

reaches the clavicle, it divides to go on both sides of the small subclavius muscle, which lies between the clavicle and the first rib.

Muscles of the Shoulder Proper

Sternocleidomastoid

Besides the two shoulder muscles already described as lying primarily in the pectoral region, there are two anteriorly located muscles connected with the clavicle. The **sternocleidomastoid,** a muscle in the neck, has two heads of *origin:* a tendinous head from the sternum and a thinner, muscular head from the medial third of the clavicle (see Fig. 5-11). The muscle runs obliquely upward and posteriorly across the neck. Its *insertion* is onto the prominent mastoid process behind the ear (see Fig. 21-9). If the sternal and clavicular attachments of this muscle are fixed, the *action* of the muscle of one side (unilateral contraction) is to pull on the skull to turn the face toward the opposite side and, at the same time, to flex the neck toward the side of the muscle acting (bringing the ear down toward the clavicle). Bilateral action (contraction of both muscles) is normally described as producing flexion of the neck, as in raising the head when the body is in a supine position (lying on the back). However, some reports have suggested that contraction of both muscles (particularly their posterior fibers) may, in addition, produce some extension of the neck at the uppermost vertebrae. If the head is fixed by contraction of other muscles attaching to the skull, the sternocleidomastoid acts on the clavicle and sternum to raise them. Through this action, it becomes an accessory respiratory muscle.

The sternocleidomastoid receives *innervation* from the accessory nerve (cranial nerve XI). This nerve runs obliquely downward and posteriorly to reach the muscle only an inch (2.5 cm) or so below the mastoid process. It supplies the muscle as it passes either through it (most common) or deep to it, and then it continues its oblique course toward the trapezius muscle. Fibers of spinal nerves, usually from C2, also enter the muscle either separately or after joining the accessory nerve. The accessory nerve is motor only, whereas the cervical nerve fibers to the sternocleidomastoid are probably all sensory.

Subclavius

The **subclavius** muscle has a short tendon of *origin* from the first rib and passes laterally and upward to a muscular *insertion* on the lower surface of the clavicle (see Fig. 5-11). Its *action* is to slightly depress the clavicle or help in raising the first rib as the clavicle is raised. Because it runs laterally to reach its insertion, it aids in retaining the sternal end of the clavicle in place within the sternoclavicular joint. Aside from these actions, the muscle also affords protection to the subclavian artery in fractures of the clavicle. Its muscular belly intervenes between the artery and the possibly sharp edges of the fractured bone. *Innervation* to the subclavius is provided by a tiny branch from the upper trunk of the brachial plexus.

Trapezius

Most of the remaining shoulder muscles can best be studied from the back. Two large, flat ones, the trapezius and the latissimus dorsi, between them cover almost the entire back, extending from the skull to the sacrum and crest of the ilium (Fig. 5-12). The **trapezius,** the more superior of these muscles, has an extensive *origin* from the midline of the back, including the ligamentum nuchae (the "ligament of the back of the neck," extending from the skull to the prominent vertebral spinous process of the lowest

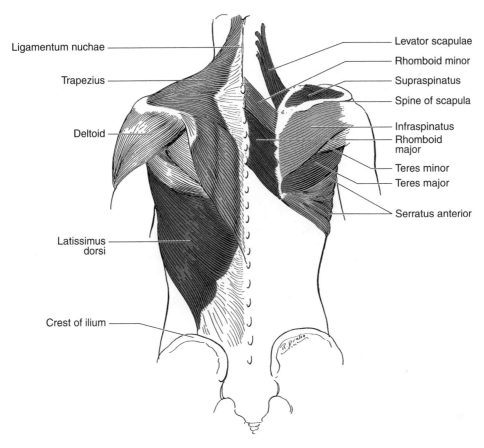

Figure 5-12 Musculature of the shoulder region (posterior view) and superficial back.

cervical vertebra at the base of the neck), the lowest cervical spinous process, and all the thoracic spinous processes. It often also attaches directly to and lateral to the external occipital protuberance of the skull. From this wide origin, the muscle converges to a more limited *insertion* on the spine of the scapula, the acromion, and the lateral third of the clavicle. The trapezius receives motor *innervation* from the accessory nerve (cranial nerve XI) and sensory fibers from spinal cord segments C3 and C4. The accessory nerve runs on the deep surface of the trapezius (in company with a branch of the transverse cervical artery) after supplying the sternocleidomastoid.

Because of its wide origin, the trapezius muscle has several different *actions*. Its superior fibers, inserting on the clavicle and acromion, can raise the point of the shoulder and are the only fibers that can do so directly. (The part inserting on the clavicle

is thin, and so it is the thickest part of the muscle that inserts on the acromion that is most effective.) Working with the inferior fibers of the muscle, which pull downward on the base of the scapular spine, the superior fibers of the trapezius help to turn the glenoid cavity upward; that is, they rotate the scapula upward. Contraction of the muscle as a whole or of only the middle fibers results in pulling the scapula posteriorly, whereas contraction of the inferior fibers alone depresses the scapula. The superior fibers can also flex the neck toward the same side, by taking their fixed point from below.

Two of the vessels to the shoulder, the transverse cervical and suprascapular arteries (see Fig. 5-9), arise in the neck, usually from the thyrocervical trunk. They run laterally and posteriorly, with the transverse cervical artery superior to the clavicle and the suprascapular artery posterior to the clavicle, and disappear deep

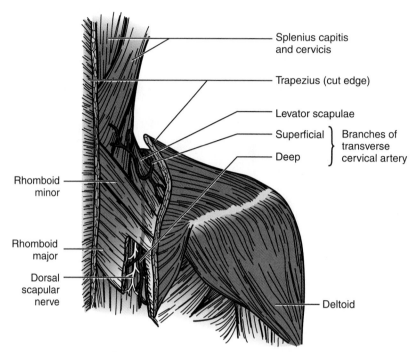

Splenius capitis
and cervicis

Trapezius (cut edge)

Levator scapulae

Superficial ⎱ Branches of
⎰ transverse
Deep cervical artery

Rhomboid
minor

Rhomboid
major

Dorsal
scapular
nerve

Deltoid

Figure 5-13 The dorsal scapular nerve and transverse cervical artery.

to the trapezius muscle. Under cover of the trapezius, the transverse cervical artery divides into a superficial branch, which runs on the deep surface of the trapezius, and a deep branch (dorsal scapular artery) that runs on the deep surface of the rhomboid muscles with the dorsal scapular nerve (Fig. 5-13). (Quite often, the artery corresponding to the superficial branch arises separately from the thyrocervical trunk and is termed the *superficial cervical artery*. The artery corresponding to the deep branch arises directly from the subclavian artery as the *descending scapular artery*.)

Latissimus dorsi

The *origin* of the **latissimus dorsi** is from about the lower six thoracic and all the lumbar and sacral spinous processes and from a posterior portion of the crest of the ilium by a broad aponeurosis of origin that covers the back muscles. Fleshy slips from the lower four ribs join the deep surface of the muscle. On occasion, in addition to its major origin, this muscle has a small origin from the inferior angle of the scapula. The fibers converge to a relatively narrow, flat tendon, which, passing across the posterior wall of the axilla, runs anteriorly around the medial surface of the humerus to an *insertion* on the medial lip and floor of the intertubercular groove. As it does so, it twists so sharply around an underlying muscle (teres major) that its original anterior surface is directed posteriorly. The *action* of the muscle is to extend, medially rotate, and adduct the arm, a movement used, for instance, in chopping wood and in the overhand swimming stroke. In contrast to the lower portion of the pectoralis major, with which it works in the first part of these movements, the latissimus dorsi carries the arm posteriorly beyond its position at the side; that is, it hyperextends the arm. Through its action on the arm, the latissimus dorsi can also depress the shoulder. Although the latissimus dorsi and the lower part of the pectoralis major form an anteroposterior sling from the trunk to the free limb, the latissimus dorsi is the more powerful and important component of this sling in extending the arm at the glenohumeral joint and depressing the shoulder.

Table 5-2	STERNOCLEIDOMASTOID, SUBCLAVIUS, TRAPEZIUS, AND LATISSIMUS DORSI			
Muscle	**Origin (Proximal Attachment)**	**Insertion (Distal Attachment)**	**Action**	**Innervation**
Sternocleidomastoid	Tendinous head from sternum; muscular head from medial third of clavicle	Mastoid process of skull	One muscle: flexion of neck toward same side (turns face to opposite side and brings ear of same side toward clavicle)	Accessory nerve (cranial nerve XI)
Subclavius	Rib 1	Undersurface of clavicle	Possibly depresses clavicle; maintains sternoclavicular joint	Nerve to subclavius
Trapezius	External occipital protuberance; ligamentum nuchae; spinous processes of seventh cervical and all thoracic vertebrae	Spine of scapula; acromion; lateral third of clavicle	Elevation of scapula (upper fibers); retraction of scapula (middle fibers); depression of scapula (inferior fibers); rotation of glenoid cavity upward	Accessory nerve (C3 and C4 sensory)
Latissimus dorsi	Spinous processes of lower six thoracic and all lumbar and sacral vertebrae; posterior part of iliac crest	Medial lip (crest of lesser tubercle) and floor of intertubercular groove of humerus	Extension, adduction, and medial rotation of arm	Thoracodorsal nerve

FUNCTIONAL/CLINICAL NOTE 5-8

Chin-up exercises are possible when the latissimus dorsi is intact but the lower part of the pectoralis major is damaged, but they become impossible if the latissimus dorsi alone is gravely weakened. Similarly, a person cannot walk on crutches unless the latissimus dorsi functions to prevent the shoulder from being pushed up by the weight on the crutch.

The *innervation* to the latissimus dorsi is through the thoracodorsal nerve, a branch from the posterior cord of the brachial plexus, which transmits fibers derived from C6, C7, and C8 (Table 5-2; see Figs. 5-7 and 5-8). It lies at first on the costal surface of the subscapularis muscle, on which it runs downward to the deep or costal surface of the latissimus. The chief vessel entering the muscle is the thoracodorsal artery, a branch of the subscapular artery that runs on the deep surface of the muscle and also helps supply the adjacent serratus anterior muscle.

Levator scapulae, rhomboid minor, and rhomboid major

Under cover of the trapezius are three smaller muscles attached to the medial border of the scapula (see Fig. 5-12). The upper one, the **levator scapulae,** typically has an *origin* from the transverse processes of the upper four cervical vertebrae, and its *insertion* is on the superior angle and upper part of the medial border of the scapula. The levator scapulae sometimes receives *innervation,* in part, by the dorsal scapular nerve but is supplied chiefly by small twigs from the third and fourth cervical nerves into its anterior surface (Table 5-3). Inferior to the levator scapulae are the rhomboid minor and rhomboid major muscles. These two muscles are not necessarily clearly distinct from each other. The *origin* of the **rhomboid minor** is from the inferior part of the ligamentum nuchae and the spinous processes of seventh cervical and first thoracic vertebrae, and its *insertion* is on the medial border of the scapula at the base of the spine. The *origin* of the **rhomboid major** is from the spinous processes of the second to the fifth thoracic vertebrae, and its *insertion* is on the rest of the medial border of the scapula, inferior to the

Table 5-3	LEVATOR SCAPULAE, RHOMBOID MINOR, AND RHOMBOID MAJOR			
Muscle	**Origin (Proximal Attachment)**	**Insertion (Distal Attachment)**	**Action**	**Innervation**
Levator scapulae	Transverse processes of upper four cervical vertebrae	Superior angle and upper part of medial border of scapula	Elevation of scapula	C3 and C4; dorsal scapular nerve
Rhomboid minor	Lower part of ligamentum nuchae; spinous processes of seventh cervical and first thoracic vertebrae	Medial border of scapula at base of spine	Elevation and retraction of scapula; downward rotation of glenoid cavity	Dorsal scapular nerve
Rhomboid major	Spinous processes of second to fifth thoracic vertebrae	Medial border of scapula below rhomboid minor	Elevation and retraction of scapula; downward rotation of glenoid cavity	Dorsal scapular nerve

Table 5-4	SERRATUS ANTERIOR			
Muscle	**Origin (Proximal Attachment)**	**Insertion (Distal Attachment)**	**Action**	**Innervation**
Serratus anterior	Ribs 1-8 on anterolateral thoracic wall	Medial border of scapula; heaviest insertion to inferior angle	Protraction of scapula; upward rotation of glenoid cavity; holds medial border against thoracic wall	Long thoracic nerve

rhomboid minor. The *action* of these three muscles is to aid in raising the scapula or fixing its medial border. Acting together, they raise primarily the medial border and produce downward rotation of the glenoid cavity; the rhomboids also retract the scapula. *Innervation* to the rhomboids is provided by the dorsal scapular nerve that arises from the anterior ramus of the C5 spinal nerve as it enters the brachial plexus (see Figs. 5-7 and 5-13). This nerve runs transversely across the neck, paralleling the transverse cervical and suprascapular arteries; passes deep to or through the levator scapulae; and then runs with the deep cervical or descending scapular artery on the deep surface of the rhomboids close to the medial border of the scapula.

Serratus anterior

The *origin* of the **serratus anterior** muscle is from the anterolateral thoracic wall by muscular slips from about the upper eight ribs. It runs posteriorly, closely apposed to the curve of the thoracic wall. Its *insertion* is on the costal surface of the entire medial border of the scapula (see Figs. 5-6, 5-8, and 5-11). The heaviest insertion, however, is on the inferior angle. Some of the lower slips run upward to reach this, whereas others, of higher origin, run downward to this insertion. The *action* of the muscle as a whole

is to protract the scapula; because it protracts the inferior angle, it is particularly important in upward rotation of the lateral angle. Because the serratus anterior curves around the thoracic wall, it also keeps the medial border of the scapula closely applied to this wall. Its inferior fibers aid in depression of the scapula. Although once regarded as a respiratory muscle because it could raise the ribs, it apparently does not function as one in normal breathing. Its *innervation* is by the long thoracic nerve, which arises from the anterior rami of C5, C6, and C7 before these enter into the formation of the brachial plexus (Table 5-4; see Fig. 5-7). The chief root of the nerve is usually from C6; contributions from either C5 or C7 may be lacking. This nerve runs posterior to the other elements of the brachial plexus and lies superficial, rather than deep, to the serratus anterior. The blood vessels supplying the muscle are those of the anterolateral thoracic wall and of the scapular region, primarily the lateral thoracic and thoracodorsal arteries (see Fig. 5-8).

Deltoid

The most prominent intrinsic muscle of the shoulder (arising from the girdle) is the **deltoid** (see Figs. 5-11 and 5-12). The *origin* of this muscle is anteriorly from

Table 5-5	DELTOID			
Muscle	**Origin (Proximal Attachment)**	**Insertion (Distal Attachment)**	**Action**	**Innervation**
Deltoid	Lateral third of clavicle; acromion; spine of scapula	Deltoid tuberosity on shaft of humerus	Abduction (middle fibers), flexion and medial rotation (anterior fibers), and extension and lateral rotation (posterior fibers) of arm	Axillary nerve

about the lateral third of the clavicle, posteriorly from the spine of the scapula, and, between these two origins, from the acromion. The origin as a whole corresponds closely to the insertion of the trapezius; it works with the upper fibers of the trapezius in abducting the arm. From this origin, the deltoid converges to its *insertion* on the deltoid tuberosity on the lateral surface of the humerus. Because the fibers of the deltoid pass in front of, lateral to, and behind the glenohumeral joint, this muscle produces several movements. The *action* of the middle fibers is to raise the arm away from the side: that is, abduct it. The anterior fibers working alone flex and medially rotate the humerus, whereas the posterior fibers extend and laterally rotate it. Finally, the lower fibers of both anterior and posterior parts of the muscle may be brought into play in forcible adduction of the arm, although this may be primarily a protective action against the downward displacement of the humerus that the more powerful adductors, the latissimus dorsi and pectoralis major, tend to produce (Table 5-5). The *innervation* of the muscle is provided by the axillary nerve (C5 and C6) and it is vascularized by the posterior circumflex humeral artery, as well as by other vessels in the area (see Figs. 5-9 and 5-10). The nerve and artery pass below the subscapularis and teres minor muscles and above the teres major and circle anteriorly close against the surgical neck of the humerus.

Supraspinatus, infraspinatus, teres minor, teres major, and subscapularis

There are five muscles that arise entirely from the scapula and insert on the humerus. Three of them attach to the greater tubercle. The *origin* of the **supraspinatus** is from the dorsal surface of the scapula above the spine (supraspinous fossa) and from the fascia covering the muscle (see Figs. 5-10 and 5-12). It passes over the top of the glenohumeral joint to an *insertion* on the upper part of the greater tubercle.

Between this muscle and the overhanging acromion there is an important subacromial (subdeltoid) bursa. The **infraspinatus** muscle has its *origin* from its covering fascia and from the infraspinous fossa, and its *insertion* is on the greater tubercle directly inferior to the insertion of the supraspinatus muscle. The *origin* of the **teres minor** is from about the upper two thirds of the posterior surface of the lateral border of the scapula and from septa between it and both the infraspinatus above and the teres major below. The *insertion* of the teres minor muscle is on the greater tubercle directly inferior to the insertion of the infraspinatus (Table 5-6).

The *action* of the supraspinatus is primarily to abduct the arm, assisting the deltoid in this movement. The infraspinatus and teres minor are primarily lateral rotators of the humerus and are also important in maintaining the head of the humerus in position during other movements of the arm. The supraspinatus and infraspinatus muscles receive *innervation* from the suprascapular nerve (C5 and C6). As this nerve reaches the superior border of the scapula it passes through the scapular notch deep to the transverse scapular ligament, runs between the bone and the supraspinatus muscle, and then continues laterally around the spine of the scapula to reach the infraspinatus muscle. The *innervation* to the teres minor is by a branch from the axillary nerve, given off as this nerve passes below the muscle on its way to the deltoid.

The suprascapular artery, arising anteriorly at the base of the neck, accompanies the suprascapular nerve to these muscles (see Fig. 5-10); it passes across the scapular notch superficial to the transverse scapular ligament but otherwise has a course similar to that of the nerve. The circumflex scapular artery rounds the lateral border of the scapula by passing through the origin of the teres minor, and ramifies in the infraspinous fossa. The suprascapular, transverse

Table 5-6	SUPRASPINATUS, INFRASPINATUS, TERES MINOR, TERES MAJOR, AND SUBSCAPULARIS			
Muscle	**Origin (Proximal Attachment)**	**Insertion (Distal Attachment)**	**Action**	**Innervation**
Supraspinatus	Supraspinous fossa of scapula	Greater tubercle of humerus	Abduction of arm	Suprascapular nerve
Infraspinatus	Infraspinous fossa of scapula	Greater tubercle of humerus below supraspinatus	Lateral rotation of arm	Suprascapular nerve
Teres minor	Upper two thirds of lateral border of scapula	Greater tubercle of humerus below infraspinatus	Lateral rotation of arm	Axillary nerve
Teres major	Inferior angle of scapula	Medial lip of intertubercular groove of humerus	Adduction, medial rotation, and extension of arm	Lower subscapular nerve
Subscapularis	Subscapular fossa of scapula	Lesser tubercle and crest of humerus	Medial rotation of arm	Upper and lower subscapular nerves

cervical (particularly its deep branch), and circumflex scapular arteries anastomose freely with each other and provide an alternative route by which blood from the subclavian artery can reach the axillary artery.

The **teres major** (see Figs. 5-10 and 5-12) is at its *origin* closely associated with the teres minor and infraspinatus, arising from septa between it and these muscles and from the posterior surface of the inferior angle of the scapula. As it passes to its insertion, it is separated from the teres minor by the long head of the triceps muscle (not shown in Fig. 5-12 but labeled in Fig. 5-10). It becomes closely associated with the tendon of insertion of the latissimus dorsi, a bursa usually intervening between the two, and passes with this latter muscle to an *insertion* on the medial lip of the intertubercular groove. The teres major receives *innervation* from the lower subscapular nerve (C5 and C6), which arises from the posterior cord of the brachial plexus. The lower subscapular nerve runs downward on the subscapularis muscle to supply the lower part of this muscle and continues into the teres major (see Fig. 5-8). In its *action*, it resembles the latissimus dorsi, being an extensor, hyperextensor, medial rotator, and adductor of the arm, but assisting the latissimus in these movements only when there is resistance to them.

The **subscapularis** muscle (see Fig. 5-26, *B*) has its *origin* from most of the costal aspect of the scapula (subscapular fossa) and passes across the front of the glenohumeral joint to an *insertion* on the lesser tubercle and its crest. A subscapular bursa, usually opening into the synovial cavity of the glenohumeral joint, intervenes between the muscle and the neck of the scapula. This muscle is *innervated* by the upper and lower subscapular nerves from the posterior cord of the brachial plexus (see Fig. 5-7). The upper subscapular nerve passes directly into the muscle, whereas the lower subscapular nerve runs caudally to supply the inferior part of the subscapularis and teres major. The *action* of the subscapularis muscle is to produce medial rotation, and it is particularly important in preventing anterior dislocation of the head of the humerus. Laxity of this muscle (or even tears) is usually found during surgery to correct recurrent anterior dislocations (see Table 5-6).

Rotator (musculotendinous) cuff

Four of the muscles (and their tendons) just described form the **rotator (musculotendinous) cuff** of the glenohumeral joint (Fig. 5-14). Posteriorly, from a superior to an inferior position, the cuff is made up of the *supraspinatus, infraspinatus,* and *teres minor* muscles. The *subscapularis* muscle forms the anterior part of the cuff. As the tendons of these muscles cross the glenohumeral joint, they are closely apposed to the joint capsule. The muscles aid in stabilizing the joint by holding the head of the humerus in the glenoid cavity. The cuff is closely associated with bursae around the joint and is subject to injury, including tearing. No tendons are present to support the inferior part of the joint and, therefore, dislocation of the humerus is possible in that area.

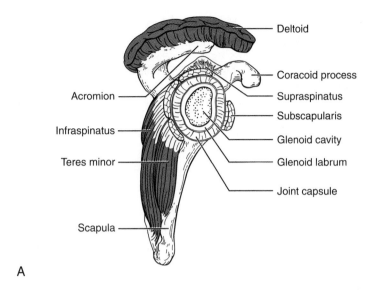

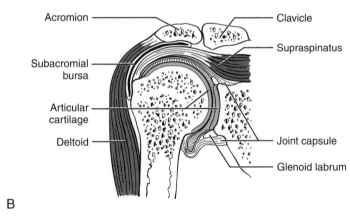

Figure 5-14 Shoulder region and glenohumeral joint. **A,** Lateral view of the shoulder with the humerus removed. The cut ends of the muscles forming the rotator cuff are illustrated. **B,** Frontal section through the shoulder region.

Muscle Variation

Except for minor variations of origin and insertion, which usually do not affect function, and the very rare absence of all or part of a muscle, the muscles of the shoulder are rather constant. Extra muscles occasionally found in this region include the **sternalis,** small paired or unpaired muscles on the anterior thoracic wall superficial to the pectoralis major, and an **axillary arch muscle.** The last one consists of muscle fibers that tend to arch across the axilla, hence its name. Although it may assume various forms and at-

tachments, one simple type is a bundle of fibers connecting the latissimus dorsi and pectoralis major.

Surface Anatomy

Some of the muscles of the shoulder are easy to identify; others are difficult or impossible to palpate. Some can be identified while performing movements designed to produce contraction of each individual muscle and of any part that acts differently from another. It should be remembered that muscular action is never any stronger than is required to bring about the desired movement, and some muscles that can help bring about the movement do not contract at all unless they are needed. Resistance to the movement, most easily produced in many cases by having the patient push against resistance offered by the observer's hand, reveals muscular contraction both more plainly and more completely. However, contraction of a muscle does not necessarily mean it is bringing about the movement, because it may be contracting synergistically to prevent some other undesired movement. Although it is not always possible to determine which muscles are prime movers and which are synergists, a knowledge of their anatomy often enables the decision to be made.

The **pectoralis major** can be easily identified on the front of the thorax. In men, it is largely responsible for the contour of the pectoral region, and in both sexes, it is the chief component of the anterior axillary fold. In muscular individuals, the slips of origin of the **serratus anterior** from the ribs are visually evident on the anterolateral thoracic wall below the pectoralis major. Both the **pectoralis minor** and the **subclavius** lie too deeply (the minor behind the major, the subclavius under cover of the clavicle) to be recognizable.

On the back, the lateral border of the upper part of the **trapezius,** as it runs from the neck to the shoulder, is both visually evident and palpable; atrophy of the muscle is easily recognized because of the change in contour in this region. Because of its flatness, however, other parts of the muscle are difficult to identify. Similarly, only a lateral part of the **latissimus dorsi,** as it extends toward the posterior axillary fold, is clearly recognizable. In the axillary fold, it is difficult or impossible to distinguish between the latissimus dorsi and the teres major because the muscles are closely apposed and have generally the same actions. The **teres major,** however, forms the larger bulk of the musculature in the fold.

The **deltoid** is easily recognizable because it gives shape to the junction of shoulder and arm; it is a particularly favorable muscle in which to demonstrate different actions of various parts. The **supraspinatus** is sometimes visible as it produces a slight outward bulging of the trapezius immediately above the scapular spine. However, it is difficult to palpate distinctly because, when it contracts in abduction, the overlying upper part of the trapezius also contracts. Because the deltoid also abducts, there is no good means of estimating the strength of the supraspinatus.

The other muscles intimately attached to the scapula—the **infraspinatus, teres minor,** and **subscapularis**—are not usually identifiable in the living person. However, because the first two are pure lateral rotators and the subscapularis is a pure medial rotator, the clinician can estimate the strength of these muscles by observing the strength of rotation of the humerus, taking care that the person being observed attempts neither flexion nor extension at the same time. With the forearm flexed at the elbow, thus eliminating pronation and supination of the forearm and hand, medial and lateral rotation of the arm can be demonstrated.

MOVEMENTS OF THE SHOULDER

Scapular Movements

Movements at the glenohumeral joint are ordinarily accompanied by movements of the scapula itself. The coordinated movement of both elements is sometimes referred to as the **scapulohumeral rhythm,** and disturbances of the normal rhythm are typical of certain lesions around the shoulder region. Many of the muscles acting across the glenohumeral joint are short ones that attach close to the proximal end of the humerus and do not have the leverage that could be obtained by a more distal insertion. Movements of the scapula increase the force of arm movements and also, by tilting the glenoid cavity in the desired direction, increase the range of movement of the free limb. As the arm is abducted, for instance, the deltoid and supraspinatus are obviously the active movers at the glenohumeral joint. Accompanying this abduction is an upward rotation of the glenoid cavity, variably reported as being one degree of rotation for every two degrees of abduction, or as two degrees for every three degrees of abduction. This upward rotation is brought about by the lower part of the serratus anterior and the upper and lower parts of the trapezius. In a similar way, movements of extension and flexion at the shoulder typically involve both scapular and humeral movement. Actually, fairly good use of the arm may persist despite the almost total destruction of the glenohumeral joint; in this case, scapular movements substitute for the normal combined action of both scapula and humerus.

Of the muscles acting on the scapula, some act directly on it through their attachment there, whereas others act primarily through their attachment to the humerus. There are only four muscles that are capable of producing **elevation of the scapula** (Fig. 5-15). The *upper fibers of the trapezius* inserting on the spine and acromion of the scapula, and on the clavicle, are solely responsible for elevation of the lateral angle of the scapula. The *levator scapulae* and the *two rhomboids* are attached in such a way that they can act only on the medial border.

FUNCTIONAL/CLINICAL NOTE 5-9

When paralysis of the trapezius muscle (injury to the accessory nerve) occurs, the lateral angle of the scapula, having nothing to support it, is dragged downward by the weight of the free limb. The weight of the entire limb is then thrown onto the levator scapulae and the rhomboids, which, reflexively increasing their activity in response to this greater stretch, contract to produce excessive elevation of the superior angle of the scapula.

In **depression of the scapula**, the *pectoralis minor, subclavius,* and *latissimus dorsi,* and *lower fibers of the trapezius, serratus anterior,* and *pectoralis major,* may all participate (Fig. 5-16). The pectoralis minor tends to rotate the scapula downward, whereas the serratus anterior rotates it upward. The subclavius, although identified as a depressor, can actually have only limited effect on the shoulder because of both its size and its very oblique position. The latissimus dorsi, through its action on the humerus, depresses the shoulder, and the lower fibers of the trapezius retract the scapula as they depress it. The inferior fibers of the pectoralis major protract the scapula as they assist in depressing it. An apparently simple movement, such as depression of the shoulder, may involve most of the muscles of the shoulder, either as prime movers, or as fixators to prevent rotation and

maintain the contact between the glenoid cavity and the head of the humerus.

Upward rotation of the scapula, necessary to allow abduction of the arm above the horizontal position, is performed by the combined actions of the *trapezius* and the *serratus anterior* (Fig. 5-17). The superior fibers of the trapezius pull upward on the clavicle and acromion; the inferior fibers pull downward on the base of the spine. Through their strong insertion on the inferior angle, the inferior fibers of the serratus anterior pull this portion of the medial border laterally and forward and are important in upward rotation of the lateral angle. Although some inferior fibers of the serratus anterior also tend to depress the scapula, this tendency is overcome, in upward rotation, by the contraction of the superior part of the trapezius. Obviously, this movement also demands a delicate distribution of action among several shoulder muscles, in order to prevent the scapula as a whole from being dragged anteriorly and inferiorly as it is rotated. Usually, upward rotation of the scapula is accompanied by elevation of this bone, assisting the arm in reaching higher.

FUNCTIONAL/CLINICAL NOTE 5-10

When the trapezius is paralyzed, there is first a depression and downward rotation produced by the weight of the arm and the pull of the serratus anterior. Only thereafter, with the levator scapulae and rhomboids stabilizing the medial border, does upward rotation occur. This partially reverses the downward rotation but does not actually turn the glenoid cavity upward, so that abduction even to the horizontal position is frequently not obtainable.

The opposite movement of **downward rotation of the scapula** is brought about through the action of the *rhomboids* and the *levator scapulae* in raising the medial border of the scapula, whereas the *pectoralis minor,* the *pectoralis major,* and the *latissimus dorsi,* aided also by the effect of gravity on the free limb, pull down the lateral angle (Fig. 5-18). Downward rotation of the scapula is usually associated with its depression, as in reaching down to pick up a suitcase.

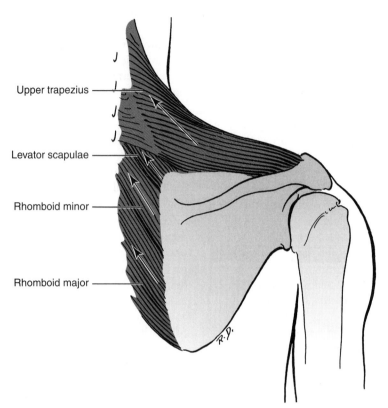

Upper trapezius

Levator scapulae

Rhomboid minor

Rhomboid major

Figure 5-15 Elevators of the scapula.

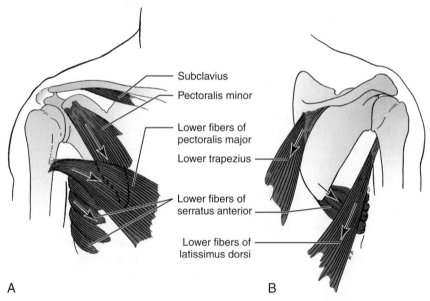

Subclavius

Pectoralis minor

Lower fibers of
pectoralis major

Lower trapezius

Lower fibers of
serratus anterior

Lower fibers of
latissimus dorsi

A

B

Figure 5-16 Depressors of the scapula. **A,** Anterior view. **B,** Posterior view.

Protraction of the scapula is brought about by the *serratus anterior* and by the *pectoralis major and minor* (Fig. 5-19). **Retraction** results from contraction of the middle fibers of the *trapezius* or to the trapezius acting as a whole, with the *rhomboids* and the *latissimus dorsi* (Fig. 5-20).

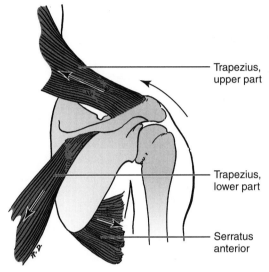

Figure 5-17 Upward rotators of the scapula.

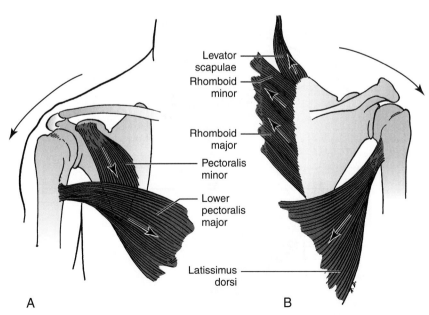

Figure 5-18 Downward rotators of the scapula. **A,** Anterior view. **B,** Posterior view.

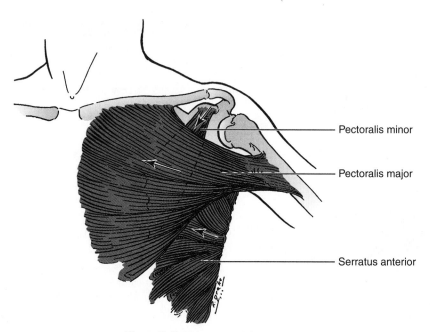

Pectoralis minor

Pectoralis major

Serratus anterior

Figure 5-19 Protractors of the scapula.

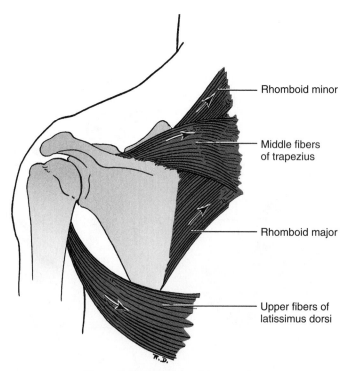

Rhomboid minor

Middle fibers
of trapezius

Rhomboid major

Upper fibers of
latissimus dorsi

Figure 5-20 Retractors of the scapula.

Humeral Movements

The musculature acting at the glenohumeral joint can be divided into two general groups: the shorter ones, which act primarily to retain and produce rotation of the humerus in the glenoid cavity, and the longer ones, which are responsible for much of the free movement between the humerus and glenoid cavity. With the arm by the side, downward displacement of the humerus is resisted by the coracohumeral ligament and assisted, if necessary, by the supraspinatus and the posterior fibers of the deltoid. During flexion or abduction, however, the ligament is relaxed, and it is the short muscles—the supraspinatus, infraspinatus, teres minor, and subscapularis—that prevent humeral displacement; they contract during all movements of flexion and abduction.

Flexion of the arm at the glenohumeral joint can be brought about (Fig. 5-21) through the action of the *anterior portion of the deltoid,* the *clavicular portion of the pectoralis major,* the *coracobrachialis* (a muscle of the arm), and the *biceps brachii* (the prominent muscle on the front of the arm). Of these, the anterior part of the deltoid is the most important. Because the biceps

brachii crosses the glenohumeral joint, it is capable of aiding in flexion of the arm at that joint. Its major function at the glenohumeral joint, however, is to assist in stabilizing the head of the humerus in the glenoid cavity during flexion of the arm. Complete flexion at the glenohumeral joint—that is, raising the limb forward until it is above the head—is not possible when the elbow is kept straight unless the flexion is accompanied by medial rotation of the humerus. Such movement can be carried out when the elbow is bent so as to diminish the pull of the biceps against the front of the humerus, where the tendon of its long head lies in the intertubercular groove. All of these muscles are supplied through C5 and C6; the coracobrachialis may also receive fibers from C7. Therefore, injury to the upper portion of the brachial plexus may markedly affect flexion at the shoulder.

Extension of the arm at the glenohumeral joint is brought about (Fig. 5-22) through the *posterior fibers of the deltoid,* the *latissimus dorsi,* the *sternocostal fibers of the pectoralis major,* the *teres major* (against resistance), and, weakly, the *long head of the triceps brachii* (the muscle on the posterior aspect of the arm). Although the lower fibers of the pectoralis major can

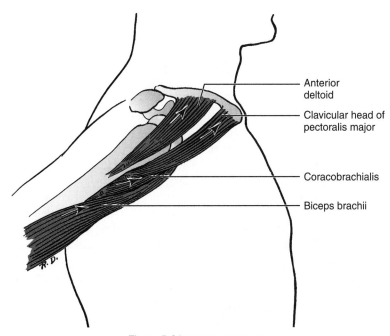

Figure 5-21 Flexors of the arm.

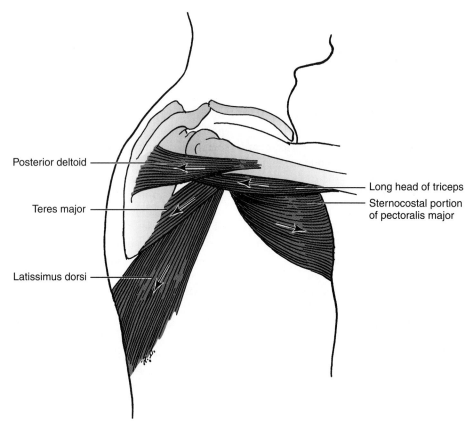

Posterior deltoid

Teres major

Latissimus dorsi

Long head of triceps

Sternocostal portion
of pectoralis major

Figure 5-22 Extensors of the arm.

assist this movement only to the extent of bringing the flexed arm downward until it reaches the side, they are nevertheless an important contributor to such extensor actions as bringing an axe downward, the pull of a swimming stroke, or chin-ups. The posterior fibers of the deltoid can draw the arm farther back than can any of the other muscles, making possible such movements as placing the hand into a back pocket. The segmental nerves involved in extension of the arm are all those contributing to the brachial plexus.

Abduction of the arm is brought about (Fig. 5-23) by the simultaneous action of the *deltoid,* especially its middle or more lateral part, and by the *supraspinatus.* With rotation of the humerus, the anterior or posterior parts of the deltoid are brought into a more lateral position so that they abduct more strongly. Abduction in lateral rotation is stronger than it is in medial rotation; because the movement is weakest from medial rotation, weakness of the deltoid is most easily demonstrated by testing abduction from this position. Of the two muscles, the more powerful deltoid can produce full abduction, to about 90 degrees when there is no accompanying scapular rotation; the supraspinatus sometimes can, but more frequently cannot, perform good abduction when the deltoid is paralyzed. Lateral rotation of the humerus always accompanies complete abduction of the arm. Apparently, this is necessary to allow the greater tubercle to slide under, rather than hit against, the acromion. The two abductor muscles are innervated exclusively through C5 and C6, and abduction, like flexion, is easily interfered with by lesions of the upper portion of the brachial plexus.

Adduction of the arm is produced mainly by the *pectoralis major, latissimus dorsi,* and *teres major.* The

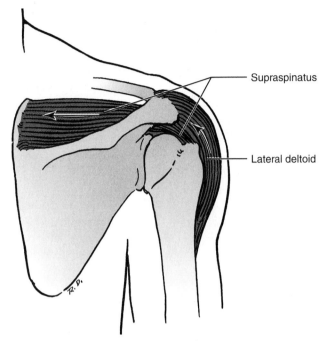

Figure 5-23 Abductors of the arm.

coracobrachialis, and, to a small extent, the *long head of the triceps,* to a small extent, also assist (Fig. 5-24). Furthermore, the *deltoid,* the chief abductor, can also aid in adduction. Because the posterior fibers of the deltoid are lower, they can assist in adduction while the arm is about 45 degrees from the side, but the anterior fibers cannot help until the arm is fairly close to the side, because only then do they lie below the axis of motion at the glenohumeral joint. (It is also possible that the anterior fibers act only when there is simultaneous flexion and that the posterior fibers contract primarily to prevent the pectoralis major and latissimus dorsi from medially rotating or depressing the humerus.) The muscles composing the adductor group are innervated through fibers arising from all elements of the brachial plexus.

Medial rotation is brought about primarily by the *subscapularis* (Figs. 5-25 and 5-26). The *pectoralis major* medially rotates as it adducts; the *latissimus dorsi* medially rotates as it flexes and extends; and the *clavicular fibers of the deltoid* medially rotate as they flex. The *teres major* muscle apparently contracts, although somewhat weakly, for pure medial rotation.

The medial rotators are innervated through all segments contributing to the brachial plexus.

Lateral rotation is carried out by the *infraspinatus* and *teres minor,* and by the *posterior fibers of the deltoid,* if extension and lateral rotation are combined (Fig. 5-27; see Fig. 5-25). These three muscles are innervated through C5 and C6.

BURSAE AND SHOULDER LESIONS

There are numerous bursae located within the shoulder region. Two of the major ones are the *subacromial bursa* (see Fig. 5-14) and the *subdeltoid bursa.* Neither communicates with the joint cavity, but the two may communicate with each other, often together being called simply the *subacromial bursa.* The true subacromial bursa rests on the upper surface of the supraspinatus muscle, intervening between it and the overlying deltoid muscle, acromion process, and coracoacromial ligament. The subdeltoid bursa is positioned more laterally under the deltoid muscle. Any upward movement of the humerus tends to force the head and greater tubercle, with the covering supraspinatus muscle, against the arch of the acromion and coracoacromial ligament. The bursae allow for movements of the proximal end of the humerus beneath overlying structures and are especially important in abduction.

NERVE INJURIES: BRACHIAL PLEXUS

In the section on the brachial plexus, temporary loss of nerve function and injury associated with various types of thoracic outlet syndrome were described. Now that the anatomy and function of the entire shoulder region have been discussed, additional injuries of the brachial plexus can be considered. By understanding the scheme of formation and branching of the plexus (see Fig. 5-7), the innervation of the skin and muscles of the region, and the functions of the muscles and movements produced, it is possible to determine the effect of a lesion of any of the components of the plexus. The plexus is formed by the anterior rami of spinal nerves C5, C6, C7, C8, and T1. The fibers of each anterior ramus become mixed with those of the others as they course through the trunks, divisions, cords,

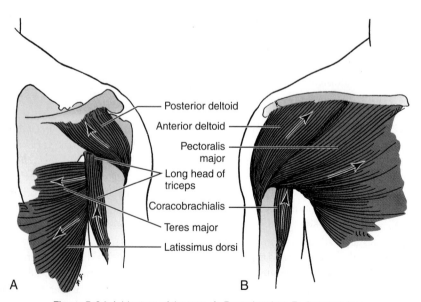

Posterior deltoid
Anterior deltoid
Pectoralis major
Long head of triceps
Coracobrachialis
Teres major
Latissimus dorsi

A   B

Figure 5-24 Adductors of the arm. **A,** Posterior view. **B,** Anterior view.

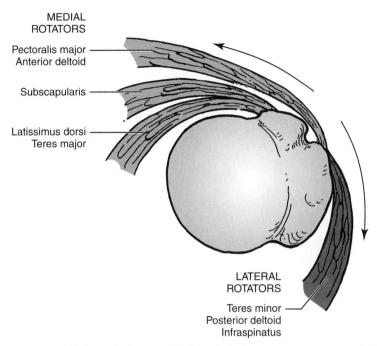

MEDIAL ROTATORS

Pectoralis major
Anterior deltoid

Subscapularis

Latissimus dorsi
Teres major

LATERAL ROTATORS

Teres minor
Posterior deltoid
Infraspinatus

Figure 5-25 Relations of the lateral *(dark shading)* and medial *(light shading)* rotators to the upper end of the humerus. Right arm, superior view.

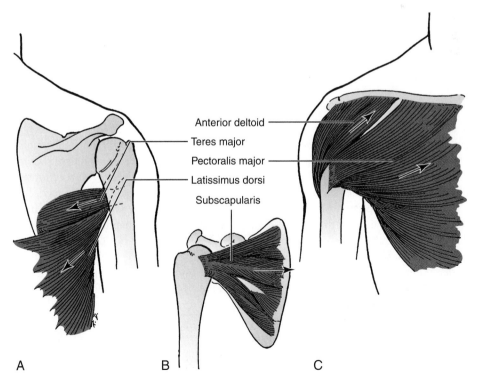

Anterior deltoid
Teres major
Pectoralis major
Latissimus dorsi
Subscapularis

A   B   C

Figure 5-26 The chief medial rotators of the arm. **A,** Posterior view. **B** and **C,** Anterior views.

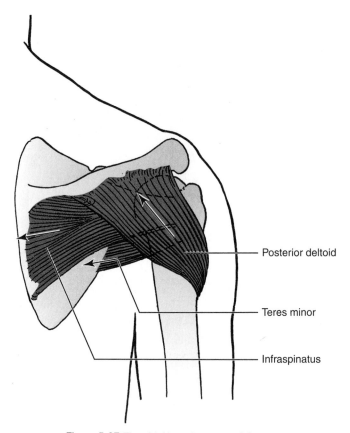

Figure 5-27 The chief lateral rotators of the arm.

- Posterior deltoid
- Teres minor
- Infraspinatus

and branches. An injury to one of the anterior rami entering the brachial plexus would be associated with different deficits than one to a branch formed after mixing of the fibers within the plexus. For instance, a complete lesion of the anterior ramus of C5 would eliminate all C5 fibers entering the plexus, and therefore these fibers would be absent from the trunks, divisions, cords, and any branch of the plexus (e.g., suprascapular, axillary, lateral pectoral) in which they would normally be included. Sensory loss would be noted in the dermatome supplied by this segment of the spinal cord. Motor loss of varying degrees would be evident in any muscle innervated by a nerve containing fibers from C5. In the case of the rhomboids, which are supplied by the dorsal scapular nerve containing fibers exclusively from C5, there would be complete loss of function. Only partial loss (muscle weakness) would be noted in muscles that receive fibers from

both C5 and other spinal cord segments. For example, in the serratus anterior, which receives fibers from C5, C6, and C7 through the long thoracic nerve, such a lesion would paralyze muscle tissue innervated by C5, but the portion of the serratus anterior receiving fibers from C6 and C7 would be unaffected. This discussion of C5 illustrates the idea of *segmental innervation* that was described in Chapter 3.

With a lesion of one of the branches of the plexus, the loss would involve only structures or areas innervated by that particular nerve. If the long thoracic nerve was severed immediately after its formation, all fibers to the serratus anterior would be lost, and the muscle would be unable to function. Such loss would be evident, as mentioned earlier in the chapter, as "winging" of the scapula when the affected individual pushes against resistance. No sensory loss would occur, because the long thoracic nerve provides no

Table 5-7   NERVES OF THE SHOULDER

Nerve	Muscle Name	Segmental Innervation*	Chief Action
Accessory cranial nerve	Sternocleidomastoid Trapezius	Cranial	Lateral flexion and rotation of head Elevation of tip of shoulder
Nerves to levator scapulae	Levator scapulae	C3, C4	Elevation of scapula
Dorsal scapular nerve	Rhomboid major and rhomboid minor	C5	Retraction of scapula
Nerve to subclavius	Subclavius	C5, C6	Depression of clavicle (possibly)
Axillary nerve	Teres minor Deltoid	C5, C6	Lateral rotation of arm Abduction of arm
Upper subscapular nerve	Subscapularis	C5, C6	Medial rotation of arm
Lower subscapular nerve	Subscapularis Teres major	C5, C6	Medial rotation of arm Extension and medial rotation of arm
Suprascapular nerve	Supraspinatus Infraspinatus	C5, C6	Abduction of arm Lateral rotation of arm
Long thoracic nerve	Serratus anterior	C5–C7	Upward rotation of scapula
Lateral pectoral nerve	Upper pectoralis major	C5–C7	Adduction-flexion of arm
Medial pectoral nerve	Lower pectoralis major Pectoralis minor	C8, T1	Adduction-extension of a flexed arm Depression of shoulder
Thoracodorsal nerve	Latissimus dorsi	C6–C8	Extension-adduction of arm

*Muscles innervated by a nerve may or may not receive fibers from all the spinal nerves contributing to the peripheral nerve, but when a nerve is distributed to only one or two muscles, as are those in this table, the segmental innervation of the muscle is the same as the segmental composition of the nerve.

cutaneous innervation. In the case of a lesion to the axillary nerve as it passes around the surgical neck of the humerus, motor innervation to the deltoid and teres minor and sensory innervation to the skin over the lower part of the shoulder and proximal part of the arm (see Figs. 6-5 and 9-6) would be lost. Because the axillary nerve contains fibers from C5 and C6 as indicated in Table 5-7, the dermatomes involved in the sensory loss are those from two spinal cord segments. These examples illustrate *peripheral nerve* innervation (see Chapter 3). Peripheral nerves formed from nerve plexuses (cervical, brachial, lumbar, and sacral) usually (but not always: i.e., the dorsal scapular nerve) contain fibers from more than one spinal cord segment as a result of mixing of fibers within the plexus.

FUNCTIONAL/CLINICAL NOTE 5-13

Obviously, more extensive deficits occur when the lesion involves several components of the brachial plexus. Injury to the upper elements of the plexus (C5 and C6), called *Erb* or *Erb-Duchenne paralysis* or *palsy*, can result when the head and neck are forcefully separated from the shoulder region, such as in a fall on the shoulder or during childbirth, when the baby's head is pulled and the shoulder is not yet free from the birth canal. Such an injury may involve all the muscles acting as flexors, abductors, and lateral rotators, whereas only some of the muscles producing extension, adduction, and medial rotation may be affected. The injured limb hangs by the side with the arm adducted and medially rotated, the forearm extended and pronated, and the hand flexed at the wrist (the "waiter's tip" position).

Injury to the lower components of the brachial plexus (C8 and T1), known as

Klumpke or *Klumpke-Dejerine paralysis* or *palsy,* is a result of exaggerated abduction of the arm, as in grabbing a bar or limb to break a fall. In this type of injury, most of the effect is on the distal part of the upper limb, particularly the hand.

ANALYSES OF ACTIVITIES AND ASSOCIATED MOVEMENTS

In the preceding discussions of movements of the scapula (e.g., upward rotation, protraction) and humerus (e.g., abduction, medial rotation), muscles that produce those specific movements have been noted. Each movement is brought about usually by two or more primary muscles. To produce a coordinated movement, however, these muscles are aided by other muscles. For instance, in abduction of the arm, the primary muscles producing this action are the supraspinatus and deltoid. Abduction, however, requires that the humeral head be held firmly in the glenoid cavity. If this did not occur, the action of the deltoid on the humerus, with the arm by the side, would raise the head of the humerus rather than abduct the limb, and as the arm is abducted, its weight would tend to dislocate the head of the humerus downward. The infraspinatus, the subscapularis, and the teres minor all contract to help retain the head of the humerus in the glenoid cavity. Finally, as has already been pointed out, abduction above the horizontal position always involves an upward rotation of the scapula; therefore, cooperation of the muscles involved in this movement is necessary. Abduction at the glenohumeral joint and rotation of the scapula go on simultaneously in an almost constant ratio (see p. 90), with no more than a little irregularity in the scapulohumeral rhythm at the beginning and end of the movements. In upward rotation of the scapula, the serratus anterior acts with the superior and inferior fibers of the trapezius. The smoothness of the movement is aided especially by the levator scapulae and, to a lesser extent, by the rhomboids. About 10 muscles assist directly in abduction of the arm. A person who has experienced a strained back may recall that even the back muscles indirectly participate during movements of the shoulder.

Activity: *Painting with a Brush.* Analyzing familiar activities can provide an integrated review of the movements occurring at various joints and the muscles involved with those movements. These activities usually involve more than one movement (such as a combination possibly of extension and medial or lateral rotation) and the involvement of numerous muscles. Consider painting a door with a brush, with a side-to-side (horizontal) stroke. Which scapular and humeral movements would take place? Which muscles would be involved? Such an analysis has to take into consideration painting technique, position of the upper limb, stroke width, and so on. The movements and major muscle involvement can be determined by observation and palpation while a person tries the activity. If the brush is held at chest level and moved repetitively from side to side in a wide stroke, movement of both the scapula and humerus will be evident. Scapular movements are not extensive, but with the wide brush stroke, the scapula would be protracted and retracted alternately. As discussed previously, protraction is brought about by the serratus anterior and pectoralis major and minor, whereas retraction is produced by the middle fibers of the trapezius, with possibly some help from the rhomboids and latissimus dorsi.

Humeral movements include flexion of the arm at the glenohumeral joint to position the upper extremity closer to the door to be painted, alternating medial and lateral rotation of the humerus as the brush is moved from side to side, and adduction and abduction to produce a wide stroke. If the arm is held firmly in an adducted position against the side, thus eliminating any abduction, only medial and lateral rotation would be necessary, but the width of the brush stroke would be diminished. Muscles involved in flexing the arm would be the anterior portion to the deltoid, the clavicular part of the pectoralis major, the coracobrachialis, and the biceps brachii. Medial rotation is produced mainly by the subscapularis; the pectoralis major and latissimus dorsi can assist in this movement as they adduct the arm. The infraspinatus and teres minor are the main lateral rotators. Adduction is produced mainly by the pectoralis major, latissimus dorsi, and teres major, whereas abduction is produced by the deltoid and supraspinatus.

Activity: *Throwing a Ball.* Another activity that has components of movement occurring at the glenohumeral joint is that of throwing a ball. Style of throwing, force of the throw, type of ball being thrown, and other details determine the specifics of the activity and the related movements. A complete analysis of throwing a ball would obviously necessitate examination of movements and muscle activity in both upper limbs, as well as in the head and neck, trunk, and both lower limbs. This analysis focuses on the throwing arm and associated glenohumeral joint.

Consider an overhand throw of a baseball. As a starting position, the ball can be held in the palm of a supinated hand, with the forearm flexed at the elbow and the arm slightly abducted. The action is initiated by extension of the arm at the glenohumeral joint, combined with abduction and lateral rotation of the arm. Once the arm is fully extended and abducted to the appropriate level, flexion at the glenohumeral joint is initiated and is accompanied by adduction and medial rotation. The ball is then released at the desired time, and the upper limb returns to an adducted position at the side of the body.

The first movements noted for throwing a ball overhand were extension, abduction, and lateral rotation of the arm, all of which occur, for the most part, together rather than consecutively (e.g., rather than having extension completed before abduction is initiated). Extension of the arm is produced primarily by the posterior fibers of the deltoid and the latissimus dorsi, with assistance from the long head of the triceps and the teres major. The pectoralis major, as mentioned previously, can assist in extension but only when the arm is in a flexed position. It can produce extension only to a position where the arm is by the side. The deltoid and supraspinatus are the primary abductors of the arm. The deltoid becomes a stronger abductor as the arm is rotated laterally by the infraspinatus and teres minor. The posterior fibers of the deltoid can assist in lateral rotation while also producing extension of the arm. Abduction past the horizontal position is possible only with upward rotation of the glenoid cavity, which is produced by the serratus anterior and trapezius.

The subsequent flexion of the arm at the glenohumeral joint is produced by the deltoid, pectoralis major, and coracobrachialis muscles. The accompanying medial rotation of the arm is brought about by the subscapularis, with assistance from the pectoralis major and deltoid as they produce flexion. The pectoralis major, latissimus dorsi, and teres major are the primary muscles involved in adduction.

Activity: *Removing a Wallet from a Back Pocket.* If movements of the entire upper limb are considered in the activity of removing a wallet

Continued

from a back pocket, it is apparent that all of the joints of the limb are involved and that the activity is really quite complex. Movements and actions discussed here include only those associated with the glenohumeral joint. It would be helpful for the reader to consider the other joints and muscles in the upper limb that are involved in this and the preceding activities as the forearm and hand are studied in subsequent chapters.

With the upper limb by the side, the initial movements at the glenohumeral joint would be extension, abduction, and medial rotation. These movements enable the flexing forearm (with the hand) to clear the side of the body. The medially rotating humerus places the forearm and hand posterior to the back. With the hand above the back pocket, extension at the elbow enables the hand to be lowered into the pocket. This is accompanied by adduction of the arm. With the wallet grasped between the fingers and thumb, the forearm is flexed at the elbow and the arm is abducted. For the wallet to be brought forward, the arm is then laterally rotated, flexed, and adducted.

In summary, the movements occurring at the glenohumeral joint while a person removes a wallet from the back pocket are (1) extension, abduction, and medial rotation; (2) adduction; (3) abduction; and (4) lateral rotation, flexion, and adduction. Extension of the arm results from contraction of the posterior fibers of the deltoid and the latissimus dorsi. (The triceps brachii also extends the arm, but this is not discussed in this chapter.) The pectoralis major is involved with extension only if the arm is in a flexed position; however, with this activity, the arm starts at a nonflexed position at the side. Abduction is brought about by the deltoid and supraspinatus; in this case, because the humerus does not have to be abducted above a horizontal position, no upward rotation of the humerus is necessary. The subscapularis would be the main muscle involved

in medial rotation with the arm in an abducted and extended position; the pectoralis major would assist in medial rotation as it is adducting the arm. The pectoralis major is assisted in adduction by the latissimus dorsi. Lateral rotation would be produced by contraction of the infraspinatus, teres minor, and posterior fibers of the deltoid. Flexion of the arm is carried out by the anterior fibers of the deltoid; because the arm is extended, the pectoralis muscle can effectively help with flexion until the arm reaches the side. The coracobrachialis can also assist in flexion. The biceps brachii, discussed in Chapter 6, can also produce flexion of the arm at the glenohumeral joint.

Considering variations in the activities just described (e.g., painting with a vertical stroke, throwing underhand, or removing a cell phone from a front pocket) or other activities, as well as observing and analyzing the movements of other people, is helpful in understanding the functional anatomy of the body. Such analysis demonstrates the complexity of the action and coordination involved in what might be considered a simple movement or activity.

Nerve supply to the muscles must be intact for normal function to occur. Any interruption of this innervation can limit or eliminate normal muscle activity, depending on the severity of the lesion. Considering an injury to a specific nerve and the effect it could have on a particular movement or activity can provide insight into clinical deficits and the problems that could arise in an individual's occupational or home-related activities. For instance, in the activities just discussed, injury to the suprascapular nerve would affect the function of both the supraspinatus and infraspinatus muscles. The supraspinatus is involved with abduction of the arm, while the infraspinatus produces lateral rotation. Therefore, these actions would be affected in some way, depending on the severity of the injury.

REVIEW QUESTIONS

1 Describe the acromioclavicular joint. Include in the description information on the ligaments present at the joint, the type of movement each ligament resists, and the sensory innervation of the joint.

2 What are the origin, insertion, action, and motor innervation of the pectoralis major muscle? What is the segmental (spinal cord level) innervation to this muscle?

3 Which muscles form the rotator cuff? What is the position of each at the glenohumeral joint?

4 The musculocutaneous nerve can receive fibers from which spinal cord segments? What are the terminal branches of the posterior cord of the brachial plexus? Which artery courses with the axillary nerve as it passes to the posterior aspect of the shoulder? A lesion of the suprascapular nerve could result in loss of motor function of which muscle or muscles? What function or functions would be weakened with such a lesion?

5 A carpenter complains of being unable to hold the upper limb above head level to pound a nail. To do so, the carpenter has used the opposite hand to support the limb at the elbow. A physical examination reveals atrophy in the muscle mass that covers the most lateral part of the shoulder and upper lateral surface of the humerus. Which muscle is probably affected? How could the functional integrity of the muscle be tested? If a nerve lesion is suspected, which nerve is involved? What sensory loss would be associated with the lesion?

6 Starting in the anatomical position, discuss the sequence of movements in the shoulder region and the muscles involved in the following activities:
a opening the clasp of a necklace
b removing a pencil from a front pants pocket
c raising a hand in class to answer a question

7 Which of the following is not a place of origin for muscle fibers of the deltoid?
a acromion
b spine of the scapula
c coracoid process
d lateral third of the clavicle

EXERCISES

1 Demonstrate the following movements:
a depression of the scapula
b retraction of the scapula
c flexion of the arm at the glenohumeral joint
d adduction of the arm
e medial rotation of the arm

2 Draw anterior and posterior views of the scapula (artistic ability is not important), labeling the major bony features, borders, and angles. On these drawings, indicate the areas of origin and insertion of muscles of the shoulder region.

3 Diagram the brachial plexus, showing the anterior rami that contribute to the plexus, pattern of fiber mixing, and formation of the branches. (Ability to remember the pattern of the plexus enhances the understanding of the innervation of the upper limb.)

4 Demonstrate by palpation:
a position of the acromion and scapular spine
b extent of the deltoid muscle
c location of the greater tubercle
d clavicular and sternal heads of the sternoclavicular muscle

6 THE ARM

CHAPTER CONTENTS

General Considerations

Bones and Joints

Fascia and Superficial Nerves and Vessels

Muscles

Nerves and Vessels

Movements at the Elbow Joint

Analyses of Activities and Associated Movements

GENERAL CONSIDERATIONS

Movements between the arm and forearm are of two types: *flexion-extension* and *pronation-supination*. The actions of flexion and extension can each be described in several ways. *Flexion,* the bending of the elbow to produce a decreased angle between the arm and forearm, can be described as *flexion of the forearm, flexion of the forearm at the elbow,* or *flexion of the elbow.* The first two descriptions are those used in this text primarily to describe joint movement and muscle action, indicating movement of the part distal to the joint. The opposite action, *extension of the forearm* or *extension of the forearm at the elbow,* increases the angle between forearm and arm. Pronation and supination are most easily described in reference to a flexed forearm held anteriorly in a horizontal position, although they actually may occur in any position of the forearm. *Pronation* is the movement of turning the palm of the hand down (causing the radius to cross over the ulna). *Supination* is the movement of turning the palm up (returning the radius to its normal position).

The **muscles** in the arm are few in number and are clearly divided into *anterior (flexor)* and *posterior (extensor)* muscle masses. The chief action of both groups is at the elbow, but some of the muscles also have some action at the glenohumeral joint.

The **nerves** to the muscles of the arm pass through the axilla with the axillary artery. Neither the median nor the ulnar nerve, the larger components from the anterior portion of the brachial plexus, provides any innervation to the muscles of the arm; they supply muscles of the forearm and hand only. The muscles of the anterior surface of the arm are supplied by the *musculocutaneous nerve* from the lateral cord of the brachial plexus (see Fig. 6-12). The *radial nerve,* from the posterior cord of the plexus, supplies the posterior musculature of the arm (see Fig. 9-6).

The **arteries** supplying blood to the muscles of the arm are predominantly *branches of the brachial artery,* the continuation of the axillary artery into the arm. These are supplemented by *branches of the axillary artery* that descend across the glenohumeral joint and by small *branches of the radial, ulnar, and interosseous arteries* in the forearm that ascend across the elbow joint.

BONES AND JOINTS
Bones

Just as the pectoral (shoulder) girdle and the proximal end of the humerus had to be studied for an understanding of the shoulder muscles, so must the humerus (Fig. 6-1) and the proximal ends of the radius and ulna, the two bones of the forearm, be studied for an understanding of the arm muscles.

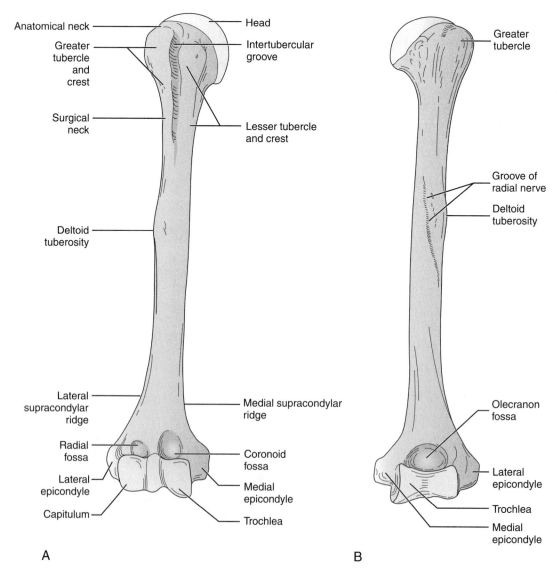

Figure 6-1 Anterior **(A)** and posterior **(B)** views of the humerus.

Humerus

On the shaft (body) of the **humerus,** only two prominent features are evident. Laterally, the *deltoid tuberosity* marks the insertion of the deltoid muscle, and posteriorly, the *groove of the radial nerve* (radial groove or sulcus) indicates the course of the radial nerve. The distal end of the humerus expands laterally and medially and at the same time becomes flattened anteroposteriorly. The sharp medial and lateral borders, or *supracondylar ridges,* give origin to some of the muscles of the forearm and end below in more rounded but prominent *medial* and *lateral epicondyles,* which are also projections for the attachment of forearm muscles. On the posteroinferior surface of the medial epicondyle is the *groove for the ulnar nerve.* The distal end of the humerus has two articular surfaces, a lateral *capitulum* for articulation with the head of the radius and a medial *trochlea* (pulley) for articulation with the ulna. Above the rounded trochlea anteriorly is the *coronoid fossa,* which receives the coronoid process of the ulna when the forearm is flexed. Posteriorly, the *olecranon fossa* receives the olecranon (the backward-projecting portion, or proximal end, of the ulna) when the forearm is extended. On occasion, the bone is completely deficient between these two fossae, and a hole appears at this place in the bone, which during life is bridged by a membrane. The concavity on the anterior surface of the humerus above the capitulum is the *radial fossa,* which receives the head of the radius when the forearm is flexed.

Ulna

The **ulna** is the more medial of the two forearm bones (Figs. 6-2 and 6-3; see also Fig. 7-2). Its proximal end, the *olecranon,* is subcutaneous, as is much of the ulna throughout its length. On the anterior surface of the ulna is the deep *trochlear notch* (incisure) for articulation with the trochlea of the humerus. The articular surface of the notch is shared by, and limited inferiorly by, the projecting *coronoid process.* On the lateral side of the coronoid process, there is a second articular surface, the *radial notch,* which receives the head of the radius. Below the coronoid process is the *ulnar tuberosity,* marking the insertion of the brachialis muscle. Distal to this, the ulna narrows to become more rounded and, finally, even triangular in cross-section in the middle of its shaft.

Radius

The proximal end of the **radius** is an expanded disc-like *head,* smooth not only on its proximal end but also on its edges. The proximal end is slightly concave and fits against the capitulum of the humerus. The circumferential part of the articular surface is in contact with the radial notch on the ulna and with a ligament (annular ligament) that holds it against this notch. The proximal end of the radius has a slightly constricted *neck* and a rather well-marked *radial tuberosity* for the insertion of the biceps brachii. Beyond this point, the radius, like the ulna, becomes rounded and then approximately triangular in cross-section.

Joints

Elbow joint

There are three joints present at what is referred to as "the" elbow joint: *humeroulnar, humeroradial,* and *proximal radioulnar.* The humeroulnar and humeroradial joints are associated with the movements of flexion and extension of the forearm at the elbow, whereas the proximal radioulnar joint works in conjunction with the distal radioulnar joint to permit pronation and supination. A single articular capsule surrounds the three joints at the elbow, and a single joint cavity is present. The *humeroulnar joint* is formed by the articulation of the trochlea of the humerus and the trochlear notch of the ulna; the *humeroradial joint* is the articulation between the capitulum of the humerus and the concave depression on the head of the radius. The *proximal radioulnar joint* is the articulation of the outer surface of the head of the radius with the radial notch of the ulna. *Sensory innervation to the joints can be provided by any of the nerves passing across the elbow (musculocutaneous, radial, median, and ulnar), but the majority of the branches are supplied by the musculocutaneous and radial nerves.*

Humeroulnar and humeroradial joints

The strength of the **humeroulnar** and **humeroradial joints,** which act as a single joint in *flexion and extension,* depends primarily on the muscles, especially the brachialis and triceps, that cross it and on the shape of the articular surfaces of the humerus and ulna. The articulation is essentially a *hinge joint.*

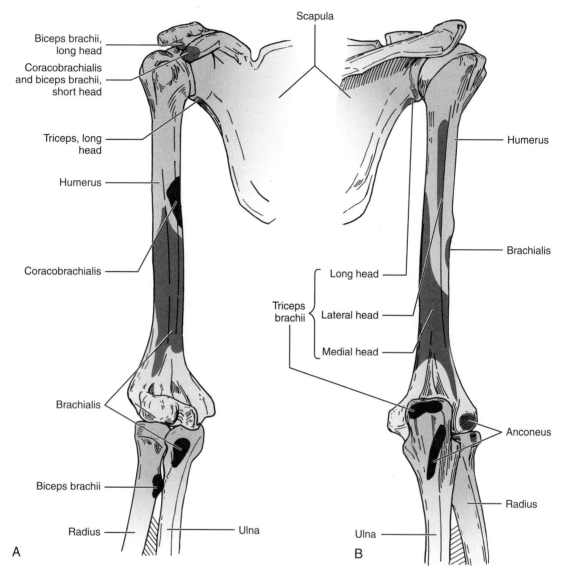

Figure 6-2 Osteological diagram of the arm and elbow region. Anterior **(A)** and posterior **(B)** views illustrating origins of muscles *(color)* and insertions of muscles *(black)*.

FUNCTIONAL/CLINICAL NOTE 6-1

Because of the shape of the trochlea, the extended forearm angles laterally and is not brought into a straight line with the humerus. This lateral deviation of the forearm at the elbow, termed the *carrying angle*, can be observed with the upper extremity held in the anatomical position. This angle is usually greater in women. The carrying angle in theory could help to keep an item being carried, such as a bucket, away from the side of the body. Usually, however, the hand is at least partially pronated, which diminishes the angle, and the arm must be abducted at the shoulder to position the bucket further laterally.

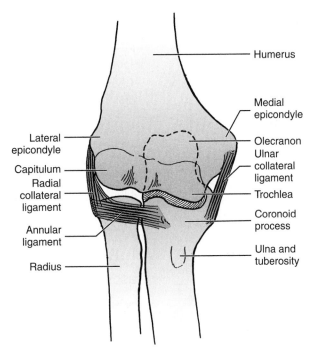

Figure 6-3 Anterior view of right elbow joint. The capsule is not shown. Note that the ulna with its posteriorly projecting olecranon forms a hinge joint with the humerus, and the head of the radius is free to rotate within the annular ligament.

The joint capsule at the elbow joint is thin, lax, and rather redundant, allowing free movement. Anteriorly and posteriorly, muscles rather than ligaments protect the capsule, but medially and laterally, special ligaments are present (Fig. 6-4; see Fig. 6-3). The *ulnar collateral ligament* arises from the medial epicondyle and fans out to insert on the coronoid process and the olecranon (see Fig. 6-4, *A*). It consists of thickened *anterior and posterior bands,* a *transverse band* that forms the lower part of the ligament (stretching from the olecranon to the coronoid process), and a thinner central part that is bounded by the other components of the ligament. The *radial collateral ligament* arises from the lateral epicondyle (see Fig. 6-4, *B*). It fans out less than does the ulnar collateral ligament and attaches mostly into the annular ligament (a strong attachment to the radius would interfere with pronation and supination).

Proximal radioulnar joint

The **proximal radioulnar joint** is one allowing rotation of the head of the radius to produce the movements of pronation and supination. The important ligament of this joint, the *annular ligament* of the radius, is attached at both ends to the coronoid process and forms about four fifths of a circle, the remaining fifth of the articular surface being provided by the radial notch of the ulna. Because the synovial membrane of the elbow joint extends downward around the neck of the radius deep to the annular ligament, the radius can rotate freely within this circle. Although a purely ringlike ligament, such as that implied by the term *annular ligament,* would allow this movement, it would offer no resistance against distal displacement of the head of the radius. Such displacement is prevented, or at least limited, by the shape of the annular ligament, which resembles a portion of a tapered cup with the bottom broken out of it more than it does a ring. The head of the radius fits within the expanded lips of the cup, with the neck of the radius being grasped by the narrowed bottom of the cup. The cup is held firmly in place through the ligament's attachment to the ulna medially and through its attachment into the radial collateral ligament laterally. A muscle of the forearm, the supinator muscle, arises partly from the annular ligament.

One other aspect of the mechanism of the radioulnar joint is important: If the radius is to move

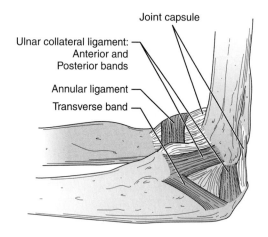

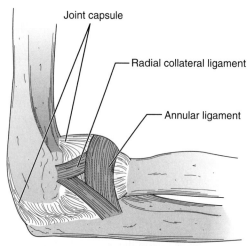

Figure 6-4 Medial **(A)** and lateral **(B)** views of the ligaments of the elbow joint. The ulnar collateral ligament **(A)** consists of thickened anterior and posterior bands, a transverse band, and a less pronounced central part *(lighter color)*.

in pronation and supination, it must be free to move about the ulna at its distal end also. There is a distal radioulnar joint cavity, located at the wrist, intervening between the distal ends of the radius and ulna. Between the two radioulnar joints, the radius and ulna are united by a flexible *interosseous membrane.* Both radioulnar joints are of the *trochoid,* or *pivot,* type.

Surface Anatomy

In examining the surface anatomy of the arm, it is necessary to consider the palpable landmarks not only of the humerus but also of the scapula and proximal region of the radius and ulna. The scapula and

proximal part of the humerus are described in Chapter 5. At the distal end of the **humerus,** the *medial* and *lateral epicondyles* and, to some extent, the corresponding *supracondylar ridges* can be palpated. The medial epicondyle is more prominent than the lateral one. At the proximal end of the **ulna,** on the posterior surface of the elbow joint, the *olecranon* can be felt just beneath the skin, and the *shaft of the ulna* can be followed distally. Laterally, on the proximal end of the **radius,** the *head of the radius* is palpable and can be rotated beneath a finger in the movements of supination and pronation.

FASCIA AND SUPERFICIAL NERVES AND VESSELS

Fascia

The **superficial fascia** (subcutaneous tissue) of the arm contains a variable amount of fat, and the superficial nerves and vessels lie within it. Deep to this, enclosing the muscles of the arm, is a tough membranous layer of fascia, the **brachial fascia** or **deep fascia** of the arm. This fascia forms a complete sheath around the arm and is penetrated by many of the superficial nerves and vessels. Anteriorly, it is loose fitting in order to allow for contraction of the muscles. Posteriorly, it is fused to the underlying muscle. The brachial fascia passes between the anterior and posterior muscle groups, most notably on the distal part of the arm, to attach to the humerus. In this manner, it forms the *medial* and *lateral intermuscular septa.*

Nerves

Numerous nerves contribute to the cutaneous innervation of the skin of the arm (Fig. 6-5). Laterally, innervation is provided by the **superior lateral cutaneous nerve of the arm** (a branch of the axillary nerve) and the **inferior lateral cutaneous nerve of the arm** (a branch of the radial nerve). Medially, skin of the proximal region of the arm is supplied by the **intercostobrachial nerve** from the second, or second and third, intercostal nerves. Much of the middle and distal areas is innervated by the **medial cutaneous nerve of the arm,** a branch directly off the medial cord of the brachial plexus. The intercostobrachial and medial cutaneous nerves of the arm usually communicate or join as they innervate the arm. Cutaneous innervation of the posterior region of the arm is provided by the **posterior cutaneous nerve of the arm,** a branch of the radial nerve. Nerves that continue into the forearm supply a variable amount of sensory innervation to the arm. The **medial cutaneous nerve of the forearm** from the medial cord perforates the brachial fascia with the basilic vein in the distal part of the arm. It supplies innervation to the skin not only on the medial side of the

arm at the elbow joint but also on the anterior surface. The **lateral cutaneous nerve of the forearm** (the continuation of the musculocutaneous nerve) penetrates the brachial fascia, passes anterior to the elbow joint just lateral to the tendon of the biceps brachii muscle, and innervates the overlying skin. Finally, the smallest of the cutaneous nerves of the arm, the **posterior cutaneous nerve of the forearm** from the radial nerve, emerges posterolaterally in the lower third of the arm to supply innervation to the skin of the region.

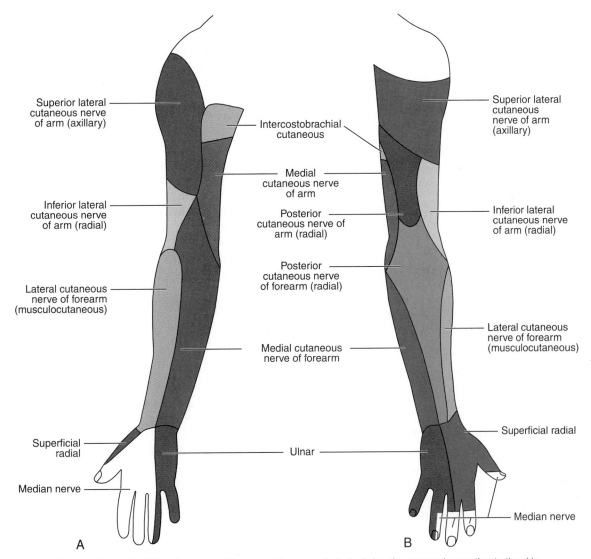

Figure 6-5 Anterior **(A)** and posterior **(B)** views of the upper limb depicting the sensory innervation to the skin.

Vessels

There are two main superficial veins in the arm (see Fig. 4-3). The **cephalic vein** lies in the superficial fascia of the forearm and arm. In the distal part of the arm, it lies along the anterolateral surface of the biceps muscle and is frequently visible through the skin. In the proximal part of the arm, the cephalic vein passes between the deltoid and pectoralis major muscles to empty into the axillary vein. The **basilic vein** also lies superficially in the forearm and the medial side of the distal part of the arm. On the anterior surface of the elbow (cubital fossa), there is usually a prominent communication, the **median cubital vein,** from the cephalic to the basilic vein. The prominence and accessibility of the superficial veins anterior to the elbow make them particularly convenient vessels for venipuncture (withdrawing blood). At about the junction of the middle and distal thirds of the arm, the basilic vein passes deep to the brachial fascia and courses proximally. As it enters the axilla, it becomes the axillary vein, which receives the deep veins and the cephalic vein.

MUSCLES

The musculature of the arm consists, anteriorly, of the biceps brachii, coracobrachialis, and brachialis (Fig. 6-6); posteriorly, it consists of the triceps brachii with its associated anconeus muscle (Fig. 6-7).

Muscles of the Anterior Arm

Biceps brachii

The **biceps brachii** has two heads, as its name implies. The *origin* of the *short head* is from the tip of the coracoid process of the scapula in common with the coracobrachialis muscle. The *origin* of the *long head* is from the supraglenoid tubercle of the scapula and traverses the cavity of the glenohumeral joint to run in the intertubercular groove between the greater and lesser tubercles. An intertubercular synovial sheath, which is continuous with the synovial lining of the glenohumeral joint, follows it downward in the intertubercular groove. The two heads unite in the distal part of the arm and form a strong tendon that passes across the front of the elbow joint to an *insertion* on the prominent radial tuberosity on the proximal end of the radius. As the tendon passes

distally, it gives off a strong expansion, the *bicipital aponeurosis*, which blends with the fascia over the flexor muscles of the forearm and passes with this fascia to the ulna. Because the tuberosity on the radius is somewhat on the ulnar surface of this bone, the *action* of the biceps is not only to produce flexion at the elbow but also to rotate the radius so as to produce supination. Both heads of the biceps are situated so as to be able to flex the arm at the glenohumeral joint, and when the humerus is laterally rotated, the long head is in a position to help in abduction. The biceps brachii is usually involved only in abduction, however, if the deltoid is paralyzed. The *innervation* of the biceps brachii is provided by the musculocutaneous nerve (Table 6-1).

Coracobrachialis and brachialis

The **coracobrachialis** has its *origin* from the coracoid process with the short head of the biceps brachii, and its *insertion* is on the anteromedial surface of the middle of the humerus. The *action* of the coracobrachialis is to flex and adduct the arm. Because it does not cross the elbow, it cannot produce movement of the forearm. The musculocutaneous nerve leaves the axilla by running through the muscle. The *origin* of the **brachialis** is from much of the lower half of the anterior surface of the humerus and from both intermuscular septa between it and the triceps. The muscle covers the front of the elbow joint, and its *insertion* is on the ulnar tuberosity just distal to the coronoid process. The *action* of the brachialis is to flex the forearm.

FUNCTIONAL/CLINICAL NOTE 6-2

When doing chin-ups (pull-ups), the most effective flexion (which would involve both the biceps and brachialis) is obtained when the forearm is supinated, the bar being grasped with the palms toward the body. If the forearm is fixed in pronation, the effectiveness of the biceps brachii is reduced by the vain attempt to supinate as it flexes. The brachialis, however, is an equally effective flexor whether the forearm is pronated or supinated, inasmuch as it inserts on the ulna.

The coracobrachialis, brachialis, and biceps brachii (see previous section)—that is, all the anterior muscles in the arm—receive *innervation* from the

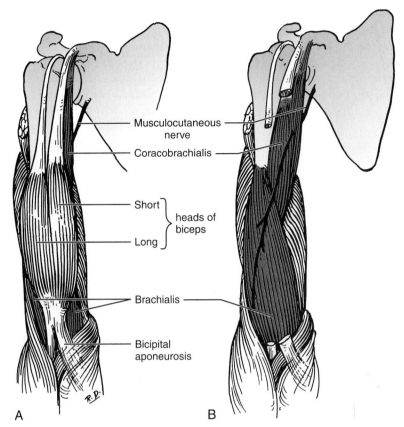

Musculocutaneous nerve

Coracobrachialis

Short ⎤
          ⎬ heads of biceps
Long ⎦

Brachialis

Bicipital aponeurosis

A   B

Figure 6-6 Anterior muscles of the right arm. **A** and **B**, The insertion of the deltoid, parts of the medial and lateral heads of the triceps, and the origins of some of the forearm muscles are also seen. **B,** The biceps is omitted to better demonstrate the brachialis.

musculocutaneous nerve (see Fig. 6-12). Before the nerve leaves the axilla by running through the cora-cobrachialis, it supplies this muscle. Because it lies between the biceps and the brachialis, it supplies innervation to both of these. The musculocutaneous nerve contains fibers from spinal nerves C5, C6, and C7. The lateral part of the brachialis often receives a branch from the radial nerve, although the functional importance of this is not clear. This branch helps supply the elbow joint and may provide only sensory fibers to the brachialis (Table 6-2).

Muscles of the Posterior Arm

Triceps brachii and anconeus
Of the three heads of the **triceps brachii** muscle (see Fig. 6-7), the *origin* of the *long head* is from the infra-glenoid tubercle on the lateral border of the scapula just inferior to the glenoid cavity. It passes distally in front of the teres minor but behind the teres major (see Fig. 5-10). The *origin* of the *lateral head* is from the humerus above and lateral to the groove of the ra-dial nerve and from the lateral intermuscular septum. It unites with the long head to form the superficial tendinous part of the insertion of the muscle. The *origin* of the *medial head* is also from the humerus but medial to and below the spiraling groove of the radial nerve. It comes to cover the entire posterior surface of the distal part of the bone, where it also arises from both intermuscular septa. It attaches into the deep surface of the combined lateral and long heads. The radial nerve and the deep brachial artery pass between the long head and the humerus and then pass posteriorly around the humerus between the origins of the lateral and medial heads. They lie approximately in the groove of the radial nerve but usually

on the uppermost fibers of the medial head rather than directly against the bone. All three heads of the triceps have an *insertion* together on the proximal end of the olecranon. The chief *action* of the triceps brachii is to extend the forearm at the elbow. Because the long head of the triceps, but not the other two heads, crosses the glenohumeral joint, the long head also aids in extension and adduction of the arm.

The **anconeus** is a small, triangular muscle that has its *origin* from the lateral epicondyle and its *insertion* on the lateral side of the olecranon and adjacent part of the ulna. Although it is too small to supply much power, its *action* is not only to extend the forearm at the elbow but also to act to stabilize the elbow joint against flexion or pronation-supination. The triceps brachii receives *innervation* from the radial nerve, which passes posteriorly under cover of this muscle to reach the lateral side of the arm. A branch of the nerve to the medial head of the muscle is continued downward to innervate the anconeus (Table 6-3).

Surface Anatomy

Of the anterior muscles of the arm, the one most easily demonstrated is the **biceps brachii.** With the forearm supinated and flexed at the elbow, the tendon of insertion of this muscle can be palpated anterior to the elbow joint. Along the medial edge of the tendon, the *bicipital aponeurosis* can be felt as it blends with the fascia of the forearm. The two heads of origin of the muscle are not easily separable, but the *short head* and the **coracobrachialis muscle** can be identified in the lower part of the axilla, where they lie posterior to the insertion of the pectoralis major. They can be distinguished from each other because the more anterior, rounded tendon of the biceps brachii is prominent in forcible flexion of the elbow, whereas the broader and posteriorly lying coracobrachialis is particularly prominent when the arm is adducted against resistance. The fact that the biceps brachii contracts strongly for combined flexion and supination of the forearm, but little or not at all for either movement alone unless it is resisted, can be demonstrated by attempting these movements. The

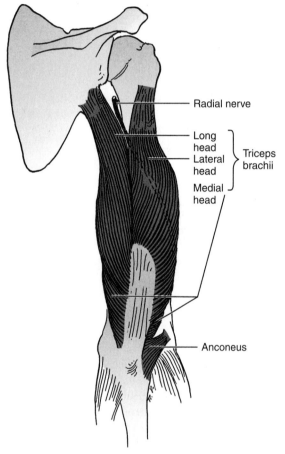

Radial nerve

Long head
Lateral head } Triceps brachii
Medial head

Anconeus

Figure 6-7 Posterior muscles of the right arm.

Table 6-1	BICEPS BRACHII			
Muscle	**Origin (Proximal Attachment)**	**Insertion (Distal Attachment)**	**Action**	**Innervation**
Biceps brachii	Short head: tip of coracoid process of scapula Long head: supraglenoid tubercle of scapula	Radial tuberosity and bicipital aponeurosis into fascia of forearm	Flexion and supination of forearm; flexion of arm	Musculocutaneous nerve

Table 6-2	CORACOBRACHIALIS AND BRACHIALIS			
Muscle	**Origin (Proximal Attachment)**	**Insertion (Distal Attachment)**	**Action**	**Innervation**
Coracobrachialis	Coracoid process of scapula	Anteromedial surface of midshaft of humerus	Flexion and adduction of arm	Musculocutaneous nerve
Brachialis	Lower half of anterior surface of humerus; intermuscular septa	Ulnar tuberosity	Flexion of forearm	Musculocutaneous nerve (lateral side may receive twig from radial nerve)

Table 6-3	TRICEPS BRACHII AND ANCONEUS			
Muscle	**Origin (Proximal Attachment)**	**Insertion (Distal Attachment)**	**Action**	**Innervation**
Triceps brachii	Long head: infraglenoid tubercle of scapula Lateral head: posterior surface of humerus above and lateral to groove of radial nerve and lateral intermuscular septum Medial head: posterior surface of humerus below and medial to groove of radial nerve and both intermuscular septa	Proximal end of olecranon of ulna	Extension of forearm; extension of arm (long head)	Radial nerve
Anconeus	Lateral epicondyle of humerus	Lateral side of olecranon of ulna	Extension of forearm; stabilize elbow joint against flexion or pronation-supination	Radial nerve

brachialis is somewhat more difficult to palpate. It is perhaps most easily recognized by palpating on the medial side of the tendon of insertion of the biceps brachii while the supinated forearm is being flexed against resistance. The **triceps brachii** can be identified when the forearm is extended against opposition, and its long head can be felt in the axilla when the arm is adducted. The anconeus is not identifiable.

NERVES AND VESSELS

Nerves

Of the four main nerves traversing the arm—median, ulnar, musculocutaneous, and radial (Fig. 6-8)—the first two give off no branches to the muscles of the arm. After their origins from the brachial plexus, these two nerves run down the medial side of the arm. The **median nerve** is at first anterolateral to, but later is medial to, the brachial artery, and the **ulnar nerve** is posterior to the brachial artery. Just above the elbow, the median nerve lies on the anterior surface of the brachialis muscle and passes with the brachial artery anterior to the elbow joint. The ulnar nerve passes down the arm posterior to the median nerve and brachial artery. It gradually diverges posteriorly, penetrates the medial intermuscular septum, and runs on the medial head of the triceps to pass posterior to the medial epicondyle.

Musculocutaneous nerve

The **musculocutaneous nerve** (see Fig. 6-8) arises from the lateral cord of the brachial plexus (C5 to C7) and passes through the substance of the coracobrachialis muscle to lie between the biceps brachii and brachialis. Just before or as it penetrates

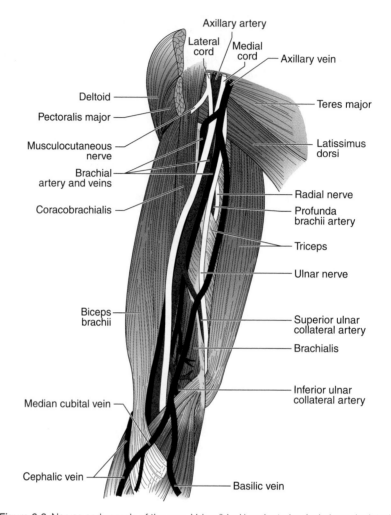

Figure 6-8 Nerves and vessels of the arm. Veins *(black)* and arteries *(color)* are depicted.

the coracobrachialis, it supplies this muscle and then gives off branches to both heads of the biceps brachii and to the brachialis. The musculocutaneous nerve continues as the *lateral cutaneous nerve of the forearm,* which passes lateral to the biceps tendon, penetrates the brachial fascia, and supplies innervation to the skin of the forearm.

Radial nerve

The **radial nerve** (see Fig. 9-6), the continuation of the posterior cord, leaves the axilla by passing posteriorly in a wide spiral course around the humerus. It first lies between the long head of the triceps brachii

and the humerus and then approximately in the groove of the radial nerve on the posterior surface of the humerus, between the origins of the lateral and medial heads of the triceps brachii (Fig. 6-9). It is accompanied in this course by the profunda brachii artery (deep artery of the arm; deep brachial artery) and veins. Emerging on the lateral side of the humerus, the radial nerve lies first between the triceps brachii and brachialis and then passes anterior to the extensor forearm group to lie between the brachioradialis and brachialis, in which position it passes into the forearm (see Fig. 9-4). Although the radial nerve is on the medial side of the arm, it usually gives off a branch to the long head of the triceps and a second branch that descends parallel to the ulnar nerve to reach the medial head of this muscle. In its course deep to the triceps brachii, it gives additional branches to all three heads of this muscle, and in the distal part of the arm, it may give a twig into the brachialis.

The radial nerve supplies the triceps brachii (and anconeus) with fibers derived primarily from spinal nerves C6, C7, and C8.

FUNCTIONAL/CLINICAL NOTE 6-3

Although injury to the radial nerve may abolish all active extension at the elbow, some of the branches to the triceps brachii usually arise before the nerve leaves the axilla. Injury to the nerve as it lies in the groove of the radial nerve affects primarily extension of the wrist and fingers, actions produced mainly by muscles of the forearm.

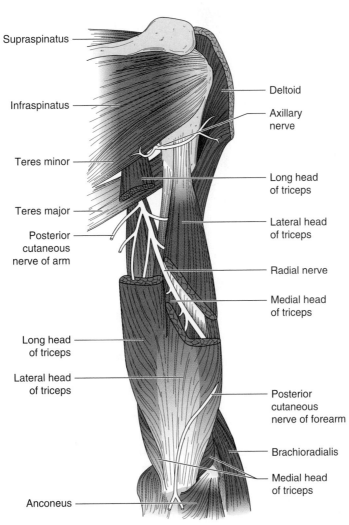

Figure 6-9 Posterior view of the arm, illustrating the course of the radial nerve.

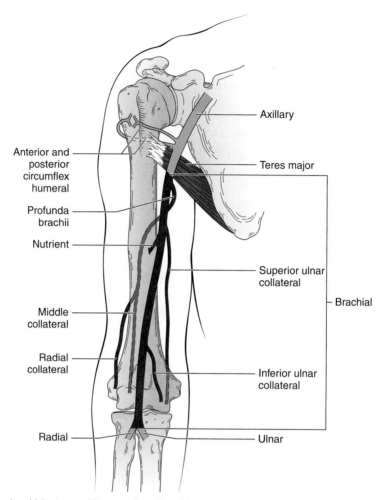

Figure 6-10 The brachial artery and its major branches. Muscular branches have not been included on the illustration.

Vessels

Brachial artery

The **brachial artery** (see Fig. 6-8), the continuation of the axillary artery, passes distally on the medial side of the arm and then runs with the median nerve in front of the elbow, lying on the brachialis muscle. It gives off branches to the muscles of the arm, including the *profunda brachii artery*, which accompanies the radial nerve in its posterior course around the humerus. Other branches (Fig. 6-10) include a *nutrient artery* to the humerus; the *superior ulnar collateral artery*, which passes posterior to the medial epicondyle along with the ulnar nerve; and the *inferior ulnar collateral artery*, which courses anterior to the medial epicondyle. The latter two branches, along with terminal branches of the profunda brachii artery (the *radial collateral artery*, which accompanies the radial nerve anteriorly across the lateral side of the elbow, and the *middle collateral artery*, which is found posterior to the lateral epicondyle), form anastomoses around the elbow with branches of arteries of the forearm (see Chapter 8 and Fig. 8-8). On occasion, the brachial artery is doubled during part or its entire course in the arm. When this occurs, one of the vessels usually lies superficial to the median nerve and is known as a *superficial brachial artery*.

Veins

The brachial artery is accompanied by two **brachial veins,** which frequently blend into one for a part of their course. The brachial veins join the axillary vein, which is a continuation of the basilic vein. In addition to the deep veins, there are two important superficial veins, the **cephalic vein** and the **basilic vein,** described previously in this chapter.

Surface Anatomy

Of the nerves and vessels of the arm, only a few can be observed or palpated. Parts of the **cephalic and basilic veins** are usually identifiable, particularly anterior to the elbow, where the **median cubital vein** can often be seen connecting them. They become more apparent when their flow is temporarily occluded by wrapping a band tightly around the arm above the elbow.

In the proximal part of the arm, the **brachial artery** can be palpated against the humerus—this is the area that is occluded by a blood pressure cuff when the blood pressure is measured—and the accompanying nerves can be rolled against the bone. The artery can also be palpated on the anterior surface of the brachialis muscle, just medial to the biceps tendon at the elbow. This is the area in which the physician listens for the sound of the blood flow resuming through the artery as the pressure of the blood pressure cuff is released. The **ulnar nerve** can be palpated as it passes posterior to the medial epicondyle. The sensation induced by pressing on or hitting the nerve here has given rise to the colloquial "funny bone" for the medial epicondyle. The "tingling" experienced in the ring and little fingers provides an indication of the cutaneous distribution of the ulnar nerve to the skin of the hand (see Fig. 6-5).

MOVEMENTS AT THE ELBOW JOINT

In considering the movements at the elbow joint, note that flexion and extension occur between the humerus and both the ulna and the radius, whereas pronation and supination involve rotation of the radius about the ulna. **Flexion** (Fig. 6-11) is brought about especially through the actions of the *biceps brachii* and *brachialis.* (Because the biceps brachii supinates as it flexes, flexion from the pronated position is carried out by the

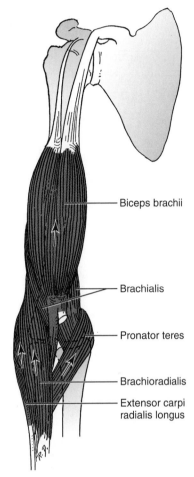

Figure 6-11 The flexors of the forearm.

Biceps brachii

Brachialis

Pronator teres

Brachioradialis

Extensor carpi radialis longus

brachialis alone, unless there is strong resistance.) A paralysis of these muscles, caused, for instance, by injury to the musculocutaneous nerve (Fig. 6-12 and Table 6-4), does not, however, abolish the ability to flex the elbow, because forearm muscles that cross the elbow anteriorly are innervated by other nerves. The most superficial muscle of the lateral forearm group, the *brachioradialis,* arises from the lateral border of the humerus, some distance proximal to the elbow, and crosses well in front of the elbow joint. It is a particularly good flexor of this joint when the hand is held so that the thumb is up (semiprone position), although it normally participates in flexion, primarily when the movement is a fast one. Other muscles on the extensor side, especially the *extensor carpi radialis longus,* may assist the brachioradialis in its flexor action but

MUSCULOCUTANEOUS NERVE

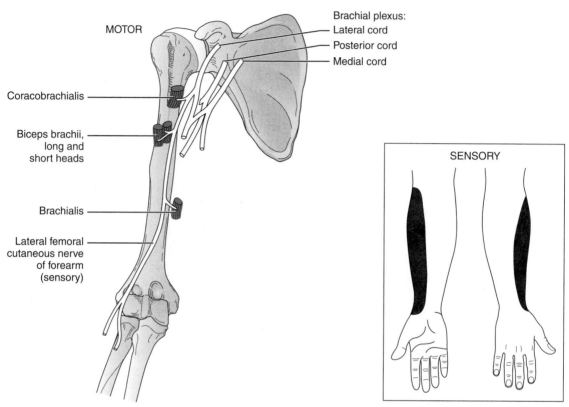

Figure 6-12 Distribution of the musculocutaneous nerve. Its cutaneous branch to the forearm, the lateral cutaneous nerve of the forearm, is included in the illustration on the left. (See Fig. 8-8 for an illustration of the anastomoses around the elbow.)

Table 6-4	NERVES OF THE ARM			
		Muscle		
Nerve and Origin*	**Name**	**Segmental Innervation**	**Chief Action**	
Musculocutaneous nerve C5–C7	Biceps brachii	C5, C6	Flexion-supination of forearm	
	Coracobrachialis	C5–C7	Adduction-flexion of arm	
	Brachialis	C5, C6	Flexion of forearm	
Radial nerve C5–C8	Triceps brachii	C6–C8	Extension of forearm	
	Anconeus	C7, C8	Extension of forearm	

*A common segmental origin or segmental innervation. The composition of both the chief nerves and their muscular branches varies somewhat among persons.

arise too low on the humerus to be as important in flexion. Of the flexor muscle mass in the forearm, the *pronator teres* has the highest origin from the humerus, although not as high as that of the brachioradialis. It is, accordingly, a much weaker flexor of the

forearm on the arm and, working alone, may or may not be able to perform this movement against gravity. Other muscles of the flexor forearm group arise from the medial epicondyle and have no significant action in flexing the elbow joint. Supination is carried out normally by the supinator muscle in the forearm, but loss of the biceps brachii markedly weakens this action.

The muscles producing **extension** of the forearm are the *anconeus* and the *triceps brachii* (see Fig. 6-7). The anconeus apparently acts first to extend or stabilize the elbow, and the various heads of the triceps brachii are recruited, as needed, for more strength: first the medial, then the lateral, then the long head.

The movements of pronation and supination can best be understood after the muscles of the forearm have been studied (see Chapter 10).

ANALYSES OF ACTIVITIES AND ASSOCIATED MOVEMENTS

The discussions in this chapter have demonstrated that the muscles of the arm have their major effect on flexion and extension of the forearm at the elbow joint. However, it has also been noted that some muscles may be capable of producing other movements. For example, because both heads of the biceps brachii and the long head of the triceps brachii originate on the scapula, and therefore cross the glenohumeral joint, they can also produce flexion and extension, respectively, of the arm at that joint. As a result of its insertion on the radial tuberosity, the biceps brachii also supinates the forearm and, in fact, provides the power for this movement.

Activity: *Picking up a Coffee Mug.* An analysis of most activities involving the upper limb illustrates the involvement usually of more than one joint and several muscles or groups of muscles. The task of picking up a coffee mug from a desk top and bringing it to the mouth to take a drink involves joints at the shoulder, elbow, wrist, and hand. Simple analysis of the movements involved while a person performs this activity provides a means of reviewing and integrating information presented in this chapter. Starting in a sitting position with the forearm resting on the arm of the desk chair and the mug located on the desk, movement must occur at the glenohumeral, elbow, and wrist joints to position the hand so that the mug can be grasped. In a continuous movement, the arm is flexed at the glenohumeral joint (and possibly abducted or adducted, depending on the position of the mug), and the forearm is extended at the elbow joint. The hand is maintained in a semiprone position. When the handle is grasped, the arm is extended

while the forearm is being flexed. Some medial rotation of the arm occurs as the mug is brought to the mouth. With the mug positioned at the mouth, the hand is slowly pronated in order to tip the mug for drinking.

Now consider the muscles of the arm that produce these movements, keeping in mind that numerous other muscles in the shoulder, forearm, and hand are also involved in this activity. Flexion at the glenohumeral joint involves the biceps brachii because both heads arise from the scapula and cross the joint; the opposite action of extension to remove the mug from the desk top involves the triceps brachii because its long head arises from the infraglenoid tubercle of the scapula. At the elbow, extension of the forearm is produced by the triceps brachii, with some assistance from the anconeus. Flexion of the forearm at the elbow as the mug is brought back and raised to the mouth results from contraction of the brachialis and biceps brachii (and also the brachioradialis in the forearm; see Chapter 9). However, the biceps brachii also supinates as it contracts. Maintaining the hand in a semiprone position and then pronating the forearm to enable drinking from the mug are coordinated actions between muscles producing pronation (pronator teres and pronator quadratus muscles in the forearm) and those producing supination (supinator muscle in the forearm and the biceps brachii).

Differences in body position, which limb is used, and the position of the object all play a role in determining the movements and muscles that are involved. For example, if the right limb is used to retrieve a mug that is located on the far right side of the desk, the arm must be laterally rotated; if the left limb is used, the arm must be medially rotated.

Continued

ANALYSES OF ACTIVITIES AND ASSOCIATED MOVEMENTS—cont'd

Activity: *Doing a Push-up.* The act of doing a push-up has components that involve muscles of the arm acting at the elbow and glenohumeral joints, as well as muscles of the shoulder region and forearm. In a push-up, the fixed point from which movement occurs is different from that in reaching for a coffee mug. In the latter, the shoulder (and trunk) is the fixed component, and the hand is free to move toward or away from the core of the body. In this scenario, the typical description of origin (proximal attachment) and insertion (distal attachment) can be applied. In contrast, in performing a push-up, the hands are fixed, and the body moves closer to or farther from the hand. This is essentially a reverse of the typical description of muscle origin and insertion.

A push-up can be initiated from a prone position on the floor or with the body elevated above the floor. Starting from the latter position, the hands are pronated and extended at the wrists, and the forearms are extended at the elbows. The arms are in a flexed position at the glenohumeral joints. Initial action is influenced primarily by gravity, but the downward movement must be controlled by muscle activity. As the body is lowered to the floor, the arms are abducted and extended at the glenohumeral joints, and the forearms are flexed at the elbows. To return the body to an elevated position, the opposite actions occur: extension takes place at the elbows and flexion, accompanied by adduction, occurring at the glenohumeral joints.

Muscles in the arm that are involved in the downward movement include the triceps brachii and anconeus of both limbs. These muscles contract eccentrically to control the rate of flexion occurring at the elbow. Shoulder muscles control abduction and extension of the arm, with assistance from the coracobrachialis and the long head of the biceps brachii, both of which cross the glenohumeral joint. Extension of the forearm at the elbow during elevation of the body is produced by the triceps brachii and anconeus

(concentric contraction). The biceps brachii and coracobrachialis assist in flexion of the arm at the glenohumeral joints. This analysis demonstrates that the same muscles in the arm contract during the downward and upward phases of the push-up, although in a different manner, either to control or produce the given movement.

Activity: *Removing a Hat.* As with the other activities described in this section, removing a hat from the head involves movement at all joints of the upper limb. With the hand at the side in a semiprone position, the forearm and hand and the arm are brought forward and upward in a smooth movement that involves flexion of the forearm at the elbow joint and flexion of the arm at the glenohumeral joint. Once the hand is raised high enough to enable grasping the hat, the hat can be removed to the front by continued flexion of the arm to lift it off the head; this is accompanied by extension of the forearm. With the hat off the head, it can be lowered by a combination of continued extension of the forearm, combined with extension of the arm at the glenohumeral joint.

Muscles of the arm that would produce flexion of the forearm are the biceps brachii and brachialis; the biceps brachii also helps bring the hand into a semiprone position. Extension of the forearm would be produced by contraction of the triceps brachii and anconeus. Most of the muscles involved with flexion and extension of the arm at the glenohumeral joint are those of the pectoral girdle that were described in Chapter 5. However, because both heads of the biceps brachii and the long head of the triceps brachii arise proximal to the glenohumeral joint, these muscles can, respectively, flex and extend the arm. With variations in this activity, additional movements may be necessary. For instance, if the hat is removed to the side, rather than to the front, the arm would have to be abducted, requiring involvement of additional muscles.

REVIEW QUESTIONS

1 Name three muscles that have an attachment to the coracoid process of the scapula.

2 What movement is possible at the proximal radioulnar joint? Which ligament is found at this joint, and how is it arranged?

3 What is the carrying angle? Is there a difference between the carrying angle in women and that in men? Explain your answer.

4 Which nerve provides sensory innervation to the skin of the distal lateral aspect of the arm? Of which nerve is it a branch? Which nerve provides sensory innervation to the skin of the medial side of the forearm?

5 How does the biceps brachii produce supination of the hand?

6 What is the origin of each head of the triceps brachii muscle? Where does the muscle insert? What is its action?

7 The radial nerve courses distally in the arm in company with which artery? What is the relationship of the radial nerve to the humerus and the triceps brachii muscle? Injury to the radial nerve as it arises from the posterior cord of the brachial plexus could result in what motor and sensory losses (or weaknesses) in the arm?

8 While being treated for a stab wound to the shoulder region (just inferior to the distal end of the clavicle), a patient reports difficulty in flexing the forearm at the elbow. Examination reveals not only noticeable weakness in flexion but also weakness in supination and loss of sensation of the skin on the lateral side of the forearm. On the basis of these findings, which nerve was probably injured? With such an injury, why may weak flexion still be possible at the elbow? Why would this injury affect supination?

9 What movements occur at the elbow joint, and which muscles of the arm are involved in performing the following activities?
a applying wax to a car by hand
b brushing your hair
c rowing a boat

EXERCISES

1 On the humerus (or a figure of the bone) identify the following:
a medial and lateral epicondyles
b deltoid tuberosity
c coronoid fossa
d capitulum
e trochlea

2 Demonstrate by palpation the following:
a coracobrachialis muscle
b bicipital tendon and aponeurosis
c pulse of the brachial artery
d ulnar nerve as it passes posterior to the elbow joint
e medial and lateral epicondyles of the humerus

7 FOREARM AND HAND: GENERAL SURVEY

CHAPTER CONTENTS

General Considerations

Movements

Nerves and Arteries

Bones and Joints

Fascia and Superficial Nerves and Vessels

GENERAL CONSIDERATIONS

The muscles of the forearm act on the elbow, wrist, and digits (fingers and thumb), whereas the muscles in the hand act on the digits alone. In the proximal part of the forearm, the muscles form fleshy masses below the medial and lateral epicondyles, but these masses rapidly taper off toward the wrist, where the muscle bellies are replaced by long tendons that continue into the hand. The reduction in bulk obtained by the transformation of the muscles into tendons allows a far greater number of muscles to have access to the hand than would otherwise be possible.

The **muscles of the forearm** can be divided into flexor and extensor groups. The *flexor group* arises largely from the medial epicondyle and occupies the medial border and anterior (flexor) surface of the forearm, from which many muscles continue into the palm of the hand. The *extensor group* is particularly prominent in the region of the lateral epicondyle and occupies the lateral border and the posterior (extensor) surface of the forearm. Many of the muscles of this group send tendons onto the posterior (dorsal) surface of the hand.

The **muscles in the hand** form two masses in the palm: the *thenar eminence* at the base of the thumb and the *hypothenar eminence* at the base of the little finger. Other muscles of the palm are situated more deeply, behind the long tendons and in association with the long bones (metacarpals) of the hand.

For the most part, the names of the muscles of the forearm and hand describe the chief action and relative location, shape, or size of each muscle:

Pronator, supinator, flexor, extensor, abductor, and *adductor* refer to movements that are described in the next section.

Radialis (radial), *ulnaris* (ulnar), *superficialis* (superficial), and *profundus* (deep) are adjectives of position.

Carpi (of the carpus or wrist), *digitorum* (of the digits or fingers), *pollicis* (of the thumb or pollex), *indicis* (of the index finger), and *digiti minimi* (of the little finger) are qualifying nouns describing the member or joint on which the muscle exerts its action.

Longus (long), *brevis* (short), *teres* (round), and *quadratus* (quadrangular) are adjectives of shape.

On the basis of this terminology, *extensor carpi radialis longus* means "long extensor of the wrist on the radial side"; *flexor digitorum profundus* is the "deep flexor of the digits"; and *pronator quadratus* means the "quadrangular pronator."

MOVEMENTS

Movements of the wrist are numerous. *Pronation* and *supination* are movements occurring at the elbow that result in turning the palm downward or upward, respectively, when the flexed forearm is held horizontally. *Flexion* at the wrist is the act of bending the palm of the hand toward the forearm (Fig. 7-1). *Extension* is the movement of straightening the flexed wrist; when this movement of extension is continued past the anatomical position, causing the wrist to bend posteriorly, it is called *hyperextension.* Obviously, flexion is freer than is extension.

In addition to flexion and extension, movements at the wrist can take place in the plane of the extended hand. These movements can be described with

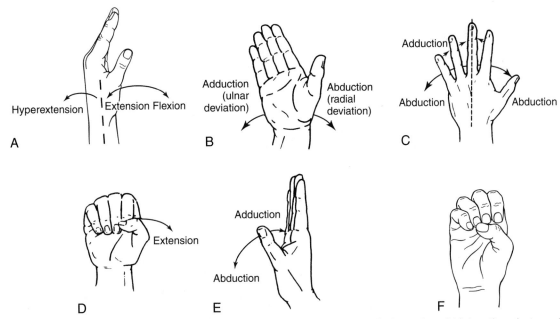

Figure 7-1 Movements at the wrist and of the digits. **A,** As indicated by the *arrows,* flexion at the wrist brings the palm toward the forearm, and extension returns the hand to the anatomical position (*dotted line* indicates the axis of the anatomical position). In hyperextension, the hand bends posteriorly. **B,** The hand is shown in adduction at the wrist; the opposite action is abduction, which is a more limited movement. **C,** The *dashed line* indicates the midline axis of the hand around which abduction and adduction of the fingers are defined. **D,** All of the digits are in flexion, and the *arrow* indicates the direction of movement for extension of the thumb. Note that this movement is in a different plane than that of extension-flexion of the fingers. **E,** Abduction of the thumb moves the thumb away from the plane of the palm, and adduction moves it toward the plane of the palm. **F,** In opposition of the thumb, the thumb is flexed and rotated medially and adducted so that it can come into contact with the tips of the fingers.

reference to their relation either to the midline of the body or to the midline of the hand itself. Movement toward the little finger side of the hand is referred to as *adduction,* or *ulnar deviation,* of the hand. Similarly, movement at the wrist toward the thumb side is *abduction,* or *radial deviation.* A greater amount of movement is possible in adduction than in abduction. Because the joint between the radius and wrist bones, although concave-convex in shape, is ellipsoidal rather than of the ball-and-socket type, rotation at the wrist is barely possible. A limited amount may accompany pronation and supination.

Movements of the thumb are best described separately from those of the four fingers. The thumb is in the normal position when its palmar surface is almost at a right angle to the palm of the hand, and movements of the thumb are described with reference to this position. In *flexion* of the thumb, the thumb is bending in a plane parallel to that of the palm (it does *not* involve doing this and at the same time rotating so that its pad comes in contact with the palmar surface of the fingers). *Extension* is, of course, the opposite movement. In *abduction,* the thumb is raised away from the other fingers, in a plane perpendicular to the palm, whereas *adduction* involves bringing it back toward the palm.

The first metacarpal (the long bone at the base of the thumb) moves with the thumb. It contributes more to these movements, except in flexion and extension of the distal joint of the thumb, than do the joints of the thumb itself. Movements of the metacarpal in flexion and extension are not single movements; they also involve rotation and usually adduction or abduction. As the thumb as a whole is flexed, it is also rotated medially and adducted so that its pad can come in contact with the pads of the fingers; this combination of movements is known as *opposition.* The movement away from opposition, involving extension, external rotation, and usually abduction, is conveniently termed *reposition.*

Movements of the four fingers include *flexion,* or closing the hand as in making a fist, and *extension,* or straightening the fingers. Some hyperextension, or *dorsiflexion,* is also possible. Also, the fingers may be spread apart in the plane of the palm, or *abducted,* or they may be brought together, or *adducted,* in this plane. For such movements, *the midline of the hand is*

considered as a line along the third metacarpal and middle finger. Because the metacarpophalangeal joints allow flexion and extension and abduction and adduction, a finger as a whole may also be *circumducted.* In addition to the previously described movements, which occur at the joints of the fingers, the little and ring fingers have metacarpals that, although far less mobile than the metacarpal of the thumb, can flex to help cup the hand.

NERVES AND ARTERIES

The muscles of the forearm are innervated by the median, ulnar, and radial nerves, and those of the hand are innervated by the median and ulnar nerves. Because both the median and the ulnar nerves are derived from the anterior divisions of the brachial plexus, they are distributed to the anterior musculature of the forearm and hand. The **median nerve** supplies most of the anterior (flexor) musculature of the forearm but only a few muscles in the hand (see Fig. 8-6). The **ulnar nerve** supplies only about one and one half muscles in the forearm but the majority of those in the hand (see Fig. 8-7). The **radial nerve,** the only derivative of the posterior division of the brachial plexus to reach either the arm or the forearm, supplies all the posterior (extensor) muscles of the forearm (see Fig. 9-6). There are normally no muscles on the posterior surface of the hand. These three nerves innervate most or all of the skin of the hand, but only the radial nerve innervates skin of the forearm (see Fig. 6-5).

The **radial and ulnar arteries,** terminal branches of the brachial artery, provide the blood supply to the forearm and hand. Both run down the anterior side of the forearm and end in the palm. The posterior side of the forearm and the dorsum of the hand are supplied by the branches of these two vessels.

BONES AND JOINTS
Bones

The proximal ends of the bones of the forearm (Fig. 7-2), the radius on the side of the thumb and the ulna on that of the little finger, are described in Chapter 6. The articulation of the *head of the radius*

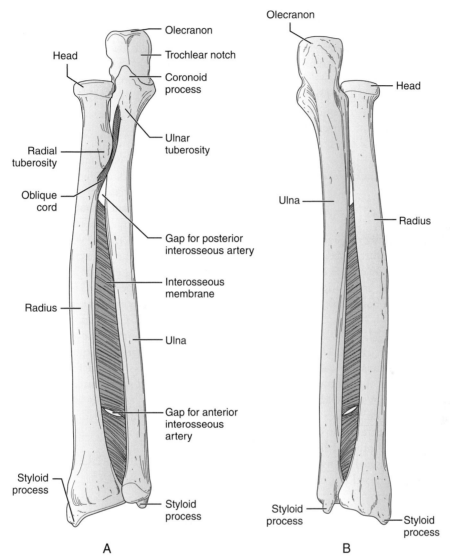

Figure 7-2 Anterior **(A)** and posterior **(B)** views of the radius and ulna.

with the ulna and the annular ligament is particularly important because this allows the radius to rotate and cross the ulna in the movement of pronation. The chief marking on the shaft of each bone is the interosseous border (medially on the radius, laterally on the ulna). Between these borders is stretched a strong **interosseous membrane** that largely fills the interval between the bones and completes the separation between anterior and posterior structures of the forearm. Above the proximal end of the interosseous membrane is a gap between the radius and ulna through which the posterior interosseous artery passes. That artery is the chief arterial supply to the posterior side of the forearm. In the distal part of the membrane is a small opening through which a branch of the anterior interosseous artery passes from the anterior to the posterior sides of the forearm.

Radius

The **radius** expands distally and ends in a cartilage-lined concavity termed the *carpal* (wrist) *articular surface.* On the medial (ulnar) side of the distal end, there is the *ulnar notch* for articulation with the ulna. More laterally, there is a bony projection, the *styloid process.*

Ulna

The distal end of the **ulna** is its *head* (thus, the head of the radius is proximal; that of the ulna is distal). Much of its circumference and its distal surface are smooth for articulation with the radius and the fibrocartilaginous disc that separates the distal radioulnar joint from the wrist joint proper (the ulna does not participate in the latter joint). The nipple-like projection from the posteromedial side of the head is the *styloid process* of the ulna.

Carpals, metacarpals, and phalanges

The wrist is formed by eight **carpals,** which are arranged in two rows. Each is named and described in detail in Chapter 11. The bones are so arranged that they form a concave anterior surface, the *carpal groove.* The bulk of the hand is formed by long bones, the **metacarpals,** which are designated by Roman numerals, that of the thumb being metacarpal I or the first metacarpal. The skeleton of the fingers is formed by **phalanges.** The three phalanges of each finger are called *proximal, middle,* and *distal* phalanges, respectively; the two of the thumb are called the *proximal* and *distal* phalanges. The digits are numbered like the metacarpals and are named. The first digit is the *thumb* (in Latin, the *pollex*), and the second to fifth digits are also called the *index, middle* (sometimes *long*), *ring,* and *little digits or fingers.* The middle finger is named according to its position as the middle digit. The skeleton of the wrist and hand is shown in Figures 11-1 and 11-2, and Figure 11-3 illustrates the joints at the wrist.

Joints

The **joints** of the wrist and fingers are also described in more detail in Chapter 11. The large joint at the wrist is the *radiocarpal joint* (between the radius and the carpal bones), but there are also *intercarpal joints* (joints among the carpals), and these contribute to mobility at the wrist. The *carpometacarpal joints* (between the bones named) of the second and third digits are essentially immovable, but the fourth metacarpal can be moved slightly and the fifth even more. The carpometacarpal joint of the thumb is very movable and responsible for much of the movement of the thumb. The *metacarpophalangeal joints* of the fingers form the knuckles and are much more movable than is that of the thumb. There are two *interphalangeal joints,* proximal and distal, for each finger, and a single joint for the thumb. Movements at these joints have already been defined.

FASCIA AND SUPERFICIAL NERVES AND VESSELS

Fascia

The **deep fascia** of the forearm (**antebrachial fascia**) resembles that of the arm in being a tough fibrous membrane that surrounds the underlying muscles. In the proximal part, it receives the bicipital aponeurosis and is the point of origin of the more superficial fibers of both flexor and extensor muscles of the forearm. Septa passing from it between the muscles provide further attachment for these muscles in the upper part of the forearm. In the lower part of the forearm, the fascia more loosely surrounds the muscles, and on the anterior surface of the wrist, it is partially split into two layers, between which pass the palmaris longus tendon and the ulnar vessels and nerve. The more superficial layer at the wrist, covering the previously mentioned structures, may be thin and poorly developed. The deeper layer of fascia at the wrist is markedly strengthened by transverse fibers that stretch across the carpal groove between its higher medial and lateral sides and thus convert the groove into the *carpal tunnel* or *canal.* These transverse fibers form the **flexor retinaculum.** Most of the tendons going into the palm of the hand pass posterior to this retinaculum and are in the carpal tunnel. On the posterior side of the wrist, the fascia is similarly thickened to form the **extensor retinaculum,** but as this stretches from one side of the wrist to the other, it is attached to the underlying bones by septa that divide the space deep to the ligament into a number of separate compartments for the tendons going onto the dorsum of the hand.

The deep fascia of the hand is continuous through the retinacula with the antebrachial fascia. That of the palm merits special description (see Chapter 11), but until the hand is studied, it need only be understood that a central part of the palmar fascia, the **palmar aponeurosis,** is particularly thick and tendinous. The major tendons, nerves, and vessels of the palm lie mostly posterior to the palmar aponeurosis.

Nerves

The cutaneous innervation of the forearm is provided by three nerves (see Fig. 6-5). Running down the back of the forearm is the **posterior cutaneous nerve of the forearm,** a branch of the radial nerve, arising above the elbow. The **lateral cutaneous nerve of the forearm,** the continuation of the musculocutaneous, supplies skin on both anterior and posterior surfaces of the lateral aspect of the forearm. The **medial cutaneous nerve of the forearm,** a nerve arising directly from the medial cord of the brachial plexus, similarly supplies skin on the anterior and posterior surfaces of the medial side of the forearm. These nerves usually end close to the wrist but may continue a variable distance into the hand, either as independent branches or by joining the radial or ulnar nerve branches to the hand.

The cutaneous innervation of the hand is provided primarily by the median, ulnar, and radial nerves (see Fig. 6-5). The **median nerve** typically innervates much of the skin on the palmar surface of the hand, including that of the thumb, index, middle, and the radial half of the ring finger (see Fig. 8-6). In addition to this palmar distribution, the median nerve sends branches toward the dorsum to supply the bases of the nails and most of the skin over the middle and distal phalanges of index and middle fingers and half of the ring finger. The **ulnar nerve** typically innervates the ulnar side of the palm of the hand, the ulnar half of the ring finger, and all the palmar surface of the little finger (see Fig. 8-7). In addition, through its *dorsal branch* to the hand, it innervates at least the corresponding fingers on their dorsal surfaces and a similar region on the back of the hand, and it frequently supplies or helps to supply innervation to the adjacent dorsal surfaces of the proximal phalanges of ring and middle fingers (see Fig. 6-5).

The **radial nerve** (see Fig. 9-6) through its *superficial branch,* innervates the remaining surface of the dorsum of the hand, including the proximal part of the dorsum of the thumb and the proximal portion of one and a half or two and a half adjacent fingers. The *digital branches* of the radial nerve do not supply the more distal portions of the fingers.

Vessels

The superficial veins of the hand form a dense network on both surfaces of the fingers. The veins on the palmar surface drain primarily posteriorly into the dorsum of the hand, where the chief venous network of the hand occurs. Superficial veins are scarce in the palm. From the extensive venous network on the dorsum, two veins, both of which have already been described in the arm, have origins and run proximally in the superficial fascia. The **cephalic vein** arises largely from the radial side of this network. It winds around the radial side of the forearm to reach the lateral side of the front of the elbow, where it communicates with the basilic vein through the median cubital vein. The **basilic vein** arises more from the ulnar portion of the dorsal veins and runs proximally on the medial border of the anterior surface of the forearm. The **median forearm vein,** usually much smaller than the preceding two but of varying size, may run up the middle of the anterior surface of the forearm to communicate with the basilic or cephalic vein or both.

REVIEW QUESTIONS

1 Which metacarpal and finger serve as the midline of the hand around which abduction and adduction of the fingers are described?

2 At which end of the ulna, proximal or distal, is its head? Is this also true of the head of the radius?

3 How many phalanges does the thumb have? How many phalanges are there in the middle finger? What are they called?

4 An incision of the skin on the lateral aspect of the forearm would stimulate sensory endings innervated by what nerve? What is the origin of this nerve?

5 What connective tissue structure spans transversely across the carpal groove and helps form the carpal tunnel?

6 What is the orientation of the fibers of the interosseous membrane between the radius and ulna? What is the functional significance of this orientation?

EXERCISES

1 Describe and demonstrate the following movements:
   a flexion and extension of the hand at the wrist
   b abduction (radial deviation) of the hand
   c abduction of the thumb
   d adduction of the fingers
   e flexion of the thumb

2 Demonstrate the following:
   a location of the hypothenar eminence
   b positions of the styloid processes of the radius and ulna
   c location of the metacarpophalangeal joints of the thumb and fingers

8 FLEXOR FOREARM

CHAPTER CONTENTS

Bones

Muscles

Nerves and Vessels

BONES

The features of the bones of the forearm are described in Chapters 6 and 7; a general description of the bones and joints of the hand and wrist is presented in Chapter 7. Before the flexor muscles of the forearm are described, consideration of the surface anatomy provides a review of many of the osteological features of the area.

Surface Anatomy

Of the bony landmarks that can be observed on the living forearm, the **ulna** is the most apparent. It is subcutaneous throughout its length and is palpable from the *olecranon* to its rounded *head* and *styloid process*, which produce a bulge on the posterior side of the forearm just proximal to the wrist. The ulna separates the anteromedial flexor muscles from the muscles on the posterior side of the forearm.

The upper part of the **radius** is covered not only laterally and posteriorly but also anteriorly by the extensor muscles. Its *head*, however, can be felt immediately below the *lateral epicondyle* of the humerus. The head of the radius is easily distinguished from the humerus by palpating the lateral side of the elbow during flexion and extension or during pronation and supination. The distal half of the radius can be palpated and traced to its expanded distal end. Its rather broad *styloid process* can best be felt on the extreme radial border of the anterior surface of the wrist, just anteromedial to the prominent tendons extending to the base of the first metacarpal and at about the level of the proximal crease in the skin at the wrist. If the styloid processes of both the radius and the ulna are palpated, it is apparent that the styloid process of the radius extends more distally than that of the ulna.

Ridges on two of the carpal bones (scaphoid and trapezium) form the rounded projection, largely distal to the distal crease of the wrist, at the base of the thenar eminence. On the ulnar side, the slightly movable **pisiform bone** (one of the carpal bones) can be felt at the level of the distal crease, whereas just distal to it, at the base of the hypothenar eminence, the unyielding projection of another carpal bone, the **hamate bone,** can be palpated. The **flexor retinaculum** stretches between the bony prominences on the radial and ulnar sides. Although it cannot be distinctly palpated, the location of its proximal edge is indicated by the distal skin crease at the wrist. The flexor tendons, palpable proximally, cannot be felt at this level.

MUSCLES

The flexor muscles of the forearm may be conveniently divided into superficial, intermediate, and deep groups. There are four muscles in the **superficial group:** *pronator teres, palmaris longus, flexor carpi radialis,* and *flexor carpi ulnaris* (Fig. 8-1). These muscles are in part fused where they arise from the medial epicondyle and share a tendon of origin called the *common flexor* tendon. They arise also from the antebrachial fascia covering them and from intermuscular septa between them. The **intermediate layer** is made up of only one muscle, the *flexor digitorum superficialis* (Fig. 8-2). The **deep group** of muscles consists of the *flexor digitorum profundus, flexor pollicis longus,* and *pronator quadratus* (Fig. 8-3). The pronator quadratus arises more distally on the forearm and is positioned posterior to the tendons of the other two muscles. The origin and insertion of each of the muscles discussed in this chapter are illustrated in Figure 8-4.

Superficial Muscles

Pronator teres

The uppermost member of the superficial group, therefore contributing to the fleshy mass distal to the medial epicondyle, is the **pronator teres** (Table 8-1).

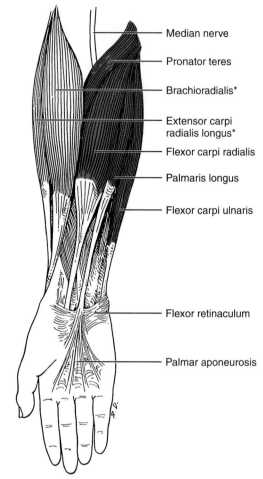

Figure 8-1 The more superficial flexor muscles of the right forearm. The muscle names with *asterisks* refer to anterior muscles of the extensor group.

Median nerve
Pronator teres
Brachioradialis*
Extensor carpi radialis longus*
Flexor carpi radialis
Palmaris longus
Flexor carpi ulnaris
Flexor retinaculum
Palmar aponeurosis

The *origin* of this muscle is by two heads: the medial epicondyle and the coronoid process of the ulna. The two heads unite and have an *insertion* on the lateral surface of the radius (near the middle of the shaft). *Innervation* to the pronator teres is provided by branches of the median nerve arising just before and, as the nerve passes, between the two heads of the muscle. Because the pronator teres is wrapped around the radius, its chief *action* is to roll the radius medially and therefore to pronate the forearm (and hand). Because of its relatively high origin on the humerus, it is also a weak flexor of the forearm.

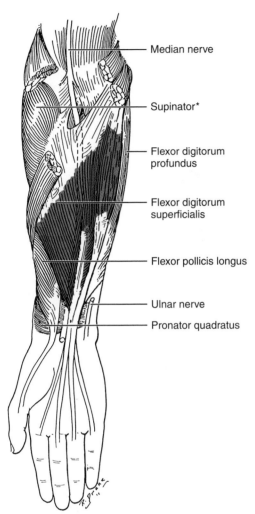

Figure 8-2 The intermediate muscle layer (flexor digitorum superficialis) of the right forearm. The supinator *(asterisk)* is part of the extensor forearm group of muscles.

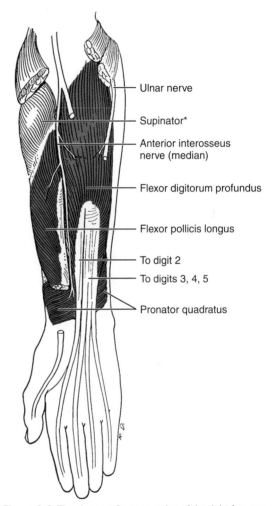

Figure 8-3 The deepest flexor muscles of the right forearm. The supinator *(asterisk)* is part of the extensor forearm group of muscles (see Chapter 9).

Palmaris longus

The middle element of the three remaining members of the superficial flexor group is the **palmaris longus.** Its *origin* is from the medial epicondyle (common flexor tendon) along with other muscles of the flexor group. The short body of the muscle is continuous with a long, narrow tendon that passes superficial to the flexor retinaculum. Its *insertion* is into the palmar aponeurosis. The *action* of the palmaris longus, although weak, is to aid in the flexion of the hand. *Innervation* is provided by a branch of the median

nerve. This muscle is subject to variation and may be absent in one or both limbs.

Flexor carpi radialis

Lying to the radial side of the palmaris longus and partly covered at its origin by the humeral head of the pronator teres is the **flexor carpi radialis.** Its *origin* is from the common flexor tendon (medial epicondyle of the humerus). The tendon of the muscle passes obliquely across the wrist and into the hand to an *insertion* upon the base (proximal end) of the second

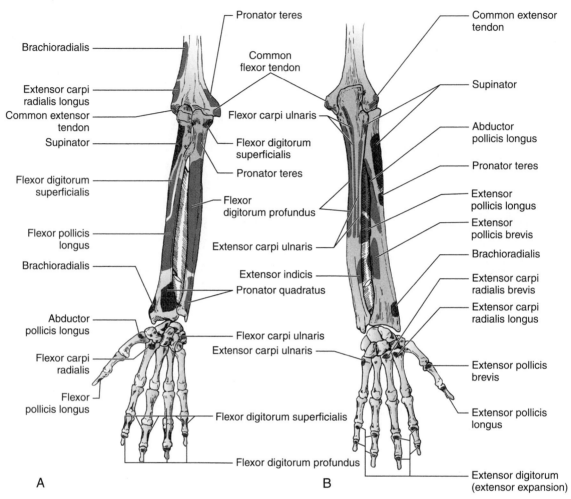

Figure 8-4 Anterior **(A)** and posterior **(B)** views of the bones of the elbow region, forearm, and hand, illustrating origins *(color)* and insertions *(black)* of flexor and extensor muscles of the forearm.

metacarpal. It may send a tendinous slip to the base of the third metacarpal. At the wrist, the tendon of the flexor carpi radialis possesses a synovial sheath that extends almost to its insertion, protecting it as it passes through the radial attachment of the flexor retinaculum (*not* deep to the retinaculum with the flexor tendons of the digits). The *action* of the muscle is to flex the hand at wrist. Because of its radial insertion, it may also produce abduction at the wrist (radial deviation), and its obliquity allows it to assist in pronation. The *innervation* of the flexor carpi radialis is by the median nerve, sometimes through two branches.

Flexor carpi ulnaris

On the ulnar side of the palmaris longus is the **flexor carpi ulnaris,** which has an *origin* both from the humerus through the medial epicondyle (common flexor tendon) and from the proximal two thirds of the posterior surface of the ulna through an aponeurosis that covers part of the deeper lying flexor digitorum profundus. Between the two heads of origin, the ulnar nerve passes into the forearm. The tendon of *insertion* of the flexor carpi ulnaris attaches to the pisiform bone (a carpal bone of the proximal row) on the ulnar side of the hand (see Fig. 11-1). Through the pisohamate and pisometacarpal ligaments (which

Table 8-1	SUPERFICIAL MUSCLES			
Muscle	**Origin (Proximal Attachment)**	**Insertion (Distal Attachment)**	**Action**	**Innervation**
Pronator teres	Medial epicondyle of humerus; coronoid process of ulna	Lateral surface of midshaft of radius	Pronation of forearm (and hand)	Median nerve
Palmaris longus	Medial epicondyle of humerus (common flexor tendon)	Palmar aponeurosis	Flexion of hand	Median nerve
Flexor carpi radialis	Medial epicondyle of humerus (common flexor tendon)	Base of second metacarpal and possibly third metacarpal	Flexion and abduction (radial deviation) of hand	Median nerve
Flexor carpi ulnaris	Medial epicondyle of humerus (common flexor tendon); proximal two thirds of posterior surface of ulna	Pisiform bone	Flexion and adduction (ulnar deviation) of hand	Ulnar nerve

Table 8-2	INTERMEDIATE MUSCLE			
Muscle	**Origin (Proximal Attachment)**	**Insertion (Distal Attachment)**	**Action**	**Innervation**
Flexor digitorum superficialis	Medial epicondyle of humerus (common flexor tendon); medial aspect of coronoid process of ulna; proximal half of radius distal to radial tuberosity	Base of middle phalanx of each of four fingers (medial four digits)	Flexion of middle phalanx of each of four fingers (medial four digits); with continued action, flexion of each proximal phalanx; aids in flexion of hand	Median nerve

connect the pisiform bone to the hamate bone and to the fifth metacarpal, respectively) the *action* of the flexor carpi ulnaris is continued across the entire wrist joint. It is, therefore, a better flexor of the hand than would appear from an inspection of its insertion. The muscle also produces adduction (ulnar deviation) at the wrist. In contrast to most of the flexor muscles of the forearm, the flexor carpi ulnaris receives *innervation* from the ulnar nerve through two to four branches.

Intermediate Muscle

Flexor digitorum superficialis

The **flexor digitorum superficialis** forms an intermediate layer between the superficial and deep groups (Table 8-2; see Fig. 8-2). Its *origin* is by two heads: a humeroulnar head with the common flexor tendon from the medial epicondyle and the coronoid process of the ulna, and a broader but thinner radial head from the upper half of the radius below the radial tuberosity. Proximally, the median nerve and ulnar artery lie between the two heads; distally, both lie deep to the muscle. The median nerve clings to the posterior surface of the muscle and runs in almost a straight course distally. The ulnar artery runs obliquely toward the ulnar side and passes deep to the flexor carpi ulnaris. Four tendons arise from the combined muscular belly, and as they reach the wrist, they are arranged in two layers. The two anterior tendons go to the middle and the ring fingers, and the posterior two go to the index and the little fingers. At the wrist, the tendons of this muscle pass deep to the flexor retinaculum, where they are

Table 8-3	DEEP MUSCLES			
Muscle	**Origin (Proximal Attachment)**	**Insertion (Distal Attachment)**	**Action**	**Innervation**
Flexor digitorum profundus	Anterior and medial surfaces of proximal two thirds of ulna; interosseous membrane; aponeurosis of flexor carpi ulnaris	Distal phalanx of each of the four fingers (medial four digits)	Flexion of distal phalanx of each of the four fingers (medial four digits); with continued action, flexion of the middle and proximal phalanges; aids in flexion of hand	Median and ulnar nerves
Flexor pollicis longus	Anterior surface of middle half of radius; adjacent interosseous membrane	Distal phalanx of thumb	Flexion of distal phalanx of thumb	Median nerve
Pronator quadratus	Distal fourth of ulna	Distal part of radius	Pronation of forearm (and hand)	Median nerve

surrounded by a large synovial sheath (the common flexor sheath, containing also the tendons of the flexor digitorum profundus) that facilitates their free movement in this position. The four tendons of the flexor digitorum superficialis diverge after passing behind the flexor retinaculum and run out along the digits to attach to their middle phalanges. In its course on the finger, each tendon is enclosed in a digital synovial sheath with the tendon of the deep flexor to that finger. Each tendon of the flexor digitorum superficialis splits around the associated tendon of the flexor digitorum profundus (see Fig. 11-8) to allow the tendons of the profundus to pass further distally on the finger. The two bands interchange some fibers behind this deep tendon, and then each has an *insertion* onto the sides of the palmar surface of the base of the middle phalanx. The primary *action* of the flexor digitorum superficialis is as a flexor of the middle phalanx. Continued action can produce flexion of the proximal phalanges, the metacarpals, and the hand. Its *innervation* is by several branches from the median nerve.

Deep Muscles

Flexor digitorum profundus

The **flexor digitorum profundus** has an extensive *origin* from the anterior and medial surfaces of the proximal two thirds or more of the ulna, the adjacent

interosseous membrane, and the aponeurosis, from which the flexor carpi ulnaris takes part of its origin (Table 8-3). Like the flexor digitorum superficialis, this muscle ends in four tendons, but in contrast to that muscle, the four tendons are arranged at the wrist in the same plane. These tendons pass into the common flexor sheath at the wrist and lie deep to both the flexor retinaculum and the superficial flexor tendons of the fingers. As the tendons diverge toward the fingers after passing beyond the flexor retinaculum, they lie immediately deep to the superficial flexor tendons. Within the synovial sheaths on the fingers, they run through the divided portions of the superficial tendons (see Fig. 11-8). After passing across the interphalangeal joints, the tendons of the flexor digitorum profundus have an *insertion* on the bases of the distal phalanges of each of the four fingers. The main *action* of the muscle is to produce flexion of the distal phalanx of each finger. It is also secondarily a good flexor at the proximal interphalangeal joint. The portion of the muscle going to the index finger is usually separate from the rest of the muscle for some distance in the distal part of the forearm. Separate tendons for the remaining fingers are usually formed just above the wrist.

The *innervation* of the flexor digitorum profundus is supplied by two nerves: a radial portion of the muscle is supplied by the median nerve (through its anterior interosseous branch), and an ulnar portion is supplied by the ulnar nerve. The exact amount of the muscle supplied by each nerve varies from one individual to another.

Flexor pollicis longus

The **flexor pollicis longus** has an *origin* from about the middle half of the anterior surface of the radius and from the adjacent interosseous membrane. Its tendon has a separate synovial sheath deep to the flexor retinaculum, on the radial side of the common flexor sheath. Its *insertion* is on the base of the distal phalanx of the thumb. The *action* of this muscle is to flex the distal phalanx of the thumb. *Innervation* is provided by the anterior interosseous branch of the median nerve.

Pronator quadratus

The **pronator quadratus** is a flat quadrangular muscle that has its *origin* from the distal fourth of the ulna. Its fibers pass mostly transversely but with a slight distal slant to their *insertion* on the distal part of the radius. The *action* of the pronator quadratus is to pronate the forearm (and therefore the hand) with assistance from the pronator teres when more speed or power is required. *Innervation* is provided by the anterior interosseous branch of the median nerve.

Surface Anatomy

Several of the muscles, tendons, and muscle masses of the flexor forearm are palpable. The depression in front of the elbow between the lateral and medial muscle masses is the **cubital fossa.** The **tendon of the biceps brachii** passes into the cubital fossa, and the **bicipital aponeurosis** can be traced medially over the medial muscle mass. The fact that the **lateral mass** is composed of extensor muscles can be easily confirmed by palpating it when the wrist is extended. Similarly, the fact that the **medial mass** is composed of flexor muscles and arises in part from the medial epicondyle can be verified by palpating it when the person's fingers are clenched, when the wrist is flexed, or when both actions are performed together. However, few of the individual muscles can be identified at this level. Perhaps the easiest muscle

to identify is the **pronator teres,** which can be felt as the medial border of the cubital fossa when the forearm is slightly flexed and strongly pronated. The posteromedial border of the **flexor carpi ulnaris** can be identified, and the muscle traced to its tendon at the wrist, by palpating deeply in front of the ulna when the hand with extended fingers is sharply adducted. Contraction of the **flexor digitorum profundus** can be recognized by palpating in the same place, between the ulna and the flexor carpi ulnaris, and strongly flexing the fingers.

Several tendons can be recognized without difficulty at the wrist. The rather thin sharp **tendon of the palmaris longus** (unless the muscle is missing) can usually be both palpated and visualized in the midline of the wrist when the hand is flexed. The tendon is particularly prominent because it passes superficial to the flexor retinaculum. Very close to it, on its radial side, is the broader **tendon of the flexor carpi radialis,** the position of which is made more apparent by flexing the hand against resistance. Although it may seem to end at the bony prominence at the base of the thenar eminence, it actually runs just medial to this. On the ulnar side of the wrist, the **tendon of the flexor carpi ulnaris** is best identified when the wrist is simultaneously slightly flexed and slightly adducted (deviated to the ulnar side) and can be traced to the pisiform bone. The **tendons of the flexor digitorum superficialis** can be palpated between, but deeper than, the tendons of the palmaris longus and flexor carpi ulnaris.

NERVES AND VESSELS
Nerves

Median nerve

Aside from cutaneous branches, there are only two nerves on the anterior aspect of the forearm: the median and the ulnar. The **median nerve** passes into the forearm with the brachial artery, lying medial to it on the surface of the brachialis muscle (Fig. 8-5). Although it supplies innervation to no muscles of the arm, branches to both the pronator teres and flexor carpi radialis may arise slightly above the elbow. As, and after, it passes between the two heads of the pronator teres, the median nerve gives off branches

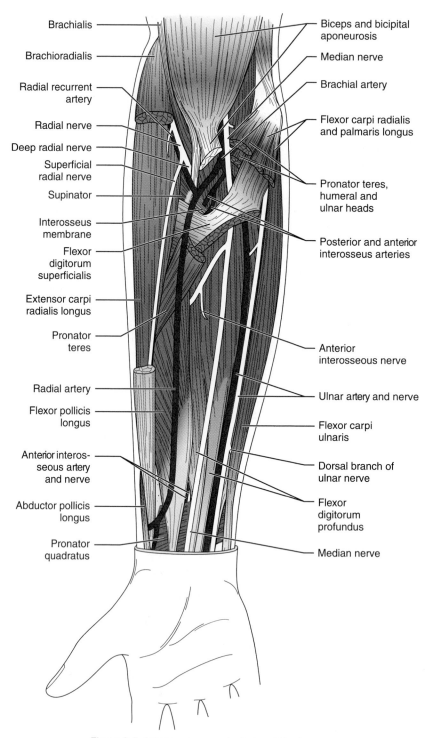

Brachialis

Brachioradialis

Radial recurrent artery

Radial nerve

Deep radial nerve

Superficial radial nerve

Supinator

Interosseus membrane

Flexor digitorum superficialis

Extensor carpi radialis longus

Pronator teres

Radial artery

Flexor pollicis longus

Anterior interosseous artery and nerve

Abductor pollicis longus

Pronator quadratus

Biceps and bicipital aponeurosis

Median nerve

Brachial artery

Flexor carpi radialis and palmaris longus

Pronator teres, humeral and ulnar heads

Posterior and anterior interosseus arteries

Anterior interosseous nerve

Ulnar artery and nerve

Flexor carpi ulnaris

Dorsal branch of ulnar nerve

Flexor digitorum profundus

Median nerve

Figure 8-5 Anterior nerves and arteries of the forearm.

to that muscle and to the palmaris longus, flexor carpi radialis, and flexor digitorum superficialis (Fig. 8-6) in no regular order. The nerve to the palmaris longus may arise with a branch to the flexor carpi radialis. The median nerve then passes between the two heads of the flexor digitorum superficialis, may give off additional branches to that muscle, and gives rise to the *anterior interosseous nerve*. This runs distally along the anterior surface of the interosseous membrane to be distributed to a lateral portion of the flexor digitorum profundus and to the flexor pollicis longus and the pronator quadratus muscles. *The median nerve supplies all the flexor forearm muscles, with the exceptions of the flexor carpi ulnaris muscle and a variable ulnar portion of the flexor digitorum profundus muscle.* The main stem of the median nerve continues distally adherent to the deep surface of the flexor digitorum superficialis and appears on the radial side of the tendons of this muscle just proximal to the wrist. It passes into the hand deep to the flexor retinaculum but superficial to the flexor tendons.

FUNCTIONAL/CLINICAL NOTE 8-1

Severing the median nerve above the elbow might be expected to prevent pronation because both pronators are innervated by it, but it only weakens the movement. Apparently, the brachioradialis muscle can pronate, whether it does so normally or not. Such sectioning has little effect on flexion of the hand because the flexor carpi ulnaris, innervated by the ulnar nerve, and the abductor pollicis longus, innervated by the radial nerve, can produce that action. The effect on the hand is discussed later.

Ulnar nerve

The **ulnar nerve** passes posterior to the medial epicondyle and enters the forearm between the two heads of the flexor carpi ulnaris. Under cover of this muscle, it gives off branches to this and to an ulnar part of the flexor digitorum profundus (Fig. 8-7) and, continuing distally, crosses superficial to the flexor retinaculum to enter the hand. Proximal to the wrist, it gives rise to a small *palmar branch* that innervates

skin of the hypothenar eminence and a larger *dorsal branch* that gives rise to the ulnar nerve's *dorsal digital branches*. As it enters the palm, the ulnar nerve divides into *superficial and deep branches*. The superficial branch gives rise to the *palmar digital branches,* whereas the deep branch disappears into the muscles of the hypothenar eminence.

FUNCTIONAL/CLINICAL NOTE 8-2

At the level of the medial epicondyle, the ulnar nerve is subject to damage by being stretched across the epicondyle, from a roughness of the ulnar groove, or from compression by a fibrous band extending between the two heads of the flexor carpi ulnaris. The condition has been treated by transplanting the nerve to a shorter course in front of the epicondyle, resecting the epicondyle, or dividing the fibrous band and a small amount of the adjacent muscle. Almost all the effects of ulnar nerve injury are in the hand. Paralysis of the flexor carpi ulnaris is hard to detect, but there may be some weakness in ulnar deviation of the hand.

Segmental innervation

Because the median nerve arises from both medial and lateral cords of the brachial plexus, it can contain fibers from all of the spinal nerves contributing to the plexus (C5 to T1). It does receive fibers from all but has relatively few motor fibers from C5. The ulnar nerve, arising from the medial cord, contains fibers from the segments contributing to the medial cord, C8 and T1, and sometimes receives some from C7 by a communication from the lateral cord. Of the flexor muscles in the forearm, the pronator teres and flexor carpi radialis are usually supplied mostly by C6 and C7 through the median nerve and the palmaris longus by C7 and C8 (Table 8-4). The flexor digitorum superficialis usually receives fibers from C7, C8, and T1. The other muscles—the flexor carpi ulnaris, the flexor digitorum profundus, the flexor pollicis longus, and the pronator quadratus—are usually innervated by fibers from C8 and T1. The flexor carpi ulnaris often gets fibers from C7.

MEDIAN NERVE

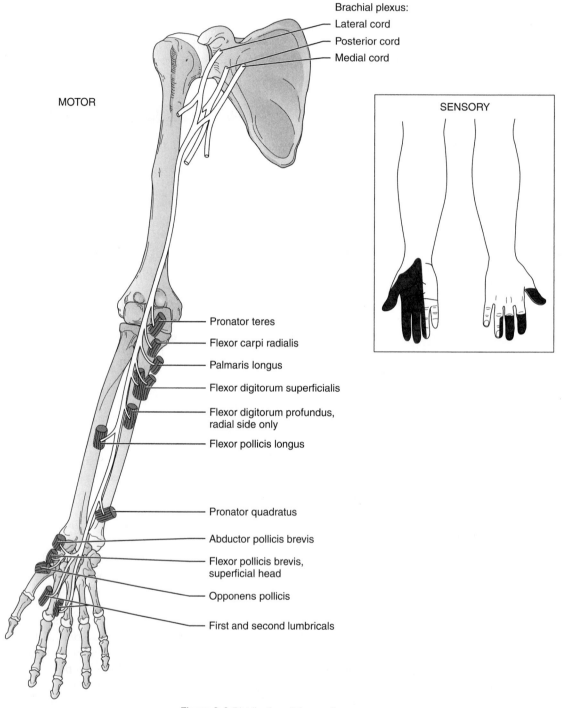

Brachial plexus:
Lateral cord
Posterior cord
Medial cord

MOTOR

SENSORY

Pronator teres

Flexor carpi radialis

Palmaris longus

Flexor digitorum superficialis

Flexor digitorum profundus, radial side only

Flexor pollicis longus

Pronator quadratus

Abductor pollicis brevis

Flexor pollicis brevis, superficial head

Opponens pollicis

First and second lumbricals

Figure 8-6 Distribution of the median nerve.

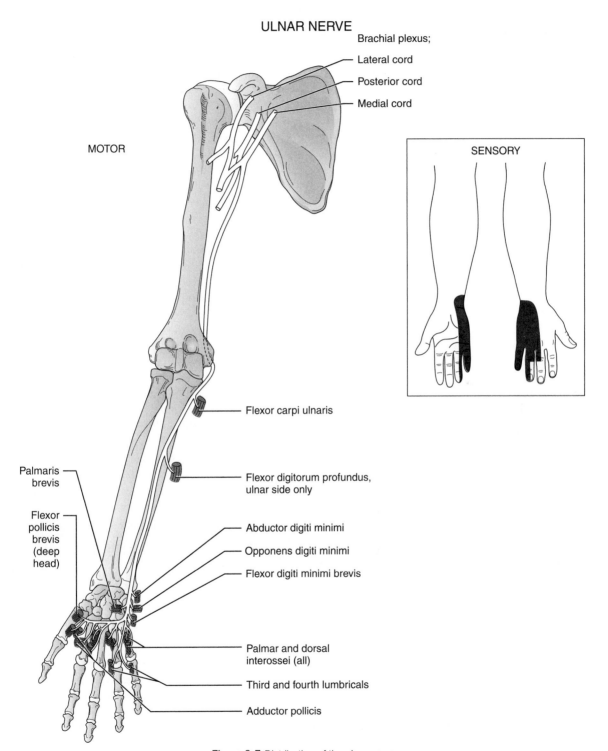

ULNAR NERVE

Brachial plexus;

Lateral cord

Posterior cord

Medial cord

MOTOR

SENSORY

Flexor carpi ulnaris

Flexor digitorum profundus, ulnar side only

Palmaris brevis

Flexor pollicis brevis (deep head)

Abductor digiti minimi

Opponens digiti minimi

Flexor digiti minimi brevis

Palmar and dorsal interossei (all)

Third and fourth lumbricals

Adductor pollicis

Figure 8-7 Distribution of the ulnar nerve.

Vessels

The brachial artery divides into the radial and ulnar arteries (Fig. 8-8) while lying anterior to the brachialis muscle and proximal to the pronator teres (see Fig. 8-5).

Radial artery

The **radial artery** courses distally and somewhat laterally. It gives off the *radial recurrent branch,* which runs anterior to the lateral aspect of the elbow to anastomose with the radial collateral branch of the profunda brachii artery. The radial artery continues distally, at first under cover of the brachioradialis but later covered only by skin and fascia, on the radial side of the anterior surface of the forearm. At the wrist, it winds dorsally deep to the extensor tendons of the thumb to follow a course that is described in connection with the hand.

Ulnar artery

The **ulnar artery** is at first larger than the radial artery. After passing behind the pronator teres, it continues between the two heads of the flexor digitorum superficialis, deep to which it gives off the *anterior and posterior ulnar recurrent arteries.* The anterior ulnar recurrent artery courses proximally, anterior to the medial epicondyle, and anastomoses with the inferior ulnar collateral artery (a branch of the brachial artery). Passing posterior to the medial epicondyle, the posterior ulnar recurrent artery anastomoses with the superior ulnar collateral artery (a branch of the brachial artery). The ulnar artery continues distally and gives off a large *common interosseous artery.* Appearing from under cover of the flexor digitorum superficialis, the ulnar artery passes distally under cover of the flexor carpi ulnaris and in company with the ulnar nerve and enters the hand superficial to the flexor retinaculum, on the radial side of the ulnar nerve. The common interosseous artery divides into *anterior and posterior interosseous* branches. The posterior interosseous artery passes between the radius and ulna, in the gap above the interosseous membrane, to supply blood to extensor muscles of the forearm. Near its origin, it gives off an *interosseous recurrent artery* that anastomoses with the middle collateral branch of the profunda brachii artery. The anterior interosseous artery passes distally with the corresponding branch of the median nerve. At the distal end of the forearm, it supplies *branches to the palmar surface of the wrist* and

Table 8-4	NERVES OF THE FLEXOR FOREARM		
	Muscles		
Nerve and Origin*	**Name**	**Segmental Innervation***	**Chief Action**
Median C5–T1	Pronator teres	C6, C7	Pronation of forearm
	Pronator quadratus	C8, T1	Pronation of forearm
	Flexor carpi radialis	C6, C7	Flexion at wrist
	Palmaris longus	C7, C8	Flexion at wrist
	Flexor digitorum superficialis	C7–T1	Flexion of middle phalanges of fingers
	Flexor pollicis longus	C8, T1	Flexion of distal phalanx of thumb
	Flexor digitorum profundus, radial part	C8, T1	Flexion of distal phalanges of second and third digits
Ulnar C8 and T1	Flexor digitorum profundus, ulnar part	C8, T1	Flexion of distal phalanges of fourth and fifth digits
	Flexor carpi ulnaris	C8, T1	Flexion-adduction at wrist

*A common segmental origin or innervation. The composition of both the chief nerves and their muscular branches varies somewhat among persons—the median nerve may contain no fibers from C5 or none from T1; the ulnar nerve frequently contains fibers from C7.

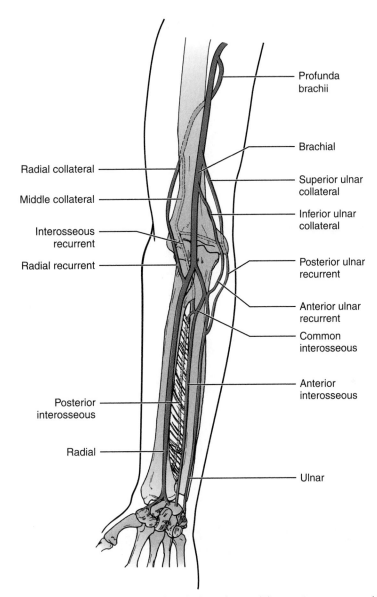

Figure 8-8 Radial and ulnar arteries and their major branches and the anastomoses around the elbow.

a larger *perforating branch* that passes through the interosseous membrane to supplement or unite with the lower end of the posterior interosseous artery.

Surface Anatomy

The superficial veins (described in Chapter 7) can often be seen fairly clearly, particularly in the area of the cubital fossa. The **basilic** *vein* (lying medially)

and **cephalic** *vein* (laterally) communicate by way of the **median cubital vein** near the cubital fossa.

The **radial artery** can be palpated, as is usually done in "checking" the pulse, by pressing it lightly against the radius, where it is superficially located in the lower part of the forearm. It lies lateral (radial) to the tendon of the flexor carpi radialis. The **ulnar artery** is difficult to palpate, but at the wrist it lies just lateral to the tendon of the flexor carpi ulnaris muscle and the pisiform bone. By knowing the locations of these vessels at the wrist and the position of the parent brachial artery just medial to the biceps tendon at the elbow, the approximate courses of the vessels can be visualized.

Of the nerves, the **ulnar nerve** can be identified posterior to the medial epicondyle just before it enters the forearm. It is under cover of or too close to the flexor carpi ulnaris to be palpable elsewhere. However, at the wrist it emerges from behind the lateral border of the tendon of this muscle and, with the ulnar artery lateral to it, passes across the radial side of the pisiform bone. It travels in practically a straight course down the forearm. The **median nerve** also runs almost straight down the middle of the forearm. Although it is not palpable, its course can be visualized because at the elbow it lies just medial to the tendon of the biceps, and at the wrist it lies posterior, or posterior and slightly lateral, to the tendon of the palmaris longus.

REVIEW QUESTIONS

1 Which muscles constitute the superficial flexor group of the forearm? Which muscles make up the deep group?

2 Provide a detailed description of both the origin and the insertion of the flexor digitorum superficialis. What is the action of the muscle? How are the tendons of the flexor digitorum superficialis arranged as they reach the wrist?

3 Which of the flexor muscles in the forearm receive motor innervation from the ulnar nerve?

4 The tendon of which muscle passes superficial to the flexor retinaculum? What is the relationship of the median nerve to the flexor retinaculum?

5 In the forearm, the brachial artery divides into which branches? Describe the course of those branches.

6 Describe the arterial anastomoses around the elbow.

EXERCISES

1 Demonstrate the palpable bony landmarks of the distal part of the arm and proximal part of the forearm.

2 Describe and demonstrate the course of the median nerve in the forearm. A complete section of the median nerve above the elbow would affect which muscles. A lesion of the median nerve in the distal third of the forearm would have what effect? Would either lesion affect the sensory innervation to the skin on the anterior surface of the forearm?

3 Identify the following on yourself or another student:
   a ulnar nerve as it passes posterior to the medial epicondyle
   b bicipital aponeurosis
   c tendon of the palmaris longus muscle, if present
   d tendon of the flexor carpi radialis muscle

9 EXTENSOR FOREARM

CHAPTER CONTENTS

Muscles

Nerves and Vessels

MUSCLES

The superficial nerves and vessels and the fascia of the posterior side of the forearm are described in Chapter 7. Of the muscles of the extensor forearm, not all are placed posteriorly. Some arise from the anterior aspect of the distal end of the humerus, pass across the anterior aspect of the elbow joint, and are visible anteriorly (e.g., see Fig. 8-1). Some muscles, however, are entirely posteriorly placed, and the insertions of the extensor muscles are almost entirely on the lateral and posterior sides of the limb (Fig. 9-1). The tendons of the extensor muscles that cross the wrist are housed in a number of separate compartments deep to a special thickening of the deep fascia, the **extensor retinaculum** (Fig. 9-2). Each compartment has a single synovial sheath; where two or more tendons share a compartment, they also share the sheath.

The extensor muscles are conveniently divided into two groups: superficial and deep. All members of the superficial group have an origin from the humerus (at or around the lateral epicondyle), but most of those of the deep group do not. In the distal part of the posterior side of the forearm, some of the members of the deep group (muscles to the thumb) become superficial and cover some of the superficial muscles. The **superficial extensor forearm muscles** are the *brachioradialis, extensor carpi radialis longus, extensor carpi radialis brevis, extensor digitorum, extensor digiti minimi,* and *extensor carpi ulnaris* (see Fig. 9-2).

The **deep extensor muscles** are the *supinator, extensor indicis,* and the three thumb muscles: *abductor pollicis longus, extensor pollicis brevis,* and *extensor pollicis longus* (Fig. 9-3).

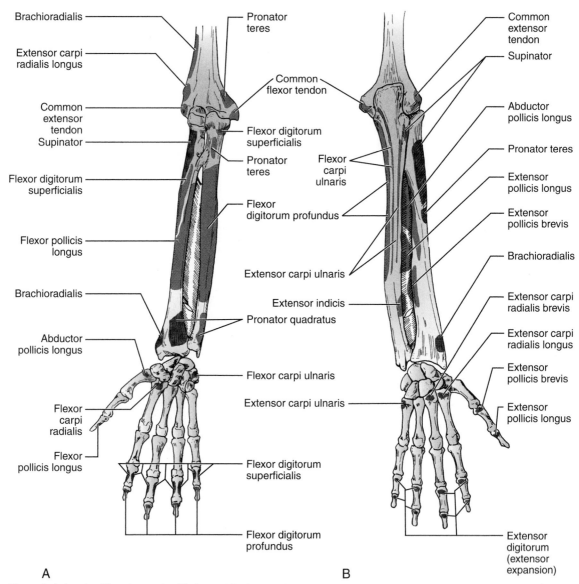

Brachioradialis
Extensor carpi radialis longus
Common extensor tendon
Supinator
Flexor digitorum superficialis
Flexor pollicis longus
Brachioradialis
Abductor pollicis longus
Flexor carpi radialis
Flexor pollicis longus

Pronator teres
Common flexor tendon
Flexor digitorum superficialis
Pronator teres
Flexor digitorum profundus
Extensor carpi ulnaris
Pronator quadratus
Flexor carpi ulnaris
Extensor carpi ulnaris
Flexor digitorum superficialis
Flexor digitorum profundus

Common extensor tendon
Supinator
Abductor pollicis longus
Pronator teres
Extensor pollicis longus
Extensor pollicis brevis
Brachioradialis
Extensor carpi radialis brevis
Extensor carpi radialis longus
Extensor pollicis brevis
Extensor pollicis longus
Extensor digitorum (extensor expansion)

Flexor carpi ulnaris
Extensor indicis

A

B

Figure 9-1 Anterior **(A)** and posterior **(B)** views of the bones of the elbow region, forearm, and hand, illustrating origins *(color)* and insertions *(black)* of flexor and extensor muscles of the forearm.

The radial nerve innervates all the muscles of the extensor surface of the forearm.

Superficial Muscles

Brachioradialis

The **brachioradialis** (barely visible in Fig. 9-2, but better seen in Fig. 8-1) is the most anterior member of the superficial group. Its *origin* is anteriorly from the lateral supracondylar ridge of the humerus and from the lateral intermuscular septum of the arm (Table 9-1). The *insertion* of the brachioradialis is on the lateral side of the distal end of the radius. Its primary *action* is to flex the forearm, and it is used particularly to add speed or power to this movement. It may pronate from a position of supination and may

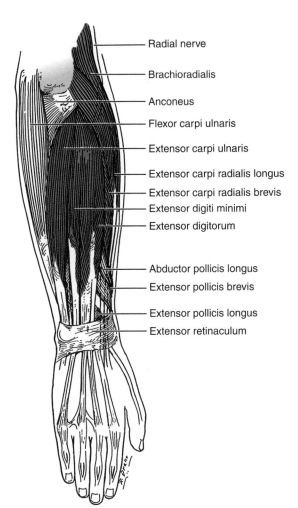

Figure 9-2 The superficial extensor muscles *(color)* of the right forearm.

Labels (from top):
- Radial nerve
- Brachioradialis
- Anconeus
- Flexor carpi ulnaris
- Extensor carpi ulnaris
- Extensor carpi radialis longus
- Extensor carpi radialis brevis
- Extensor digiti minimi
- Extensor digitorum
- Abductor pollicis longus
- Extensor pollicis brevis
- Extensor pollicis longus
- Extensor retinaculum

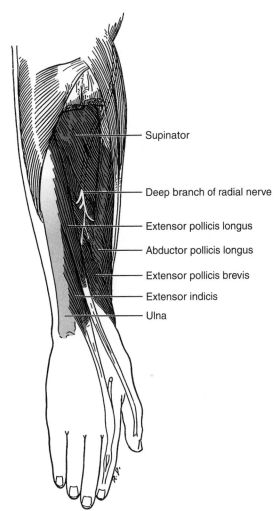

Figure 9-3 The deeper extensor muscles *(color)* of the right forearm.

Labels (from top):
- Supinator
- Deep branch of radial nerve
- Extensor pollicis longus
- Abductor pollicis longus
- Extensor pollicis brevis
- Extensor indicis
- Ulna

supinate from one of pronation. It is not efficient and may not be normally used in either action, but, apparently, it can pronate better than it can supinate.

Extensor carpi radialis longus and extensor carpi radialis brevis

Partly under cover of the brachioradialis, the **extensor carpi radialis longus** has its *origin* largely from the lateral supracondylar ridge of the humerus and the lateral intermuscular septum (see Fig. 9-2). Its lowest fibers arise from the lateral epicondyle by a common extensor tendon, which it shares with other muscles of the superficial group. Closely associated with it is

the **extensor carpi radialis brevis.** Its *origin* and that of the remaining superficial muscles are not only from the epicondyle but also from intermuscular septa and the covering antebrachial fascia. The two muscles can be traced distally, deep to the extensor muscles of the thumb and then deep to the extensor retinaculum (sharing a common compartment and synovial sheath), to their *insertions* on the bases of the second metacarpal (for the longus) and third metacarpal (for the brevis). The *action* of both muscles is to extend the hand, and the extensor carpi radialis longus, at least, helps abduct it. In extending the hand, the extensor carpi radialis brevis apparently acts alone unless more speed

Table 9-1	SUPERFICIAL MUSCLES OF THE EXTENSOR FOREARM			
Muscle	**Origin (Proximal Attachment)**	**Insertion (Distal Attachment)**	**Action**	**Innervation**
Brachioradialis	Lateral supracondylar ridge of humerus; lateral intermuscular septum of arm	Lateral side of distal end of radius	Flexion of forearm	Radial nerve
Extensor carpi radialis longus	Lateral supracondylar ridge and lateral intermuscular septum; epicondyle of humerus (common extensor tendon)	Base of second metacarpal	Extension and abduction (radial deviation) of hand	Radial nerve
Extensor carpi radialis brevis	Lateral epicondyle of humerus (common extensor tendon); intermuscular septa; antebrachial fascia	Base of third metacarpal	Extension of hand	Radial nerve
Extensor digitorum	Lateral epicondyle of humerus (common extensor tendon); intermuscular septa; antebrachial fascia	Middle and distal phalanges of each of four fingers (medial four digits)	Extension of each of four fingers (medial four digits)	Radial nerve
Extensor digiti minimi	Lateral epicondyle of humerus (common extensor tendon) and intermuscular septa in common with the extensor digitorum	Middle and distal phalanges of little finger	Extension and abduction of little finger	Radial nerve
Extensor carpi ulnaris	Lateral epicondyle of humerus (common extensor tendon); proximal half of posterior border of ulna	Base of fifth metacarpal	Extension and adduction (ulnar deviation) of hand	Radial nerve

or power is required. Probably the long extensor, and perhaps the short one, can contribute to flexion of the forearm.

Extensor digitorum

The **extensor digitorum** occupies much of the posterior surface of the forearm. Its *origin* is from the lateral epicondyle, intermuscular septa, and the antebrachial fascia, and it splits into three or four tendons as it reaches the wrist. These tendons pass deep to the extensor retinaculum in a synovial sheath common to them and another muscle, the extensor indicis. On the hand, they diverge to the four fingers, but the tendons are united by obliquely placed bands that limit the independent movement of any one tendon. The tendon of the little finger is typically small and may not be present.

The extensor tendon to the index finger and, if present, that to the little finger unite with the tendons of the extensor indicis and the extensor digiti minimi,

respectively. On the fingers, the tendons receive the insertions of the interossei and of the lumbrical muscles in the hand. The *insertion* of the extensor digitorum is on both middle and distal phalanges (see Chapter 12 for a more detailed description). Expansions from the tendons form the posterior capsules of the metacarpophalangeal and interphalangeal joints. The *action* of the extensor digitorum is to extend all joints of the fingers, but it can extend the interphalangeal joints only when the metacarpophalangeal joints are kept from hyperextending.

Extensor digiti minimi

Closely associated with the extensor digitorum and appearing indeed as an ulnar portion of this muscle is the **extensor digiti minimi.** Its *origin* is in common with that of the extensor digitorum. The tendon of the extensor digiti minimi diverges at the wrist and passes through its own compartment deep to the extensor retinaculum. On the dorsum of the hand, its tendon is usually doubled. The radial, or undivided, tendon receives the extensor digitorum tendon to the little finger, or a slip from the tendon to the ring finger, and the combined tendons have *insertions* on the middle and distal phalanges of the little finger. The *action* of the muscle is to extend and to abduct the little finger.

Extensor carpi ulnaris

The **extensor carpi ulnaris** has an *origin* in part from the lateral epicondyle and more extensively from somewhat more than the proximal half of the posterior border of the ulna. Its tendon passes in its own compartment deep to the extensor retinaculum and then to an *insertion* on the base of the fifth metacarpal. The *action* of the extensor carpi ulnaris is to aid in extension and adduction (ulnar deviation) of the hand.

Deep Muscles

Supinator

Of the deep muscles, the **supinator** is the most proximal (Table 9-2). Its *origin* is from the posterolateral surface of the ulna just distal to the radial notch, from the lateral epicondyle, and from the radial collateral and annular ligaments. It passes obliquely (in a distal and lateral direction) across the arm to an *insertion* on the lateral and adjacent posterior and anterior aspects of the radius for a considerable distance below the radial head. The deep radial nerve separates its fibers into a superficial and a deep lamina. As its name indicates, the *action* of the muscle is to supinate the forearm and, therefore, the hand.

Abductor pollicis longus, extensor pollicis brevis, and extensor pollicis longus

Of the three muscles of the thumb, the first two emerge between the extensor digitorum and the radial extensors and cross superficial to the latter. The **abductor pollicis longus** has *origins* in three places: the posterior surfaces of both the ulna and the radius below the insertion of the supinator and the intervening interosseous membrane. Its *insertion* is on the front (radial side) of the base of the first metacarpal. Often the tendon splits to attach also to the trapezium or to fascia or muscles of the thenar eminence. The **extensor pollicis brevis** is partly covered by the abductor longus. Its *origin* is from the radius and the

Table 9-2	DEEP MUSCLES OF THE EXTENSOR FOREARM			
Muscle	**Origin (Proximal Attachment)**	**Insertion (Distal Attachment)**	**Action**	**Innervation**
Supinator	Posterolateral surface of ulna below radial notch; lateral epicondyle; radial collateral and annular ligaments	Lateral and adjacent posterior and anterior aspects of proximal shaft of radius	Supination of forearm (and hand)	Radial nerve
Abductor pollicis longus	Posterior surface of ulna and radius; interosseous membrane	Base of first metacarpal	Abduction and extension of thumb; abduction and flexion of hand at wrist	Radial nerve
Extensor pollicis brevis	Posterior surface of radius; interosseous membrane	Proximal phalanx of thumb	Extension of proximal phalanx and metacarpal of thumb; abduction of hand at wrist	Radial nerve
Extensor pollicis longus	Posterior surface of middle third of ulna; interosseous membrane	Distal phalanx of thumb	Extension of proximal and distal phalanges of thumb; extension and adduction of metacarpal of thumb	Radial nerve
Extensor indicis	Posterior surface of ulna; interosseous membrane	Extensor expansion of index finger	Extension and adduction of index finger	Radial nerve

interosseous membrane below the radial origin of the long abductor, and its *insertion* is on the proximal phalanx of the thumb. The long abductor and this muscle usually share a compartment and synovial sheath deep to the extensor retinaculum. The **extensor pollicis longus** takes *origin* from about the middle third of the ulna and the adjacent interosseous membrane, largely distal to the origin of the long abductor. Its tendon crosses the wrist, obliquely, to proceed along the thumb to an *insertion* on the distal phalanx. It also crosses superficially to the radial extensors, but at the wrist rather than in the forearm.

The *action* of the abductor pollicis longus is to extend and externally rotate the first metacarpal, restoring (repositioning) this bone to its normal position after opposition of the thumb. By virtue of its location at the wrist, it is also both an abductor and a flexor of the hand. The *action* of the extensor pollicis brevis is to extend both the proximal phalanx and the metacarpal of the thumb. The *action* of the extensor pollicis longus is to extend both phalanges and to extend and to adduct the metacarpal. The extensor pollicis brevis may also help to abduct the hand at the wrist, and the extensor pollicis longus helps extend it.

Extensor indicis

The **extensor indicis** has its *origin* from the ulna and interosseous membrane distal to the origin of the extensor pollicis longus. Its tendon runs laterally across the wrist, within the synovial sheath for the extensor digitorum, to join the medial side of this muscle's radial tendon at the distal end of the second metacarpal. The *insertion* of the extensor indicis is into the extensor expansion or aponeurosis. The *action* of this muscle, like that of the extensor digitorum, is to extend all joints of the index finger; it also adducts this finger.

Surface Anatomy

The muscular bulge that forms the lateral border of the cubital fossa is produced by three muscles: *brachioradialis, extensor carpi radialis longus,* and *extensor carpi radialis brevis.* The **brachioradialis** can be differentiated by forceful flexion of the forearm with the thumb up; it then stands out at the elbow lateral to the biceps tendon. Contraction of the **extensor carpi radialis longus** and **extensor carpi radialis brevis** can

be palpated when the wrist is extended. On the posterior side of the limb, the muscle belly of the **extensor digitorum** can be felt when the fingers are extended, and its tendons and those of the extensors of the index and little fingers can be palpated and frequently visualized beneath the skin of the dorsum of the hand.

There are five tendons palpable or visually evident at the wrist. Beginning on the ulnar side, the first tendon is the **extensor carpi ulnaris**, largely covering the styloid process of the ulna. The second is the **extensor digitorum** in the middle of the wrist. The third, the **extensor pollicis longus,** runs obliquely from the posterior surface of the wrist onto the dorsum of the thumb, at the junction of posterior and lateral (radial) surfaces of the wrist. Anterior to the extensor pollicis longus, and almost at the junction of the lateral and anterior surfaces of the wrist, are the fourth and fifth tendons, those of the **extensor pollicis brevis** and **abductor pollicis longus**.

The depression on the radial side of the wrist, which is accentuated by extension and abduction of the thumb, is often called the **anatomical snuffbox**. It is bounded posteriorly by the *tendon of the extensor pollicis longus* and anteriorly by those of the *extensor pollicis brevis and abductor pollicis longus*. The tendon of the extensor pollicis brevis overlies that of the long abductor at the wrist, but it is thinner and, when the thumb is extended, can usually be traced some distance along the metacarpal. The broader tendon of the long abductor inserts on the base of the metacarpal and is best visualized by slight flexion and abduction (radial deviation) of the hand. The **radial artery** can frequently be palpated in the anatomical snuffbox as it runs onto the dorsal surface of the hand. The **scaphoid** and **trapezium** are located in the floor of the snuffbox and can be palpated there; tenderness in the snuffbox upon palpation may indicate fracture of, in particular, the scaphoid bone.

NERVES AND VESSELS
Nerves

Radial nerve

The **radial nerve** emerges from its position deep to the triceps brachii on the lateral side of the distal part of the arm to lie between the brachialis muscle and first the brachioradialis and then the extensor carpi radialis longus muscle (Fig. 9-4). In this position, it gives off branches to both the brachioradialis and the extensor carpi radialis longus; the nerve supply to the brevis arises more distally from the radial nerve proper or from one of the two chief branches of this nerve. Soon after it enters the forearm, the radial nerve splits into superficial and deep branches.

The *superficial branch* of the radial nerve lies under cover of the brachioradialis muscle for much of its course. It emerges from deep to the tendon of this muscle in the distal part of the forearm to be distributed both to skin on the dorsum of the hand and to a variable number of joints.

The *deep branch* of the radial nerve (Fig. 9-5) plunges into the supinator muscle, supplying innervation to

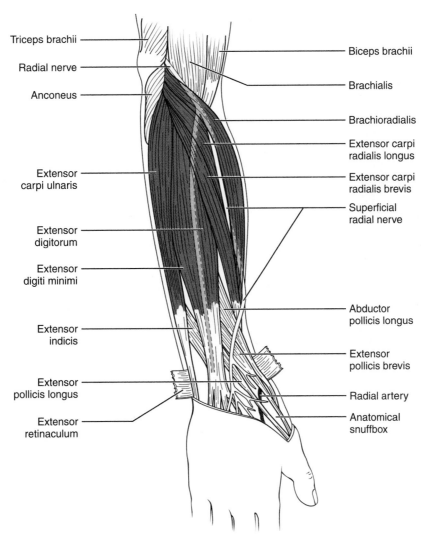

Figure 9-4 Posterior aspect of the forearm. The course of the radial nerve and its superficial and deep branches are illustrated *(dotted lines* indicate the course of the nerves deep to the muscles). The brachioradialis is reflected laterally to show a portion of the superficial radial branch that lies between it and the extensor carpi radialis. Most of the extensor retinaculum is not depicted, but two parts remain to indicate its position. The superficial extensor muscles are *shown in color.*

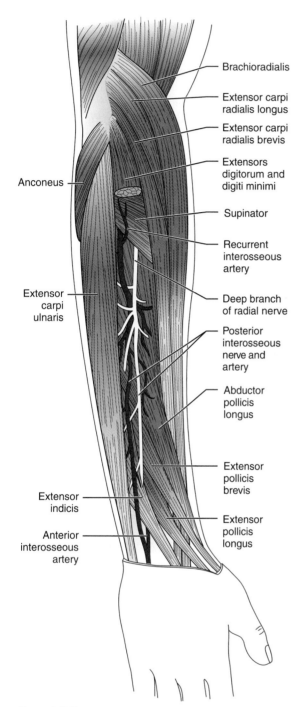

Brachioradialis

Extensor carpi radialis longus

Extensor carpi radialis brevis

Extensors digitorum and digiti minimi

Supinator

Recurrent interosseous artery

Deep branch of radial nerve

Posterior interosseous nerve and artery

Abductor pollicis longus

Extensor pollicis brevis

Extensor pollicis longus

Anconeus

Extensor carpi ulnaris

Extensor indicis

Anterior interosseous artery

Figure 9-5 Nerves and arteries of the posterior aspect of the forearm. The extensor digitorum and extensor digiti minimi are omitted in order to show the deep branch of the radial nerve and deep arteries.

this as it passes through, and then follows the muscle around the radius to reach the posterior aspect of the forearm. Here, under cover of the superficial posterior extensor muscles, it divides into a number of branches to the remaining extensor muscles, just as it emerges at the lower border of the supinator. The continuation of the deep radial nerve, called the *posterior interosseous nerve,* extends distally in company with the posterior interosseous artery across the superficial surface of the abductor pollicis longus and gives off one or more branches into each of the long thumb muscles and the extensor of the index finger. A small branch continues deep to the extensor pollicis longus, on the interosseous membrane, to the wrist joint. The distribution of the radial nerve is shown diagrammatically in Figure 9-6.

FUNCTIONAL/CLINICAL NOTE 9-1

The radial nerve is especially susceptible to injury when fracture of the shaft of the humerus occurs, because of its close association with that bone. This usually occurs when the fracture is in the distal third of the bone, in which case the triceps brachii is spared because it receives its innervation more proximally. The nerve may also be entrapped by fibrous bands associated with the lateral head of the triceps brachii or with the entrance of the deep branch into the supinator. In the former case, many of the nerve branches to the muscle are spared; in the latter, as would also happen in a fracture of the proximal third or half of the radius, the brachioradialis and the two radial extensors would also be spared.

Paralysis of all of the extensors of the wrist and digits (produced by a complete lesion to the radial nerve in the arm) results in **wristdrop,** which is evident when the forearm and hand are pronated and held horizontally with the fingers relaxed (see Fig. 11-17, *C*). In this position, the hand hangs loosely downward. Making a fist or trying to grasp an object in this position pulls upon the extensor tendons, tightening them and producing some passive extension at the wrist, but a firm grip is not possible without further extension at the wrist. If the forearm and hand are supinated rather than pronated, action of the flexors of the fingers (and the grip) would be improved as a result of increased extension at the wrist caused by gravity. In wristdrop, the phalanges cannot be extended because their extensors are also paralyzed. However, if the metacarpophalangeal joints are fixed in extension, muscles in the palm can extend the remaining phalanges.

A hand with wristdrop is useless; therefore, if the nerve does not regenerate, it is necessary to restore extension at the wrist by other means. This can be done by transferring flexor tendons to the dorsum to extend both wrist and fingers. One flexor of the wrist, however, must always be left in position; otherwise, the wrist is so sharply extended that a good grasp is impossible.

If the lesion to the radial nerve is above the origin of the superficial branch, there is some loss of sensation on the dorsum of the hand. This is always somewhat limited and is situated between the first and second metacarpals.

Segmental innervation

The radial nerve, arising as it does from the posterior cord of the brachial plexus, can receive fibers from all the anterior rami entering into the brachial plexus. Actually, however, the posterior division of the lower trunk (C8 and T1) to the posterior cord is usually small, and the radial nerve often receives only C8 fibers through it. The radial nerve contains fibers derived mostly from C5, C6, C7, and C8, and the number coming into the nerve from C5 appears to be variable. The brachioradialis and the supinator are supplied primarily from C5 and C6, especially the latter. The extensor carpi radialis longus and brevis regularly receive fibers from C6 and C7 and often from either C5 or C8 or from both. The extensor digitorum, extensor digiti minimi, and abductor pollicis longus are supplied with fibers from approximately C6, C7, and C8, mainly

C7. The remaining muscles—extensor carpi ulnaris, extensor indicis, extensor pollicis longus, and extensor pollicis brevis—all receive fibers from C7 and C8.

FUNCTIONAL/CLINICAL NOTE 9-2

On the basis of the segmental distribution of nerve fibers in the radial nerve, it is evident that lesions of the brachial plexus that involve C6, C7, and C8 markedly affect the extensor forearm muscles. If the deficit is great enough, wristdrop may be apparent. Segmental innervation is summarized in Table 9-3.

Vessels

Posterior interosseous artery

The more anterior extensor muscles are supplied by a recurrent branch from the radial artery that runs up along them and the radial nerve anterior to the lateral epicondyle, but the **posterior interosseous artery** (see Fig. 9-5) is the chief vessel supplying blood to the extensor muscles on the posterior side. After leaving the common interosseous artery on the anterior side of the forearm, it passes between the radius and ulna to reach the posterior aspect deep to the supinator muscle. It then courses distally on the interosseous membrane, giving off branches to the various muscles. At the wrist, it may be reinforced by the perforating branch of the anterior interosseous artery, and the latter vessel or the common terminal stem formed by the two arteries supplies branches to the dorsal aspect of the wrist.

Surface Anatomy

None of the nerves of the extensor forearm are palpable. The course of each was described previously. The **venous plexus on the dorsum of the hand** is usually evident. These veins are tributaries of the cephalic and basilic veins. The **radial artery** is palpable in the anatomical snuffbox. Its pulse is normally taken anterior to this area, just lateral to the tendon of the flexor carpi radialis.

RADIAL/AXILLARY NERVES

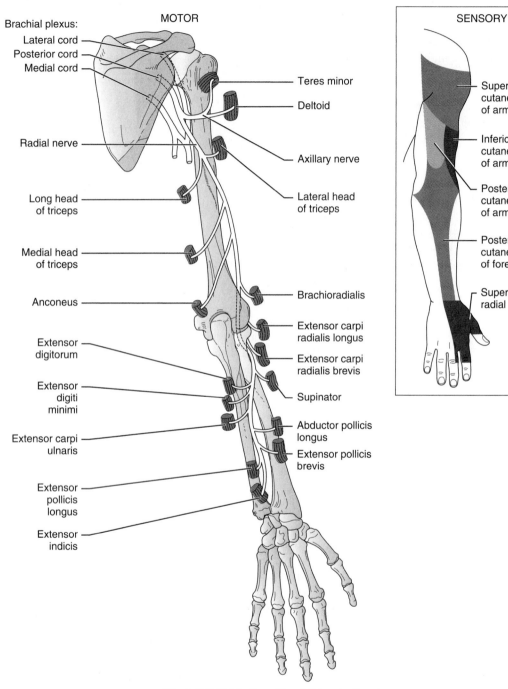

MOTOR

SENSORY

Brachial plexus:
Lateral cord
Posterior cord
Medial cord

Radial nerve

Long head
of triceps

Medial head
of triceps

Anconeus

Extensor
digitorum

Extensor
digiti
minimi

Extensor carpi
ulnaris

Extensor
pollicis
longus

Extensor
indicis

Teres minor

Deltoid

Axillary nerve

Lateral head
of triceps

Brachioradialis

Extensor carpi
radialis longus

Extensor carpi
radialis brevis

Supinator

Abductor pollicis
longus

Extensor pollicis
brevis

Superior lateral
cutaneous nerve
of arm (axillary)

Inferior lateral
cutaneous nerve
of arm (radial)

Posterior
cutaneous nerve
of arm (radial)

Posterior
cutaneous nerve
of forearm (radial)

Superficial
radial nerve

Figure 9-6 Distribution of the radial and axillary nerves.

Table 9-3	NERVES OF THE EXTENSOR FOREARM		
	Muscle		
Nerve and Origin*	**Name**	**Segmental Innervation***	**Chief Action**
Radial	Brachioradialis	C5, C6	Flexion at elbow
C5–C8	Extensor carpi radialis longus and brevis	C6, C7	Extension-abduction at wrist
	Extensor carpi ulnaris	C7, C8	Extension-adduction at wrist
	Supinator	C5, C6	Supination of forearm
	Extensor digitorum	C6–C8	Extension of all joints of second to fifth digits
	Extensor digiti minimi	C6–C8	Extension of all joints of fifth digit
	Extensor indicis	C7, C8	Extension of all joints of second digit
	Extensor pollicis longus	C7, C8	Extension of both phalanges and extension and adduction of metacarpal of thumb
	Extensor pollicis brevis	C7, C8	Extension of proximal phalanx and metacarpal of thumb; abduction at wrist
	Abductor pollicis longus	C6–C8	Extension and abduction (reposition) of thumb; flexion and abduction at wrist

*A common segmental origin or innervation. The composition of both the radial nerve and its muscular branches varies among persons. The radial nerve may receive fibers from T1 and may receive few or no motor fibers from C5.

REVIEW QUESTIONS

1 What is the action of the brachioradialis muscle at the elbow? Does it have any action at the wrist? Why?

2 Name the muscles that comprise the deep extensor group of the forearm. What is the action of each muscle?

3 What is wristdrop? What nerve and muscles are involved?

4 Is a firmer grip possible with the hand flexed or extended at the wrist? Why?

5 Sensory innervation to the skin on the dorsum of the hand between the first and second metacarpals is provided by what specific branch of the radial nerve?

6 What is the primary arterial supply to the extensor muscles of the forearm?

7 Which tendons define the borders of the anatomical snuffbox? Which carpal bones can be palpated within the snuffbox?

8 What is the segmental innervation of the following muscles?
   a extensor digiti minimi
   b extensor carpi radialis longus
   c abductor pollicis longus

EXERCISES

1 On a skeleton, demonstrate the origin and insertion of each muscle comprising the superficial extensor group of the forearm.

2 Identify the palpable tendons on the posterior and lateral aspects of the wrist and the posterior aspect of the hand.

10 RADIOULNAR AND WRIST MOVEMENTS

CHAPTER CONTENTS

Movements at the Radioulnar Joints

Movements at the Wrist Joint

Analyses of Activities and Associated Movements

The descriptions provided in the preceding chapters demonstrate that the forearm muscles may act on the elbow joint, the wrist joint, or the fingers and thumb. The part played by the brachioradialis and other forearm muscles in flexion at the elbow has been described, and movements of the fingers can best be considered after the muscles of the hand have been studied. In this chapter, the movements of pronation and supination of the forearm and movements of the hand at the wrist are considered.

MOVEMENTS AT THE RADIOULNAR JOINTS

These movements are those of pronation and supination, which are used in such common actions as in turning a doorknob or a screwdriver. **Pronation** is produced by a number of muscles (Fig. 10-1). The *pronator quadratus* pronates alone until further strength or speed is needed, at which time the *pronator teres* also contracts. The *flexor carpi radialis* apparently pronates after it has first flexed the wrist. Based upon its anatomy, the *brachioradialis* is capable of bringing the hand to an intermediate (semi-prone) position from either a pronated or supinated position.

Normally, the brachioradialis contributes little to pronation, but it is a better pronator than it is a supinator. It participates in pronation only when the movement is resisted or when the pronator teres and pronator quadratus are paralyzed.

FUNCTIONAL/CLINICAL NOTE 10-1

The pronator quadratus, pronator teres, flexor carpi radialis, and palmaris longus muscles are innervated by the median nerve; therefore, lesions of the median nerve above the elbow markedly weaken pronation but do not abolish it.

Supination is a much stronger movement than pronation, because it is brought about not only by the *supinator* but also by the *biceps brachii* (Fig. 10-2). The supinator may act alone, but the biceps brachii supplies most of the power. The biceps brachii is most effective when the forearm is flexed, contracting for supination of the extended forearm only when the movement is resisted. The brachioradialis and, to a lesser extent, the extensor carpi radialis longus are anatomically positioned to assist in supination. However, their affects are limited.

FUNCTIONAL/CLINICAL NOTE 10-2

The greater strength supplied by the biceps brachii is reflected in the design of screws. A right-handed person must supinate to drive the screw into wood.

The muscles producing supination are supplied by either the musculocutaneous nerve (to the biceps brachii) or the radial nerve. Because most of the muscles receive fibers from spinal nerves C5 and C6, much of the strength of this important movement may be expected to be lost in damage to the upper trunk or lateral cord of the plexus. The supinator and extensor carpi radialis longus may also receive fibers from other cervical nerves, especially C7, and therefore may retain some function in a lesion of the upper trunk.

MOVEMENTS AT THE WRIST JOINT

These movements have already been defined as **flexion, extension, abduction** (radial deviation), and **adduction** (ulnar deviation). The amount of

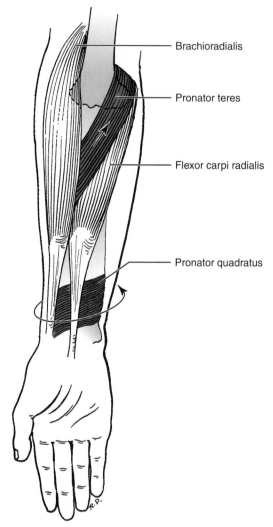

Figure 10-1 Pronators of the forearm. The most important pronators are highlighted with *color*. Note their general direction of pull, resulting from the fact that they run obliquely from ulnar to radial side.

movement in any of these directions varies greatly from one person to another, varies appreciably according to whether the hand is pronated or supinated, and may even vary somewhat between the two hands of the same person. Because of the ellipsoidal nature of the radiocarpal joint, rotation there is minimal.

With the single exception of the flexor carpi ulnaris, all the muscles acting primarily upon the wrist pass across the carpals to attach to the metacarpals.

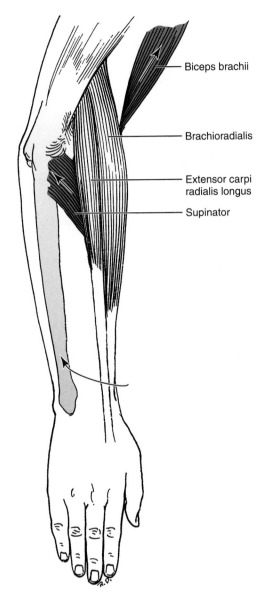

Biceps brachii

Brachioradialis

Extensor carpi radialis longus

Supinator

Figure 10-2 Supinators of the forearm (the most important supinators are hightlighted with *color*). The prevailing direction of these is an oblique one from ulnar to radial side. The obliquity of the brachioradialis and extensor carpi radialis longus is increased considerably by pronation; therefore, these muscles can presumably supinate no farther than to about the neutral position between pronation and supination. They certainly contribute little strength, and whether they are normally used in supination is doubtful. The biceps brachii is a strong supinator because of its insertion on the anteromedial surface of the radius.

The flexor carpi ulnaris may be considered as inserting upon the fifth metacarpal through a pisometacarpal ligament that represents a distal part of the tendon. Therefore, all of these muscles exert an action not only on the radiocarpal joint but also across the intercarpal joints. The joint between the two rows of carpals (midcarpal joint; see Chapter 11) is particularly important, for the additional movement occurring between the proximal and distal rows increases the total amount of movement at the wrist considerably. Therefore, the midcarpal joint contributes more to flexion than does the radiocarpal joint, and it also contributes appreciably to extension. The midcarpal joint contributes almost all of the limited movement of abduction. Only in adduction (ulnar deviation) does the midcarpal joint fail to contribute significantly to the movement of the radiocarpal joint.

Flexion of the hand is brought about primarily through the *flexor carpi radialis* and *flexor carpi ulnaris*. Also assisting in this action are the *palmaris longus* and *abductor pollicis longus* (Fig. 10-3). The *flexor digitorum superficialis* and *flexor digitorum profundus* assist in wrist flexion only if the digits are kept extended. Their range of action is too short to allow them to flex the fingers and wrist simultaneously.

Extension of the hand is brought about by the *extensor carpi radialis longus, extensor carpi radialis brevis* and *extensor carpi ulnaris;* pure extension may be produced by the extensor carpi radialis brevis alone. For more power, both the extensor carpi radialis longus and extensor carpi ulnaris both contract, each overcoming the tendency of the other to abduct or adduct the hand, respectively (Fig. 10-4). The *extensor digitorum, extensor digiti minimi, extensor indicis,* and *extensor pollicis longus* can assist in wrist extension if the fist is clenched.

Abduction of the hand at the wrist (radial deviation) is brought about by the *extensor carpi radialis longus* and *flexor carpi radialis*. The *abductor pollicis longus, extensor pollicis brevis, extensor carpi radialis brevis,* and *extensor pollicis longus* may also participate in abduction (Fig. 10-5). **Adduction** (ulnar deviation) is brought about by the combined actions of the *extensor carpi ulnaris* and *flexor carpi ulnaris* (see Fig. 10-5).

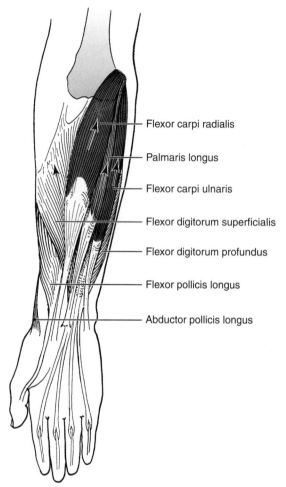

Flexor carpi radialis

Palmaris longus

Flexor carpi ulnaris

Flexor digitorum superficialis

Flexor digitorum profundus

Flexor pollicis longus

Abductor pollicis longus

Figure 10-3 Flexors at the wrist. The flexor carpi radialis and the flexor carpi ulnaris are the muscles most directly involved with flexion *(dark color)*. The palmaris longus and abductor pollicis longus assist in this movement *(light color)*; the flexor digitorum superficialis and flexor digitorum profundus can assist best in flexion at the wrist if the digits are extended.

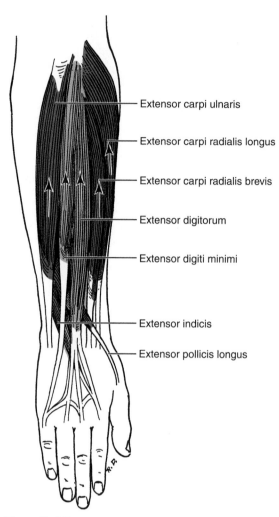

Extensor carpi ulnaris

Extensor carpi radialis longus

Extensor carpi radialis brevis

Extensor digitorum

Extensor digiti minimi

Extensor indicis

Extensor pollicis longus

Figure 10-4 Extensors at the wrist. The muscles highlighted are involved primarily in extension, and the *light colored* muscles may assist in this movement.

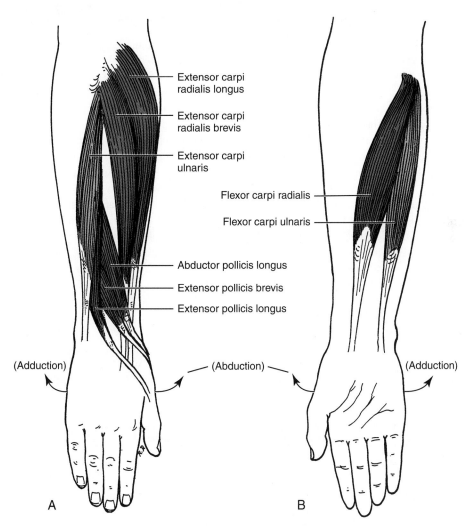

Figure 10-5 Abductors *(dark colored)* and adductors *(light colored)* at the wrist. **A,** Posterior view. **B,** Anterior view.

FUNCTIONAL/CLINICAL NOTE 10-3

The flexors of the wrist joint are innervated by all three nerves of the forearm: median (to most of the muscles), ulnar (flexor carpi ulnaris and part of the flexor digitorum profundus), and radial (abductor pollicis longus). The abductor pollicis longus can flex the wrist when it alone is acting; therefore, even combined injury to both median and ulnar nerves may not totally abolish wrist flexion. The flexors of the wrist, however, receive most of their innervation from C7, C8, and T1. Consequently, injuries to the lower part of the brachial plexus affects wrist flexion more markedly than do injuries to the upper part of the plexus.

All the extensors of the wrist are supplied by the radial nerve with fibers from C6, C7, and C8. If all the wrist extensors are paralyzed by a lesion of the radial nerve or posterior cord (a condition called *wristdrop*, described in Chapter 9), the wrist can nonetheless be straightened by making a fist. Such flexion of the fingers would create tension on the extensor tendons, thereby causing the hand to be extended at the wrist.

Abduction at the wrist involves both the median and radial nerves, whereas adduction at the wrist involves ulnar and radial nerves. The abductors as a group are supplied by most segments contributing to the brachial plexus; both the two adductors (extensor carpi ulnaris and flexor carpi ulnaris) may receive fibers from C8, but they otherwise have no innervation in common.

As a group, the forearm muscles acting across the wrist (as well as the intrinsic muscles of the hand) receive most of their innervation through the lower portion of the brachial plexus. *Erb (Erb-Duchenne) paralysis* (see Chapter 5), or injury to the upper portion of the plexus (C5 and C6), affects especially muscles of the shoulder and arm. *Klumpke (Klumpke-Dejerine) paralysis*, involving injury to C7, C8, and T1, affects most of the muscles of the forearm and hand and is characterized by severe disabling of the wrist and fingers.

ANALYSES OF ACTIVITIES AND ASSOCIATED MOVEMENTS

Activity: *Hammering a Nail.* The movements at the radioulnar joints (pronation/supination) and those at the wrist joint (flexion/extension and abduction/adduction) have been described in the previous sections. Most activities are the result of more than one movement and the coordinated involvement of several muscles. Consider movements and muscles of the forearm involved in hammering a nail. Gripping the handle of the hammer involves flexion of the fingers, opposition of the thumb (which is produced by a combination of flexion, abduction, and adduction of the thumb), and some extension of the hand at the wrist to enable proper action of the flexors of the fingers to produce a firm grip. Muscles of the forearm that are involved in flexion of the fingers are the flexor digitorum superficialis and flexor digitorum profundus. Opposition of the thumb is produced by the flexor pollicis longus in the forearm and several muscles of the hand, which are discussed in Chapter 11. Extension at the wrist is produced mainly by the extensor carpi radialis longus, extensor carpi radialis brevis, and extensor carpi ulnaris.

Once the hammer is firmly gripped, the hand would normally be maintained in a midposition between pronation and supination, requiring action by both the pronators (primarily the pronator quadratus, but possibly the pronator teres) and the supinators (supinator and biceps brachii). Holding the hammer in this position requires action by the abductors of the wrist to resist the force of gravity. Using the hammer to drive the nail requires alternate adduction and abduction at the wrist (as well as movement at the shoulder and elbow, which is not reviewed here). Adduction is produced by contraction of the extensor carpi ulnaris and flexor carpi ulnaris, whereas abduction is the result of action of the extensor carpi radialis longus and flexor carpi radialis, with possible assistance from several other muscles (see Fig. 10-5).

Activity: *Beating an Egg.* Another activity that illustrates a combination of movements of the radioulnar and wrist joints is that of manually beating an egg. Depending on the technique used, if movement involved primarily the hand rather than the forearm and arm, it would be possible to utilize all movements discussed in this chapter. Manipulating a utensil in a clockwise motion, with the right hand starting in a pronated position, the hand is adducted and flexed and then abducted and extended with each stroke. A varying amount of supination can also be involved as the hand is adducted and flexed; pronation accompanies abduction and extension.

The flexor carpi ulnaris (with the extensor carpi ulnaris) produces adduction of the hand at the wrist. It also, along with the flexor carpi radialis, produces flexion at the wrist. The flexors must overcome any extension resulting from contraction of the extensor carpi ulnaris. As mentioned previously in this chapter, the flexor digitorum superficialis and flexor digitorum profundus can aid in wrist flexion when the fingers are maintained in extension. In beating an egg, the fingers are flexed to hold the utensil, and the flexors of the fingers are therefore not significantly involved with flexion at the wrist.

With the subsequent abduction and extension of the wrist, the extensor carpi radialis longus and extensor carpi radialis brevis can produce a combination of both movements. The flexor carpi radialis takes part in abduction, while the extensor carpi ulnaris assists with extension. In this phase of the movement, any flexion resulting from

contraction of the flexor carpi radialis is overcome by the action of the extensors.

In this analysis, the technique of beating an egg involves movements occurring primarily at the wrist. If a more exaggerated technique is used, additional movements could involve the entire upper limb. These may include abduction, flexion, and extension at the shoulder, possibly some medial and lateral rotation of the humerus, and flexion and extension at the elbow joint.

Activity: *Opening and Closing a Jar Lid.* Several movements at the radioulnar and wrist joints are involved in opening and closing the lid of a jar. When opening the jar, one hand is used to stabilize the jar and the other turns the lid. The jar can be supported from below with a supinated hand or from the side with a hand in a semipronated position. To remove the lid, the hand is placed over the jar in a pronated position and the lid is firmly grasped by the fingers and thumb. For the flexors of the digits to provide a firm enough grasp, the hand must be extended somewhat at the wrist. The lid is rotated counterclockwise by pronation, accompanied by abduction at the wrist. Closing the lid requires the opposite movements of supination and adduction at the wrist.

Pronation is brought about by the pronator quadratus and pronator teres, whereas supination is produced by the supinator and the biceps brachii; the pronator teres and biceps brachii are the more powerful of the muscles in their respective movements. Abduction of the hand at the wrist results mainly from the contraction of the flexor carpi radialis and extensor carpi radialis longus. Adduction of the hand is produced by the flexor carpi ulnaris and extensor carpi ulnaris. The extensor carpi radialis longus, extensor carpi radialis brevis, and extensor carpi ulnaris cause extension at the wrist, which aids the flexors in gripping the jar lid.

REVIEW QUESTIONS

1 What muscles are involved in flexion of the hand at the wrist joint? What is the effect on this movement if the median nerve is completely severed in the middle of the arm? What would be the effect on flexion at the wrist joint if the ulnar nerve was injured in the distal part of the arm? What would be the effect if the injury to the ulnar nerve was in the distal part of the forearm?

2 What two nerves provide motor innervation to the muscles that produce adduction at the wrist joint?

3 Describe the radioulnar and wrist movements and muscles involved in the following:
   a bringing the hand to the forehead (from the anatomical position), as in a salute
   b screwing a light bulb into a lamp socket
   c brushing your teeth

4 What movements are involved at the elbow and glenohumeral joints with each of the activities listed in question 3?

EXERCISES

1 Demonstrate the movements of supination and pronation. As these are demonstrated, consider the muscles that are involved, the nerves that provide motor innervation to the muscles, and an explanation of the relationship of the radius to the ulna during the movements.

2 Place a hand over the extensor muscles of the forearm and, as the wrist is abducted, palpate the contraction of the muscles in this area. Which muscles are contracting to produce this movement?

11 THE HAND

CHAPTER CONTENTS

General Considerations

Bones and Joints

The Palmar Fascia

The Flexor Synovial Sheaths, Tendons, and Lumbrical Muscles

Fascial Spaces of the Palm

Muscles

Nerves and Vessels

Dorsum of the Hand

Nerve Injuries

GENERAL CONSIDERATIONS

The hand is an anatomically complex structure. Within it are concentrated not only the previously considered tendons of the long muscles but also a large number of intrinsic muscles confined to the hand, together with important nerves and vessels. Movements of the digits are discussed in more detail in Chapter 12, and the nerve supply to the muscles is shown diagrammatically in Figures 8-6 and 8-7.

The terms *lateral* and *radial* are used to describe the thumb side of the hand, and *medial* and *ulnar* are used to describe the little-finger side of the hand, just as they distinguish these sides of the forearm. Instead of being described as having anterior and posterior surfaces, however, the hand is described as having *palmar* and *dorsal (posterior) surfaces.* The *thenar eminence* is the prominence that the thumb muscles form on the lateral side of the hand, and the *hypothenar eminence,* on the medial side, is that formed by the muscles of the little finger.

BONES AND JOINTS
Bones

In the hand, *carpal bones* compose the carpus or wrist (Figs. 11-1 and 11-2). The *metacarpals* form the skeleton of the major part of the hand, and the *phalanges* are the bones of the digits.

Carpal bones
The eight carpal bones are arranged in two rows (see Figs. 11-1 and 11-2). The three large bones of the *proximal row,* beginning laterally, are the **scaphoid,**

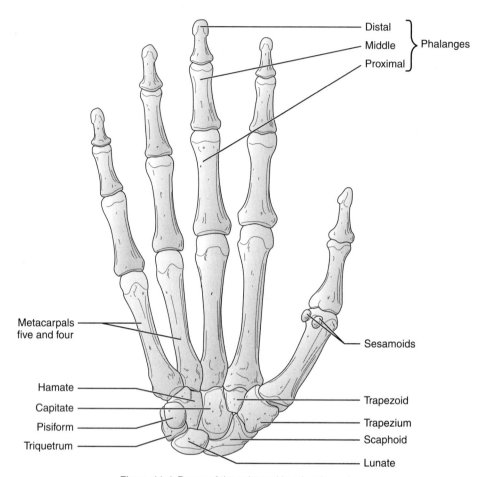

Figure 11-1 Bones of the wrist and hand, palmar view.

lunate, and **triquetrum;** the smaller **pisiform** bone sits on the palmar surface of the triquetrum. The *distal row,* from lateral to medial, consists of the **trapezium, trapezoid, capitate,** and **hamate.** Some of the carpals, such as the scaphoid, lunate, pisiform, and hamate, can be recognized easily by their shape, whereas the identification of others involves more attention to details. The scaphoid, lunate, and triquetrum articulate with the radius and the articular disc on the ulna and form a convex surface on which movement at the wrist occurs. The carpals also articulate with each other. As a whole, the dorsal surface of the carpus is convex, the palmar surface concave. This concavity, which accommodates the median nerve and the long flexor tendons to the hand, is called the *carpal groove.*

Metacarpals, phalanges, and sesamoid bones
The carpals articulate distally with the elongated **metacarpals.** Distal to the metacarpals are the **phalanges,** two for the thumb and three for the other digits. The proximal end of each metacarpal and phalanx is its *base,* the distal end is its *head,* and the *shaft (body)* intervenes between base and head. Two **sesamoid bones,** one on each side of the anterior surface of the metacarpophalangeal joint of the thumb, articulate with the head of the first metacarpal.

Joints

The joints at the wrist are actually multiple and include the distal radioulnar joint, radiocarpal joint (often thought of as "the" wrist joint), the intercarpal

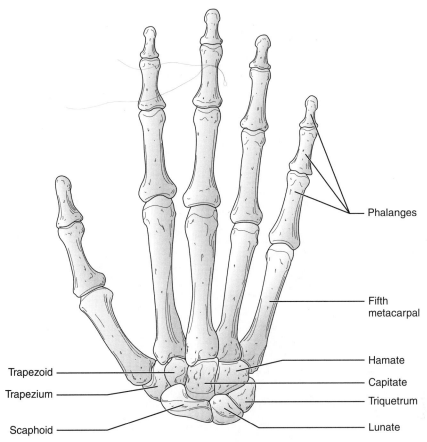

Figure 11-2 Bones of the wrist and hand, dorsal view.

Labels on figure:
Phalanges
Fifth metacarpal
Hamate
Capitate
Triquetrum
Lunate
Trapezoid
Trapezium
Scaphoid

joints, the midcarpal joint, and the carpometacarpal joints (Fig. 11-3). The metacarpophalangeal joints and the interphalangeal joints are also discussed in this section.

Distal radioulnar joint

The proximal and distal radioulnar joints are *pivot (trochoid)* joints between the radius and ulna that make possible movements of pronation and supination. The proximal radioulnar joint was discussed in Chapter 6. The **distal radioulnar joint** is L-shaped. The vertical portion of its synovial cavity is interposed between the distal ends of the radius and ulna, and the transverse portion lies between the distal end of the ulna and its articular disc. A weak joint capsule surrounds the joint.

Radiocarpal joint

The *condylar (ellipsoidal)* **radiocarpal joint** is between the articular surface of the radius (and the distal surface of the ulnar articular disc) and the scaphoid, lunate, and triquetrum. The movements here, and those at the midcarpal joint (discussed later in this chapter), are discussed in Chapter 10. The joint capsule is reinforced by special ligaments, of which the radial and ulnar collateral ligaments are narrow bands on the sides of the joint indicated by their names. The *radial collateral ligament* is attached to the styloid process of the radius and to a tubercle on the scaphoid, with some fibers reaching the trapezium (Fig. 11-4). The *ulnar collateral ligament* extends from the styloid process of the ulna to the nonarticular part of the medial surface of the triquetrum and

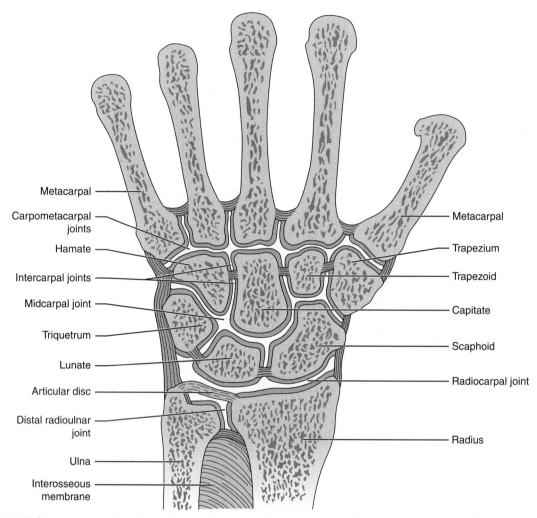

Figure 11-3 The bones and the joint cavities of the right wrist. The radiocarpal and inferior radioulnar joint cavities are separate and distinct; the midcarpal joint is continuous with the intercarpal joints between the proximal and distal rows of the carpals; and the carpometacarpal joints, except for that of the thumb, are continuous with the intermetacarpal joints and with the distal parts of the intercarpal joints, but they have no communication with the midcarpal joint. Note that the pisiform bone is not depicted because it is not in the plane of this illustration.

to the pisiform. There is a small *palmar ulnocarpal ligament* extending from the distal end of the ulna to the lunate and triquetrum; it tends to blend with both the ulnar collateral ligament and the larger *palmar radiocarpal ligament.* The latter ligament extends obliquely medially from the radius to all the bones of the proximal row and to the capitate in the distal row. There is also a *dorsal radiocarpal ligament,* attached to the proximal row of bones. Because the fibers of both radiocarpal ligaments extend toward the ulna as they pass from the radius to the proximal row of carpal

bones, they ensure that the hand moves with the radius during pronation and supination. During pronation, the fibers of the dorsal radiocarpal ligament carry the hand with the radius, and during supination, those of the palmar radiocarpal ligament do so.

Intercarpal and midcarpal joints
The carpals in each row are bound together by small *intercarpal ligaments* on both their palmar and dorsal surfaces and also by *interosseous intercarpal ligaments* (situated between the palmar and dorsal ligaments)

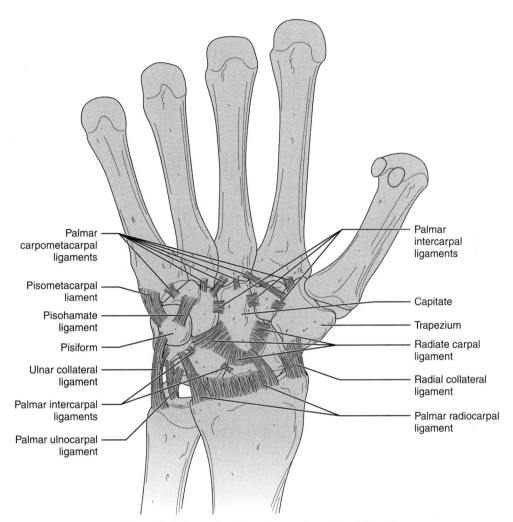

Figure 11-4 Ligaments of the palmar surface of the right wrist.

that interrupt the continuity of the intercarpal joint cavities. Attached to the pisiform are the *pisohamate* and *pisometacarpal ligaments,* generally considered extensions of the tendon of the flexor carpi ulnaris (which also attaches to the pisiform). The **intercarpal joints** between members of the proximal row of carpals, and also those between members of the distal row of carpals, allow only a little gliding movement between adjacent bones in one row.

Between the two rows lies a larger intercarpal joint cavity, the **midcarpal joint.** This joint allows the distal row of carpals to move rather freely on the proximal row. It is a single cavity that separates the two rows of bones (see Fig. 11-3). It sends some

expansions between the members of the proximal carpal row to form the intercarpal joints. Shorter expansions between the members of the distal row form proximal portions of the intercarpal joints of this row. *Interosseous ligaments* intervene between the radiocarpal joint and the intercarpal joints of the proximal row, and the intercarpal joints of the distal row are divided into proximal and distal parts by similar interosseous ligaments. Therefore, the proximal portions of the distal intercarpal joints are continuous with the midcarpal joint, and the distal portions are proximal extensions from the *carpometacarpal joints.* Because of these interosseous ligaments, there is usually no communication between the midcarpal joint and either the radiocarpal or carpometacarpal joint (see Fig. 11-3).

Carpometacarpal joints

The **carpometacarpal joint of the thumb** is a separate synovial cavity; because of its *saddle or sellar* shape, the first metacarpal can undergo movements of abduction, adduction, flexion, extension, and rotation. The **carpometacarpal joints of the other four digits** constitute a single cavity, which not only provides proximal extensions to help form the joint cavities between the carpals of the distal row but also sends similar extensions distally to form the intermetacarpal joints. The metacarpals of the second and third digits articulate with the distal carpals and with each other in such a way that almost no movement of them is possible.

FUNCTIONAL/CLINICAL NOTE 11-1

The metacarpal of the ring (fourth) finger is slightly more mobile than those of the index (second) and middle (third) fingers, and that of the little finger is even more mobile (although less so than that of the thumb). This mobility helps account for the firmness with which many tools, such as a hammer, are held, with the grip primarily on the ulnar side.

Metacarpophalangeal joints

The *condylar-type* **metacarpophalangeal joints** allow not only flexion and extension but also free movement of the fingers from side to side when the fingers are extended. However, when the fingers are flexed, such side-to-side movement becomes almost impossible. This is because of the *collateral ligaments* (Fig. 11-5, *B*), one on each side of the joint, which extend obliquely distally and palmar-ward from the dorsum of the side of the metacarpal to the palmar aspect of the side of the proximal phalanx.

FUNCTIONAL/CLINICAL NOTE 11-2

The collateral ligaments become tight during flexion and check the rocking movement of the digits at this joint.

In addition to the collateral ligaments, each metacarpophalangeal joint is protected on its palmar surface by a dense fibrocartilaginous pad called the *palmar ligament*. Dorsally, the joint is protected by an expansion of the long extensor tendon called the *extensor expansion* or *extensor hood* (see Fig. 11-5, *B*). The heads of the metacarpals of the four fingers are also connected by strong transverse bands, the *deep transverse metacarpal ligaments,* which attach also to the palmar ligaments. There is no such band between thumb and index finger; its presence would restrict the mobility of the first metacarpal.

Interphalangeal joints

The **interphalangeal joints** differ from the metacarpophalangeal joints in that they are hinge joints and allow only flexion and extension (see Fig. 11-5, *A* and *B*). The collateral ligaments of these joints are similar to those of the metacarpophalangeal joints. The *palmar ligaments* of the interphalangeal joints are, however, of particular importance, as they prevent hyperextension of these joints. If one of them is ruptured, the associated phalanx may become locked in hyperextension.

Innervation

The joints at the wrist are innervated by the *median nerve through its anterior interosseous branch, the radial nerve by way of its posterior interosseous branch, and the ulnar nerve through its deep and dorsal branches.* Innervation to the metacarpophalangeal and interphalangeal joints is provided primarily by the *palmar digital nerves* adjacent to the joints, through either the median or ulnar nerves. The *dorsal digital branches* may also contribute some innervation to the joints.

Surface Anatomy

Because of the overlying muscles, tendons, retinacula, and palmar aponeurosis (anteriorly), it is difficult to palpate all of the bony features of the wrist and hand. On the palmar surface of the wrist, the prominences raised by the **scaphoid** and **trapezium** can be palpated laterally. These bones form the floor of the anatomical snuffbox along with the styloid process of the radius proximally and the base of the first metacarpal distally. The **pisiform** (on which the

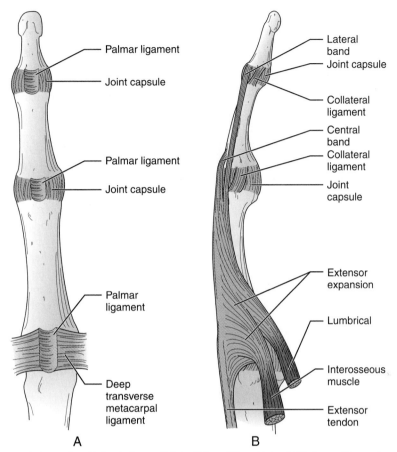

Figure 11-5 Metacarpophalangeal and interphalangeal joints. Palmar **(A)** and lateral **(B)** views of the metacarpophalangeal joint with the extensor tendon and extensor expansion in place.

flexor carpi ulnaris inserts) and the **hamate** can be located medially. On the dorsum of the hand, the **metacarpals** can be palpated. The **phalanges** are also palpable because the extensor tendons on them are very flat. On the palmar surface, the bones are not distinctly palpable, because of the flexor tendons and connective tissue pads on their anterior surfaces.

The **styloid processes** of the radius (laterally) and the ulna (medially) can be palpated at the wrist. The styloid process of the radius is positioned more distally than that of the ulna. Abducting and adducting the hand demonstrates the greater mobility possible in adduction. Of the joints of the hand, it is possible to locate and demonstrate the range of motion of the **metacarpophalangeal and interphalangeal joints** of all of the digits.

THE PALMAR FASCIA

The heavy fibrous **palmar aponeurosis** bridges the center of the palm of the hand and receives the insertion of the palmaris longus muscle. It is continuous with the distal edge of the **flexor retinaculum,** the strong transverse thickening of the antebrachial fascia at the wrist that converts the carpal groove into a *carpal tunnel* or canal. Distally, the aponeurosis gives rise to slips to each finger. These slips not only attach to the metacarpals and palmar ligaments around the fibrous sheaths for the long flexor tendons and to the front of the sheaths but may also extend to the proximal phalanges.

Medially and laterally, the palmar aponeurosis sends septa to attach to the first and fifth metacarpals. These septa pass medial to the thenar muscles and lateral to the hypothenar ones, forming the walls of a **central palmar compartment.** A less dense fascia covers the muscles of the thenar and hypothenar eminences.

Within the central palmar compartment, which is bordered by the palmar aponeurosis and the intermuscular septa, lie the tendons of the long flexor muscles of the fingers, short muscles associated with these tendons, arterial arches that supply blood to the hand and fingers, and branches of the median and ulnar nerves.

THE FLEXOR SYNOVIAL SHEATHS, TENDONS, AND LUMBRICAL MUSCLES

The **synovial sheaths** (variably termed *the synovial tendon sheaths, tendinous sheaths,* or *tendon sheaths*) of the palmar surface of the hand provide free movement for the long flexor tendons and are situated both at the wrist and on the digits themselves (Figs. 11-6 and 11-7). At the wrist there are two synovial sheaths, one that surrounds the tendon of the flexor pollicis longus and one surrounding the tendons of both the

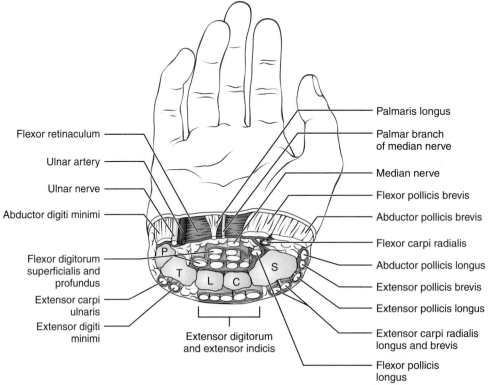

Figure 11-6 Anatomical relationships of structures at the wrist. The flexor retinaculum and the arrangement of tendons, synovial sheaths, and median nerve within the carpal tunnel are illustrated. *P,* pisiform; *T,* triquetrum; *L,* lunate; *C,* capitate; *S,* scaphoid.

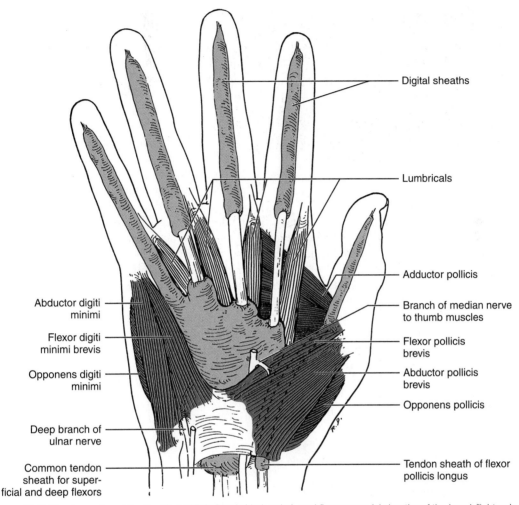

Digital sheaths

Lumbricals

Adductor pollicis

Branch of median nerve
to thumb muscles

Flexor pollicis
brevis

Abductor pollicis
brevis

Opponens pollicis

Tendon sheath of flexor
pollicis longus

Abductor digiti
minimi

Flexor digiti
minimi brevis

Opponens digiti
minimi

Deep branch of
ulnar nerve

Common tendon
sheath for super-
ficial and deep flexors

Figure 11-7 Short muscles of the thumb and little finger *(dark color),* and flexor synovial sheaths of the hand *(light color).*

flexor digitorum superficialis and flexor digitorum profundus. The **synovial sheath of the flexor pollicis longus,** sometimes called the *radial bursa,* is the most radial of the two. It is continued around the tendon almost to the tendon's insertion on the distal phalanx of the thumb. The part of the sheath on the thumb is called the **synovial sheath of the thumb;** it is simply a continuation of the sheath from the wrist. The much larger sheath on the ulnar side of the wrist is the **common flexor sheath** (common flexor synovial sheath); it is sometimes termed the *ulnar bursa.* It surrounds the tendons of both the flexor digitorum superficialis and flexor digitorum profundus. This sheath also begins

just proximal to the flexor retinaculum and, in passing deep to it, occupies most of the space within the carpal tunnel. The larger part of the common flexor sheath stops at about the middle of the palm of the hand, but an ulnar portion typically continues out around the long flexor tendons to the little finger. Therefore, the **synovial sheath of the little finger** is a direct continuation of the common flexor sheath (see Fig. 11-7). In contrast, the **synovial sheaths for the flexor tendons to the index, middle, and ring fingers** usually begin blindly near the bases of the fingers, distal to the common flexor synovial sheath, and they normally have no connection with the sheath at the wrist.

Because of this discontinuity, infections within the synovial sheaths on the index, middle, and ring fingers can extend proximally toward the wrist only by rupture of the sheaths. Infections within the synovial sheath of the little finger or that of the thumb, however, routinely manifest at the wrist because of the continuity between these sheaths and those at the wrist.

At the wrist and in the palm, the synovial sheaths are thin and are supported by the overlying flexor retinaculum and palmar aponeurosis. On the digits, however, each synovial sheath acquires a heavy outer fibrous layer, the **fibrous sheath,** which extends from the metacarpal heads to the distal phalanx. The fibrous sheath of each digit attaches along the radial and ulnar margins of the phalanges, and with the underlying bone it creates an *osseofibrous tunnel* that contains the synovial sheath and corresponding tendon or tendons. Anterior to the joints (where it might

interfere with movement), the sheath is thinner, and its fibers are arranged predominantly obliquely, in a cruciate (crossed) pattern. Elsewhere, the sheath is thicker and has an annular arrangement, with the fibers running directly from the radial to the ulnar side of the phalanx. The arrangement of the annular bands has been described as forming a series of pulleys that hold the flexor tendons close to the bone and facilitate movements of the tendons.

Within the synovial sheaths on the fingers, each tendon of the flexor digitorum superficialis divides to allow the corresponding flexor digitorum profundus tendon to pass through (Fig. 11-8). The superficial tendon is attached by remains of its mesotendon, the *short and long vincula,* to the proximal phalanx, but the insertion of the tendon is on the base of the middle phalanx. Similarly, the flexor digitorum profundus tendon has vincula attaching to the middle phalanx, but its real insertion is on the base of the distal phalanx. The vincula (especially the short ones) serve primarily as pathways for vessels to enter and leave the tendons.

Associated with the tendons of the flexor digitorum profundus in the hand are four small

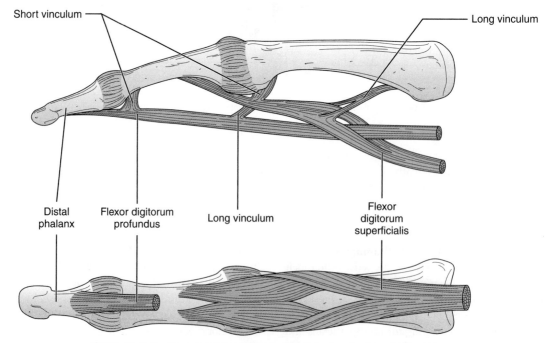

Figure 11-8 The flexor tendons of a finger, lateral *(top)* and palmar *(bottom)* views.

Table 11-1 LUMBRICALS				
Muscle	**Origin (Proximal Attachment)**	**Insertion (Distal Attachment)**	**Action**	**Innervation**
Lumbricals (4)	Tendons of flexor digitorum profundus	Extensor expansion of medial four digits on the proximal phalanges	Extension of interphalangeal joints of medial four digits; flexion of metacarpophalangeal joints	Median nerve (lateral two); ulnar nerve (medial two)

lumbrical ("wormlike") muscles (Table 11-1; see Fig. 11-7). These muscles have *origins* from the tendons of the flexor digitorum profundus (as the tendons diverge toward the fingers). These muscles then pass over the palmar surfaces of the deep transverse metacarpal ligaments, curve dorsally on the radial side of each of the four medial digits, and have their *insertion* into the expanded extensor tendons on the proximal phalanges. (The expanded tendons of the extensor muscles are known as the *extensor expansions* or *extensor hoods*.) The *action* of these muscles, through their attachment to the extensor expansions, is to aid in all movements of extension of the interphalangeal joints; secondarily, they can also aid in flexing the metacarpophalangeal joints. Although there may be some variability, the first two lumbricals (counting from the radial side) typically receive *innervation* from the median nerve, while the ulnar nerve innervates the third and fourth lumbricals.

FASCIAL SPACES OF THE PALM

Deep to the flexor tendons and their associated lumbrical muscles is an area of loose connective tissue. It is bounded on the radial side by the septum passing from the palmar aponeurosis to the first metacarpal and on the ulnar side by the similar septum passing to the fifth metacarpal. Distally, the space ends near where the digital part of the synovial sheaths of the flexor tendons begin. Most accounts describe a septum that tends to separate this subtendinous area into two compartments, of which the more ulnar is known as the **midpalmar space** and the more radial as the **thenar space.** These spaces are bounded superficially by the associated flexor tendons and palmar fascia and deeply by the fascia on the interosseous muscles and the adductor pollicis muscle.

(A different description is that there is only one palmar fascial space, although it is subdivided distally into compartments for the flexor tendons, lumbrical muscles, and digital nerves and vessels.)

FUNCTIONAL/CLINICAL NOTE 11-5

The palmar fascial spaces are of importance in infections of the hand, because a considerable amount of pus can collect in the very loose connective tissue that they contain. They may be infected directly through penetrating wounds of the hand or indirectly through rupture of flexor synovial sheaths into them.

MUSCLES
Muscles of the Thumb

The four short muscles of the thumb (pollex) interact with the long muscles to greatly increase the usefulness of the thumb. Three of the muscles, the *abductor pollicis brevis, opponens pollicis*, and a major part of the *flexor pollicis brevis*, form the **thenar eminence** (Table 11-2; see Fig. 11-7). The fourth, the *adductor pollicis*, lies deeply in the palm posterior to the long flexor tendons, where it forms the posterior wall of the thenar fascial space. It is associated with the deep part of the flexor pollicis brevis.

Abductor pollicis brevis
The **abductor pollicis brevis** is a flat muscle that has its *origin* from the flexor retinaculum and the scaphoid and trapezium and *insertion* on the radial side of the base of the proximal phalanx (Fig. 11-9). A portion of the muscle usually inserts on the tendon

Table 11-2	MUSCLES OF THE THUMB			
Muscle	**Origin (Proximal Attachment)**	**Insertion (Distal Attachment)**	**Action**	**Innervation**
Abductor pollicis brevis	Flexor retinaculum; scaphoid and trapezium	Base of proximal phalanx	Abduction of thumb	Median nerve
Opponens pollicis	Flexor retinaculum; trapezium	First metacarpal	Opposition of thumb	Median nerve
Flexor pollicis brevis	Superficial head: flexor retinaculum (and possibly trapezium) Deep head: trapezoid and capitate	Base of proximal phalanx	Flexion of thumb; aids in opposition and adduction	Median nerve (superficial head); ulnar nerve (deep head)
Adductor pollicis	Transverse head: third metacarpal Oblique head: capitate, trapezoid, and trapezium and bases of first three metacarpals	Base of proximal phalanx	Adduction and flexion of thumb	Ulnar nerve

of the extensor pollicis longus. Its *action* is as a true abductor of the thumb in the sense that it moves the thumb almost perpendicularly away from the plane of the palm. Because the abductor pollicis brevis lies closer to the palmar than the dorsal surface on the side of the metacarpophalangeal joint, it is also a flexor at this joint. Because of its partial insertion onto the long extensor tendon, it can also aid in extending the distal phalanx.

Opponens pollicis

The **opponens pollicis** is largely covered by the abductor pollicis brevis. Like that muscle, its *origin* is from the flexor retinaculum and the trapezium but its *insertion* is along most of the length of the first metacarpal on its radial side. Its *action* is to draw the first metacarpal across the palm of the hand, rotating this bone as it contracts, producing the movement known as *opposition of the thumb.*

Flexor pollicis brevis

The **flexor pollicis brevis** typically has two heads of origin, one superficial and one deep. The large and constant superficial head has its *origin* predominantly from the flexor retinaculum, as do the muscles already described, and possibly the trapezium. The deep

head, which may be small or absent, arises, if present, from the floor or dorsal wall of the carpal tunnel, from one or more of the carpal bones of the distal row (usually the trapezoid and the capitate), and is closely associated with some of the origin of the adductor pollicis. The two heads unite deep to the tendon of the flexor pollicis longus. *Insertion* of the muscle is close to the abductor pollicis brevis on the radial side of the base of the proximal phalanx, but it is actually more on the palmar surface than is the insertion of the other muscle. In reaching this insertion, it attaches in part to the more lateral of the two sesamoid bones of the metacarpophalangeal joint of the thumb (see Fig. 11-1). The *action* of the flexor pollicis brevis is not only to flex the metacarpophalangeal joint but also to aid in adduction and opposition of the thumb.

Adductor pollicis

The **adductor pollicis** also has two heads, one transverse and the other oblique. The transverse head has its *origin* from the palmar surface of the shaft of the third metacarpal, while the oblique head has its origin from the ligamentous floor of the carpal tunnel over the distal parts of the capitate, trapezoid, and trapezium, and the adjacent bases of the first

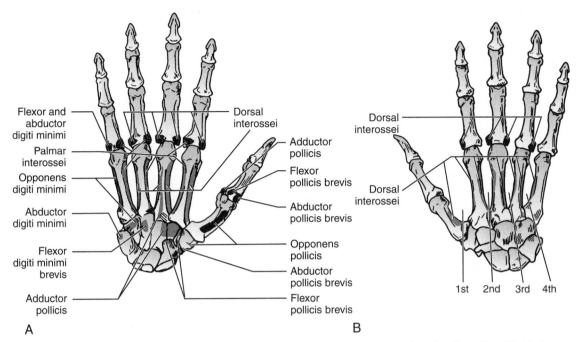

Flexor and
abductor
digiti minimi

Palmar
interossei

Opponens
digiti minimi

Abductor
digiti minimi

Flexor
digiti minimi
brevis

Adductor
pollicis

Dorsal
interossei

Adductor
pollicis

Flexor
pollicis brevis

Abductor
pollicis brevis

Opponens
pollicis

Abductor
pollicis brevis

Flexor
pollicis brevis

Dorsal
interossei

Dorsal
interossei

1st   2nd   3rd   4th

A

B

Figure 11-9 Palmar **(A)** and dorsal **(B)** views of the bones of the hand, illustrating origins *(color)* and insertions *(black)* of muscles of the hand. The position of each of the four dorsal interossei is indicated in part *B*.

three metacarpals. Both heads are triangular. The transverse head extends almost transversely, while the oblique head almost parallels the first metacarpal. The two heads come together to an *insertion* on the ulnar side of the palmar surface of the base of the proximal phalanx of the thumb. Their tendon of insertion attaches in part to the ulnar sesamoid of the metacarpophalangeal joint of the thumb, and a smaller part continues to the long extensor tendon. The *action* of the adductor pollicis is to adduct and flex the thumb at the carpometacarpal joint and to flex the metacarpophalangeal joint.

Innervation of the thumb muscles

Innervation to the muscles of the thumb is provided by the median or ulnar nerve or both. As the median nerve emerges from deep to the flexor retinaculum, it gives off a motor branch. The exact distribution of this branch varies. Through it, however, the median nerve commonly supplies innervation to the abductor pollicis brevis and opponens pollicis and to the large superficial head of the flexor pollicis brevis. The adductor pollicis and the deep head of the flexor pollicis

brevis are usually innervated by the deep branch of the ulnar nerve, which runs transversely across the hand to end in these muscles.

Muscles of the Little Finger

Palmaris brevis, abductor digiti minimi, flexor digiti minimi brevis, and opponens digiti minimi

Lying in the fascia over the hypothenar eminence is the small **palmaris brevis** (a general muscle of the hand described here because of its location). It is a transversely arranged muscle that has its *origin* from the medial border of the palmar aponeurosis and *insertion* into the skin of the ulnar border of the hand (Table 11-3). The palmaris brevis receives *innervation* from the superficial branch of the ulnar nerve. Its *action* is to tense the skin covering the hypothenar eminence and, in this way, to aid in producing a better grip by the hand.

The muscles of the little finger (see Fig. 11-7) are only three in number, and movements of this finger are less complex than those of the thumb. The most superficial muscle on the ulnar border of the palm

Table 11-3	MUSCLES OF THE LITTLE FINGER			
Muscle	**Origin (Proximal Attachment)**	**Insertion (Distal Attachment)**	**Action**	**Innervation**
Palmaris brevis	Palmar aponeurosis, medial border	Skin on ulnar side of hand	Stabilization of skin of palm for gripping	Ulnar nerve
Abductor digiti minimi	Pisiform	Base of proximal phalanx of little finger	Abduction of little finger	Ulnar nerve
Flexor digiti minimi brevis	Flexor retinaculum; hook of hamate	Proximal phalanx of little finger	Flexion of little finger	Ulnar nerve
Opponens digiti minimi	Flexor retinaculum; hook of hamate	Fifth metacarpal	Opposition of little finger to thumb	Ulnar nerve

is the **abductor digiti minimi,** which has its *origin* largely from the pisiform and *insertion* on the ulnar aspect of the base of the proximal phalanx (see Fig. 11-9). The **flexor digiti minimi brevis** takes *origin* from the flexor retinaculum and the projecting hamulus or hook of the hamate bone. It joins the abductor to have an *insertion* with it on the proximal phalanx but more onto the palmar surface than does the abductor digiti minimi. The **opponens digiti minimi** lies deep to these muscles. Its *origin* is from the flexor retinaculum and the hook of the hamate, and its *insertion* is onto the ulnar border of almost the entire length of the shaft of the fifth metacarpal.

The *action* of the abductor digiti minimi is to abduct the little finger, with the action aided possibly by the flexor digiti minimi brevis. Both the abductor digiti minimi and the flexor digiti minimi brevis flex the little finger at the metacarpophalangeal joint. The opponens digiti minimi assists in opposition of the little finger to the thumb and also in cupping the hand and in grasping tools firmly. *Innervation* to all three of these muscles is supplied by the deep branch of the ulnar nerve as it passes among them to reach a deep position in the palm of the hand.

The Interossei

The interossei are deep-lying muscles that are largely situated, as their name implies, between the bones (the metacarpals) of the hand. The adductor pollicis lies anterior to the interossei on the radial side of the third metacarpal, but the interossei on the ulnar side of this bone form most of the posterior wall of the midpalmar fascial space. At

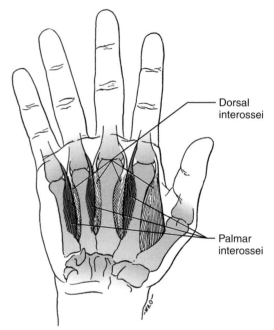

Dorsal interossei

Palmar interossei

Figure 11-10 The dorsal and palmar *(color)* interosseous muscles.

their proximal ends, the interossei are crossed by the deep branch of the ulnar nerve as it passes laterally from the hypothenar muscles and by the deep palmar arterial arch, which enters the palm through the most radial interosseous and runs medially across the hand (see Fig. 11-13). Branches from both the arch and the nerve run distally on the surfaces of the interossei.

The interossei are divided into two groups, palmar and dorsal (Fig. 11-10 and Table 11-4). In contrast to the lumbricals, with which they have certain

Table 11-4	INTEROSSEI			
Muscle	**Origin (Proximal Attachment)**	**Insertion (Distal Attachment)**	**Action**	**Innervation**
Palmar interossei (3 in number)	Shaft of metacarpal: one each to index, ring, and little fingers	Extensor expansion of finger of origin	Adduction of the respective finger (index, ring, and little fingers); flexion of metacarpophalangeal joints; extension of interphalangeal joints	Ulnar nerve
Dorsal interossei (4 in number)	Adjacent surfaces of two metacarpals	First: proximal phalanx on radial side of index finger. Second, third, and fourth: proximal phalanx on radial side of middle, ulnar side of middle, and ulnar side of ring fingers, respectively, and extensor expansion	Abduction of index, middle, and ring fingers; flexion of metacarpophalangeal joints; extension of interphalangeal joints (depending on insertion, first one may not extend interphalangeal joints)	Ulnar nerve

actions in common, all the interossei pass dorsal to the deep transverse metacarpal ligaments as they run distally to their insertions. Furthermore, they are arranged about the midline of the hand, which runs through the long axis of the middle finger, in such a way that they abduct and adduct the fingers around this midline.

Palmar interossei

The **palmar interossei** are the adductors. Because there are three fingers and a thumb to be adducted toward the middle digit, it takes four muscles to carry out this movement. The thumb, however, has an adductor of its own, the adductor pollicis. Therefore, there are only *three palmar interossei*. These *insert* on the index, ring, and little fingers and are sufficient to carry out the movement of adduction by working with the adductor of the thumb. The three palmar interossei have *origins* from the second, fourth, and fifth metacarpals, respectively, of the three fingers on which they insert. They pass across the metacarpophalangeal joints on the side nearest the middle digit, and their tendons then pass dorsally to *insertions* into the extensor expansions on the proximal phalanges. The *action* of these muscles is to adduct the index, ring, and little fingers. They also flex the

metacarpophalangeal joints and, thereafter, can help extend the interphalangeal joints.

Dorsal interossei

The **dorsal interossei** are arranged to abduct the fingers from the midline of the hand. There are two arranged about the middle finger, so that this finger may be abducted in either a radial or ulnar direction. It takes four more abductors to move the remaining four digits, but both the little finger and thumb have abductors of their own. Therefore, there are only *four dorsal interossei* in all, one for the index and one for the ring finger, in addition to the two attaching to the middle finger. The four dorsal interossei have *origins* from the adjacent surfaces of two metacarpals. The first dorsal interosseous arises from the first and second metacarpals, the second from the second and third metacarpals, and so forth. The first dorsal interosseous has usually a strong *insertion* on the radial side of the base of the proximal phalanx of the index finger and little or no attachment to the extensor expansions. The second and third interossei are attached in part to the base of the proximal phalanx of the middle finger on its radial and ulnar sides, respectively, but also send strong connections to the extensor expansion. The fourth dorsal interosseous arises from the fourth and fifth metacarpals, and, passing on the ulnar side of the metacarpophalangeal joint of the ring finger, inserts like the preceding muscles into both the proximal phalanx and the extensor expansion of this finger. The *action* of the four dorsal interossei, in conjunction with the abductors of the thumb and little finger, is to abduct all the digits. With the usual exception of the first dorsal interosseous, they are also, like the palmar interossei, extensors of the interphalangeal joints when the metacarpophalangeal joints are flexed. With the palmar interossei, they are the primary flexors at the metacarpophalangeal joints.

The deep branch of the ulnar nerve usually supplies *innervation* to all the interossei. The only common exception is the first dorsal interosseous, which in a small percentage of cases is supplied partially or completely by the median nerve.

Surface Anatomy

The muscles of the thenar eminence as a group are recognizable, but they are difficult to distinguish with certainty from each other. The **abductor pollicis brevis** can be outlined reasonably well when the thumb is strongly abducted (raised away from the palm). The **flexor pollicis brevis** can be recognized more vaguely, deep to and on the ulnar side of the abductor, as it is made to contract for flexion of the proximal phalanx. The contraction is much stronger if the thumb is opposed, but it is then impossible to know how much of the contraction is caused by the flexor and how much by the underlying opponens pollicis. The opponens pollicis cannot be identified, nor can the adductor pollicis with any certainty, although the adductor (along with the first dorsal interosseous muscle) forms part of the muscle mass between the first and second metacarpals. On the dorsum of the hand, between these metacarpals, the **first dorsal interosseous** can be palpated distinctly when the index finger is abducted. It is the only interosseous that can be plainly recognized.

Of the muscles of the hypothenar eminence, the **abductor digiti minimi** can usually be identified along the ulnar border of the hand when the finger is abducted, but the other muscles cannot be recognized. As discussed in Chapter 12, weakness or

paralysis of individual muscles of the hand, especially those of the thenar group, is often difficult to assess accurately because of the number of muscles that may assist in carrying out a specific movement.

On the dorsum of the hand, the tendons of the **extensor digitorum** can be observed. With flexion and extension of the fingers, the interconnections between the tendons are often evident. The tendons of the **extensor indicis** and **extensor digiti minimi** lie medial to (on the ulnar side of) the respective tendons of the extensor digitorum to the index and little fingers. They can often be palpated and become more evident with movement of the fingers.

The tendons outlining the anatomical snuffbox, the depressed area on the radial side of the wrist at the base of the thumb, can be palpated and identified when the thumb is extended. The more anterior boundary is formed by the tendons of the **abductor pollicis longus** and the **extensor pollicis brevis;** the tendon of the abductor ends at the base of the first metacarpal, whereas that of the extensor can be palpated to its insertion on the proximal phalanx. The tendon of the **extensor pollicis longus** forms the posterior boundary.

NERVES AND VESSELS
Nerves

Median nerve

Before reaching the hand, the **median nerve** gives off numerous branches within the forearm. At the elbow and proximal part of the forearm, *muscular branches* are provided to the pronator teres, flexor carpi radialis, palmaris longus, and flexor digitorum superficialis. The *anterior interosseous branch* innervates the radial side of the flexor digitorum profundus, the flexor pollicis longus, and the pronator quadratus and the joints of the wrist. The *palmar cutaneous branch* is given off just proximal to the flexor retinaculum. This branch passes superficial to (or possibly penetrates) the flexor retinaculum to innervate skin of the palm and thenar eminence (see later "Cutaneous Innervation" section). It communicates with the palmar cutaneous branch of the ulnar nerve.

The median nerve enters the palm deep to the flexor retinaculum, between this and the common flexor synovial sheath. Close to the distal edge of the retinaculum it gives off *common palmar digital branches,* which divide into *proper palmar digital nerves* (Figs. 11-11 and 11-12). Motor branches to the first two lumbricals usually arise from the nerves to the index and middle fingers. A large *muscular branch* provides innervation to the abductor pollicis brevis and opponens pollicis and most of the flexor pollicis brevis.

Ulnar nerve

After providing innervation to the flexor carpi ulnaris and the ulnar side of the flexor digitorum profundus, the **ulnar nerve** gives off two cutaneous branches in the distal part of the forearm. The *palmar cutaneous branch* innervates skin of the palm and communicates with the palmar cutaneous branch of the median nerve. The *dorsal branch* passes between the tendon of the flexor carpi ulnaris and the ulna to reach and innervate skin on the dorsal aspect of the hand (see later "Cutaneous Innervation" section).

The ulnar nerve enters the hand in company with the ulnar artery, passing superficial to the flexor retinaculum. Close to the distal border of the retinaculum, it divides into superficial and deep branches. The *superficial branch* supplies the palmaris brevis muscle and divides into two sensory branches, the *proper palmar digital branch* to the ulnar side of the little finger and the *common palmar digital* (see Fig. 11-12). The latter divides into the *proper palmar digital nerves* to adjacent sides of the little and ring fingers. The *deep branch* (Fig. 11-13) passes deeply among and innervates the hypothenar muscles and then runs across the palm of the hand in company with the deep palmar arterial arch. The deep branch also innervates the third and fourth lumbricals and all the interossei and ends in muscles of the thumb, usually innervating only the adductor and the deep portion of the short flexor. In its deep palmar course, it also sends branches to a variable number of the metacarpophalangeal joints.

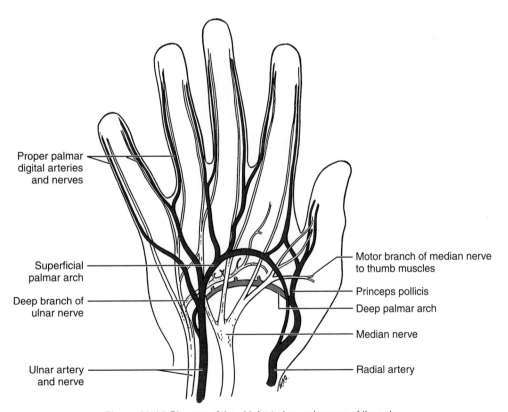

Proper palmar digital arteries and nerves

Superficial palmar arch

Deep branch of ulnar nerve

Ulnar artery and nerve

Motor branch of median nerve to thumb muscles

Princeps pollicis

Deep palmar arch

Median nerve

Radial artery

Figure 11-11 Diagram of the chief arteries and nerves of the palm.

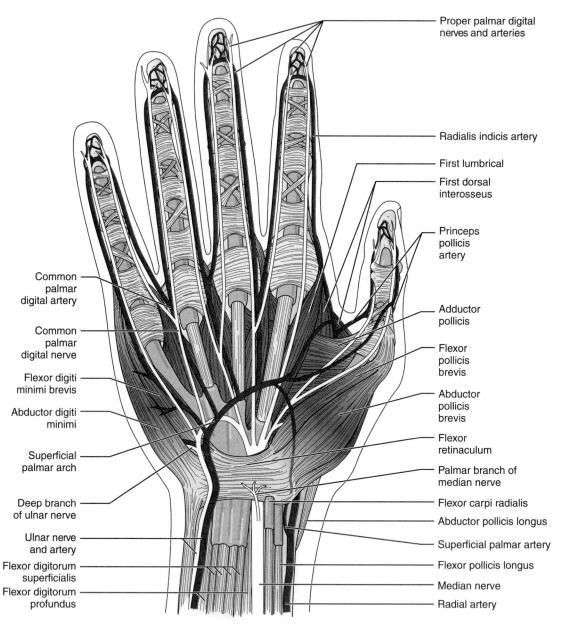

Proper palmar digital
nerves and arteries

Radialis indicis artery

First lumbrical

First dorsal
interosseus

Princeps
pollicis
artery

Adductor
pollicis

Flexor
pollicis
brevis

Abductor
pollicis
brevis

Flexor
retinaculum

Palmar branch of
median nerve

Flexor carpi radialis

Abductor pollicis longus

Superficial palmar artery

Flexor pollicis longus

Median nerve

Radial artery

Common
palmar
digital artery

Common
palmar
digital nerve

Flexor digiti
minimi brevis

Abductor digiti
minimi

Superficial
palmar arch

Deep branch
of ulnar nerve

Ulnar nerve
and artery

Flexor digitorum
superficialis

Flexor digitorum
profundus

Figure 11-12 Muscles, nerves, and arteries of the palm after removal of the palmar aponeurosis.

Table 11-5 summarizes the segmental innervation of the muscles of the hand.

Cutaneous innervation

The pattern of cutaneous innervation of the hand does vary, but all sensory input to the hand is from the median, ulnar, and radial nerves. As described previously, the median nerve has one cutaneous branch to the hand, the palmar cutaneous branch, which originates in the forearm, whereas the ulnar nerve has two (palmar cutaneous and dorsal). The rest of the cutaneous branches arise in the hand. As the median and ulnar nerves enter the hand (see Fig. 11-12), they are still large trunks, and many of the fibers of each are sensory

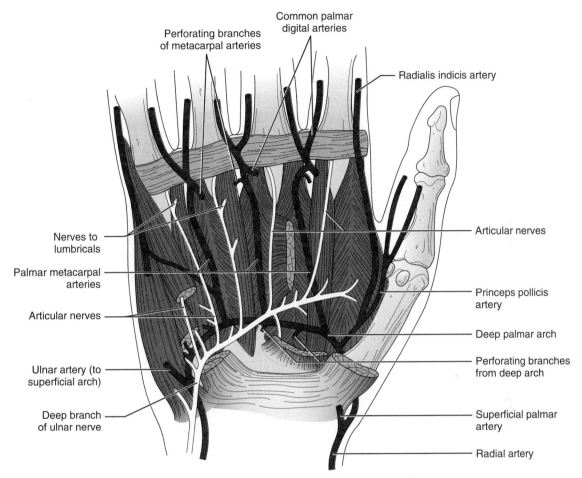

Figure 11-13 The deep arteries and nerves of the palm.

fibers for the skin of the palm and digits (Fig. 11-14). The proper palmar digital nerves accompany the corresponding arteries. The **median nerve** usually *supplies the skin on the palmar surfaces of the thenar eminence and thumb* (except for the lateralmost part of the eminence, which is supplied by the radial nerve), *midpalm, index and middle fingers, and half of the ring finger,* and it also sends branches to *the more distal portion of the dorsum of these fingers and usually the thumb.* The continuation of the **ulnar nerve** into the palm typically *innervates the skin on the hypothenar eminence and adjacent palm and the little finger and half of the index finger anteriorly.* Considerable variability exists in interpretation of the pattern of sensory innervation to the skin of the dorsum of the hand by the ulnar and radial nerves.

The dorsal branch of the ulnar nerve, arising above the wrist, *innervates the same areas of skin posteriorly as do the palmar branches of the ulnar nerve anteriorly, or even possibly portions of two and a half fingers posteriorly* (see Figs. 6-5 and 11-14 for comparison of two different patterns). The **radial nerve** *supplies skin on the lateral side of the thenar eminence and proximal portions of the dorsum of the thumb and remaining fingers: that is, of about two and a half or more digits* (see Fig. 11-14).

Vessels

The ulnar and radial arteries, each accompanied by smaller paired veins, are still large vessels when they reach the hand (see Fig. 11-11). The branches of

Table 11-5   NERVES OF THE HAND

| Nerve and Origin* | Muscle | | |
	Name	Segmental Innervation	Chief Action
Median C5–T1	Abductor pollicis brevis	C8, T1	Abduction of thumb
	Flexor pollicis brevis, superficial head	C8, T1	Flexion at metacarpophalangeal joint of thumb
	Opponens pollicis	C8, T1	Opposition of thumb
	Lumbricals, first and second	C8, T1	In second and third digits, extension at interphalangeal joints and flexion at metacarpophalangeal joints
Ulnar C8, T1	Flexor pollicis brevis, deep head	C8, T1	Flexion at metacarpophalangeal joint of thumb
	Adductor pollicis	C8, T1	In thumb, adduction of metacarpal and flexion at metacarpophalangeal joint
	Palmaris brevis	C8, T1	Wrinkling and stabilization of skin of hypothenar eminence
	Abductor digiti minimi	C8, T1	Abduction of fifth digit
	Flexor digiti minimi brevis	C8, T1	Flexion at metacarpophalangeal joint of fifth digit
	Opponens digiti minimi	C8, T1	Cupping of hand
	Lumbricals, third and fourth	C8, T1	In fourth and fifth digits, extension at interphalangeal joints and flexion at metacarpophalangeal joints
	Palmar interossei	C8, T1	Adduction of second, fourth, and fifth digits; flexion at their metacarpophalangeal joints; extension at their interphalangeal joints
	Dorsal interossei	C8, T1	Abduction of second, third, and fourth digits; other actions similar to palmar interossei

*The common segmental origins; see footnote on Table 8-4.

the arteries are in general divisible into ones that lie superficial to the flexor tendons (primarily from the ulnar artery) and those that lie between the tendons and the interossei (mainly from the radial artery).

Ulnar artery

The **ulnar artery** passes into the hand superficial to the flexor retinaculum and forms an arch, the **superficial palmar arch,** across the hand (see Figs. 11-11 and 11-12). This arch lies between the palmar aponeurosis and the long flexor tendons. It ends in the muscles of the thumb, where it is usually completed by a branch from the radial artery. From the arch it gives off a *proper palmar digital artery* to the ulnar side of the little finger and three *common palmar digital arteries,* which, after being joined near the heads of the metacarpals by branches from the deep

arch, divide between the fingers to supply branches, the *proper palmar digital arteries,* to the adjacent sides of the little and ring fingers, ring and middle fingers, and middle and index fingers. The radial side of the index finger and both sides of the thumb are regularly supplied with blood by branches from the radial artery. These branches may or may not be joined by one or more branches from the superficial palmar arch.

Radial artery

The **radial artery** enters the palm by a more indirect course. Just distal to the area in which it is usually palpated in taking the pulse, the radial artery gives off a *superficial palmar branch* into the thumb muscles (this is the branch that may complete the superficial arch) and then turns sharply dorsally deep to the long

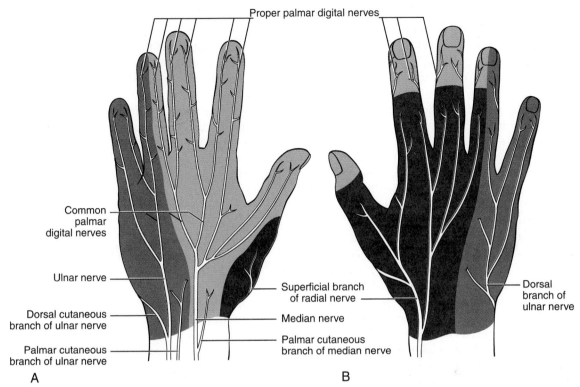

Figure 11-14 Cutaneous innervation of the palmar **(A)** and dorsal **(B)** surfaces of the right hand. The dorsal branch of the ulnar nerve may supply up to two and one half fingers posteriorly (see Fig. 6-5).

abductor and the extensor tendons of the thumb to reach the dorsum of the hand. Here the artery gives off a small *dorsal carpal branch* that helps give rise to *dorsal metacarpal and dorsal digital arteries* and then passes into the palm of the hand by traversing the space between the two heads of the first dorsal interosseous muscle (see Fig. 11-13). As it passes through the muscle, it gives off the *princeps pollicis artery,* which supplies the thumb and may help supply the radial side of the index finger. After reaching the palm of the hand, it continues as the **deep palmar arch** toward the ulnar side, lying against the palmar surfaces of the interossei, at first deep to the adductor pollicis and then on the floor of the midpalmar fascial space. This arch is often completed by the small deep branch of the ulnar artery, which may join the arch after it supplies blood to muscles of the little finger. The *palmar metacarpal branches* of the deep arch join the common palmar digital branches of the superficial arch to help supply blood to the digits. The

radialis indicis artery, to the radial side of the index finger, arises variably from the radial artery, princeps pollicis artery, first palmar metacarpal artery, or some combination of these. It may also receive a contribution from the superficial palmar arch.

Surface Anatomy

None of the nerves and vessels of the hand is visually evident or palpable, except for the superficial venous network on the dorsum. It is not difficult, however, to locate the major nerves and vessels in relation to the surface. The course of the **median nerve** in the wrist and hand can be visualized by noting its relation to the tendons in the wrist and the flexor retinaculum. Because of its depth, the median nerve is not palpable, but its position at the wrist can be approximated. Just proximal to the flexor retinaculum, it lies between, but deep to, the tendons of the palmaris longus and flexor carpi radialis muscles. It is in this location that the palmar cutaneous branch is given off. This branch lies superficial to the flexor retinaculum, whereas the median nerve passes deep to it. At the distal edge of the flexor retinaculum, the median nerve gives rise to its branches within the hand.

In the distal part of the forearm the **ulnar nerve** gives rise to its dorsal branch and enters the hand just lateral to the pisiform bone and superficial to the flexor retinaculum. Its superficial and deep branches arise just distal to the pisiform and flexor retinaculum. The digital branches project distally to the sides of the fingers it innervates, while the deep branch tends to parallel the deep palmar arch.

Because the **ulnar artery** passes into the palm on the radial side of the pisiform, its course can be approximated by drawing a line distally to about the proximal palmar crease; the **superficial arch** follows this crease across the palm. The **radial artery,** after passing through the anatomical snuffbox, dives palmar-ward between the bases of the first and second metacarpals. The **deep arch** lies an inch or more proximal to the superficial arch, at about the level of the palm where the thenar and hypothenar eminences come together.

DORSUM OF THE HAND
Extensor Tendons and Synovial Sheaths

The extensor tendons to the dorsum of the hand are held in place at the wrist by the extensor retinaculum. They are provided with synovial sheaths as they pass between extensor retinaculum and the underlying bones of the wrist. Each sheath may accommodate one or more than one tendon (Fig. 11-15). Pairs of tendons that share a single sheath include the *abductor pollicis longus* and *extensor pollicis brevis;* the *extensor carpi radialis longus* and *extensor carpi radialis brevis;* and the *extensor digitorum* and *extensor indicis.* In contrast to the palm, these synovial sheaths are not continued much beyond the distal edge of the extensor retinaculum, and so the long tendons lie, for the most part, in direct contact with the loose connective tissue of the dorsum. There are no intrinsic muscles of the dorsum of the hand. Therefore, the tendons

to the digits lie almost directly on the metacarpal bones and the dorsal surfaces of the dorsal interossei. On both the dorsum of the hand and the digits, the tendons are subcutaneous. With the limited extent of the synovial sheaths, blood vessels can enter the extensor tendons over much of their surfaces, instead of being limited to the narrow entrance afforded by a mesotendon or a vinculum, as in many of the flexor tendons. Also, the extensor tendons are much more intimately associated with the metacarpophalangeal and interphalangeal joint cavities than are the flexor tendons. The extensor tendons and expansions from them form the chief dorsal protection of these joints, and if the extensor tendons are torn away, the joint cavities are usually exposed.

Cutaneous Innervation

The cutaneous nerves to the dorsum of the hand are shown in Figure 11-16. The *dorsal branch of the ulnar nerve* innervates one and a half to two and a half fingers. The *superficial branch of the radial nerve* supplies the proximal portions of the dorsum of the thumb, index, and middle fingers, and the *posterior cutaneous nerves* of the forearm may pass for variable distances onto the hand. The sensitive tissue deep to the nails is in every case innervated by *dorsal branches of the proper palmar digital nerves.* The *palmar branches of the median nerve* also innervate most of the skin over the two distal phalanges of the index and middle fingers and the radial portion of the ring finger.

Vessels

Because there is relatively little tissue to be supplied with blood on the dorsum of the hand, the blood vessels are small. The dorsal carpal branch given off by the radial artery before it passes into the palm joins twigs from the interosseous and ulnar arteries to form a *dorsal carpal arch (rete).* This gives off four small *metacarpal arteries* that, after being joined by small perforating branches from the deep palmar arch and the palmar metacarpal vessels, divide into *dorsal digital arteries* to the adjacent sides of two digits. There are also branches to the radial side of the dorsum of the thumb and the ulnar border of the little finger. The dorsal digital arteries are minute and can rarely

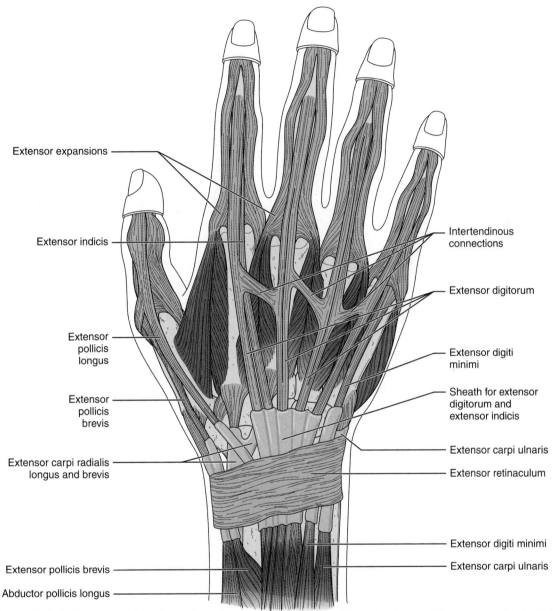

Extensor expansions

Extensor indicis

Extensor pollicis longus

Extensor pollicis brevis

Extensor carpi radialis longus and brevis

Extensor pollicis brevis

Abductor pollicis longus

Intertendinous connections

Extensor digitorum

Extensor digiti minimi

Sheath for extensor digitorum and extensor indicis

Extensor carpi ulnaris

Extensor retinaculum

Extensor digiti minimi

Extensor carpi ulnaris

Figure 11-15 Tendons, synovial sheaths and muscles of the dorsum of the wrist and hand. Dorsal interossei are unlabeled but are shown between the metacarpals.

be traced beyond the first interphalangeal joint. Much of the blood supply of the dorsum of the fingers is received from the *proper palmar digital arteries.*

There are both deep and superficial veins in the dorsum of the hand. The deep veins correspond in name to the arteries and have communications with the veins of the palm. The superficial veins form a *dorsal venous plexus (network),* which drains predominantly into the *cephalic vein* laterally and the *basilic vein* medially.

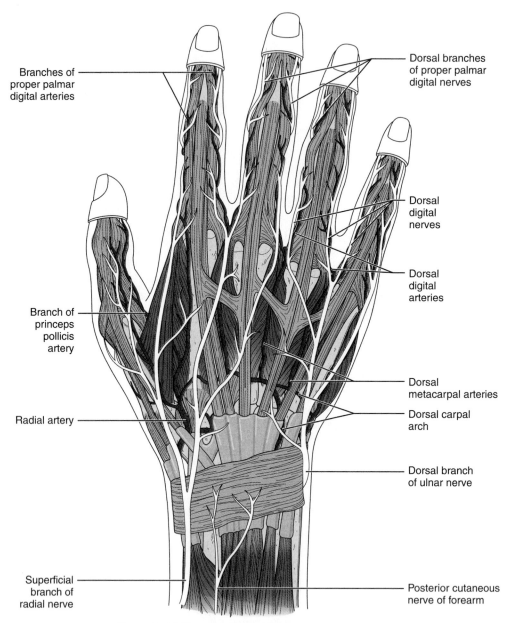

Figure 11-16 Nerves and arteries of the dorsum of the hand.

Branches of proper palmar digital arteries

Dorsal branches of proper palmar digital nerves

Dorsal digital nerves

Dorsal digital arteries

Branch of princeps pollicis artery

Dorsal metacarpal arteries

Dorsal carpal arch

Radial artery

Dorsal branch of ulnar nerve

Superficial branch of radial nerve

Posterior cutaneous nerve of forearm

NERVE INJURIES

In considering nerve injuries, it is important to consider the branching pattern of the nerve and the sensory and/or motor distribution of those branches. The location of the lesion determines whether specific branches are involved or spared. Branches given off distal to a lesion are affected, while those proximal to the injury are not affected.

Median Nerve

The effects of median nerve injuries on movements at the elbow and wrist are described in Chapter 8. The effect on the hand varies somewhat with the level of the lesion. A *lesion above the elbow* eliminates all innervation provided by the median nerve. The effect on the hand is evident in loss of all cutaneous innervation provided by the median nerve and motor innervation to the flexor digitorum superficialis, part of the flexor digitorum profundus, the flexor pollicis longus, and the majority of the thenar muscles (abductor pollicis brevis, superficial head of the flexor pollicis brevis, and opponens pollicis). Such a lesion would abolish flexion of at least the distal phalanx of the thumb and flexion of the index and middle fingers. The ulnar side of the flexor digitorum profundus is supplied by the ulnar nerve. In most cases, this muscle is able to flex the three medial digits: either because the ulnar nerve helps innervate the parts of the muscle going to these digits or because the tendons separate so low that contraction of the part going to the little finger, or to the little and ring fingers, pulls also on the tendon to the middle finger. Therefore, loss of median nerve innervation to the long flexors typically results only in inability to flex the middle and distal phalanges of the index finger and the distal phalanx of the thumb.

A *lesion specifically of the anterior interosseous branch* would affect only flexion of the distal phalanges of the thumb and one or two adjacent fingers, as a result of loss of the flexor pollicis longus and the radial side of the flexor digitorum profundus, respectively. Because this branch provides no sensory innervation to the skin of the hand, no cutaneous loss would be evident. A *lesion of the median nerve distal to the origin of the anterior interosseous branch* would affect only the thenar muscles, as would a lesion at the wrist. Sensory loss could involve the entire area of the palm and digits innervated by the median nerve. However, if the injury is distal to the origin of the palmar cutaneous branch, the skin of the midpalm would still be innervated.

FUNCTIONAL/CLINICAL NOTE 11-6

As the median nerve passes between the flexor tendons and the unyielding flexor retinaculum, it is subject to compression by anything that decreases the space in the carpal tunnel. Such compression may result from a carpal dislocation, but it is more commonly related to rheumatoid thickening of the synovial membrane of the synovial sheaths. The resulting condition (sensory changes, pain, perhaps atrophy of the thenar eminence) is called **carpal tunnel syndrome.** Surgery to correct this syndrome consists of slitting the flexor retinaculum. (The flexor tendons remain in place when the digits are flexed, because the wrist must be extended for digital flexion to occur.)

Loss of the thenar muscles innervated by the median nerve would be expected to abolish opposition because the abductor pollicis brevis and opponens pollicis are the principal muscles involved, but occasionally it does not. There are at least two reasons why opposition and abduction of the thumb are not always lost with a complete lesion (severing) of the median nerve. One is that the "rule" that this nerve innervates the abductor pollicis brevis, opponens pollicis, and superficial head of the flexor pollicis brevis is only generally true. Any or all of these muscles may be innervated by the ulnar nerve or may receive through the ulnar nerve median nerve fibers that have joined the ulnar in the forearm. (Here the level of the lesion, whether above or below the communication, would obviously make a difference.) The second reason is that the abductor pollicis longus (innervated by the radial nerve) and the deep head of the flexor pollicis brevis (ulnar nerve), or the abductor pollicis longus and the adductor pollicis (ulnar nerve), can often substitute satisfactorily for the opponens pollicis and abductor pollicis brevis. Although tendon transfers to produce flexion of the distal phalanges, and perhaps opposition, are usually necessary with high lesions of the median nerve, they are less often necessary with lesions at the wrist. In any case, if the nerve is completely interrupted and regeneration does not occur, the loss of sensation is very disabling.

With loss of the thenar muscles in a median nerve lesion, the abductor pollicis longus, extensor pollicis longus, and extensor pollicis brevis, which are all innervated by the radial nerve, gradually rotate the first metacarpal into the plane of the palm. This condition is referred to as **ape hand** (Fig. 11-17, *A*).

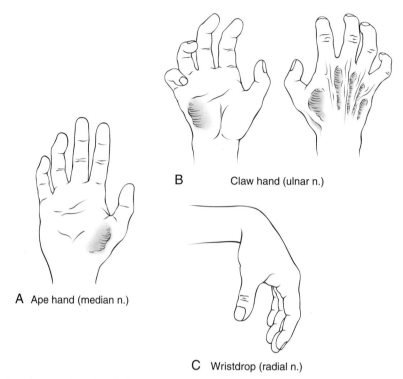

B   Claw hand (ulnar n.)

A   Ape hand (median n.)

C   Wristdrop (radial n.)

Figure 11-17 Hand postures resulting from lesions of the ulnar **(A)**, median **(B)**, and radial **(C)** nerves. With the ulnar nerve lesion, note the atrophy of the hypothenar eminence and of the interossei on the posterior surface of the hand. With a median nerve lesion, atrophy is evident in the thenar eminence.

Ulnar Nerve

There is little difference in the hand between the results of a lesion of the ulnar nerve at the elbow or one at the wrist. In a more *proximal lesion,* ulnar deviation would be affected as a result of paralysis of the flexor carpi ulnaris. Loss of the part of the flexor digitorum profundus innervated by the ulnar nerve would produce a variable disability in flexing the distal phalanges of the fourth and fifth digits, because the portion of the muscle acting on these digits may or may not be partly innervated by the median nerve. The findings in the hand are the same for both lesions.

In a severe *proximal or distal lesion,* some wasting of the hypothenar muscles and weakness in abduction-adduction of the fingers would occur as a result of the effect on the interossei. In complete paralysis of the interossei, the movements of abduction and adduction can still be produced, but only secondarily by other muscles. Although the extensor digitorum abducts as it extends, and the long flexors of the fingers adduct as they flex, normal abduction and adduction of the fingers is not possible with loss of the interossei. The most important loss is that of the flexing action of the interossei at the metacarpophalangeal joints. Because of this, the extensors draw the proximal phalanges into as much extension as the ligaments of the joints allow. With their pull concentrated on the proximal phalanges, the extensors lose their effect on the other two phalanges, and the flexor digitorum superficialis and flexor digitorum profundus, which become stretched, flex them. This condition is referred to as a **claw hand** (see Fig. 11-17, *B*). The greater the ligamentous laxity at the metacarpophalangeal joints is, the greater is the clawing. Clawing is usually less pronounced in the index and middle fingers because the lumbricals can flex the proximal metacarpals and extend the distal ones, and those of the index and middle fingers are commonly innervated by the median nerve.

Median and Ulnar Nerves

Combined injuries of the median and ulnar nerves have a devastating effect on the hand. A *lesion at the wrist* paralyzes all intrinsic muscles of the hand. Although the long flexors would still be functional, fine movement in the hand is eliminated. A more *proximal lesion*, again depending on the location, would also affect the muscles of the flexor forearm. In both cases, the extensors would be functional as a result of their innervation by the radial nerve. Sensory loss to the skin of the hand would be quite severe; some nerve branches would be spared with a lower lesion.

Radial Nerve

Lesions of the radial nerve are discussed in Chapter 9, but additional information on how lesions would specifically affect the hand is provided here. Although the radial nerve innervates no muscles in the hand, many of those that it innervates in the forearm act on the hand. The nerve also provides sensory innervation to some of the skin on the dorsum of the hand. A complete lesion (severing) of the radial nerve in the distal part of the arm, before it provides branches to any of the forearm muscles, would produce **wrist-drop** (see Fig. 11-17, *C*), as a result of the loss of all muscles capable of producing extension of the wrist.

Within the proximal part of the forearm, the nerve divides into deep and superficial branches. A lesion of the deep branch would affect only muscles, and the deficit would be determined by location of the injury. A more distal injury may have only minimal or no effect on movements within the hand. Only sensory loss would be noticed with a lesion of the superficial branch.

The effects on movement of the hand with a radial nerve injury are varied and depend on the location and severity of the lesion. A lesion may weaken or abolish extension at the metacarpophalangeal joints. However, extension of the interphalangeal joints of the fingers by the lumbricals and interossei (as a result of ulnar nerve innervation) and of the interphalangeal joint of the thumb by virtue of the attachment of the abductor pollicis brevis (which receives median nerve innervation) to the long extensor tendon may still be possible. If the lesion is high enough to affect the extensors of the wrist, an effective grip is prevented by the flexion of the wrist accompanying digital flexion.

REVIEW QUESTIONS

1 Describe in detail the anatomy of the radiocarpal joint. What movements are possible at this joint?

2 What is the arrangement of the synovial sheaths in the palm of the hand? On the basis of the arrangement of the synovial sheath of the flexor tendons of the little finger, how far can an infection, produced by a penetrating wound to the tip of the finger and confined to the sheath, spread within the hand?

3 Describe in detail the origin, insertion, action, and innervation of the adductor pollicis muscle.

4 What is the arrangement of the tendons of the flexor digitorum superficialis and flexor digitorum profundus muscles on the phalanges, and where do they insert?

5 What is the function of the lumbrical muscles? What is their innervation?

6 Compare the similarities and differences of the anatomy and function of the palmar and dorsal interossei muscles.

7 Atrophy of the hypothenar eminence could indicate injury to which nerve? If this nerve was completely severed in the distal forearm, what muscles and movements in the hand would be affected?

8 Which nerve or nerves provide sensory innervation to the following?
   a nail bed of the index finger
   b skin of the palmar surface of the tip of the ring finger
   c skin of the palmar surface of the tip of the little finger
   d skin over the hypothenar eminence
   e skin over the dorsal aspect of the metacarpophalangeal joint of the thumb

9 From which artery does the superficial palmar arch arise? What are the major branches of this arch? Which artery forms the deep palmar arch? The princeps pollicis is a branch of which artery?

10 What are the anatomical relationships of the tendons, nerves, and vessels within the carpal tunnel? What nerves pass superficial to the flexor retinaculum?

11 Explain the terms *claw hand* and *carpal tunnel syndrome.*

12 A patient was admitted to the emergency room after tripping and pushing his hand through a glass pane of a door. He suffered a deep laceration on the medial side of the wrist near the pisiform bone. Upon examination, it was noted that no general sensation was present on the skin of the palmar area of the hand normally innervated by the ulnar nerve, which indicated involvement of that nerve in the injury. However, sensory innervation to the skin on the dorsum of the hand normally innervated by the ulnar nerve was still intact. How can this be explained?

EXERCISES

1 On a skeleton, identify the individual carpal bones.

2 Demonstrate on your hand or that of a fellow student the following:
   a pisiform bone
   b position of the scaphoid bone
   c location of the flexor retinaculum
   d tendon of the extensor pollicis longus
   e first dorsal interosseous muscle

12 MOVEMENTS OF THE DIGITS

CHAPTER CONTENTS

Flexion of the Fingers

Extension of the Fingers

Abduction and Adduction of the Digits

Movements of the Little Finger

Movements of the Thumb

Types of Grips Involved in Grasping

Analyses of Activities and Associated Movements

Movements of the fingers and thumb involve complicated integrations of the actions of muscles originating in the forearm, as well as those intrinsic to the hand. These individual movements are used in various combinations to perform the very complex actions that are possible with the hand.

FLEXION OF THE FINGERS

Flexion of the fingers is brought about by the action of the flexor digitorum profundus and flexor digitorum superficialis and muscles in the palm (Fig. 12-1). The *flexor digitorum profundus,* through its attachment on the distal phalanges, is a flexor primarily at the distal interphalangeal joints. By continued action, it also flexes the proximal interphalangeal joints and, finally, the metacarpophalangeal joints. The action of this muscle on the proximal interphalangeal joints depends, however, on these joints' being already in slight flexion. If, as a result of rupture of the palmar ligament of the joint, the proximal interphalangeal joint is in slight extension, contraction of the muscle increases this extension, and the joint is locked in an extended position. Normally, the integrity of the palmar ligaments allows the flexor digitorum profundus to act not only on the distal interphalangeal joints but also on the other more proximal joints, and although other muscles can assist, it alone is commonly used in making a fist. It is so efficient in flexing the proximal interphalangeal joints that it was once routine for it to be left as the sole flexor of these joints, the flexor digitorum superficialis being removed, when the flexor tendons on the fingers were injured.

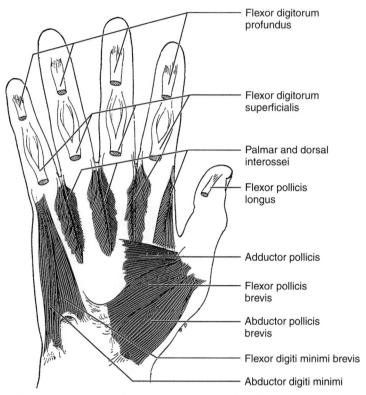

Figure 12-1 The flexors of the interphalangeal and metacarpophalangeal joints. (The lumbricals, secondary flexors at the metacarpophalangeal joints, are omitted.)

The *flexor digitorum superficialis*, through its attachment to the middle phalanges, acts on the proximal interphalangeal joints, and by continued action, it also aids in flexing the metacarpophalangeal joints. The *lumbricals* flex the metacarpophalangeal joints only after they have extended the interphalangeal ones. Their primary function seems to be the latter action, for they assist in this regardless of the direction of movement at the metacarpophalangeal joints. The *interossei*, however, are regularly active during flexion of the metacarpophalangeal joints, whether the joints are held in flexion or are being flexed. They are the primary flexors of these joints.

The long flexors, so essential to the power of grip of the fingers and hand, are at a mechanical advantage only when the wrist is extended. Consequently, flexion at the wrist markedly interferes with flexion of the fingers. For this reason, when extensive paralysis of flexor muscles necessitates transferring extensor tendons to the palm and joining them to the distal ends of flexor tendons, at least one good wrist extensor should be left intact. Similarly, if the wrist is to be fused to make it immobile, it is always fixed in slight extension to enable the long flexors to function efficiently.

EXTENSION OF THE FINGERS

Extension of the fingers usually involves the cooperation of two sets of muscles. The tendons of the first set, the *extensor digitorum tendons* with the associated *extensors of the little and index fingers*, expand over the metacarpophalangeal joints of each of the fingers, covering the joint capsules. They are attached to the palmar ligaments in such a way that, once they have moved proximally a certain distance, they extend the metacarpophalangeal joints even though their actual insertions are on the middle and distal phalanges. The extensor digitorum and the special extensors of the index and little fingers that join it are the sole extensors of the metacarpophalangeal joints. Distal to these joints, however, the extensor tendons are joined by a second set of tendons, those of the *lumbricals* and the *interossei* (Fig. 12-2). Over the proximal phalanx, the tendons blend together to form a single tendon that is often referred to as the *extensor expansion* or *extensor hood.* This divides into a central band that inserts on the middle phalanx and into two lateral bands that converge to an insertion on the distal phalanx. The extensor digitorum, lumbricals, and interossei all cooperate in extending the middle and distal phalanges. The lumbricals typically contract with the extensor digitorum when all joints are extended at once, and presumably both help extend the interphalangeal joints and prevent hyperextension at the metacarpophalangeal ones. The lumbricals and the interossei extend the interphalangeal joints when the metacarpophalangeal ones are flexed or are being flexed, but extension by the interossei seems to be secondary to their flexor action at the metacarpophalangeal joints.

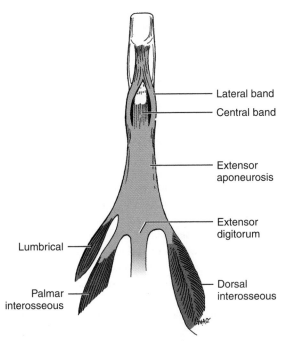

Figure 12-2 The extensors of a typical finger. The ring finger is illustrated. Other fingers have slightly different arrangements of the interossei, and some, of course, have proper extensors. The principle, however, is the same for the four fingers.

— Lateral band
— Central band
— Extensor aponeurosis
— Extensor digitorum
— Dorsal interosseous

Lumbrical —
Palmar interosseous —

The bands uniting the extensor tendons on the dorsum of the hand (the "intertendinous connections" in Fig. 11-15) limit independent extension of the individual fingers at the metacarpophalangeal joints. This is particularly true of the middle and ring fingers. The index and little fingers are less hampered in independent extension because of the individual extensors with which they are also provided.

ABDUCTION AND ADDUCTION OF THE DIGITS

Abduction of the digits results from contraction of the *dorsal interossei* and the *abductors of the thumb and little finger* (Fig. 12-3). **Adduction** is brought about by the *palmar interossei* and the *adductor of the thumb* (Fig. 12-4). The *flexor digitorum superficialis* and *flexor digitorum profundus* also adduct the fingers as they flex them, whereas the *extensor digitorum* abducts the fingers as it extends them. These long tendons, however, act on all four fingers at once and do not allow for individual abduction and adduction of a given finger. The *extensor indicis* can independently adduct the index finger, and the *extensor digiti minimi* can abduct the little finger.

MOVEMENTS OF THE LITTLE FINGER

Flexion of the little finger at the metacarpophalangeal joint can be produced by both the *flexor digiti minimi brevis* and *abductor digiti minimi*. Both muscles also abduct the little finger. **Opposition of the little finger,** which produces a certain amount of rotation of the fifth metacarpal, is produced by the *opponens digiti minimi.*

MOVEMENTS OF THE THUMB

Movements of the thumb are more complicated than are movements of the fingers as a whole. Most of the short muscles of the thumb contract during any movement of that part, either to directly assist or to steady the movement. The diagnosis of injury to the musculature or nerves of the thumb is complicated in clinical practice because the innervation of the muscles of the thumb may vary. A given muscle is

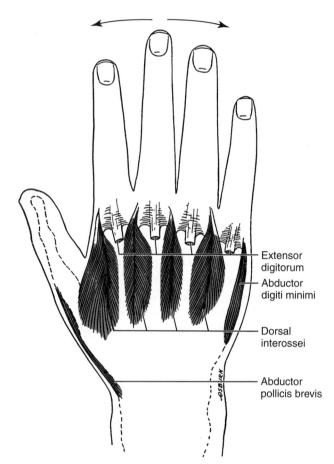

Figure 12-3 Dorsal view of the chief abductors of the right digits.

supplied in some cases by the median nerve and in others by the ulnar nerve or by a combination of both.

Flexion of the thumb at the interphalangeal joint can be brought about only by the *flexor pollicis longus*. Flexion at the metacarpophalangeal joint of the thumb is more limited and is usually accompanied by marked movement of the metacarpal. The *flexor pollicis brevis* and *adductor pollicis* produce flexion at the metacarpophalangeal joint and, if they move the metacarpal, also produce adduction and opposition of the thumb. The *abductor pollicis brevis* also aids in flexion at this joint.

In contrast to the fingers, the most movable joint of the thumb is the saddle-shaped carpometacarpal joint. **Opposition,** involving movement of the metacarpal at this joint, is the most useful movement

of the thumb. Such movement is necessary for holding a small object, such as a pin, between the thumb and index finger, or for grasping a baseball firmly, and it helps in handling such tools as a hoe or hammer; in the latter case, the firmer part of the grip is on the ulnar side of the hand. Opposition is carried out by the *opponens pollicis, flexor pollicis brevis,* and *abductor pollicis brevis,* with the first two contributing most if firm pressure is necessary. This movement is aided also by the *flexor pollicis longus* and *adductor pollicis.*

Pure **adduction of the thumb** involves the movement of the thumb toward the palm of the hand at right angles to the plane of the palm (see Fig. 1-3, *F*). This movement can be brought about only through the combined actions of the *adductor pollicis* and the *extensor pollicis longus.* The adductor acting alone

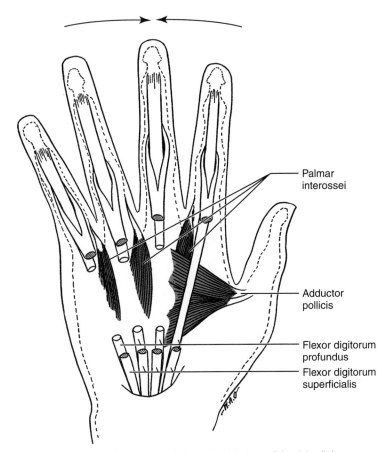

Figure 12-4 Plantar view of the chief adductors of the right digits.

tends to pull the thumb across the palm, as well as to adduct it. Pure **abduction of the thumb** is brought about by the action of the *abductor pollicis brevis*. The *abductor pollicis longus* abducts, extends, and externally rotates at the carpometacarpal joint, bringing about a movement (reposition) that is the reverse of opposition.

Extension at the interphalangeal joint of the thumb (see Fig. 1-3, *E*) is produced by the *extensor pollicis longus* and *abductor pollicis brevis* and, if the movement is resisted, by the *adductor pollicis* (both the abductor and the adductor muscles insert in part into the long extensor tendon). Extension at the metacarpophalangeal joint is carried out by the *extensor pollicis brevis*, which may also join the long extensor and thereby help extend the distal phalanx. Flexion and extension at the carpometacarpal joint

of the thumb are usually accompanied by rotation of the metacarpal.

TYPES OF GRIPS INVOLVED IN GRASPING

This chapter has focused on the various individual movements of the digits and the muscles that produce them. These movements can be combined to accomplish complex activities. The act of grasping and holding an object *(prehension)* is an example. The type of grip necessary to pick up, hold, and manipulate an object varies with the size and shape of that object and the force necessary to hold it to perform the activity. There are two main categories of grip, power and precision, each of which can be subdivided into various types (Fig. 12-5).

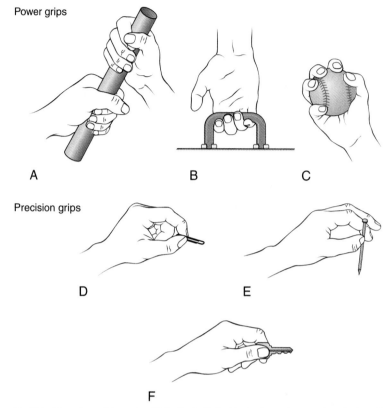

Power grips

A   B   C

Precision grips

D   E

F

Figure 12-5 Power grips (**A** to **C**) and precision grips (**D** to **F**). **A,** Cylindrical grip, as in grasping the handle of a broom. **B,** Hook grip, as in grasping the handle of a briefcase. **C,** Spherical grip, as in holding a baseball. **D,** Tip-to-tip grip, as in holding a paper clip. **E,** Pad-to-pad grip, as in holding a nail. **F,** Pad-to-side grip, as in holding a key.

Power Grips

As the name implies, a power grip is the more powerful of the two. It usually involves the fingers and the thumb and may or may not involve contact of the object with the palm. Not all power grips are the same. For example, in holding a tennis racket, the digits are positioned differently than when grasping a baseball or the handle of a suitcase.

The type of power grip used in holding a broom handle, a steering wheel, or a tennis racket is called a **cylindrical grip** (see Fig. 12-5, *A*). The fingers are flexed tightly around the handle, with more flexion and rotation occurring at the more medial digits. The thenar eminence is drawn toward the handle to provide a secure grip, and the thumb either overlaps the fingers for the strongest grasp or is placed along the length of the object. The hand is often adducted at

the wrist to better align the item being held with the long axis of the forearm, such as in holding a screwdriver. The long flexors provide power to the grip, and the thenar and hypothenar muscles come into play for the movements of abduction, opposition, and flexion of the thumb and little finger, respectively. This type of activity involves muscles that are innervated by the median or the ulnar nerve or both, and for a strong grip, the wrist must be partially extended by muscles innervated by the radial nerve. A similar type of grip is used to hold a large glass of water, but because of the larger size of the object, the grasp must be modified, with no overlap of the fingers by the thumb.

In the case of a **hook grip** (see Fig. 12-5, *B*), as in carrying a suitcase or bucket, the fingers are flexed at the interphalangeal joints by contraction of the long flexors, and the metacarpophalangeal joints are typically maintained in extension. In this way, a "hook" is created to hold the handle, and the handle is supported on the middle phalanges. The hook grip does not usually involve the thumb and palm.

The type of power grip used to grasp a baseball, an orange, or a doorknob is termed a **spherical** (or **ball**) **grip** (see Fig. 12-5, *C*). With this grip, the metacarpophalangeal and interphalangeal joints of the fingers and thumb are flexed and the digits are abducted so that they can better surround the object. The palm may not be in contact with the object being grasped.

Precision Grips

The second major category of grip, the *precision grip,* uses less power but has more refined muscle action, involving both muscles originating in the forearm and the intrinsic muscles of the hand. In precision grips, the hand is usually fixed at the wrist and the thumb is in opposition to one or two fingers, particularly the index and middle fingers. Such grips are used to pick up, hold, and manipulate small items. Precision grips can be categorized by describing the surface contact areas on the thumb and fingers. Three of the major

precision grips are tip-to-tip, pad-to-pad, and pad-to-side.

In a **tip-to-tip (pincer) grip** (see Fig. 12-5, *D*) the tips of the thumb and finger grasp the object, such as in picking up a paper clip. To accomplish this task, the metacarpophalangeal and interphalangeal joints of the thumb and finger are flexed. For the **pad-to-pad (pinch) grip** (see Fig. 12-5, *E*), the pad (pulp) of the index (and possibly that of the middle finger) is in opposition to the pad of the thumb, such as in holding a nail while it is being hammered or in grasping a cracker. This is similar to the tip-to-tip grip. However, the interphalangeal joint of the thumb and the distal interphalangeal joint of the finger are extended so that the pads make contact with the item being grasped.

With a **pad-to-side grip** (see Fig. 12-5, *F*) an object such as a key (pad-to-side grip is also called a *key grip*) or a large piece of paper can be held between the thumb and lateral or radial side of the index finger. The metacarpophalangeal and interphalangeal joints of the thumb and index finger are flexed with this type of grip. The pad-to-side grip permits less precise manipulation than the preceding two grips.

ANALYSES OF ACTIVITIES AND ASSOCIATED MOVEMENTS

Activity: *Picking up a Bowling Ball.* In picking up a bowling ball, the thumb and middle and ring fingers are inserted into the holes in the ball, and the index and little fingers remain on the ball's outer surface. The thumb is partially abducted and extended at the metacarpophalangeal joint. The interphalangeal joint is slightly flexed so that the long axis of the thumb is in a straight line to enable insertion of the thumb into the ball. Abduction and extension of the thumb at the metacarpophalangeal joints are produced in this case by the abductor and extensor pollicis brevis muscles. The flexor pollicis longus flexes the interphalangeal joint.

Both the middle and ring fingers flex at the metacarpophalangeal joints but extend at the interphalangeal joints. Combined action of the lumbricals and interossei at these fingers can bring about these movements.

To remain on the surface of the ball while the other digits are inserted into the holes, the index and little fingers are extended at the metacarpophalangeal and interphalangeal joints. The extensor indicis and extensor digiti minimi muscles are the primary muscles involved. Although the extensor digitorum also has tendons to these fingers, contraction of this muscle involves extension of all fingers, with no specific action at the index and little fingers.

Once the thumb and two fingers are inserted, all the fingers flex at the interphalangeal joints (accompanied by a variable amount of flexion at the metacarpophalangeal joints). This flexion enables the palmar surface of the tip of each digit to press against the ball, either on the surfaces of the holes or outer surface of the ball. When sufficient pressure is created, the ball can then be picked up. The flexion is the result of contraction of the appropriate flexor that inserts on the distal phalanx of each digit.

Continued

ANALYSES OF ACTIVITIES AND ASSOCIATED MOVEMENTS—cont'd

Activity: *Adjusting the Time on a Watch.* Manipulating the stem of a watch to change the time or wind the mechanism requires the use of a precision grip. Once the stem is pulled outward, it is gripped in either a pad-to-pad or pad-to-side grip. In a pad-to-pad grip, the stem sits between the pads of the index finger and thumb; in a pad-to-side grip, the stem is placed between the lateral side of the index finger and the pad of the thumb. With either grip, both digits can move, or one can remain stable as the other digit works against it.

To grasp the stem of the watch, the interphalangeal and metacarpophalangeal joints of the index finger are flexed by the flexor digitorum superficialis and flexor digitorum profundus. Assistance in flexion at the metacarpophalangeal joint is provided by the interossei. The thumb is opposed to the index finger through the combined actions primarily of the opponens pollicis, flexor pollicis brevis, and abductor pollicis brevis. If contact is made with a pad-to-pad grip, the distal interphalangeal joint of the index finger is extended to produce the grip; in a pad-to-side grip, the interphalangeal joints remain flexed. The stem is then rotated by very limited flexion and extension of the distal phalanges of one or both digits. This action is produced by the long flexors and extensors of the respective digits.

Activity: *Using Forceps or Tweezers to Remove a Splinter.* To remove a splinter of wood from the skin of a finger tip, a forceps or tweezers can be grasped between the pads of the index finger and thumb in a pad-to-pad (pinch) grip. Movements involved in grasping a forceps in this way are flexion at the metacarpophalangeal joint of the thumb and the index finger; flexion of the proximal interphalangeal joint and extension of the distal interphalangeal joint of the index finger; and extension of the interphalangeal joint of the thumb. With the splinter positioned between the tips of the forceps, the tips of the forceps can be brought together with the following movements: additional flexion of the metacarpophalangeal joints of the thumb and index finger; slight abduction of the index finger; and possibly flexion of the proximal interphalangeal joint of the index finger.

Muscles involved with flexion at the metacarpophalangeal joints are the flexor pollicis brevis and adductor pollicis for the thumb and the flexor digitorum superficialis (and possibly the interossei) for the index finger. Flexion of the proximal interphalangeal joint of the index finger is produced by the flexor digitorum superficialis, whereas extension at the distal interphalangeal joint of this finger is produced by the extensor digitorum and extensor indicis muscles. The interphalangeal joint of the thumb is extended by the extensor pollicis longus. The first dorsal interosseous has been described as assisting in flexion of the metacarpophalangeal joint of the index finger; it also produces slight abduction of this finger as the forceps are closed. It can be palpated in the tissue between the thumb and index finger as it contracts.

Variations in gripping the forceps, amount of force applied, and so forth can modify the movements and the muscles that are involved. The forceps could be held in more of a tip-to-tip or a pad-to-side grip between the thumb and the side of the middle phalanx of the index finger. Observe and palpate the area as this activity is performed, and then modify the technique to determine differences in movements and muscles involved.

REVIEW QUESTIONS

1 Why is independent extension of the middle and ring fingers so limited at the metacarpophalangeal joints?

2 Which muscles are responsible for abduction of the fingers? Which muscles produce adduction?

3 What is the extensor expansion? What are the relationships of the lumbricals and interossei to the expansion?

4 Discuss the movements and muscles involved in the following:
   a making a fist
   b picking up a coin from a table
   c holding a pencil
   d making a hook grip to lift a bucket

5 Explain the anatomy of a cylindrical grip.

EXERCISES

1 Demonstrate the action of the flexor digitorum profundus if the lumbricals and interossei were unable to produce flexion at the metacarpophalangeal joints.

2 Demonstrate the movements of the thumb.

SECTION 3 The Back

13 THE BACK

CHAPTER CONTENTS

General Considerations

Vertebral Column

Vertebrae

Joints of the Vertebral Column

Movements and Stability

Musculature of the Back

The Meninges and the Spinal Cord

Analyses of Activities and Associated Movements

GENERAL CONSIDERATIONS

The skeleton and musculature of the back are largely responsible for the support and movements of the trunk. The back also supports and stabilizes the upper limbs and head so that they can move smoothly and evenly or support strains on them. Because the weight borne by the back increases from the cervical to the lumbar regions, and because greater leverage is also exerted in the lumbar region, it is obvious that the lower part of the back is subjected to great stress. The enormous strains on the lower back account for the commonness of pain in this region. Because of the importance of the musculature of the back and of the bony vertebral column in stabilizing the body as a whole, a back disability affects not only the back but also the body as a whole. It may make any posture or movement painful or difficult.

VERTEBRAL COLUMN

The vertebral column (Fig. 13-1), often called the "spinal column" or the "spine", consists of a series of bones, the *vertebrae*, usually numbering 33 at birth. Of these, there are in the adult typically 7 separate **cervical vertebrae** in the neck or cervical region, 12 **thoracic vertebrae** connected with the ribs, and 5 **lumbar vertebrae** in the lower part of the back. Usually the next 5 are fused together to form the **sacrum,** and the remaining 3 or 4, rudimentary in character, form the **coccyx.**

The vertebral column serves two chief functions: *supporting the trunk* and *protecting the spinal cord.* The **movements of the vertebral column** are *flexion* (forward bending), *extension, lateral flexion,* and *rotation.* These are accomplished with varying amounts of freedom of movement in the various regions of the vertebral column, and certain movements are quite regularly a combination of two of these primary movements.

If the vertebral column is viewed as a whole (see Fig. 13-1) in an articulated skeleton, it becomes obvious that the length of the column is not dependent purely on the length of the vertebral bodies; it is also determined by the **intervertebral discs** that lie between adjacent vertebrae (see later "Intervertebral discs" section, Fig. 13-1, and Fig. 13-7). These discs are responsible for approximately 25 percent of the total length of the vertebral column above the sacrum.

In early fetal life, the vertebral column as a whole is somewhat C-shaped (concave forward), whereas at birth, a slight flexure is present between the lumbar and sacral parts of the column (Fig. 13-2, *A* and *B*). The *thoracic and sacral curvatures* of the adult represent the remains of the original curve (see Fig. 13-2, *C*). The *cervical and lumbar curvatures* of the column in the adult are oriented so that their concavities are directed posteriorly. These two reverse curves develop as a means of better balancing the weight of the body on the vertebral column. The cervical curvature develops as the infant tries to hold up the head, and the lumbar curvature develops during the stages of

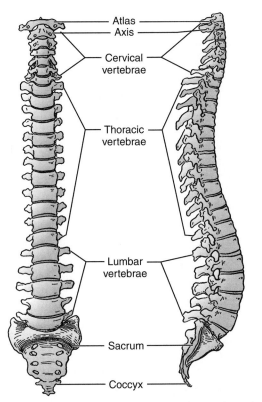

Figure 13-1 The vertebral column as a whole, anterior and lateral views. Discs are highlighted in *color.*

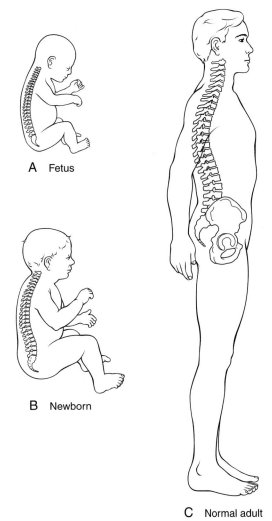

Figure 13-2 Normal curvatures of the vertebral column.

learning to sit, stand, and walk. The lumbar curvature results from unequal growth of the anterior and posterior borders of both the bodies of the vertebrae and discs; the cervical curvature to the discs alone. The part that the discs play in the curvatures is strikingly shown by comparison of an articulated vertebral column with one strung on a string. The general forward concavity of the latter is reminiscent of the stoop associated with aging, which also results in part from changes in the intervertebral discs.

VERTEBRAE

Typical Vertebra

Before describing vertebrae in different regions of the column (cervical, thoracic, and so forth), it is helpful to present features common to most vertebrae: in essence, describing a "typical" vertebra. A typical vertebra (in Fig. 13-3, *B* and *C*, include features of a typical vertebra) consists of several named parts fused together to form a single bone. The heavy, approximately cylindrical base of the vertebra is called

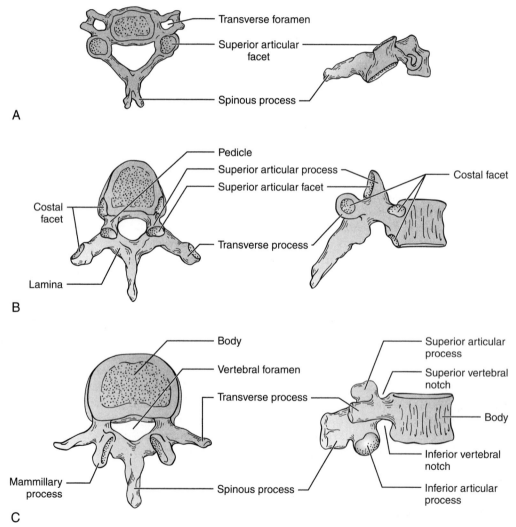

Figure 13-3 Superior *(left)* and lateral *(right)* views of a representative vertebra from the cervical **(A)**, thoracic **(B)**, and lumbar **(C)** regions.

the *body.* It is largely spongy bone covered generally by a thin layer of cortical or dense bone. However, the superior and inferior surfaces of the bodies are mostly covered by a thin layer of hyaline cartilage that persists throughout life and is responsible for the growth in length of the vertebrae during the period of growth. On the posterior surface of the body are two projections, paired pillars or *pedicles* (roots of the arch), which extend posteriorly to connect to the *laminae.* The pedicles and laminae together form the *vertebral arch.* Between the vertebral arch and body is the *vertebral foramen.* Successive vertebral foramina form the *vertebral canal,* in which the spinal cord and associated structures lie.

In most vertebrae, the pedicle has a deep *inferior vertebral notch* on its lower border. The inferior vertebral notch and the less pronounced *superior vertebral notch* on the upper border of the pedicle below (see Fig. 13-3, *C*) form an *intervertebral foramen* through which a spinal nerve makes its exit from the vertebral canal.

At about the junction of the pedicle and lamina, there are paired *superior* and paired *inferior articular processes,* or *zygapophyses,* which bear smooth facets for articulation with the vertebrae above and below. The exact position and the planes of articulation of these processes vary with the region of the particular vertebra. Projecting laterally from about the point of union of the pedicle and lamina on either side is a *transverse process* for the attachment of muscles and, in the thoracic region, for articulation with ribs. The *spinous process* (often called *spine*), also for the attachment of muscles, is a midline posterior projection from the laminae.

Regional Vertebrae

The vertebrae have regional differences, and so it is usually possible to recognize the group to which any one of them belongs. Some of them are so specialized that they can be individually recognized without difficulty.

Cervical vertebrae

The **cervical vertebrae** as a whole (see Fig. 13-3, *A*) are characterized by the fact that each of their transverse processes contains a foramen, the *transverse foramen.* The right and left vertebral arteries pass through the transverse foramina of the upper six cervical vertebrae (on their respective sides) as they course to the cranial cavity. The seventh cervical vertebra may or may not have complete transverse foramina. The *bodies* are relatively delicate, their greatest dimension being their width. The articular processes are short; the facets on the *superior articular processes* face upward and backward, and those on the *inferior articular processes* face downward and forward.

The first two cervical vertebrae (Fig. 13-4, *A* and *B*) are different from the rest. The first cervical vertebra, known as the **atlas** because it supports the "globe" of the head, is distinguished by the fact that it has *no body* but rather an *anterior arch* where a body would be expected. A *lateral mass* lies to each side of the anterior arch, and each has *articular facets* (foveae) on its superior and inferior surfaces. The superior articular facets are concave and articulate with the occipital condyles of the skull, while the inferior articular facets are flatter and articulate with the second cervical vertebra. The atlas's *transverse processes* are long, and it has no true spinous process but simply a *tubercle* where the process would be.

The second cervical vertebra, or **axis,** is characterized by a toothlike process, the *dens,* which projects upward from its body. This process articulates with the anterior arch of the atlas and is held firmly in position by ligaments (see Fig. 13-4, *C*). In this way, the dens acts as a pivot around which the atlas rotates. The dens may represent what could be considered the body of the atlas that, during development, fuses with the axis.

The remaining cervical vertebrae show a gradual increase in size caudally, but otherwise, there are no particularly individual characteristics. The spinous processes of the middle cervical vertebrae are usually bifid (forked). The seventh cervical vertebrae, or **vertebra prominens,** may be somewhat transitional between a typical cervical and a typical thoracic vertebra, and it regularly has a rather long spinous process with a somewhat bulbous tip.

Thoracic vertebrae

As the vertebral column is followed downward, the bodies of the **thoracic vertebrae** (see Fig. 13-3, *B*) continue the gradual increase in size that is observed

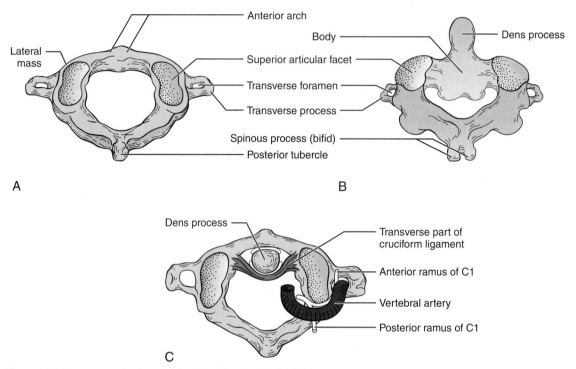

Figure 13-4 Posterosuperior views of the atlas **(A)** and axis **(B). C,** Superior view of the atlanto-axial joint. Note the course of the vertebral artery on the right (that on the left has not been included) as it passes out of the transverse foramen. It would continue superiorly into the foramen magnum in the base of the skull.

in the cervical region. The *superior* and *inferior articular facets* are almost in the frontal plane, especially in the midthoracic region; the superior facets face posteriorly, the inferior ones anteriorly. In contrast to the transverse processes of the cervical vertebrae, those of the thoracic vertebrae have no foramina. On the anterolateral surfaces of the ends of the transverse processes of the upper 10 thoracic vertebrae are smooth articular surfaces, *costal facets* (foveae), for articulation with the ribs. Similar costal facets occur on the sides of the vertebrae at about the junction of the pedicle and body. The 1st, 10th, 11th, and 12th vertebrae usually have a complete costal facet on their upper edges for articulation with the head of a rib. On the others the costal facets are shared by two adjacent vertebrae, so that most of the thoracic vertebrae have half-facets (superior and inferior articular surfaces) situated at both the upper and lower borders of the bone. The *spinous processes* of thoracic vertebrae tend to be long and slender and directed markedly downward so that they overlap each other. Those of the lower thoracic vertebrae are broader and directed more posteriorly, in this way being transitional between typical thoracic and typical lumbar vertebrae.

Lumbar vertebrae

The bodies of the **lumbar vertebrae** are more massive than those of the thoracic region, and the *spinous processes* appear much heavier and broader when viewed from the side (see Fig. 13-3, *C*). In contrast to the cervical and thoracic vertebrae, the height of each *lamina* is less than that of the body, so that a considerable space exists between adjacent laminae. The *transverse processes* tend to be long and slender. The facets of the *superior articular processes* are directed upward and posteriorly but largely medially, and those of the *inferior articular processes* are directed downward and anteriorly but largely laterally; therefore, these joints approach the median plane. On the posterior surfaces of the superior articular processes, there are large irregular protuberances, the *mammillary bodies,* for additional attachment of muscles.

Sacral vertebrae

The five sacral vertebrae are, in the adult, fused to form a single bone, the **sacrum** (Fig. 13-5). On its pelvic (anteroinferior, concave) surface are four slight ridges that mark the lines of fusion between the five elements forming the bone. Laterally, in line with these ridges, are the *anterior sacral foramina* through which the anterior rami of the first four sacral nerves make their exit. The modified *transverse processes* separating these foramina fuse again laterally to form the heavy lateral portions of the sacrum that articulate with the hip bones.

The posterior surface of the sacrum is convex and much roughened by the attachment of muscles. The irregular posterior projection in the midline, the *median crest,* represents rudimentary *spinous processes.* Laterally, the *posterior sacral foramina* provide an exit for the posterior rami of the first four sacral nerves. The vertebral canal of the sacrum is more appropriately called the *sacral canal.* At the caudal end of the sacrum, the posterior part of the sacral canal is commonly deficient, being bridged during life by ligaments. This deficient area is the *sacral hiatus.*

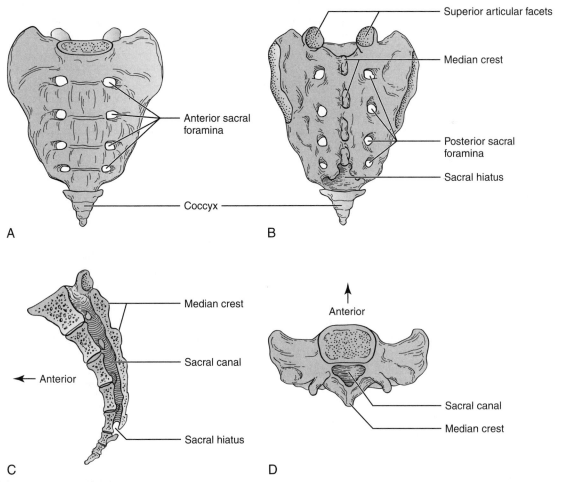

Figure 13-5 Sacrum and coccyx. **A,** Anterior view. **B,** Posterior view. **C,** Lateral view of sagittally sectioned sacrum. (The sacral canal is the lower end of the vertebral canal.) **D,** Superior view.

Coccyx

The **coccyx** (see Fig. 13-5) consists of three or four elements, typically three, which are hardly recognizable as vertebrae. They essentially represent the rudiments of vertebral bodies. The *first coccygeal vertebra* is best developed and usually remains separate from the rest throughout life, whereas the others are usually fused together.

Surface Anatomy

The **curvatures** of the vertebral column can be observed and palpated. Passing a finger down the midline along the vertebral spine enables visualization of the posteriorly directed concavities of the cervical and lumbar regions and the posteriorly directed convexity of the column in both the thoracic and sacral regions. Any lateral deviation from the midline or exaggerated curvatures can be observed in this way.

The bones of the back are often difficult to observe or palpate because of the overlying superficial muscles (latissimus dorsi and trapezius), the muscles attached to the medial border of the scapula (levator scapulae and rhomboids), and the back muscles to be described in this chapter. In studying the back, it is important to be aware of a few landmarks on the skull. Laterally, just posterior to the external ear, the **mastoid process** of each side can be palpated as it projects inferiorly from the base of the skull. On the midline of the posterior aspect of the skull, the **external occipital protuberance** can be felt. The **superior nuchal lines** (which can best be observed on a skull) extend laterally from the protuberance.

In palpation of the cervical region of the vertebral column, many of the features of the vertebrae are obscured by the overlying musculature on the back of the neck and the ligamentum nuchae that extends from the skull along the spinous processes of the cervical vertebrae (see next section). Having only a posterior tubercle, rather than a spinous process, the atlas cannot be palpated in the midline. The **spinous process of the axis**, however, can be felt in the posterior midline of the neck about two fingerbreadths inferior to the external occipital protuberance. The next prominent **spinous process** is that of the **seventh cervical vertebra.** It becomes more apparent when the neck is flexed and the head is bent forward.

Because of the obvious protrusion of its spinous process, the seventh cervical vertebra is termed the *vertebra prominens.* Laterally, in the neck, the **transverse process of the first cervical vertebra** can be felt just posterior and inferior to the mastoid process. The transverse processes of the other cervical vertebrae are more difficult to distinguish, but some may be palpable deep within the musculature of the neck.

In the thoracic region, the rather sharp **spinous processes of the thoracic vertebrae** can be seen or palpated and become more prominent with flexion of the trunk. It must be remembered that the spinous processes of the thoracic vertebrae, particularly in the midthoracic region, are long and inclined inferiorly. In this manner, each overlaps the body of the vertebra below. For instance, the spinous process of the seventh thoracic vertebra (the tip of which is at the level of the inferior angle of the scapula) lies posterior to the body of the eighth thoracic vertebra.

The broader **lumbar spinous processes** can usually be identified. These and the lower thoracic ones lie in an increasingly deep groove formed by the increasingly heavy mass of the back muscles. A line projected across the midline between the highest point of the iliac crest (see Chapter 15) on each side passes across the **spine of the fourth lumbar vertebra.** This spine is a good landmark for determining the location for a lumbar puncture, for withdrawing cerebrospinal fluid, or for administering a spinal anesthetic (see "Spinal Cord" section).

The **sacrum** can be palpated. The **second sacral vertebra** is located at the level of the **posterior superior iliac spine** of the bony pelvis. The **coccyx** can be palpated at the tip of the vertebral column. Just above the coccyx, depending on the amount of overlying tissue, the **sacral hiatus** may be palpable. Through this hiatus, anesthetic agents can be injected into the epidural space (see "Meninges" section).

JOINTS OF THE VERTEBRAL COLUMN

The joints connecting most of the vertebrae are of two kinds: *synovial,* of the plane type, formed by the apposition of the articular processes; and *cartilaginous,* between the bodies, formed by the union of the intervertebral discs with the bodies.

Synovial Joints between Articular Processes

The synovial joints formed by the articular processes (zygapophyses) allow only simple gliding movements. Although the articular capsules of these joints are lax, allowing more movement than might be expected from examination of the bony elements alone, the directions in which the articular surfaces face are significant factors in determining what type of movement (flexion-extension, lateral bending, or rotation) is possible between any two adjacent vertebrae. Branches of the posterior rami of spinal nerves innervate these joints. Arthritic changes in the joints and undue strain placed on them as a result of abnormal postures or movements are common causes of back pain.

There are numerous ligaments between the arches of the vertebrae that can be considered "accessory" ligaments of the synovial joints (Fig. 13-6). These are the **supraspinous** (supraspinal) ligament, stretched across the tips of the spinous processes; the **interspinous** (interspinal) ligament, between one spinous process and the next; and the **ligamenta flava** (singular: ligamentum flavum), paired ligaments that connect adjacent laminae and almost completely fill the spaces between them. In addition to the ligaments associated with the vertebral arches there are **intertransverse ligaments** that extend between transverse processes. These are variable in structure and prominence, but are most developed in the lumbar region.

The supraspinous and interspinous ligaments blend together where they are adjacent. In the neck,

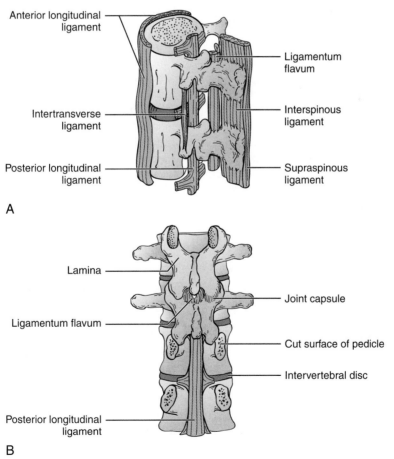

Figure 13-6 The chief ligaments of the vertebral column. **A,** Posterolateral, somewhat superior view. **B,** Posterior view with the vertebral arch omitted on lower vertebrae to expose the posterior longitudinal ligament.

between the seventh cervical vertebra and the skull, the supraspinous ligament is represented by the **ligamentum nuchae,** strong superficially where it gives rise to muscles but extending deeply as a thin midline septum between other muscles of the two sides.

Each of the paired ligamenta flava extends from the anterior surface of one lamina to the posterior surface of the next lamina below. The pairs are separated from each other by a midline gap through which pass veins that connect a venous plexus inside the vertebral canal with one around the spinous processes. Laterally, the ligamenta flava blend with the capsules of the synovial joints. The ligamenta flava, therefore, form a part of the posterior wall of the vertebral canal. In the cervical and thoracic regions, where the laminae overlap or almost overlap, these ligaments are largely hidden in posterior view by the laminae, but in the lumbar region, they fill an appreciable space between laminae.

FUNCTIONAL/CLINICAL NOTE 13-1

Flexion further widens the spaces between laminae; therefore, when a needle is to be introduced between two laminae in the lumbar region (the procedure of *lumbar puncture*), this can be done most easily when the back is flexed. The needle is then pushed through a ligamentum flavum.

The supraspinous and interspinous ligaments are largely collagenous. The ligamenta flava are composed primarily of yellow elastic tissue (*flavum* means "yellow"); therefore, they stretch during flexion of the back, remain taut, and do not fold during extension.

Cartilaginous Joints between Vertebral Bodies

Anterior longitudinal ligament

The bodies are firmly united to each other by strong collagenous ligaments that partly cover the intervertebral discs (see Fig. 13-6). Anteriorly, there is a broad band, the **anterior longitudinal ligament,** that stretches from the sacrum to the occipital bone of the skull. The anterior longitudinal ligament is

particularly strong, because it is thick and consists of fibers of varying length. The deepest fibers extend only from one vertebra to the next. Other fibers extend across a single vertebra, or across two or three, and the most superficial fibers extend over four or five vertebrae.

FUNCTIONAL/CLINICAL NOTE 13-2

The anterior longitudinal ligament gives important support to the vertebral column and is of great clinical importance in fractures of this column. Such fractures usually involve crushing of the anterior portion of one or more bodies but without injury to the anterior longitudinal ligament. In these cases, flexion allows further crushing of the vertebra or vertebrae involved and posterior displacement at the level of injury with consequent danger to the spinal cord. In hyperextension, however, the pull of the taut anterior longitudinal ligament realigns the fragments and holds them in position. The potential splinting action of this important ligament may be used in the treatment of such a fracture of the vertebral column. First aid that allows flexion may produce irreparable injury. Fractures or fracture-dislocations of the cervical vertebrae are particularly dangerous because a displacement here can easily cause death. When such fractures are suspected, first aid consists of being sure that there is no movement of the head and neck.

Posterior longitudinal ligament

On the posterior aspect of the vertebral bodies, and therefore within the vertebral canal, is a second longitudinal band, the **posterior longitudinal ligament** (see Fig. 13-6). This commences as a broad band attached to the occipital bone, and it remains fairly broad throughout most of the cervical region. In the thoracic and lumbar regions, it becomes narrowed over the centers of the bodies and expanded over the intervertebral discs so as to resemble a series of hourglasses. It is firmly attached to the intervertebral discs and the adjacent portions of the bodies, but it is separated from the middle of each body by veins

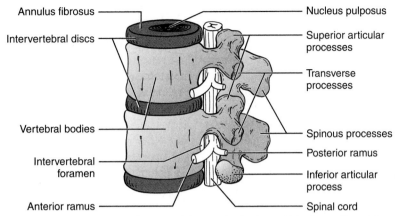

Annulus fibrosus
Intervertebral discs
Vertebral bodies
Intervertebral foramen
Anterior ramus

Nucleus pulposus
Superior articular processes
Transverse processes
Spinous processes
Posterior ramus
Inferior articular process
Spinal cord

Figure 13-7 Lateral view of a segment of the lumbar part of the vertebral column. Note the position of the spinal nerve (not labeled) within the intervertebral foramen. The ligaments of the column have not been included.

and small arteries that leave and enter the vertebra. The posterior longitudinal ligament also consists of long and short fibers. The longest fibers are placed most superficially and extend over a number of vertebrae, whereas the shortest fibers extend only from one vertebra to the next.

Intervertebral discs

The most important connections between the vertebral bodies are the **intervertebral discs** (Fig. 13-7). Besides helping to bind vertebrae together, the discs act as shock absorbers between adjacent vertebrae and allow a small amount of movement between any two adjacent vertebral bodies. The movement at one disc, when added to the similarly small movement between other vertebrae, accounts for the rather surprising mobility of the vertebral column as a whole. In the cervical and lower lumbar regions, the discs also contribute to the curvatures typical of those parts of the column as a result of their greater thickness anteriorly.

Each intervertebral disc consists of two portions: an annulus fibrosus, or outer fibrous layer, and a nucleus pulposus, or soft center. In some descriptions, the thin cartilaginous plate that separates the spongy bone of the vertebral body from the nucleus pulposus is considered a third part of the disc, although developmentally it is the epiphyseal plate of the vertebral body.

The **annulus fibrosus** (see Fig. 13-7) consists of a number of layers of dense fibrous tissue and

fibrocartilage that are firmly attached to the ends of the bodies adjoining the disc. The fibers of each of these layers run obliquely, but those of any two adjacent layers run at an angle to each other so that their fibers cross like the limbs of an X. When the annulus is compressed, the Xs become shorter and broader; when the compression is relieved, the Xs become taller and narrower.

The **nucleus pulposus** (see Fig. 13-7) is a semigelatinous mass situated somewhat eccentrically, slightly closer to the posterior edge of the disc. When the bodies and discs are cut (longitudinally along the column), the nucleus pulposus bulges outward, giving evidence of the disc's elasticity and of the compression to which it has been subjected. Even in the supine position, when the vertebral column is not supporting the weight of the body, the disc is maintained under pressure by the ligaments connecting the arches.

The nucleus pulposus contains a very high percentage of water—from 70% to more than 80%—and is essentially incompressible. Its softness, however, allows it to change shape easily, and the change in shape accounts for the compressibility of the intervertebral disc as a whole. Therefore, when a vertebral column is bent in any direction, the nucleus pulposus becomes somewhat wedge-shaped, with its thin edge in the direction of bending. The part of the annulus fibrosus toward this side bulges out, and that on the opposite side is stretched by its attachments to adjacent vertebrae.

FUNCTIONAL/CLINICAL NOTE 13-3

Because the central part of each disc, the nucleus pulposus, has such a high water content, the discs are subject to dehydration as a result of the pressure placed on them. When fresh discs are placed in a mechanical press, water droplets can be squeezed out of them. Standing and moving have the same effect. Water is squeezed out in minute quantities and absorbed into the blood stream. As the discs lose water, they of course become thinner, and sufficient dehydration can occur during a day's activity to result in a loss of height of $^3/_4$ inch (19 mm) in a man. During rest in bed, when the pressure on the discs is least, water is reabsorbed from the blood stream by the discs, and the original height is regained. Over the years, a little less water is reabsorbed than is lost, so the water content of the discs becomes somewhat less with age, and the discs become slightly thinner. This is one reason (in addition to the increased stoop with age) why older persons are typically shorter than they were as young adults.

Dehydration results in only an imperceptible change in the thickness of any one disc. Marked narrowing of a disc (visible in a radiograph because the intervertebral discs do not interfere with the X-ray beams as do the adjacent vertebral bodies) is a sign of massive loss of the substance of the disc. This may be an indication of a **herniated** or **protruded disc** (sometimes called a *ruptured* or *slipped disc*), in which the nucleus pulposus herniates through a break in the annulus fibrosus. Degenerative changes begin to appear in the discs in early adulthood, and a weakened annulus fibrosus subjected to excessive strain will bulge or break. Although massive herniation of the disc substance may cause narrowing of the intervertebral space, relatively small herniations that produce no apparent narrowing may cause distressing symptoms and markedly incapacitate the individual.

Because the annulus is thinner posteriorly, herniation of the disc is more likely to occur posteriorly. It is posterior or posterolateral

protrusions that cause symptoms and are recognized clinically. Large posterior herniations may exert pressure on the spinal cord and cause paralyses and anesthesias similar to those produced by tumors in the vertebral canal.

The most common herniations, however, are posterolateral ones, around or through the thin lateral edge of the posterior longitudinal ligament, which reinforces the annulus more strongly close to the midline than elsewhere. Such posterolateral herniations, more common in the lower lumbar and lower cervical regions than elsewhere, are very likely to press on the dural sleeves and roots of a spinal nerve just before it leaves the vertebral canal. Pain is the most common result of such pressure and is interpreted as coming from the area to which that nerve is distributed. The full extent of the sensory loss may be masked because of the overlap between spinal nerves. The same is true of motor loss due to the multiple segmental innervation of muscles.

Pain produced by the pressure of a herniated disc on a nerve root or spinal nerve produces pain in the area innervated by the compressed nerve fibers. This is termed **radicular pain.** Therefore, herniated lower cervical discs usually produce pain that seems to come from the hand, which is supplied mainly by the lower cervical nerves. Herniated lower lumbar discs produce pain radiating to the lower part of the leg and to the foot. Such pain seems to extend along the sciatic nerve, the large nerve passing down the back of the thigh to the leg and foot. Therefore, sciatic pain (commonly known as *sciatica*) is suggestive of a herniated lower lumbar disc. Flexing the thigh at the hip while the leg is held straight at the knee may draw the nerve roots contributing to the sciatic nerve forward, pressing them more firmly against a herniated disc, if one is present. In consequence, this straight-leg raising test can be expected to reproduce or accentuate sciatic pain that is caused by a herniated disc.

The pain produced by a herniated disc also produces reflex spasm of the muscles of the back, usually more on one side than on the other, so that the back is somewhat laterally flexed. Flexion is often away from the side of herniation, but sometimes it is toward that side or even alternates from side to side.

In addition to the pain produced by pressure upon a nerve root, herniation of a disc may produce local pain, apparently as a result of stretching posterior fibers of the annulus and fibers of the posterior longitudinal ligament. Spasm of the back muscles and strain on the synovial joints between the affected vertebrae are other sources of pain.

Atlanto-occipital and Atlanto-axial Joints

In addition to the joints just described between typical vertebrae, there are special joints at the upper end of the cervical column to facilitate movements of the head. The **atlanto-occipital joints** are formed between the articular facets on the upper surface of the atlas and the rounded occipital condyles of the skull. The atlanto-occipital joints are surrounded by articular capsules that are rather weak and do not contribute much to stability of the joint. The atlas and skull are also united by anterior and posterior atlanto-occipital membranes, which bridge the gap between the first cervical vertebra and the skull. The *anterior atlanto-occipital membrane* is essentially the continuation upward to the skull of a portion of the anterior longitudinal ligament; the *posterior atlanto-occipital membrane* is broader and thinner and runs only from the posterior arch of the atlas to the occipital bone. The suboccipital and other muscles attaching to the skull, and the shape of the joint itself, provide strength to the atlanto-occipital joint. This joint allows for a flexion-extension movement of the head, such as that involved in nodding.

The **atlanto-axial joints** (between the atlas and axis) consist of two laterally placed synovial joints and a median-positioned articulation of the dens of the axis with the atlas (see Fig. 13-4, *C*). The lateral joints between the inferior articular facets of the atlas and the superior facets of the axis are essentially similar to those found elsewhere in the vertebral column, whereas the articulation of the dens is unique. The dens projects cephalically from the body of the axis to lie posterior to the anterior arch of the atlas. (There is no intervertebral disc at this joint.) It is held in place against the atlas by the **cruciate** (meaning "shaped like a cross") **ligament,** the strongest part of which is the *transverse ligament* of the atlas. From the transverse ligament, vertical fibers extend cephalically to attach to the occipital bone and caudally to the body of the axis, forming the *longitudinal band.* The cruciate ligament is covered posteriorly by the **tectorial membrane,** which is the cephalic extension of the posterior longitudinal ligament. Between the anterior surface of the dens and arch of the atlas, and between the posterior surface and transverse ligament of the atlas, are synovial joints that allow the atlas to rotate on the dens as a pivot. The atlanto-axial articulation allows for considerably more rotation than can be found between other cervical vertebrae. It is responsible for much of the freedom of the movement of shaking the head, as in signifying "No." The dens can also slip downward and upward between the atlas and the transverse ligament; thus, the atlanto-axial articulation also contributes to flexion and extension of the neck.

FUNCTIONAL/CLINICAL NOTE 13-4

The lateral atlanto-axial joints are not strong enough to prevent gradual anterior dislocation of the atlas and skull on the axis. Therefore, when the dens is fractured, congenitally absent, or destroyed by disease, displacement does occur. The vertebral foramen of the atlas is so much larger than the spinal cord at this level that considerable displacement may occur before the cord is damaged, but pressure on the cord eventually produces increasing paralysis and loss of sensation. Interruption of the spinal cord at this high level is incompatible with life. (The phrenic nerve, which provides motor innervation to the diaphragm, receives its fibers from spinal cord segments C3 to C5. In a high

Continued

lesion of the spinal cord, therefore, loss of fibers from these segments would result in paralysis of the diaphragm.) The usual cause of death by hanging is fracture of the axis with dislocation between the axis and the third cervical vertebra and severance of the cord.

MOVEMENTS AND STABILITY

Movements

The movements of the skull on the atlas and of the atlas on the axis have been briefly discussed. The movements of the remainder of the vertebral column are limited not only by the various ligaments, which attach the vertebrae to one another, but also by the positions of the articular facets, the shape and slant of the spinous processes, the relative sizes of the intervertebral disc, and various other factors (such as the presence of the rib cage in the thoracic part of the column). Movement between any two adjacent vertebrae is exceedingly limited in all portions of the vertebral column. However, the total amount of movement in a given region may be considerable.

In the **cervical region**, all movements are quite free. The intervertebral discs are relatively thick in comparison to the heights of the vertebral bodies and are wedge-shaped, being thicker anteriorly. Anteroposteriorly, the vertebral bodies are convex on their superior surface and concave on their inferior surface, an arrangement that enhances the movements of flexion and extension. Laterally, the superior surface of the body is concave, whereas the inferior surface is convex. This structural arrangement facilitates lateral flexion. The oblique slope of the articular facets enables flexion and extension, lateral flexion when accompanied by rotation, and fairly free rotation. Approximately half of the rotation possible in the cervical region takes place at the atlanto-axial joint articulation.

In the **thoracic region**, the intervertebral discs are relatively thin, and the flatness or only slight concavity of both upper and lower ends of the bodies further limits the usefulness of the discs in allowing free movements. Flexion and extension are also limited by the orientation of the articular facets, which lie almost in the frontal plane. Furthermore, movement in the thoracic region is hindered by the attachment of the ribs, and extension is hampered by the overlapping of the spinous processes. Lateral flexion, with the ribs being brought closely together on one side and spread somewhat on the other, is the freest movement in this region, but rotation is more limited.

In the **lumbar region**, the bodies of the vertebrae, particularly those of the lower ones, are wedge-shaped, having a greater height anteriorly than posteriorly. The discs are also wedge-shaped (thicker anteriorly). Therefore, both the bodies and discs contribute to the lumbar curvature. The thickness of the intervertebral discs, the posterior direction of the spinous processes, and the almost sagittal orientation of the facets of the articular processes in the upper lumbar region (those of the lower lumbar vertebrae are nearly in the frontal plane) enable good flexion and extension. Lateral movement is also rather free, with the inferior facets of a vertebra sliding down on one side and up on the other; therefore, the upper portion of the trunk can be circumducted by these movements in the lumbar region. Rotation in the lumbar region varies among individuals, but it is always very limited, for the articular processes soon lock together. Movements of the lumbar portion of the vertebral column are particularly free in the lower lumbar segments.

Stability

The **stability** of the vertebral column depends on a number of factors. Of these, the relationship to a vertical line representing the center of gravity, the **line of gravity** (see Fig. 1-5), is one of the most important. When weight is properly balanced on the vertebral column, minimal muscular activity is necessary. A constantly maintained position in which the weight is not reasonably well balanced results in structural changes and a permanent deformity in the growing child and constant muscular strain in the adult.

The line of gravity should lie in the median (midsagittal) plane of the body. If it does not—for instance, because of unequal lengths of the lower limbs (which

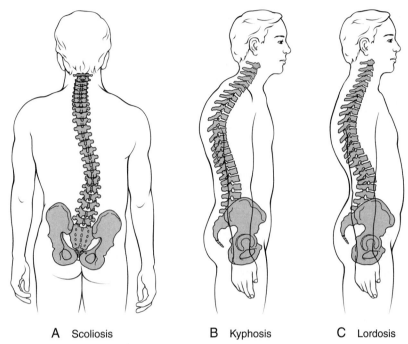

A   Scoliosis   B   Kyphosis   C   Lordosis

Figure 13-8 Abnormal curvatures of the vertebral column. **A,** The scoliosis represented is the result of a shortened right lower limb. Scoliosis could also result from unequal growth of the two sides of the vertebral bodies. **C,** The lordosis accompanies a slight downward rotation of the bony pelvis.

would result in a lateral tilt of a straight vertebral column)—the only way in which balance can be restored is by a lateral bending toward the side of the long limb (Fig. 13-8, *A*). Lateral deviation of the vertebral column is called **scoliosis.** Similarly, if a structural scoliosis develops as a result of unequal growth of the two sides of the vertebral bodies, it throws the center of gravity to one side. This change in the position of the center of gravity must be compensated for by curving some other part of the vertebral column to the opposite side. The primary scoliotic curve is thought to result often from weakness of the muscles of the back on the convex side. If uncorrected, it becomes progressively worse until growth ceases. The lateral curvature is regularly accompanied by a rotation of the vertebrae forming the curve, with their bodies turning toward its convexity and their spinous processes toward its concavity. If it is in the lumbar region, pain usually results from the rotation because, as already mentioned, little rotation is possible here. If it is in the thoracic region, the entire chest becomes markedly distorted.

The weight of the head and trunk is more nearly balanced in the frontal plane in several situations: when the line of gravity *passes posterior to the bodies of most of the cervical vertebrae but through the bodies at the junction of the cervical and thoracic parts of the column* (in this relationship, the posterior curve of the cervical column buttresses the weight of the head); when the line *passes again through the bodies at the thoracolumbar junction (passing anterior to the bodies of most of the thoracic vertebrae)*; and when it *passes not too far from the center of the body of the fourth lumbar vertebra.* This distribution of weight approaches the ideal, except that the greater weight in front of most of the thoracic vertebral bodies tends to increase the thoracic curvature. Because of the limited movements of flexion and extension of the thoracic column, this cannot be corrected by posture. Fortunately, however, it is largely the vertebrae and their ligaments, rather than the back muscles, that prevent further flexion here, although with paralysis of the back muscles in this region, flexion does become increasingly severe. **Kyphosis** (hunchback) is an increase in the anterior curvature of the thoracic region (see Fig. 13-8, *B*). It commonly results from a collapse of one or more vertebral bodies or, if congenital, from absence of one or more bodies. A mild degree of collapse accounts for the stoop associated with aging.

Because the lumbar portion of the column supports all the weight above it, it is this part of the column that commonly adjusts to forward and backward shifts in the line of gravity. Kyphosis, for instance, shifts the line anteriorly, and the resulting tendency to fall forward is most easily overcome by an increase in the lumbar curvature, **lordosis**, so that it better buttresses the weight thrown upon it (see Fig. 13-8, *C*). The lordotic curve is then a compensatory one for the kyphotic curve. In the same way, a temporary lordosis develops in later stages of pregnancy, to counteract the anterior movement of the line of gravity produced by the weight of the fetus and surrounding fluids and tissues. If, however, the center of gravity is moved posteriorly, the lumbar curve becomes somewhat flattened.

The lumbar curve also compensates for the obliquity of the upper end of the sacrum, which always slants downward and forward. The inferior articular processes and almost frontal orientation of the facets of the fifth lumbar vertebra help to stabilize the articulation with the sacrum. They, along with the ligaments and muscles, essentially keep the fifth lumbar vertebra and column from sliding downward and forward on the sacrum.

The sacrum is slightly more oblique in women than in men, and consequently, the lumbar curve is slightly greater in women than in men. Similarly, downward rotation of the pelvis, which increases the sacral obliquity, is accompanied by an increased lumbar curve. An upward rotation of the pelvis is accompanied by a decreased lumbar curve. A permanent abnormal increase in sacral obliquity is accompanied by a permanent lordosis.

Compensatory changes of the lumbar curve are brought about by the back muscles, and once they occur, they tend to stabilize the column. Movements of the trunk from the most stable position shift the relations of the line of gravity. As soon as the movements occur, the muscles acting on the column must become active. The muscles activated are usually back muscles because common shifts in the line of gravity occur anteriorly or to one side. Ultimately, the back muscles are primarily responsible for stability of the vertebral column. When these are paralyzed, it is impossible to maintain balance, because although ligaments and articular facets help check extreme movements, they must allow an appreciable amount of movement, far more than enough to upset the line of gravity.

Causes of Low Back Pain

There are apparently a number of causes of **low back pain**, but a factor common to much of such pain is the strain that may be put on the lumbar portion of the vertebral column and its muscles. The farther the line of gravity is shifted forward, the more active muscles of the back become. Therefore, bad posture is a common and correctable cause of low back pain. Because muscles use the vertebral column as a lever, the forces involved are much greater than the actual weight borne by the lumbar part of the column.

Measurements of pressure on the discs below the third and fourth lumbar vertebrae have shown that in the erect standing position, the weight borne by them is in the range of 200 to 300 lb (91 to 136 kg). The leverage is such that weights of 22 lb (10 kg) held in each hand may produce an added load of 230 lb (104 kg) on the disc when the person leans forward approximately 20 degrees. Tension exerted by the ligamenta flava, approximately 30 lb (14 kg), and that caused by the minimal muscular activity in quiet standing, must be added to the weight of the body above the level of measurement. When the person leans forward, the musculature becomes more active, increasing pressure on the disc, and with further leaning, the pressure increases still more. When these statistics are considered, it is apparent how the muscles of the lower part of the back may be strained and why degenerative changes in the discs, particularly common in the lumbosacral area, can lead to herniations that cause disabling low back pain. Using the back as a lever in picking up objects can put enormous strain on the vertebral column and its musculature. Strain can be minimized when lifting if the individual crouches, holds the back as straight vertically as possible, and uses the strong muscles of the gluteal region, thigh, and calf to do the lifting.

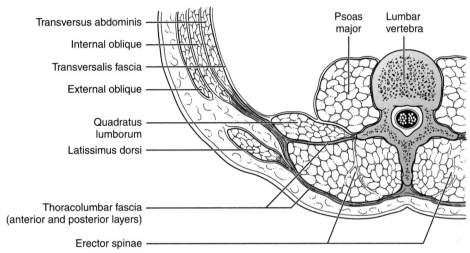

Transversus abdominis

Internal oblique

Transversalis fascia

External oblique

Quadratus
lumborum

Latissimus dorsi

Thoracolumbar fascia
(anterior and posterior layers)

Erector spinae

Psoas
major   Lumbar
vertebra

Figure 13-9 Cross-section of the lumbar region, illustrating the thoracolumbar fascia *(highlighted with color).*

Asymmetry of articular facets, most common at the lumbosacral junction, is another cause of low back pain, presumably because the strains of movement are unequally distributed between the two sides. Still other causes referable to the vertebral column are variations and abnormalities; these most frequently affect the last lumbar vertebra.

Structural abnormalities can occur in the lumbar vertebrae. The important types of congenital abnormalities are nonfusion of the two sides of the laminae, which results in **spina bifida,** and separation of the inferior articular processes from the rest of the vertebrae, a condition known as **spondylolysis.** Spina bifida varies in severity. It may be evident as an incomplete vertebral arch, but it may also involve the meninges and spinal cord. Its presence weakens the back, primarily because of the lessened area provided for the attachment of muscles.

Spondylolysis can be either unilateral or bilateral. Because the inferior articular processes of the fifth lumbar vertebra form the chief anchorage of this vertebra to the first sacral segment, bilateral spondylolysis produces pronounced weakness in the lower part of the back. With the loss of the anchoring effect of its inferior articular processes, the fifth lumbar vertebra and, therefore, all the vertebral column above it may slide anteriorly on the sacrum (a condition called **spondylolisthesis**), throwing the entire column out of line.

MUSCULATURE OF THE BACK

With the exception of a few small anterolateral muscles, the *posterior muscles of the back are innervated by the posterior rami of the spinal nerves.* These muscles were originally segmental, extending from one vertebra to the next. In the course of ontogenetic and phylogenetic development, the more superficial fibers have united to form longer bundles extending over a number of segments. Therefore, the musculature of the back is formed by a number of incompletely separated layers of muscles, distinguishable in part by the direction of their fibers and in part by their length. The longer muscles are placed superficially, the intermediate muscles more deeply, and the shortest muscles lie immediately against the vertebrae. The muscles of the back are rather completely covered by the musculature of the upper limb (see Fig. 5-12), which has spread over the back to attain attachment to the spinous processes. In addition, the thick **thoracolumbar fascia,** a combination of aponeurosis and deep fascia, covers the muscles in the lower part of the back (Fig. 13-9).

The true back muscles are composed of numerous converging and diverging fascicles that are arbitrarily grouped together and described as individual muscles (Fig. 13-10). They are, in fact, not muscles in the sense of a muscle in the limbs. They could be subdivided very easily into many more component

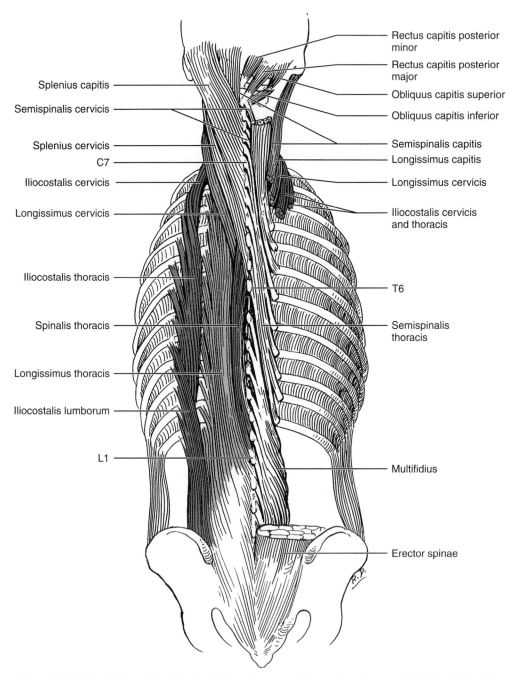

Splenius capitis

Semispinalis cervicis

Splenius cervicis

C7

Iliocostalis cervicis

Longissimus cervicis

Iliocostalis thoracis

Spinalis thoracis

Longissimus thoracis

Iliocostalis lumborum

L1

Rectus capitis posterior minor

Rectus capitis posterior major

Obliquus capitis superior

Obliquus capitis inferior

Semispinalis capitis

Longissimus capitis

Longissimus cervicis

Iliocostalis cervicis and thoracis

T6

Semispinalis thoracis

Multifidius

Erector spinae

Figure 13-10 The chief muscles of the back. The subgroups of the erector spinae are highlighted with *color*.

Table 13-1 SPLENIUS MUSCLES				
Muscle	**Origin**	**Insertion**	**Action**	**Innervation**
Splenius capitis	Ligamentum nuchae; spinous processes of seventh cervical and first three or four thoracic vertebrae	Mastoid process and occipital bone of skull	Rotation of head and cervical vertebral column to same side Bilateral action: extension of head	Posterior rami of middle cervical spinal nerves
Splenius cervicis	Spinous processes of third to sixth thoracic vertebrae	Transverse processes of upper two to four cervical vertebrae	Rotation of head and cervical vertebral column to same side Bilateral action: extension of head and vertebral column	Posterior rami of lower cervical spinal nerves

groups than are usually named, or they could be classified into only a few large groups. From the functional standpoint, there is little reason to subdivide back musculature in any detail because the muscles usually work together in large groups. Subdivision and naming of the back muscles are largely efforts to systematize them for descriptive purposes.

Splenius Muscles

In the cervical region, deep to the trapezius and rhomboids, there are two back muscles that can easily be seen to form a special group because of the direction of their fibers. These are the splenius capitis and the splenius cervicis (Table 13-1). In contrast to the other back muscles, which either run approximately parallel to the midline of the vertebral column or run toward it as they are traced upward, the splenius muscles arise medially and pass laterally as they are traced cephalically. The **splenius capitis** has its *origin* from the lower half of the ligamentum nuchae and the spinous processes of the seventh cervical vertebra and upper three or four thoracic vertebrae, and its *insertion* is laterally on the mastoid process and occipital bone of the skull (see Fig. 21-1). The **splenius cervicis** has its *origin* from the spinous processes of about the third to sixth thoracic vertebrae, and its *insertion* is laterally on the upper two to four cervical transverse processes. The splenius capitis and splenius cervicis receive *innervation* (respectively) from the posterior rami of the middle and inferior cervical spinal nerves. The *action* of the muscles of one side (when acting together) is to rotate the head and cervical vertebral column toward the same side.

When they act bilaterally, they aid in extension of the neck.

Serratus Posterior Muscles

In the upper and lower thoracic regions, there are two muscles that cover the true back muscles. They lie between the true back muscles and the muscles of the upper limb but belong to neither group. These are the superior and inferior serratus posterior muscles, connected with movements of the ribs (Table 13-2). The **serratus posterior superior** has its *origin* from the lower part of the ligamentum nuchae and the spinous processes of the seventh cervical and upper two or three thoracic vertebrae. Its *insertion* is on the upper ribs, usually the second to the fifth. This muscle receives *innervation* from branches of the first three or four intercostal nerves and therefore from anterior rami of spinal nerves. Its *action* is to assist in elevating the ribs and therefore increasing the size of the thorax.

The **serratus posterior inferior** has its *origin* from the lower two thoracic and upper two lumbar spinous processes, and its *insertion* on the lower three or four ribs. Its *innervation* is from the ninth to twelfth intercostal nerves, and its *action* is to draw the lower ribs downward to enlarge the thoracic cavity and steady these ribs against upward pull of the diaphragm.

Erector Spinae

The main mass of the back muscles can be more easily studied by beginning in the lumbar region and following the muscle groups toward the head. The heavy

Table 13-2	SERRATUS POSTERIOR MUSCLES			
Muscle	**Origin**	**Insertion**	**Action**	**Innervation**
Serratus posterior superior	Ligamentum nuchae; spinous processes of seventh cervical and upper two or three thoracic vertebrae	Upper ribs, usually second through fifth	Elevation of ribs	Anterior rami of upper three or four thoracic spinal nerves (intercostal nerves)
Serratus posterior inferior	Spinous processes of lower two thoracic and upper two lumbar vertebrae	Lower three or four ribs	Pulls lower ribs inferiorly	Anterior rami of lower thoracic (9th to 12th) spinal nerves (intercostal nerves)

musculotendinous mass over the upper sacral and the lower lumbar vertebrae represents the origin of a large segment of the back musculature, known as the **erector spinae** (see Fig. 13-10) because of its *action* in extending the vertebral column (Table 13-3). This muscle group has a common tendinous and fleshy origin from the posterior surface of the sacrum, the iliac crest, and the spinous processes of the lumbar and last two thoracic vertebrae. At its origin, it is not divisible into subgroups. As the erector spinae is followed upward, however, it divides into three series of muscles, of which only the lateral two are well developed.

All parts of the erector spinae receive *innervation* from posterior rami of spinal nerves.

Iliocostalis

The most lateral upward continuation of the erector spinae is the iliocostalis system. This lateral system is in turn described as being subdivided into three linear but overlapping parts: iliocostalis lumborum, iliocostalis thoracis, and iliocostalis cervicis. Each of these muscles has numerous segmental origins and insertions, and the insertions of one muscle markedly overlap the origins of the next muscle above it. The iliocostalis system could, therefore, be considered as one continuous muscle or as the three muscles described here, or it could be still further subdivided into about 18 overlapping muscles or muscle fascicles.

The **iliocostalis lumborum,** although sharing the common tendon, has its *origin* especially from the iliac crest and the sacrum. Its *insertion* is by a series of slips into the lower borders of the lower six or seven ribs.

The **iliocostalis thoracis** consists of a number of fascicles that take *origin* from the upper borders of the lower six or seven ribs, medial to the insertions of the iliocostalis lumborum. The *insertion* is on the lower borders of the upper six ribs.

The **iliocostalis cervicis** has its *origin* from the angles of the upper six ribs, medial to the insertions of the iliocostalis thoracis. Its *insertion* is on the transverse processes of about the fourth to sixth cervical vertebrae.

Longissimus

The second and more medial division of the erector spinae is the longissimus. It is divided into the longissimus thoracis, longissimus cervicis, and longissimus capitis; in other words, it is described as the longest muscle and is divided into thoracic, cervical, and head portions. Like the iliocostalis, each division of the longissimus is composed of a number of fascicles. These fascicles, as well as the divisions, overlap each other in such a way that the muscle has attachments on almost every segment.

The fascicles making up the **longissimus thoracis,** the lowest of the three divisions of this muscle, take *origin* from the common tendon of the erector spinae. The *insertion* is into the lower nine or ten ribs and the adjacent transverse processes of the vertebrae.

The **longissimus cervicis** has its *origin* from the transverse processes of the upper four to six thoracic vertebrae, and its *insertion* is onto the transverse processes of the second to sixth cervical vertebrae.

The **longissimus capitis** has its *origin* medial to the upper end of the longissimus cervicis, partly with the tendons of that muscle and partly from the articular processes of the lower four cervical vertebrae. It runs slightly laterally to an *insertion* onto the mastoid process of the skull.

Table 13-3 ERECTOR SPINAE MUSCLES

Muscle	Origin	Insertion	Action	Innervation
Erector spinae (component muscles listed below in anatomical order)*	Common tendon of origin: posterior surface of sacrum, iliac crest, spinous processes of lumbar and last two thoracic vertebrae (specific origins given below)	As described for each muscle	Bilateral action: extension of vertebral column Unilateral action: to bend vertebral column toward same side (lateral flexion) (Note: this is action for all muscles of this group)	Posterior rami of spinal nerves in area of muscle (Note: this is innervation for all muscles of this group)
Iliocostalis lumborum	Iliac crest; sacrum	Lower borders of lower six or seven ribs		
Iliocostalis thoracis	Upper borders of lower six or seven ribs	Lower borders of upper six ribs		
Iliocostalis cervicis	Angles of upper six ribs	Transverse processes of fourth to sixth cervical vertebrae		
Longissimus thoracis	Intermediate part of common tendon	Lower nine or ten ribs; adjacent transverse processes of vertebrae		
Longissimus cervicis	Transverse processes of upper four to six thoracic vertebrae	Transverse process of second to sixth cervical vertebrae		
Longissimus capitis	Tendons of origin of longissimus cervicis; articular processes of lower four cervical vertebrae	Mastoid process of skull		
Spinalis thoracis	Common tendon; spinous process of lower two thoracic and upper two lumbar vertebrae	Spinous processes of upper thoracic vertebrae (varies from four to eight)		
Spinalis cervicis	Ligamentum nuchae; spinous processes of seventh cervical and upper one or two thoracic vertebrae	Spinous process of axis (and possibly third and fourth cervical vertebrae)		

*The spinalis capitis is considered as the medial part of semispinalis capitis (see Table 13-4).

Spinalis

The most medial and last division of the erector spinae is the spinalis muscle. This is always poorly developed and is usually represented mostly by the **spinalis thoracis**, a slender muscle in the midthoracic region. Its *origin* is from the common tendon and lower two thoracic and upper two lumbar spinous processes. Its *insertion* is on upper thoracic spinous processes.

A slip of muscle representing a **spinalis cervicis** may be present in the cervical region, where its *origin* is from the ligamentum nuchae and spinous processes of the seventh cervical and first (and possibly second) thoracic vertebrae. The muscle's

Table 13-4	TRANSVERSOSPINALIS MUSCLES			
Muscle	**Origin**	**Insertion**	**Action**	**Innervation**
Semispinalis thoracis	Transverse processes of lower six thoracic vertebrae	Spinous processes of lower two cervical and upper four thoracic vertebrae	Extension of vertebral column	Posterior rami of cervical and thoracic spinal nerves
Semispinalis cervicis	Transverse processes of upper five or six thoracic vertebrae	Spinous processes of second (axis) to fifth cervical vertebrae	Extension of vertebral column	Posterior rami of cervical and thoracic spinal nerves
Semispinalis capitis	Transverse processes of upper six or seven thoracic vertebrae; articular processes of lower three cervical vertebrae	Occipital bone (between superior and inferior nuchal lines)	Extension of head	Posterior rami of cervical and thoracic spinal nerves
Multifidus	Sacrum and posterior superior iliac spine; mammillary processes of lumbar vertebrae; transverse processes of thoracic vertebrae; articular processes of lower cervical vertebrae	Spinous processes of lumbar through second cervical vertebrae: Fascicles span two to four segments of the column	Bilateral: extension of vertebral column Unilateral: lateral flexion and rotation (to opposite side) of the vertebral column	Posterior rami of spinal nerves
Rotatores	Sacrum and transverse processes of lumbar through lower cervical vertebrae	Spinous processes of lumbar through second cervical vertebrae: Fascicles span one to two segments of the column	Rotation (to opposite side) and extension of vertebral column	Posterior rami of spinal nerves

insertion is on the spinous process of the axis and possibly the processes of the third and fourth cervical vertebrae.

The **spinalis capitis** is not a separate muscle; it is a smaller medial part of the semispinalis capitis, which is one of the muscles included in the following discussion.

Transversospinalis Muscles

Because of their origins and insertions, the semispinalis, multifidus, and rotatores (rotators) are grouped together as the **transversospinalis muscle group** (Table 13-4). All the elements of this muscle group tend to slant inward, and the deeper any component lies, the greater is the slant and the shorter are the muscle bundles.

Semispinalis

When the erector spinae is removed, a deeper, more continuous set of fibers is seen. This is the semispinalis muscle, divided into the semispinalis thoracis, semispinalis cervicis, and seminspinalis capitis according to the insertion of the muscle bundles (Fig. 13-11). Much of the semispinalis consists of muscle fibers that arise from transverse processes and run upward and medially to attach to spinous processes. In contrast to the overlying erector spinae, these fibers are directed not so much upward as both upward and inward, taking an oblique course toward the midline. Fascicles of which this muscle is composed are of varying lengths, because the fibers that arise from any one transverse process attach to about four spinous processes, some of them running for as much as eight segments.

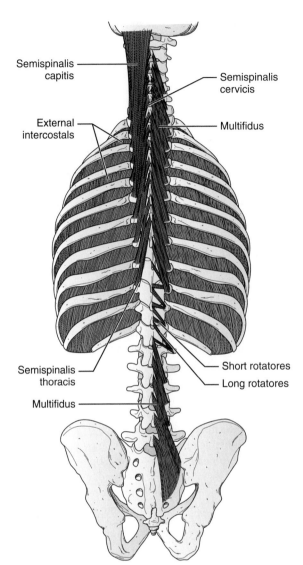

Semispinalis
capitis

Semispinalis
cervicis

External
intercostals

Multifidus

Semispinalis
thoracis

Short rotatores

Long rotatores

Multifidus

Figure 13-11 The semispinalis muscles *(left)* and the
multifidus and rotator muscles *(right)*.

The **semispinalis thoracis** takes *origin* from the
transverse processes of the lower six thoracic vertebrae, and its *insertion* is onto the spinous processes
of the last two cervical and upper four thoracic vertebrae. The *action* of this muscle is to extend the vertebral column.

The **semispinalis cervicis** has its *origin* from the
transverse processes of the upper five or six thoracic
vertebrae, and its *insertion* is onto the spinous processes of the axis through the fifth cervical vertebrae,

with the heaviest insertion upon the axis. The *action*
of this muscle is also to extend the vertebral column.

Lying deep to the splenius muscles, the **semispinalis capitis** takes *origin* from transverse processes of the
upper six or seven thoracic vertebrae and the articular
processes of the lower three cervical vertebrae. It covers the semispinalis cervicis and runs almost straight
upward to an *insertion* on the occipital bone of the
skull (between the superior and inferior nuchal lines).
The *action* of this muscle is to extend the head. The
medial part of this muscle, usually having some origin
from spinous processes, is called the **spinalis capitis.**

All three semispinalis muscles receive *innervation*
from the posterior rami of the cervical and thoracic
spinal nerves.

Multifidus

Deep to the semispinalis are the **multifidus** muscles,
which resemble the semispinalis except that the muscle fascicles are shorter, being only two to four segments in length (see Figs. 13-10 and 13-11). They
are, therefore, more obliquely placed in relation to the
vertebral column. The fascicles take *origin* from the
sacrum and posterior superior iliac spine; mammillary
processes of the lumbar vertebra; transverse processes
of the thoracic vertebrae; and articular processes of
the lower cervical vertebrae. The muscle fascicles
run upward and medially to *insertions* on the spinous
processes of the lumbar vertebrae through the second
cervical vertebra. These muscles form a continuous
mass from the upper end of the sacrum to the second
cervical vertebra. The multifidus are particularly heavy
in the lumbar region, thinner in the thoracic region,
and thicker again in the upper cervical region, but
they do not extend to the skull. The bilateral *action*
of the multifidus is to extend the vertebral column;
unilaterally, they produce rotation to the opposite side
and laterally flex the column. The multifidus receive
innervation from the posterior rami of spinal nerves.

Rotatores

The **rotatores** (rotators) extend from the level of the
sacrum to that of the second cervical vertebra. The
rotatores are obliquely set and shorter than the shortest fibers of the multifidus. They are small muscles
that can be divided into two groups: short and long
rotatores. Each has a single *origin* from a transverse

Table 13-5	SEGMENTAL MUSCLES			
Muscle	**Origin**	**Insertion**	**Action**	**Innervation**
Interspinales	Spinous processes of vertebrae (absent in much of thoracic region)	Spinous processes of vertebrae (span between adjacent vertebrae)	Extension of vertebral column	Posterior rami of cervical spinal nerves
Intertransversarii	Transverse processes of vertebrae (absent in most of thoracic region)	Transverse processes of vertebrae (span between adjacent vertebrae)	Lateral flexion of vertebral column (unilateral action)	Posterior and anterior rami of spinal nerves

process and a single *insertion* onto the base of a spinous process. The *short rotatores* pass only from one vertebra to the next above; the *long rotatores* pass from one vertebra to the second above. The *action* of the rotatores is to rotate and extend the vertebral column. The rotatores receive *innervation* from the posterior rami of the spinal nerves.

Segmental Muscles

The muscles of the segmental group (Table 13-5) arise from one vertebra and insert on the next vertebra. Although the short rotatores qualify for this group, the long rotatores do not. Therefore, the rotatores as a whole are considered instead to belong to the transversospinalis muscle group (described in the preceding section). Only two muscles make up the segmental group. The **interspinales** are between spinous processes and are not present throughout most of the thoracic region. The **intertransversarii** span between adjacent transverse processes but are poorly developed or absent in the thoracic region. They are doubled in the lumbar region, where there are *medial and lateral intertransversarii,* and also in the cervical region, where there are *anterior and posterior intertransversarii.*

Suboccipital and Deep Neck Muscles

In the uppermost part of the neck, just below the skull, there are several short muscles that extend between the axis and the occipital bone, between the atlas and the occipital bone, or between the axis and atlas. The posterior group of muscles (the obliquus capitis, inferior and superior, and the rectus capitis posterior, major and minor) is included in Figure 13-10. These muscles are grouped together as the suboccipital

muscles (Table 13-6). They lie deep to the other muscles of the back and receive *innervation* from the posterior ramus of the first cervical nerve (C1).

The **obliquus capitis inferior** has its *origin* from the spinous process of the axis and *inserts* on the transverse process of the atlas. Its *action* is to rotate the atlas, causing the head to turn toward the same side.

The **obliquus capitis superior** takes *origin* from the transverse process of the atlas (adjacent to where the obliquus capitis inferior inserts), and its *insertion* is onto the occipital bone. Its *action* is to extend and tilt the head laterally toward the same side.

The **rectus capitis posterior major** has its *origin* from the spinous process of the axis, whereas the **rectus capitis posterior minor** has its *origin* from the posterior tubercle of the atlas. Both pass upward and laterally to *insertions* on the occipital bone. The *action* of both muscles is to extend the head, and the rectus capitis posterior major, by lying more laterally, can also rotate the head toward the same side.

Several other muscles lie lateral and anterior to the vertebral column in the neck. All receive *innervation* from anterior rami of cervical spinal nerves. Two long muscles, the longus colli (*collum,* like *cervix,* means "neck") and the longus capitis, lie on the anterior surfaces of the vertebral bodies. The **longus colli** has several parts. The lower, lateral fibers take *origin* from the bodies of the first to the third thoracic vertebrae, and their *insertion* is on the transverse processes of the fifth and sixth cervical vertebrae. The superior, lateral fibers have an *origin* from transverse processes of cervical vertebrae three to five and an *insertion* on the anterior surface of the atlas. The vertical, more medial fibers take *origin* from the bodies of the upper three thoracic and lower three cervical vertebrae. Their *insertion* is on the bodies of the

Table 13-6	SUBOCCIPITAL AND DEEP NECK MUSCLES			
Muscle	**Origin**	**Insertion**	**Action**	**Innervation**
Obliquus capitis inferior	Spinous process of axis	Transverse process of atlas	Rotation of atlas (turn head to same side)	Posterior ramus of C1
Obliquus capitis superior	Transverse process of atlas	Occipital bone	Extension and lateral bending of head	Posterior ramus of C1
Rectus capitis posterior major	Spinous process of axis	Occipital bone	Extension of head; rotation of head to same side	Posterior ramus of C1
Rectus capitis posterior minor	Posterior tubercle of atlas	Occipital bone	Extension of head	Posterior ramus of C1
Longus colli	Bodies of first to third thoracic vertebrae; transverse processes of third to fifth cervical vertebrae; bodies of upper three thoracic and lower three cervical vertebrae	Transverse processes of fifth and sixth cervical vertebrae; anterior surface of atlas; bodies of second to fourth cervical vertebrae (respectively with listed origins)	Flexion; possibly lateral flexion of neck	Anterior rami of C2–C6
Longus capitis	Transverse processes of third to sixth cervical vertebrae	Occipital bone	Flexion of head and upper cervical vertebrae	Anterior rami of C1–C3
Rectus capitis anterior	Lateral mass of atlas	Occipital bone	Stabilization of atlanto-occipital joint; flexion of head	Anterior rami of C1 and C2
Rectus capitis lateralis	Transverse process of atlas	Occipital bone	Stabilization of atlanto-occipital joint; lateral flexion of head	Anterior rami of C1 and C2

second to the fourth cervical vertebrae. The muscle's *action* is to flex (and possibly laterally flex) the neck. *Innervation* is provided by fibers from the anterior rami of C2 to C6.

The **longus capitis** lies laterally to the longus colli. Its *origin* is from the transverse processes of the third through sixth cervical vertebrae, and its *insertion* is on the occipital bone. Its *action* is to flex the head and upper part of the cervical vertebrae. *Innervation* is provided by branches of the anterior rami of C1 to C3.

Two smaller muscles lie more superiorly. The **rectus capitis anterior** lies deep to the longus capitis. Its *origin* is from the lateral mass of the atlas, and its *insertion* is on the occipital bone. The *action* of the muscle is to stabilize the atlanto-occipital joint and flex the head. The **rectus capitis lateralis** has its *origin* from the transverse process of the atlas, and its *insertion* is on the occipital bone. Its *action* is to stabilize the atlanto-occipital joint and laterally flex the head. Both muscles receive *innervation* from fibers of the anterior rami of C1 and C2 (see Table 13-6).

Also situated in the neck, and acting as flexors, lateral flexors, and rotators of the neck, are the scalene muscles, which are described with other muscles of the neck in Section V of this book.

Associated Muscles

There are no muscles attached anteriorly to the thoracic region of the vertebral column. However, in the lumbar region, the **psoas major,** which is considered a limb muscle (see Chapter 16), takes its origin anteriorly from bodies and transverse processes and has a direct *action* upon the vertebral column.

FUNCTIONAL/CLINICAL NOTE 13-5

Both psoas major muscles become active, taking their fixed points from below when a person leans posteriorly from a sitting position, and the muscle on the opposite side becomes active when the person leans to one side. Similarly, the two muscles can help flex a partially flexed vertebral column. However, when the individual is supine and attempts to flex the lumbar column, as in sitting up without the use of the hands, the first action of the psoas major is to pull the lumbar column anteriorly and increase the lumbar curvature. Only secondarily does it flex the lumbar column on the pelvis and the pelvis on the femurs. Thus, in exercising the anterior abdominal muscles with a sit-up exercise, the individual should start by curling the head, shoulders, and trunk upward; otherwise, the stronger psoas major will do all the work.

A posterior abdominal muscle, the **quadratus lumborum** (see Chapter 23) attaches to the transverse processes of the lumbar portion of the vertebral column; it is a lateral flexor of the column.

Summary of Muscle Action

The true back muscles are primarily extensors and rotators of the vertebral column. The various muscles act specifically on the parts indicated by their names—muscles called *capitis* move the head, those called *cervicis* move the neck, and so forth—but many movements of the vertebral column involve simultaneous contraction of many muscles.

Almost all the muscles of the back, acting bilaterally, extend the vertebral column or the head. This is true of the three major groups. The *splenius muscles,* acting unilaterally, rotate the head and neck toward the same side (that is, turn the face toward that side). The *erector spinae* is a strong extensor; it has also been regarded as a lateral flexor and as a rotator to the same side. Lateral flexion, however, is performed primarily by the quadratus lumborum and the anterolateral abdominal muscles, and rotation is performed by the latter and by the transversospinalis. The slight activity of the erector spinae as these movements are started has been interpreted as helping to prevent concomitant flexion rather than assisting in the movement. The *transversospinalis system* rotates to the opposite side, if acting unilaterally. The multifidus, at least, are bilaterally active in extension. The interspinales are obviously only extensors, and the intertransversarii are only lateral flexors. The activity in the deeper muscles has been interpreted as being concerned primarily with fine adjustments between vertebrae rather than with movement of the vertebral column as a whole.

FUNCTIONAL/CLINICAL NOTE 13-6

The chief function of the muscles of the back, when a person is erect, is to resist gravity. Regardless of what muscles start the movement, once the vertebral column is bent far enough to sufficiently increase the gravitational force, the muscles of the back that resist this movement (rather than muscles that promote it) must actively contract in order to prevent falling and to make the movement smooth and controlled. When flexion is complete, these muscles relax, leaving support to the ligaments. To start extension, these muscles must become active.

As mentioned previously, muscles other than those of the back, even muscles that have no attachment to the vertebral column, also play a very important part in movements of the back. The anterolateral abdominal muscles are the chief flexors and lateral flexors of the trunk and are also important in rotation. A muscle of the neck, the sternocleidomastoid, flexes, laterally flexes, and rotates the head.

Surface Anatomy

The "true" muscles of the back are covered in part by other muscles and fascia. The **trapezius muscle,** which arises from the base of the skull and the spinous processes of the cervical and thoracic vertebrae, can be palpated as it passes to its insertion on the spine of the scapula, acromion process, and clavicle. It covers the upper region of the back. The **latissimus dorsi** is overlapped superiorly by the trapezius and covers the inferior region of the back. Followed laterally, it forms the majority of the posterior wall of the axilla. The thick **thoracolumbar fascia** covers the erector spinae muscle in the lumbar and lower thoracic regions.

Individual muscles of the back cannot be easily palpated, but the mass of the **erector spinae** is most obvious in the lumbar region as it arises from the iliac crest and the lumbar vertebrae. In the thoracic region, muscles are thinner and less prominent. In the cervical region, they are thicker but lie beneath the trapezius and muscles that attach to the medial border of the scapula. No nerves or vessels of the region can be palpated or observed.

THE MENINGES AND THE SPINAL CORD

Meninges

The spinal cord, continuous superiorly with the brain, lies within the vertebral canal. The spinal nerves arising from it make their exit between adjacent vertebrae, usually through the intervertebral foramina. The spinal cord is separated from contact with the bony vertebral canal and its connecting ligaments by a layer of fatty connective tissue and by the **meninges,** or special coverings of the cord. The fatty connective tissue contains vertebral venous plexuses that help to drain the vertebral column and spinal cord and connect with veins around the outer surface of the column. The tissue also contains small arterial branches that supply blood to vertebrae, connective tissue, meninges, and, to a variable extent, the spinal cord. The space occupied by this tissue is called the **epidural space.** Injections of anesthetic agents are sometimes made into it, as in the technique of providing **epidural anesthesia** or **caudal analgesia** for reducing the pain of childbirth.

The outer covering of the spinal cord is the **dura mater,** a tube of tough connective tissue that is continuous with a similar layer within the skull and tapers

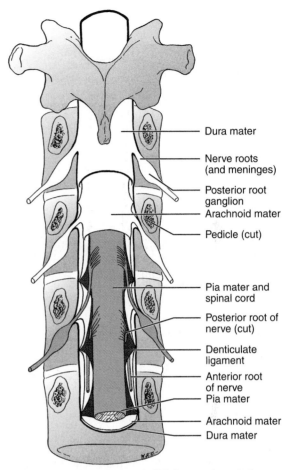

Dura mater

Nerve roots (and meninges)

Posterior root ganglion

Arachnoid mater

Pedicle (cut)

Pia mater and spinal cord

Posterior root of nerve (cut)

Denticulate ligament

Anterior root of nerve

Pia mater

Arachnoid mater

Dura mater

Figure 13-12 The spinal cord within its coverings. At the top, the cord is illustrated within an intact vertebral canal; below, the posterior portions of the vertebrae are omitted in order to show the dura mater; farther down, the dura mater is omitted in order to show the arachnoid mater; and at the bottom, this membrane in turn is omitted in order to show nerve roots, the denticulate ligaments *(dark color)*, and the pia mater *(light color)*.

to a point near the level of the second sacral vertebra (Figs. 13-12 and 13-13). Beyond this, it is drawn out into a slender thread, the **filum terminale-dural part,** which anchors the lower end of the dura mater to the posterior surface of the coccyx. The dura mater also sends tubular sheaths that form sleeves around the roots of the spinal nerves as these leave the dural sac proper.

Immediately inside the dura mater, and separated from it only by a slitlike subdural space containing just enough fluid to keep the adjacent surfaces

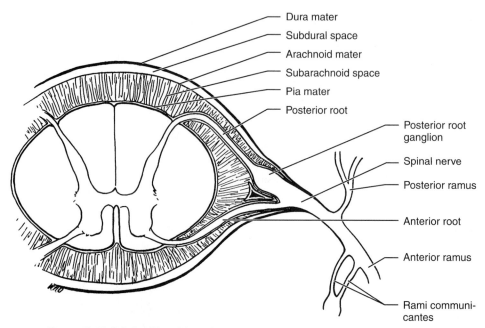

Dura mater
Subdural space
Arachnoid mater
Subarachnoid space
Pia mater
Posterior root

Posterior root
ganglion

Spinal nerve

Posterior ramus

Anterior root

Anterior ramus

Rami communi-
cantes

Figure 13-13 Relationships of the spinal cord and meninges, illustrated in cross-section.

moist, is the **arachnoid mater** (see Fig. 13-12). This tubular membrane is much thinner than the dura mater. Its outer surface is smooth, but its inner surface, although lined by flattened cells, gives off numerous strands called *trabeculae,* which are also covered by flattened cells. The trabeculae, which derive their name from their spiderweb-like appearance, cross the underlying space to blend with the innermost layer of the meninges, the pia mater. The arachnoid mater terminates at the same level as the dura mater.

The **pia mater** is also thin but is so tightly attached that it appears as the spinal cord's outer surface. There is no space between it and the cord, although pieces of it can be stripped off the cord with some difficulty. The pia mater contains numerous small blood vessels that supply the spinal cord.

The dural and arachnoidal tubes or sacs surround the spinal cord very loosely, so that there is a relatively large space, the **subarachnoid space** (see Fig. 13-13), between the arachnoid and the pia mater. During life, this space is filled with the **cerebrospinal fluid,** which is largely formed in the brain, fills the cavities of the brain, and surrounds the brain and

spinal cord. Anesthetic agents are introduced into the subarachnoid space in the procedure known as *spinal anesthesia.*

The cord and its closely attached pia mater are bathed in cerebrospinal fluid, and the cord is suspended within this protective medium not only by the arachnoid trabeculae but also by the **denticulate ligaments**. These are particularly tough lateral ligaments developed from the pia mater that project from the right and left sides of the spinal cord between each two adjacent spinal nerves, for the length of the spinal cord (see Fig. 13-12). There are 20 to 21 pointed processes on each side from the lateral free edge of the ligament that penetrate the arachnoid mater and attach into the dura mater. Viewed from behind or in front, therefore, a denticulate ligament looks somewhat like a saw.

The dura mater and arachnoid mater send sleeves outward around each posterior root and each anterior root of each spinal nerve as the nerve turns laterally to leave the dural-arachnoidal tube, and the pia mater also follows out on the surfaces of the nerve roots. These layers become continuous with the ordinary connective tissue of the nerve near the level of the spinal ganglia, but the subarachnoid space surrounds the roots up to this point.

Spinal Cord

The **spinal cord** varies from oval to almost round in cross-section. It tends to be larger at its upper end than at its lower, because its upper end contains more fibers that are either going to or coming from the brain. However, the number of cells at a given level also affects its size, and so the levels of the cord that must supply more muscle and skin—namely, the levels that supply the limbs—show localized enlargements (cervical and lumbar enlargements or swellings).

Just as the dural and arachnoidal sacs (once about as long as the vertebral column) are drawn into a thread at their lower ends, so is the spinal cord. Even more than the meninges, it fails to grow as fast as the vertebral column, and in the adult its lower end usually lies near the *lower border of the first lumbar vertebra.* From the tapered lower end of the cord, called the **conus medullaris,** there is a threadlike strand of tissue, the **filum terminale-pial part,** that represents the drawn-out original end of the cord; it runs down to attach to the ends of the dural-arachnoidal sacs and the filum of the dura mater that anchors them to the coccyx. The filum terminale-pial part consists mainly of glial cells from the cord, covered by a layer of pia mater.

Because the spinal cord has been pulled up more than the dura mater and arachnoid mater during growth, the lower part of the arachnoidal sac, between about the second lumbar and second sacral vertebral levels, contains no spinal cord. It contains only the filum terminale-pial part and the roots of spinal nerves (which have to run caudally from the spinal cord to their levels of exit between vertebrae). This collection of nerve roots around the filum terminale-pial part is the **cauda equina** (meaning "horse's tail"). The pia mater–covered roots within this lower extent of the subarachnoid cavity float in the cerebrospinal fluid. It is in this location, between lower lumbar vertebrae, that **lumbar punctures** (for withdrawing cerebrospinal fluid for examination or for introducing medicine or anesthetic agents into the subarachnoid cavity) are made. Punctures at higher levels risk damage to the spinal cord, but caudal to the end of the spinal cord, the nerves slip away from the needle.

Tracts

The **tracts** of the spinal cord consist of groupings of nerve fibers of similar function. Some of them shift position, and others are found in only one part of the cord. Each varies in size according to the level of the cord being considered, and there is much overlap between tracts.

The tracts of the spinal cord connect different parts of the cord to each other; they ascend to the brain (sensory tracts) or descend from the brain (motor tracts; see Chapter 3). The tracts are located in the anterior, lateral, and posterior funiculi (columns) of the white matter that are adjacent to and partially partitioned by the gray matter. The fibers interconnecting the segments of the spinal cord (fasciculus proprius) surround the gray matter of the cord. Collateral fibers given off from the long tracts arising in the cord also connect the various levels.

The chief long **ascending tracts** (right side of Fig. 13-14) can be categorized as those that conduct impulses to the subconscious level and those that conduct to the conscious level. In the lateral funiculi, the two *spinocerebellar tracts* (posterior and anterior or dorsal and ventral) are in the former category. They arise from cells in the gray matter, transmitting proprioceptive information (i.e., information on movement and position) from muscles in the limbs and trunk to the cerebellum. In the cerebellum, this input is used to help control muscle activity at a subconscious level. The *cuneocerebellar tract* serves the same function but transmits information only from the upper limb and neck.

The major tracts that conduct to the conscious level are the cuneate fasciculus (fasciculus cuneatus) and gracile fasciculus (fasciculus gracilis) in the posterior funiculus (posterior column) and the spinothalamic tract or tracts in the anterior and lateral funiculi. The *cuneate fasciculus*, located in the cord above the T6 vertebra, receives input from the upper part of the body, whereas the *gracile fasciculus* receives information from the lower part. These fasciculi are composed of fibers that are central processes of cells of the posterior root ganglia of the same side, and they transmit impulses concerned with touch,

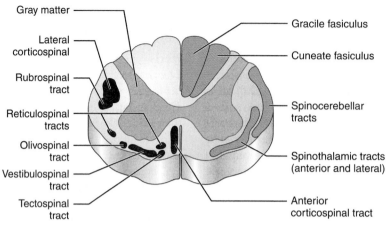

Gray matter

Lateral corticospinal

Rubrospinal tract

Reticulospinal tracts

Olivospinal tract

Vestibulospinal tract

Tectospinal tract

Gracile fasiculus

Cuneate fasiculus

Spinocerebellar tracts

Spinothalamic tracts (anterior and lateral)

Anterior corticospinal tract

Figure 13-14 Some of the major tracts of the spinal cord. Ascending tracts are illustrated on the *right (light color),* and descending tracts are illustrated on the *left (dark color).*

pressure, and proprioception. The information they carry is also essential to recognition of vibratory stimulation, as from a tuning fork placed on the shin, and judgment of the texture and shape of an object placed in the hand. They are concerned with all sensations except those of pain and temperature. Although the cuneate and gracile fasciculi conduct impulses from the same side of the body, these are relayed by cells whose fibers cross to the opposite side in the brain.

The *spinothalamic tracts* are sometimes regarded as a single structure because they blend with each other rather than being widely separated. They are often described as lateral and anterior (ventral), in which case the anterior spinothalamic tract is described as a pathway for touch and pressure and the lateral tract is the one for pain and temperature. The fibers of both tracts originate in the gray matter of the opposite side, cross anterior to the central canal of the cord, and then turn upward. Surgeons sometimes purposely interrupt this tract to alleviate pain on the opposite side in a procedure called *cordotomy.*

The major **descending** or **motor tracts** (left side of Fig. 13-14) are the *corticospinal* (pyramidal), *vestibulospinal,* and *reticulospinal tracts.* The *rubrospinal tract* is an important tract in many lower animals but is small in humans.

There are two *corticospinal* or *pyramidal tracts:* one lateral and one anterior (ventral). Both originate in

the cerebral cortex or pallium. The lateral corticospinal tract is much larger and more important, and most of its fibers cross in a lower part of the brain stem as they run toward the cord. One cerebral hemisphere controls primarily the opposite side of the body, just as it receives afferent impulses primarily from this opposite side.

The vestibulospinal, reticulospinal, and other tracts, such as the rubrospinal, tectospinal, and olivospinal, are grouped together as *extrapyramidal fibers:* that is, fibers that do not traverse the part of the brain known as the pyramids, as do the corticospinal (pyramidal) fibers. The corticospinal fibers were once regarded as being the sole pathway by which the brain could initiate voluntary movements, and the spastic paralysis typical of severe upper motor neuron lesions was attributed solely to interference with pyramidal function. There are few places, however, where corticospinal (pyramidal) fibers can be injured without affecting extrapyramidal ones; therefore, both sets are usually injured together. Either system can be responsible for most movements, and the deficit resulting from a pure pyramidal lesion is not a spastic paralysis but only a loss of delicate movements, such as those of the fingers and thumb. The extrapyramidal system is responsible primarily for postural adjustments of the trunk and limbs, and both systems usually cooperate in performing most other movements of the limbs.

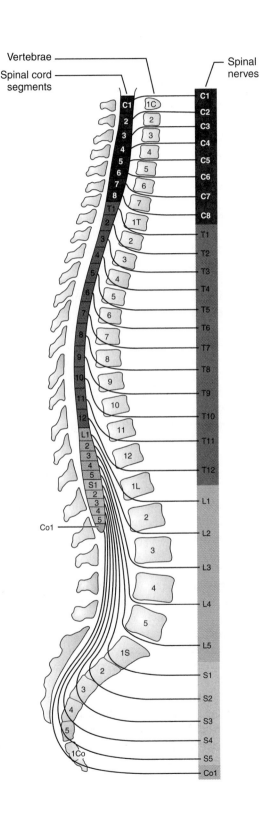

Vertebrae

Spinal cord segments

Spinal nerves

Spinal nerves

The general composition of the **spinal nerves** is discussed in Chapter 3. The **posterior roots** (sensory or dorsal roots) of the spinal nerves join the posterolateral aspect of the spinal cord, whereas the **anterior roots** (motor or ventral roots) arise anterolaterally. Lateral to the denticulate ligaments, the posterior and anterior roots of each spinal nerve parallel each other and enter into their dural-arachnoidal sleeves very close together. As already noted, the sleeves terminate at about the level of the posterior root ganglia, and the two roots join at the distal end of the ganglion to form the typical mixed spinal nerve (see Fig. 13-13).

The 31 pairs of spinal nerves are divided into 8 cervical, 12 thoracic, 5 lumbar, 5 sacral, and a single coccygeal. All are named according to their relations to the vertebrae. *The first cervical nerve exits between the skull and the first cervical vertebra, and the eighth cervical nerve exits between the seventh cervical and the first thoracic vertebrae. Below the cervical region, each nerve leaves the vertebral canal below the vertebra of the same name and number: The eighth thoracic nerve leaves below the eighth thoracic vertebra, the fifth lumbar nerve below the fifth lumbar vertebra, and so forth* (Fig. 13-15). Except between the skull and the atlas, and between the atlas and axis, the nerves leave through intervertebral foramina, which are bordered above and below by the pedicles of the vertebrae, anteriorly by the vertebral bodies and intervertebral discs, and posteriorly by the articular processes (see Fig. 13-7). Ganglia of the nerves lie regularly at the level of the intervertebral foramina, and the posterior and anterior roots of a nerve unite just as the nerve is making its exit from the vertebral canal. (In the lumbar region, in particular, the nerve lies close against the pedicle of the vertebra just above it and on the lower end of the vertebra, rather than actually below it.)

Figure 13-15 Relation of the spinal cord and nerve roots to the vertebral column. Note that the spinal cord is shorter than the vertebral column, so that even in the lower cervical and upper thoracic region, the nerve roots run downward to their exits. The lumbar, sacral, and coccygeal roots of the spinal nerves are especially long. Below the end of the cord, these roots constitute the cauda equina. The cord typically ends at the lower border of the first lumbar vertebra, but it may end at a higher level or at a lower level, as illustrated here.

The part of the spinal cord that gives rise to a pair of spinal nerves is known as a **spinal cord segment.** If the spinal cord were as long as the vertebral column, the location of spinal cord segments and vertebrae would correspond; the nerve roots of each nerve would run almost directly laterally and unite to form the nerves, and the nerves would exit through the adjacent intervertebral foramen. However, only the upper cervical nerve roots have this relationship. Because the cord ends near the lower border of the first lumbar vertebra, the spinal cord segments lie progressively farther from the intervertebral foramina through which their respective spinal nerves exit (see Fig. 13-15). Therefore, the more caudally the segment is positioned along the cord, the longer the roots must be to exit from the vertebral canal. For example, the L5 segment of the spinal cord lies within the canal near the level of the upper border of the first lumbar vertebra. Its nerve roots must travel inferiorly through the subarachnoid cavity to reach the intervertebral foramina below the fifth lumbar vertebra. Nerve roots of the sacral and coccygeal segments would have even a longer course. The caudally directed posterior and anterior roots of the lumbar, sacral, and coccygeal nerves form the **cauda equina** in the lower part of the subarachnoid space. Diagrams such as Figure 13-13, which show very short posterior and anterior roots, are approximately accurate only for upper cervical nerves. The roots of the sacral nerves are several inches long.

FUNCTIONAL/CLINICAL NOTE 13-7

Because of the discrepancy in length between the spinal cord and vertebral column, the clinician must bear in mind that injury at a given vertebral level affects a different segmental level of the cord, and several spinal nerves may be injured simultaneously (see Fig. 13-5). For instance, injury at the lower border of the 10th thoracic vertebra affects the spinal cord segment that lies at this level, usually the 12th. Furthermore, any or all nerves that arise at or above this level but leave the vertebral column below it may also be injured: in this case, the 10th, 11th, and 12th thoracic nerves.

A herniated intervertebral disc in the lower lumbar region, however, lies too low to affect the spinal cord itself; it is also usually laterally situated and typically involves the roots of a single spinal nerve inside the vertebral canal.

Each spinal nerve is formed by the union of the posterior and anterior roots. As the nerve exits from the intervertebral foramen, it divides into its two main branches, a **posterior ramus** (*ramus* means "branch") and an **anterior ramus.** The posterior ramus then turns posteriorly into the back muscles to innervate them and continues to the skin of the back, while the anterior ramus continues laterally and anteriorly. (In the sacral region, where the transverse processes of the sacral vertebrae have fused together, posterior rami exit through the posterior sacral foramina of the sacrum, and anterior rami exit through the anterior sacral foramina.) A few of the posterior rami exchange branches with each other, but for the most part, they remain segmental. In contrast, many of the anterior rami enter into plexuses, in which the identity of the contributing nerves is lost. Therefore, the anterior rami of the upper cervical nerves form the **cervical plexus,** those of the lower cervical nerves and the first thoracic form the **brachial plexus,** and most of the anterior rami of the lumbar and sacral nerves form the **lumbosacral plexus** (which is subdivided into lumbar and sacral plexuses). The anterior rami of the thoracic nerves are separated from each other by the ribs; because they lie between the ribs, these anterior rami are known as **intercostal nerves.** Whether they do or do not enter a plexus, the anterior rami of the spinal nerves supply most of the muscle and skin of the body—essentially everything except the back muscles and the skin covering them.

It is also the anterior rami that are connected to the sympathetic system. The nerves that contain preganglionic **sympathetic fibers** (all 12 thoracic and the first 2 lumbar) give off a branch to the sympathetic trunk containing these fibers, and all the spinal nerves receive from the sympathetic trunk a branch containing postganglionic fibers (see Chapter 3 for more information on the sympathetic nervous system). The postganglionic fibers are distributed through both posterior and anterior rami to blood vessels, certain other smooth muscles, and sweat glands. The connections between a spinal nerve and the sympathetic trunk are known as **rami communicantes.** All thoracic and the first two lumbar nerves should have two rami communicantes, as in Figure 13-3: one composed of preganglionic fibers and one composed of postganglionic ones (i.e., one leaving the nerve to go to the sympathetic trunk, the other leaving the trunk to join the nerve), and all the other spinal nerves should have only one, composed of postganglionic fibers. There actually is much variation in the number of rami communicantes, inasmuch as the preganglionic and postganglionic fibers sometimes run together in a single branch or, more frequently, there is more than one postganglionic ramus connecting a spinal nerve to the sympathetic trunk.

The second, third, and fourth sacral spinal nerves contain preganglionic **parasympathetic fibers** (see Chapter 3 for more information on the parasympathetic nervous system). These fibers leave the spinal nerves by way of the *pelvic splanchnic nerves,* and they synapse on or near the structure that they are innervating. This innervation is provided to the terminal part of the digestive tract and the pelvic viscera. The sacral nerves do receive postganglionic rami communicantes from the sacral part of the sympathetic trunk and conduct these fibers to the blood vessels and sweat glands of the lower limb.

ANALYSES OF ACTIVITIES AND ASSOCIATED MOVEMENTS

Movement and stability of the vertebral column were considered earlier in this chapter. The column is capable of flexion, extension, lateral flexion, and rotation. The amount of movement possible between two adjacent vertebrae is rather limited, but the additive movement of several vertebrae in a region or of the entire column is considerable. In an erect position, with the weight of the body properly balanced, the vertebral column requires only minimal muscular activity to maintain it as a stable structural unit. Any force to which the body is subjected, or any movement of the body, necessitates additional muscular activity to compensate for the shift in position or weight distribution and the resulting shift in the line of gravity. One example provided is the increased curvature of the lumbar region to compensate for the weight gain that occurs during the later stages of pregnancy. The same effect would occur with gaining weight and having additional fat deposited within the anterior abdominal wall.

Activity: *Picking Up a Toolbox.* Analysis of normal activities can provide some insight into the functional anatomy of the back. Consider the movements that occur in the back in picking up a large toolbox or shopping bag that is positioned immediately beside the left foot. Starting in the anatomical position and using the left hand to pick up the toolbox, flexing the vertebral column laterally to the left side (with accompanying movement in the lower limbs) enables the hand to be positioned to grasp the handle. In the back, the erector spinae, multifidus, and intertransversarii of the left side contract to produce lateral flexion, but the muscles on the right side also contract to control the movement. Once the handle is grasped, the muscles of the right side contract to bring the body to an erect position. Increased muscular activity is necessary to maintain the erect position because of the added weight on the left side and the shift of the line of gravity to the left. Other muscles of the trunk that could be involved in this activity include the external and internal oblique and the rectus abdominis. If the right hand is used to grasp the handle, the vertebral column is rotated and flexed, as well as laterally flexed to some extent, to bring the right hand to the left side.

The same activity could be performed with less movement of the vertebral column and less strain on the back. If flexion occurs in both lower limbs at the hip and knee joints, the trunk could be

Continued

ANALYSES OF ACTIVITIES AND ASSOCIATED MOVEMENTS—cont'd

lowered without lateral flexion. Normally, however, there is some flexion of the vertebral column to compensate for the shift in position. Although the back must be returned to an erect position and then be stabilized to support the weight of the toolbox, the muscles of the lower limb would do much of the work of lifting the box. This same type of movement would be used if two items (one on each side of the body) were picked up. If this is done, the distribution of weight between the right and left sides determines muscle activity once the body returns to the erect position. Uneven weights necessitate additional muscle compensation.

Activity: *Raising the Head after Falling Asleep in Class.* Although gravity alone can cause flexion of the neck to allow the head to drop forward during a peaceful nap in class, muscle activity is required to return the head to an upright position. Unless the head falls forward to the desktop (which could involve flexion of the entire vertebral column), the movement occurs primarily within the neck region. Extension of the cervical part of the column and head would involve a multitude of muscles. Muscles that specifically produce extension of the head when working in pairs include, among others, the rectus capitis posterior major and minor, splenius capitis, longissimus capitis, and semispinalis capitis. Those that are capable of extension of the cervical part of the vertebral column are the splenius cervicis, iliocostalis cervicis, longissimus cervicis, spinalis cervicis, and semispinalis cervicis. In addition, the deeper muscles, such as the multifidus, rotatores, interspinales, and intertransversarii muscles in the cervical region, when acting bilaterally, can all participate in extension of the vertebral column.

As is apparent from this discussion, the simple act of "dozing off" necessitates a considerable amount of muscle activity to undo.

Activity: *Turning the Head while Backing Up a Car.* The considerable mobility of the head and the cervical part of the vertebral column are used to carry out this activity. To turn the head to look out the side or back window requires rotation of the head that involves the vertebrae and muscles of the cervical region. Much of the movement occurs at the atlanto-axial joint as the anterior arch of the atlas rotates on the dens process of the axis. As mentioned previously, the movement occurring at the atlanto-occipital joint would enable flexion and extension rather than rotation, and the head and atlas therefore act as a unit during rotation at the atlanto-axial joint. More rotation can be achieved by involving additional cervical vertebrae and, if necessary, the thoracic vertebrae. Laterally flexing the cervical part of the vertebral column to the opposite side as the head is rotated may enhance the amount of rotation possible in the cervical region.

Muscles of the back involved in rotation of the head at the atlanto-axial joint include the rectus capitis posterior major and obliquus capitis inferior on the side to which the head is being rotated. The splenius capitis, by its insertion on the mastoid process, rotates the head to the same side, and the splenius cervicis, with attachment to the upper cervical vertebrae, rotates these vertebrae and assists with rotation of the head. The rotatores and multifidus muscles of the opposite side can also assist in rotation of the lower cervical and thoracic vertebrae.

REVIEW QUESTIONS

1 How many vertebrae make up the vertebral column? List the anatomical features that are specific to the vertebrae in the cervical, thoracic, and lumbar regions and would enable identification of these vertebrae. What features are unique to the atlas and the axis?

2 What are the three major groups of muscles that constitute the erector spinae? For each of these groups, provide an account of their component parts and their origins and insertions. What is the function of these muscles? What nerves provide motor innervation to the muscles?

3 Describe the arrangement of the multifidus muscles. What provides innervation to these muscles?

4 What are the three meninges of the spinal cord? What is their arrangement and extent within the vertebral canal?

5 At what vertebral level does the spinal cord normally end in the adult? Where is fluid withdrawal from or injection of medication into the subarachnoid space usually performed? Why? What is the cauda equina?

6 Spinal nerves from the following spinal cord segments pass between which vertebrae as their fibers enter the vertebral canal or pass to the periphery?
   a C2
   b C8
   c T2
   d L5

7 Discuss the movements and muscles of the back involved in the following activities:
   a shoveling snow
   b paddling a canoe
   c floating on the back

8 Describe the structure of an intervertebral disc. What is the function of the disc? What changes in the disc occur with age?

9 Describe in detail the joints that exist between two adjacent thoracic vertebrae.

10 Is the brachial plexus formed by anterior or posterior rami of spinal nerves? What forms the intercostal nerves? Does a typical posterior ramus contain sensory fibers, motor fibers, or a mix of sensory and motor nerve fibers? What nerve fiber types are found in the posterior roots?

EXERCISES

1 Using two disarticulated thoracic vertebrae, demonstrate the movements possible between them. How would these movements differ from those between vertebra in the cervical and lumbar regions? Why?

2 Demonstrate on an articulated vertebral column how a herniated disc could affect the spinal cord and spinal nerves.

3 On an articulated skeleton, demonstrate the origin and insertion of each muscle within the suboccipital region of the neck. What is the function of each muscle?

SECTION 4

The Lower Limb

14 GENERAL SURVEY OF THE LOWER LIMB

CHAPTER CONTENTS

General Considerations

Development

Skeleton

Muscles

Nerves

Arteries

Veins

GENERAL CONSIDERATIONS

The parts and regions of the lower limb are the **gluteal region** (buttock), **hip** (coxa: general area around hip joint), **thigh** (the noun *femur* is used only to apply to the bone, although the adjective *femoral* is used in the sense of the thigh as a whole), **knee** (genu) and **popliteal region** (region behind the knee), **leg** (crus), **ankle** (tarsus), and **foot** (pes).

DEVELOPMENT

The lower limb develops in much the same manner as the upper limb. It projects first as a mesenchymal bud covered by a thin layer of epithelium and develops flexures that represent the positions of the knee, ankle, and digits on the foot. As in the upper limb, the cartilaginous skeleton and the muscles develop from the mesenchyme of the bud while the vessels and nerves grow into the bud. Because the base of the bud is broader than that of the upper limb, more spinal nerves grow into the lower limb: typically all the lumbar nerves and the first three or four sacral nerves.

The big-toe side of the limb (Fig. 14-1) is at first directed cranially, like the thumb side of the upper limb, and the little-toe side is directed caudally. If the limb could be abducted at this stage, the posterior or extensor surface would face posteriorly, and the anterior or flexor surface would face anteriorly. These relations, however, are not long maintained; the limb soon begins to rotate medially, gradually bringing the extensor side of the limb into an anterior instead of a posterior position. This rotation is obvious from the fact that, in the adult, the muscles on the anterior surface of the thigh (extending also onto the lateral surface) extend the leg at the knee, and those on the posterior side of the leg plantar flex the foot and flex the toes. Limb rotation is not complete at birth, and so an infant can "clap" the feet together, but it is completed as the child learns to stand and walk.

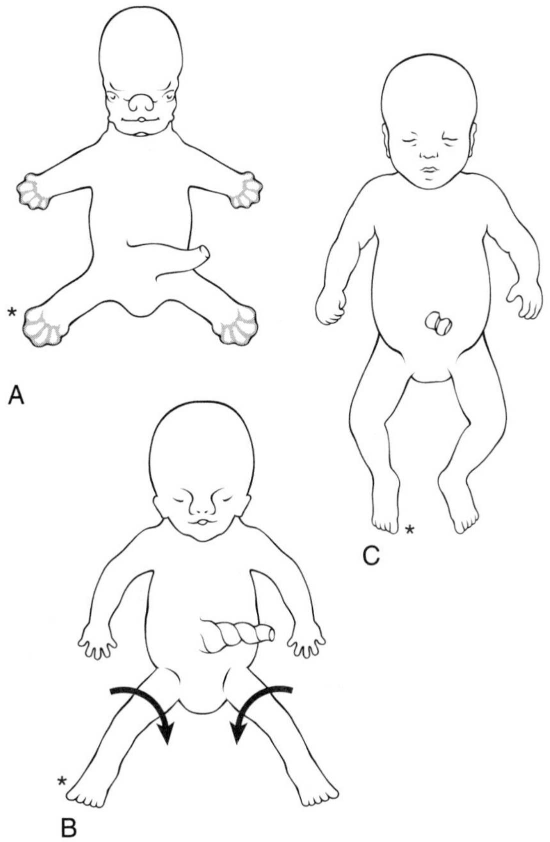

SKELETON

The skeleton of the lower limb is divided into the girdle and the skeleton of the free limb (Fig. 14-2). The girdle, often called the **pelvic girdle,** consists of

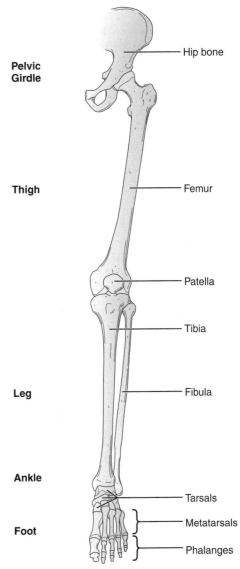

Figure 14-1 Development and rotation of the lower limb.
A, Lower limbs during embryonic development. The toe rays have just appeared, and the big toe is on the cranial side of the developing foot *(asterisk).* **B,** With further development, the limbs elongate and begin to rotate in a medial direction. The big toe still lies on the cranial (lateral) side of the foot. **C,** Continued rotation brings the big toe into a medial position.

Figure 14-2 The skeleton of the lower limb.

two **hip** (coxal or pelvic) **bones.** In contrast to the girdle of the upper limb, that of the lower limb is firmly attached to the axial skeleton (the sacral part of the vertebral column) at the *sacroiliac joint.* In addition, the two hip bones articulate anteriorly through the *pubic symphysis* and form a strong arch completed posteriorly by the vertebral column. Only slightly movable at the vertebral column, this arch transmits the weight of the body from the vertebral column to the femurs and constitutes the **bony pelvis.** In addition to the weight they receive from the vertebral column, the flared hip bones directly support some of the weight of the viscera. Muscles spanning across the pelvic floor, from one hip bone to either the other or to the sacrum, bridge the pelvic outlet (lower end of the bony pelvis) and help support the weight of the viscera.

Each hip bone bears a deep cup-shaped fossa, the *acetabulum,* that articulates with the rounded head of the femur. The hip joint is a *ball-and-socket joint.* The **femur** is the bone of the thigh, corresponding to the humerus in the arm. The tibia and fibula are the two bones of the leg corresponding to the radius and ulna in the forearm. The **tibia** is the larger bone situated on the medial side of the leg, and a portion of it is subcutaneous throughout its entire length. The **fibula** is the smaller bone on the lateral side of the leg. Its upper and lower ends are subcutaneous, but most of its body is buried in the leg muscles. In the upper limb, the ulna forms the chief articulation at the elbow, whereas the radius forms the chief articulation at the wrist. In contrast, in the lower limb, the tibia articulates at both knee and ankle and transmits most of the weight. The fibula serves for the attachment of many muscles and enters into the articulation of the ankle but not that of the knee. The *knee joint,* formed between the articular surfaces of the lower end of the femur and the upper end of the tibia, is largely a *hinge joint.* This is even truer of the *ankle joint,* formed by the lower ends of the tibia and fibula and the uppermost tarsal or ankle bone.

The seven **tarsals** are arranged to transmit weight both to the heel and to the ball of the foot; between these two weight-bearing points is the *longitudinal arch of the foot.* Although the ankle joint proper allows little movement except flexion and extension, movement between the various tarsals allows some

inversion and eversion of the foot and additional flexion and extension. *Inversion of the foot* is the movement that, if successful, would allow turning the sole of the foot inward so that the two soles could be placed together; it corresponds to supination of the hand. *Eversion of the foot* turns the foot outward so that the weight falls on the inner rather than the outer border of the foot; it corresponds to pronation of the hand. These movements in the lower limb are not performed through movements of long bones, as in the upper limb, but occur at the ankle and in the foot. Inversion and eversion of the foot are typically combined with other movements, but a foot in which eversion predominates is usually referred to by clinicians as a *pronated foot,* and one in which inversion predominates is similarly referred to as a *supinated foot.* Adjectives that have similar meanings when applied to the foot but that are also applicable to other parts of the lower limb are *valgus* and *varus.* Both mean "bent," but *valgus* denotes an outer or lateral bending and *varus* denotes an internal or medial bending. Therefore, *pes valgus* denotes a foot bent outward, hence an everted or pronated foot, and because the arch then usually flattens, is also applied to flatfoot. *Coxa vara* denotes a femur in which the angle between the neck and body of the femur is lessened, this internal bending shortening the limb in comparison with the normal side. *Genu valgum* denotes an exaggeration of the normal outward divergence of the leg at the knee, hence "knock-knee."

Much of the instep of the foot is formed by long **metatarsals.** The metatarsals articulate with the proximal **phalanges** of the digits. The big toe has two phalanges; the remaining toes each have three. The distal phalanges of the toes, with the exception of the big toe, are rather small bones. The phalanges of the toes as a whole are not as well developed as those in the hand.

The skeletons of the upper and lower limbs are built essentially on the same plan. Each limb has a girdle, followed by a single bone, the femur or humerus. The tibia and fibula correspond to the radius and ulna, the tarsals correspond to the carpals, and the metatarsals and phalanges of the foot obviously correspond to the metacarpals and phalanges of the hand.

Many other comparisons between the two limbs can be drawn, especially in regard to the muscles. However, when the lower limb undergoes torsion about the long axis to obtain a better weight-bearing position, the knee joint bends backward, while the elbow bends forward. As is clear from its development, the posterior (extensor) surface of the arm is comparable with the anterior (extensor) surface of the thigh, and the anterior surface of the leg corresponds to the extensor surface of the forearm. Furthermore, the dorsum of the hand and the dorsum (upper surface) of the foot correspond to each other, so that, in the pronated position of the hand, thumb and big toe correspond, and the little finger and little toe correspond.

MUSCLES

Although extrinsic muscles of the shoulder girdle are extremely important in suspending and moving that girdle, extrinsic muscles running from the axial skeleton to the girdle of the lower limb would be of little use because of the very limited mobility of the sacroiliac joint. The girdle of the lower limb is so well stabilized that it gives origin to various muscles acting on the trunk. Although the pelvic girdle is, in turn, acted upon by a few of these muscles, none of these are, properly speaking, limb muscles. Of the lower limb muscles, only one, the psoas major, arises from the axial skeleton. It passes across the girdle to attach to the skeleton of the free limb. The other muscles of the hip region arise from the bony pelvis. Those in closest association with the girdle cover the posterior and lateral surfaces of the hip to form the musculature of the gluteal region, and these muscles act primarily across the hip joint.

Some of the **muscles of the thigh** act primarily at the knee joint, but those attached to the girdle have an action at the hip. These may or may not extend across the knee to have an action at this joint also. The muscles in the thigh are divisible into *anterior, anteromedial,* and *posterior groups.* The tendons of some of the posterior thigh muscles are easily felt behind the knee as they border the popliteal fossa, the depression behind the knee.

The **muscles of the leg** act primarily at the ankle and on the toes. They are divisible into *muscles of the calf* and *muscles of the anterolateral part of the leg.* Some

of the muscles of the calf also extend across the knee joint and have an action there. In a manner similar to that of forearm muscles, many of the muscles of the leg continue into the foot by means of long tendons. Some of them are associated with the **short muscles of the foot** in movements of the toes, whereas others act upon the foot as a whole rather than on only the toes.

NERVES

Nerves of the lower limb (Fig. 14-3) are derived from two plexuses, the lumbar and the sacral. Together they are referred to as the **lumbosacral plexus.** The **lumbar plexus** arises primarily from the *anterior rami of the first four lumbar nerves.* Its two chief branches to the lower limb are the **femoral** and **obturator nerves,** which pass to the front and anteromedial sides of the thigh, respectively, to innervate the muscles there (see Figs. 16-10 and 16-11). The **sacral plexus** is formed by the union of the *anterior rami from the fifth lumbar and first three sacral nerves, usually joined by branches from the fourth lumbar and fourth sacral nerves.* Most branches of the sacral plexus pass posteriorly between the sacrum and the hip bone. The smaller branches supply muscles of the gluteal region, but the largest portion of the sacral plexus is continued down the posterior aspect of the thigh as the **sciatic nerve,** the largest nerve in the body. As the sciatic nerve runs down the thigh, it innervates the posterior muscles there and then divides a little above the knee into common fibular (peroneal) and tibial nerves. The **common fibular nerve** winds around the lateral surface of the leg to supply anterolateral leg muscles and continues onto the dorsum of the foot. The **tibial nerve** runs down the posterior aspect of the leg and continues into the plantar aspect (sole) of the foot.

ARTERIES

The great arterial stem of the lower limb is the **femoral artery,** which is situated anteriorly in the thigh (see Fig. 14-3). The femoral artery is the continuation of the external iliac artery, which is in turn the continuation and larger branch of the common iliac artery. The two common iliac arteries are formed

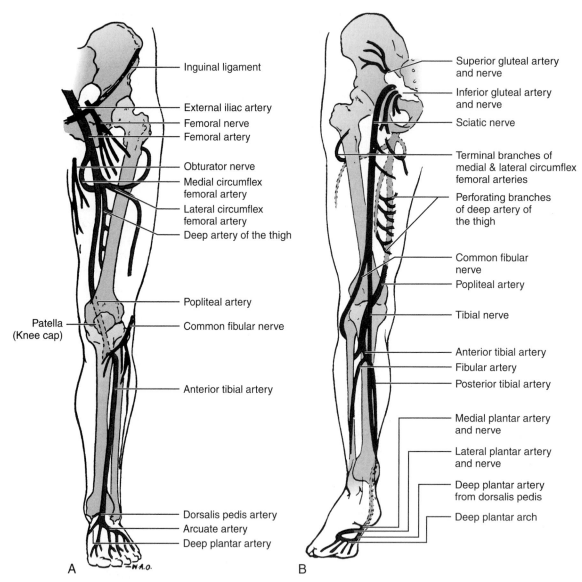

Figure 14-3 Chief vessels and nerves of the left lower limb. **A,** Anterior view. **B,** Posterior view.

by the bifurcation of the lower end of the aorta. The femoral artery runs down the anteromedial aspect of the thigh, but above the knee, it passes posteriorly around the medial surface of the femur to reach the popliteal fossa, there becoming the **popliteal artery.** In the upper part of the leg, the popliteal artery divides into anterior and posterior tibial arteries. The **posterior tibial artery** continues posteriorly down the leg to the plantar aspect of the foot, and the **anterior tibial artery** passes between the tibia and fibula to reach the anterolateral portion of the leg and continues onto the dorsum of the foot. The muscles of the gluteal region are supplied with blood by arteries that are associated with the sacral plexus. These arteries arise not from the external but from the internal iliac artery, which is the chief artery to the pelvis.

VEINS

Venous drainage of the lower limb is provided by superficial and deep veins. The superficial veins (Fig. 14-4) are located in the subcutaneous tissue. There are two major superficial veins, the great and small saphenous veins. The **great saphenous vein** begins on the medial side of the foot at the dorsal venous arch. It passes proximally anterior to the medial malleolus at the ankle, posterior to the medial condyle of the femur at the knee, and along the medial and then anterior aspects of the thigh. Along its course, the great saphenous vein receives tributaries from the leg and thigh and communicates with the deep veins by way of perforating veins that pass through the deep fascia. It also communicates with the small saphenous vein, including a connection by way of the accessory saphenous vein, if that vein is present. The great saphenous vein joins the femoral vein just below the inguinal ligament (see Chapter 16) and there receives tributaries from the anterior abdominal wall and pudendal region.

The **small saphenous vein** begins on the lateral side of the foot. After passing posterior to the lateral malleolus, it courses along the midline of the posterior aspect of the leg and joins the popliteal vein within the popliteal fossa. It receives tributaries from the superficial veins of the leg, communicates with the great saphenous vein, and also communicates with the deep veins through perforating veins.

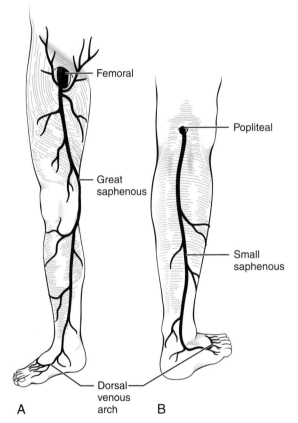

Figure 14-4 Major superficial veins of the lower limb. **A,** Anteromedial view. **B,** Posterolateral view. A small part of the femoral and popliteal veins are illustrated to show the termination of the great saphenous and small saphenous veins, respectively.

FUNCTIONAL/CLINICAL NOTE 14-1

The position of the great saphenous vein anterior to the medial malleolus is basically constant. In this area, it can be used if entry into the venous system is necessary. When the valves of the great saphenous vein and its tributaries are not functioning properly, varicosities may develop and would be evident as varicose veins within the subcutaneous tissue. The great saphenous vein can also be used as a graft in coronary bypass surgery.

The deep veins accompany the arteries of the lower limb and are named according to the artery with which they travel.

REVIEW QUESTIONS

1 The hip joint is what type of joint? What type is the knee joint?

2 Name the bones of the leg. What is their relationship to the knee and ankle joints?

3 The sacral plexus is formed by which anterior rami? What forms the lumbar plexus?

4 Just above the knee, the sciatic nerve divides into what two branches?

5 Which artery provides blood to the lower limb? As it passes posterior to the knee, it continues as what artery?

6 Which superficial vein begins on the medial side of the foot? Where does this vein end?

EXERCISES

1 On an articulated skeleton identify the following:
   a hip bones
   b acetabulum of the femur
   c fibula
   d tarsal bones

2 On your lower limb, demonstrate the course of the great saphenous vein.

15 THE BONY PELVIS, FEMUR, AND HIP JOINT

CHAPTER CONTENTS

Bones and Joints of the Bony Pelvis

Femur and Hip Joint

Movements

BONES AND JOINTS OF THE BONY PELVIS

Bones

The bony pelvis is formed by the paired **hip bones** and by the **sacrum** and **coccyx.** Each hip bone consists of three separate bones in the fetus and infant. Although these three bones—the *ilium, ischium,* and *pubis*—are so fused in the adult that it is difficult to see any signs of their junction, their names are still retained in describing the hip bone, as if they were separate bones.

Ilium

The **ilium** is the superior element of the hip bone (Figs. 15-1 to 15-3). Its *wing* (ala) forms the lateral projection of the hip, and the smooth inner and outer surfaces of this wing provide attachment to muscles of the limb. The upper free edge of the wing, the *iliac crest,* is palpable laterally and posteriorly and provides attachment to abdominal muscles. The crest ends anteriorly in the *anterior superior iliac spine* and posteriorly in the *posterior superior iliac spine.* On the anterior border of the wing of the ilium, below the anterior superior iliac spine, is the *anterior inferior iliac spine.* On the posterior border, below the posterior superior iliac spine and just above the smooth concavity (greater sciatic notch) on this border, is the *posterior inferior iliac spine.*

On a level with the posterior inferior iliac spine, the ilium bears on its medial aspect a smooth articular surface shaped somewhat like an ear and therefore called the *auricular surface.* Above and also posterior to the auricular surface is a larger rough area that

245

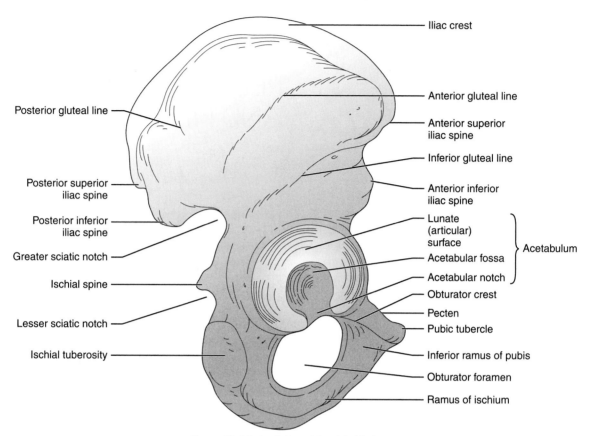

Figure 15-1 Lateral view of the right hip bone.

serves for the attachment of heavy ligaments forming an important part of the sacroiliac joint. Below the posterior inferior iliac spine and the auricular surface of the ilium is the deep *greater sciatic notch*. The lower and narrower part of the ilium, the *body*, extends inferiorly to about the level of a line drawn through the junction of the upper one third and the lower two thirds of the *acetabulum*, or hip socket.

Ischium

Of the two inferior elements of the hip bone, the **ischium** is the more posterior. Its *body* forms the posterior half of the lower two thirds of the acetabulum. Its *ramus* forms the posterior wall and a part of the inferior wall of the *obturator foramen*, the large hole in the hip bone. The ramus extends forward at the lower border of this foramen to join the pubis. On its posterior edge, the ischium bears the pointed

ischial spine. Above this spine, the posterior border of the ischium forms the lower part of the greater sciatic notch, a feature noted on the ilium. Below the ischial spine is a smaller notch, the *lesser sciatic notch*. The heavy flattened posterior expansion of the ischium is the *ischial tuberosity*.

Pubis

The **pubis** is the more anterior of the two lower parts of the hip bone. Its *superior ramus* forms approximately the anterior half of the lower two thirds of the acetabulum, and its *inferior ramus* curves posteriorly and downward to join the ischial ramus and complete the wall of the obturator foramen. Its *body*, at the junction of the superior and inferior rami, has on its anterior superior surface a thickening, the *pubic crest*, that ends laterally in a more marked *pubic tubercle*. Its medial surface is an articular one that enters into the pubic symphysis.

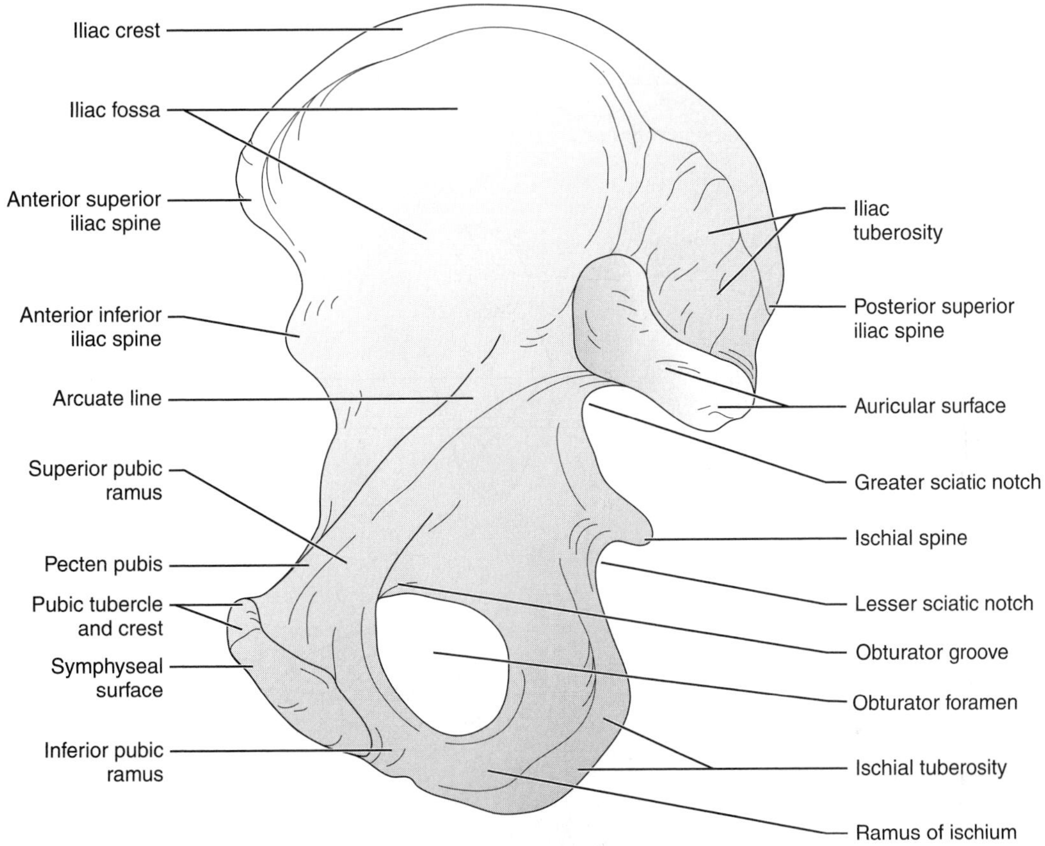
Iliac crest
Iliac fossa
Anterior superior iliac spine
Anterior inferior iliac spine
Arcuate line
Superior pubic ramus
Pecten pubis
Pubic tubercle and crest
Symphyseal surface
Inferior pubic ramus
Iliac tuberosity
Posterior superior iliac spine
Auricular surface
Greater sciatic notch
Ischial spine
Lesser sciatic notch
Obturator groove
Obturator foramen
Ischial tuberosity
Ramus of ischium

Figure 15-2 Medial view of the right hip bone.

Hip bone

As previously noted, each **hip bone** is formed by the fusion of the *ilium, ischium,* and *pubis.* All three elements of the hip bone help form the deep receptacle for the head of the femur, the *acetabulum.* Only a part of its surface is smooth and obviously adapted for articulation; a deeper, rougher portion is occupied by fat and a ligament. The lower edge of the acetabulum is deficient, making the fossa resemble a cup with a portion of the lip broken out.

The *obturator foramen* lies between the acetabulum and the conjoined ischial and inferior pubic rami. In the dried condition, this is a large foramen. In life, however, the foramen is almost completely closed by a membrane that gives attachments to muscles on both of its surfaces, hence the name *obturator* (closed or occluded) foramen.

The word *pelvis* literally means "basin." The pelvis consists not only of the two hip bones (the girdle) but also of the intervening segments of the vertebral column, the sacrum and coccyx (see Fig. 15-3). (In order to form a better idea of this structure, it is helpful to study an articulated pelvis with ligaments in place.)

The pelvis actually contains two cavities. The flared wings of the ilia form a lower boundary to the abdominal cavity proper, and the cavity here is known as the *greater (false or major) pelvis.* The *lesser (true or minor) pelvis* is the lower part of the cavity that is surrounded by the sacrum, pubes, ischia, and the lower parts of the ilia. The lesser pelvis has an inlet above, open into the abdominal cavity, and an outlet below that is bridged during life by muscles of the pelvic diaphragm.

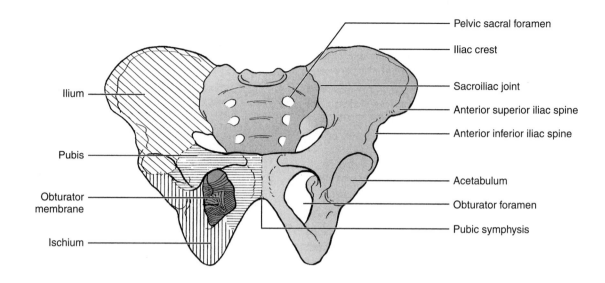

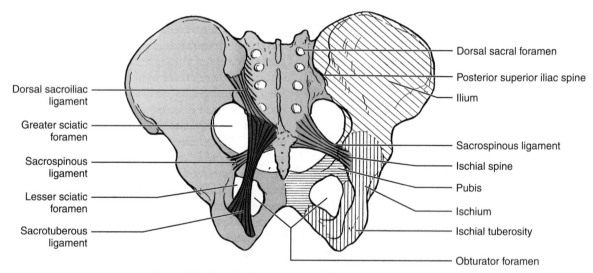

Figure 15-3 Anterior **(A)** and posterior **(B)** views of the bony pelvis.

The two hip bones are firmly attached posteriorly to the sacrum through the sacroiliac articulations. In addition, the wide interval between the lower part of each hip bone and the coccyx and lower part of the sacrum is bridged by two strong fibrous bands, the sacrotuberous and sacrospinous ligaments (see Fig. 15-3, *B*). The *sacrotuberous ligament* is a broad band stretching from the sacrum and coccyx to the ischial tuberosity. The *sacrospinous ligament* is a shorter band, largely covered posteriorly by the sacrotuberous ligament, which extends from the sacrum and coccyx to the ischial spine. The sacrospinous ligament converts the greater sciatic notch into a *greater sciatic foramen*. The sacrotuberous ligament forms a lower boundary for the lesser sciatic notch, converting this notch into a *lesser sciatic foramen*.

Joints

Pubic symphysis

The pubis of each hip bone is united anteriorly with its counterpart at the **pubic symphysis.** The *interpubic disc,* a heavy fibrocartilaginous pad, is firmly attached to the adjacent ends of the two pubes at the symphysis. The attachment of this disc to the pubis is strengthened by ligaments surrounding it. The pubic symphysis is barely movable during most of life, but in women it becomes much more movable during pregnancy.

Sacroiliac joint

The **sacroiliac joint** consists of a relatively small joint cavity between the sacrum and ilium and very powerful ligaments connecting these two bones (Fig. 15-4). The joint cavity is said to become partially or completely obliterated with age, particularly in males. Obliteration of the cavity is one of the most frequent findings in rheumatoid arthritis of the vertebral column, but it is not clear to what extent this should be regarded as a normal accompaniment of age and to what extent it is more strictly a pathological process. The *anterior sacroiliac ligament* is relatively thin and lies across the front of the joint. The *posterior sacroiliac ligament* is strong and blends deeply with the still stronger *interosseous sacroiliac ligament,* which is attached to the roughened areas behind and above the joint cavity. In addition to these ligaments, the pelvis is braced through its attachment to the sacrum by the *sacrotuberous* and *sacrospinous ligaments* (see Fig. 15-3), and to the last lumbar vertebra by matching *iliolumbar ligaments.*

The weight of the body bearing upon the sacrum tends to force the upper end of the sacrum inferiorly and anteriorly between the ilia, and its lower end tends to swing posteriorly. The wedge-shaped sacrum would then tend to spread the two ilia farther apart or to escape posteriorly and inferiorly from between the ilia. These movements of the sacrum, however, exert a greater pull on the interosseous and posterior sacroiliac ligaments (particularly the former), and this results in more firm apposition at the sacroiliac joint. The sacrospinous and sacrotuberous ligaments also tend to resist rotation of the sacrum. The pubic symphysis serves as the tie beam to resist flattening of the pelvis and consequent movement at the sacroiliac joint. Movement at the sacroiliac joint is also minimized by the fact that the opposed surfaces of the sacrum and ilium in the adult are wavy rather than flat. This joint is an exceedingly strong one and allows little movement. During pregnancy, however, the ligaments of the sacroiliac joint (like those at the pubic symphysis) become loosened, and movement at the joint increases.

FEMUR AND HIP JOINT

The bone of the thigh, the **femur** (Fig. 15-5; see also Fig. 15-4), has a rounded upper end, or *head,* that is attached to the shaft by a *neck* that does not continue in the direction of the shaft but rather projects medially at an angle of inclination, averaging 126 degrees. A large protuberance, the *greater trochanter,* projects upward where the neck joins the shaft; the greater trochanter is in line with the shaft. On the posteromedial side at the junction of neck and shaft is a smaller protuberance, the *lesser trochanter.* The two trochanters are connected on the posterior side of the femur by an *intertrochanteric crest.* The anterior surface of the upper part of the shaft of the femur is smooth, but the posterior surface below the trochanters is roughened, with two ridges that

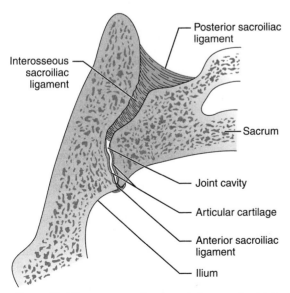

Figure 15-4 Transverse section through the sacroiliac joint.

Posterior sacroiliac ligament

Interosseous sacroiliac ligament

Sacrum

Joint cavity

Articular cartilage

Anterior sacroiliac ligament

Ilium

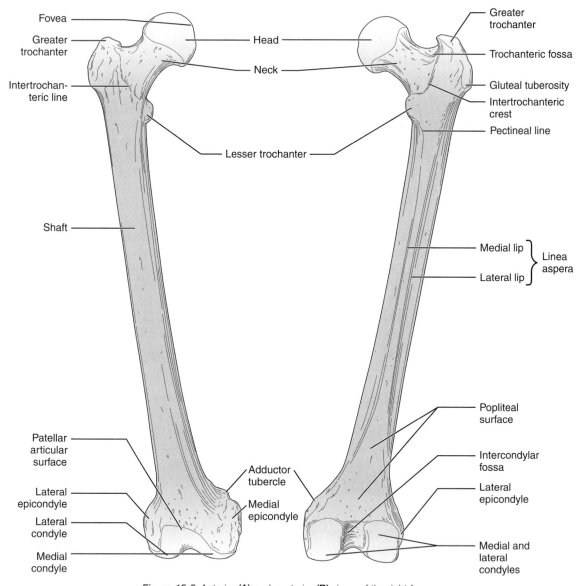

Fovea

Greater trochanter

Intertrochan-teric line

Shaft

Patellar articular surface

Lateral epicondyle

Lateral condyle

Medial condyle

Head

Neck

Lesser trochanter

Adductor tubercle

Medial epicondyle

Greater trochanter

Trochanteric fossa

Gluteal tuberosity

Intertrochanteric crest

Pectineal line

Medial lip

Lateral lip

Linea aspera

Popliteal surface

Intercondylar fossa

Lateral epicondyle

Medial and lateral condyles

Figure 15-5 Anterior **(A)** and posterior **(B)** views of the right femur.

run distally from the approximate regions of the lesser and greater trochanters to converge to form a roughened ridge, the *linea aspera,* with *medial* and *lateral lips.* The lower end of the femur is enlarged and has two rounded articular surfaces, the *condyles,* for articulation at the knee joint. The roughened medial and lateral surfaces of the condyles are the *epicondyles,* for the attachment of muscles. The medial epicondyle has an additional projection, the *adductor tubercle.*

Anteriorly, the articular surfaces of the two condyles come together to form a surface for articulation with the **patella** (knee cap). Posteriorly, they are separated by a deep *intercondylar fossa.* The flat surface of the femur above the intercondylar fossa and between the two diverging lower ends of the linea aspera is the *popliteal surface.*

The acetabulum receives the rounded head of the femur to form the **hip joint,** which is the best example in the body of a *ball-and-socket joint*. In comparison with the glenohumeral joint, the *hip joint has gained stability at the expense of some freedom of movement*. The deep ball-and-socket joint at the hip cannot allow movement as free as that which can occur between the very shallow glenoid cavity and the head of the humerus. At the same time, this deep joint allows for a great deal of stability in the various positions in which the lower limb is placed. The lower limb must exert its weight-bearing function during many phases of its movement.

The smooth articular surface of the head of the femur occupies considerably more than a hemisphere and ends at the neck, but it is interrupted at one point by a pit, or fovea, into which the ligament of the head of the femur attaches. The similarly smooth articular surface of the acetabulum forms an inverted U (see Fig. 15-1); the open end of the U is continuous with

the acetabular notch, and its cavity is occupied by a pad of fat. The acetabulum is made deeper by a fibro-cartilaginous mass, the *acetabular labrum* (Fig. 15-6), attached to its edge. The labrum bridges the notch as the *transverse acetabular ligament*. The free edge of this acetabular rim extends beyond the equator of the femoral head and, therefore, holds the head tightly within the acetabulum.

The strength of the hip joint is derived primarily from the shape of the articular surfaces and from the ligaments of this joint (Fig. 15-7), rather than from associated muscles. In contrast to the weak joint capsule of the glenohumeral joint, the joint capsule of the hip joint is very strong. It attaches lower on the anterior aspect of the femur than it does posteriorly. The capsule is composed mainly of longitudinally oriented fibers, but some deeper lying circular fibers are present. These latter fibers are most apparent

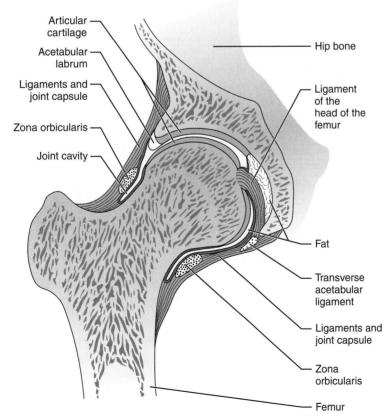

Articular cartilage
Acetabular labrum
Ligaments and joint capsule
Zona orbicularis
Joint cavity

Hip bone
Ligament of the head of the femur
Fat
Transverse acetabular ligament
Ligaments and joint capsule
Zona orbicularis
Femur

Figure 15-6 Frontal section through the hip joint. The articular cartilage *(light color)* is shown covering the articular surfaces. The synovial membrane, unlabeled, is shown in red. The zona orbicularis consists of circular fibers within the joint capsule.

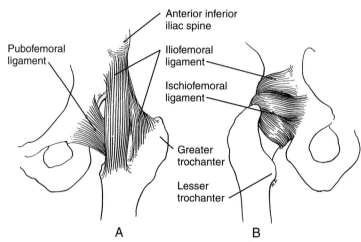

Figure 15-7 Anterior **(A)** and posterior **(B)** views of the left hip joint. Ant. inf., anterior inferior.

around the neck of the femur, where they form the *zona orbicularis*. The most prominent features of the capsule are three thickenings, the iliofemoral, pubofemoral, and ischiofemoral ligaments, that run a somewhat spiral course from the hip bone to the femur. The *iliofemoral ligament* is attached to the ilium below the anterior inferior iliac spine and covers most of the front of the joint. From this origin, two main bands tend to diverge to their attachments on the front of the femur. The iliofemoral ligament (ligament of Bigelow) is shaped like an inverted Y. The fibers of the ligament spiral somewhat medially as they run distally. This same twist is maintained by the other two ligaments of this joint. The iliofemoral ligament, in consequence of its position in front of the hip joint, *prevents undue extension at this joint. Because the weight of the body on the femur tends to keep the extended hip joint extended, the special function of the iliofemoral ligament is the maintenance of the erect posture without constant muscular action.*

The *pubofemoral ligament* arises from the pubic portion of the acetabular brim and therefore from the anteroinferior aspect of the joint. *The ligament helps to prevent excess abduction of the femur and also assists the iliofemoral ligament in checking extension at the hip.* Between the upper edge of the pubofemoral ligament and the medial edge of the upper part of the iliofemoral ligament, the capsule of the hip joint has a weak triangular area. The tendon of the iliopsoas muscle protects this area during life.

The *ischiofemoral ligament* not as well developed as the pubofemoral and iliofemoral ligaments. It arises from the ischial rim of the acetabulum and covers the lower posterior aspect of the joint. The upper fibers pass almost transversely toward the neck of the femur, whereas the lower ones pass slightly upward to their attachment there. The spiral of this ligament is decreased by flexion at the hip and increased by extension. The tightening of the ligament during extension *helps to make the extended position of the joint the most stable one.*

All three of these ligaments also have a common action in tending to limit medial rotation of the femur, inasmuch as this movement would increase their spiral. Lateral rotation tends to unwind their spiral and is checked entirely by muscles. All the parts of the capsule are relaxed during flexion and lateral rotation of the thigh; therefore, dislocation of the hip can take place more easily in this position.

Within the hip joint there is a flattened band, the *ligament of the head of the femur* (once known as the *ligamentum teres* or *round ligament*), which is attached to the nonarticular surface in the acetabulum and to the pit on the head of the femur (see Fig. 15-6). This ligament should help check abduction but never becomes tense enough to do so. In newborns and young infants, a normal ligament does check posterosuperior displacement of the head of the femur, a condition sometimes found in neonatal life.

Innervation to the hip joint is provided by the femoral nerve (either through direct branches or from its muscular branches), *the obturator nerve, the accessory obturator nerve* (when present), *the superior gluteal nerve, and the nerve to the quadratus femoris muscle.* The first three nerves are derived from the lumbar plexus, and the latter two are from the sacral plexus.

The arterial supply to the upper end of the femur (trochanters, neck, and head) is provided mainly by the medial and lateral circumflex femoral arteries (see Fig. 14-3), the superior gluteal artery (and possibly the inferior gluteal artery), and the obturator artery. The distribution to the head is of particular interest. Although a small part of the arterial supply enters through the ligament of the head of the femur (a branch of the obturator artery), most of the vessels to the neck and head pierce the capsule of the joint at its attachment to the femur and run proximally along the neck. Fractures of the femoral neck often tear the vessels and make healing of the fracture difficult.

MOVEMENTS

Movements of the Pelvis

Movements of the pelvis involve simultaneous movement of the lumbar portion of the vertebral column and movement at the hip joint. **Upward rotation** is the movement in which the anterior part of the pelvis is raised, and it involves a decrease in the lumbar curvature. **Downward rotation** is an increased tilting of the pelvis, accompanied by an increase in the lumbar curvature (lordosis). **Lateral rotation,** to the same or the opposite side, involves swinging the pelvis and the body as a whole upon one femoral head; this movement is of particular importance in walking. **Lateral tilting** of the pelvis raises one side higher than the other and involves a lateral bending of the lumbar part of the vertebral column.

Movements at the Hip Joint

There are seven types of movements at the hip joint. **Flexion** at the hip joint is the movement of bringing the thigh forward and upward toward the abdomen; **extension** is a backward movement of the thigh. **Abduction** is the drawing of one limb laterally and away from the other; **adduction** is bringing of the limbs together (see Fig. 1-4). **Circumduction** is a combination of all four of these movements. **Medial (internal) rotation** is a rotation of the limb so that the knee cap points inward; **lateral (external) rotation** is the movement in the opposite direction, so that the knee is turned outward. (Because the head and neck of the femur are not in the long axis of the limb, the "rotation" is actually a swinging on the head of the femur, as a gate swings back and forth on a hinge.)

REVIEW QUESTIONS

1 Describe in detail the anatomy of the hip joint. What are the specific functions of each of the three ligaments of the joint capsule?

2 What is the typical value of the angle between the shaft and neck of the femur?

3 What fibrocartilaginous structure lies on the outer edge of the acetabulum? What is the name given to the part of this structure that lies across the notch in the acetabulum?

4 Describe the anatomy of the sacrotuberous and sacrospinous ligaments and their relationship to the greater and lesser sciatic notches and foramina.

5 What is the greater (false) pelvis? What is the lesser (true) pelvis?

1 On a hip bone, identify its parts and the extent of each part.

2 On the ilium, identify the following:
   a iliac crest
   b anterior superior iliac spine
   c wing
   d posterior inferior iliac spine

3 Demonstrate flexion, adduction, and lateral rotation at the hip joint.

16 THE THIGH AND KNEE

CHAPTER CONTENTS

General Considerations

Bones and Joints

Fascia and Superficial Nerves and Vessels
  of the Thigh

Lumbar Plexus

Muscles

Anteromedial Nerves and Vessels

GENERAL CONSIDERATIONS

Many of the muscles of the thigh extend across both hip and knee joints and therefore have actions on both joints. The movements at the hip are briefly discussed in Chapter 15 and are considered in more detail in Chapter 17. The **movements at the knee** are largely *hinge-type movements,* consisting of flexion and extension. *Flexion* is the bending of the knee, bringing the calf of the leg toward the posterior surface of the thigh, and *extension* is the straightening of the knee. A slight hyperextension at this joint is normal in some people. In the partially flexed condition, a small amount of rotation between the tibia and femur may occur. This movement is limited to about 40 degrees and is not very obvious on inspection of the movements of the joint.

The few important **landmarks of the thigh** are, anteriorly, the *anterior superior iliac spine,* the *pubic tubercle,* the inguinal ligament extending between these two points, and the *patella* and adjacent enlarged *ends of the femur.* Except for the inguinal ligament, all of these structures are described in Chapter 15. The *inguinal ligament* is the lower edge of the aponeurosis of the most external of the flat muscles of the abdomen, and it marks the boundary between abdomen and thigh. It lies deep to the crease between the two parts, and as it runs between the ilium and pubis, it is slightly convex downward. Laterally, the landmarks include only the *greater trochanter* and, posteriorly, the *ischial tuberosity.* The hollow behind the knee is the *popliteal fossa.*

The **muscles of the thigh** are conveniently divided into three groups: an *anterior group* (originally *dorsal,* developmentally), concerned especially with flexion at the hip and extension at the knee; an *anteromedial* or *adductor group* (originally *ventral*), concerned especially

255

with adduction and flexion of the thigh; and a *posterior group* (also originally largely *ventral*), concerned with extension at the hip and flexion at the knee. Although there is some overlap in the functions and innervations of these groups, it is usually convenient to think of each group as having certain chief actions and having its own particular nerve supply. **Nerves** supplying innervation to the muscles of the thigh are the *femoral nerve* to the anterior group, the *obturator nerve* to the anteromedial group, and the *sciatic nerve* to the posterior group. The posterior muscles, nerves, and vessels are described in Chapter 17.

Although the large nerves of the thigh enter it anteriorly, anteromedially, and posteriorly, there is only one important set of **vessels** to the thigh: the femoral vessels, which lie anteriorly at the groin with the femoral nerve. The *femoral artery* is a continuation of the external iliac artery; the change in name occurs at the inguinal ligament. The *femoral vein,* similarly, continues above the inguinal ligament as the external iliac vein. A little above the knee, the femoral vessels pass through a gap in one of the muscles, close to the bone, to attain a position in the popliteal fossa. There the vessels continue as the *popliteal vessels.*

BONES AND JOINTS
Bones

The femur, the bone of the thigh, is discussed in Chapter 15, but its distal end should be studied in more detail as the knee joint is studied. Because some of the muscles of the thigh cross the knee joint to attach to bones of the leg, the proximal ends of these bones must also be studied, although a more complete description of them is provided in Chapter 19.

Femur

In brief, the expanded distal end of the **femur** has rounded *medial* and *lateral* condyles for articulation with the tibia. Anteriorly, where the articular surfaces of the condyles merge, there is an *articular surface for the patella.* The *intercondylar fossa* of the femur provides attachment to ligaments that lie within the knee joint, and the *medial* and *lateral epicondyles* provide attachment not only to muscles but also to the two important external ligaments of the knee joint.

Tibia

The expanded proximal end of the **tibia** is formed by two *tibial condyles* that have almost flat upper articular surfaces that receive the weight transmitted from the femoral condyles (see Figs. 14-2 and 19-1). The articular surfaces are separated by a nonarticular area to which internal ligaments of the knee joint attach. The sides of the tibial condyles receive the attachment of the lower part of the capsule of the knee joint and certain muscles and ligaments. On the lower surface of the lateral condyle, there is an *articular facet* for articulation with the head of the fibula. On the anterior border of the shaft of the tibia below the condyles is a roughened raised area, the *tibial tuberosity,* to which the patellar ligament attaches. (This ligament is really the lower end of the tendon of the muscle that extends the leg at the knee, the quadriceps muscle.)

Fibula

The upper end of the slender **fibula** is the *head,* which rises to a pointed apex. It articulates with the lower surface of the lateral tibial condyle, and it does not enter into the knee joint.

Patella

The **patella** (commonly called the *knee cap*) is triangular, with its apex directed downward. Posteriorly, it has on its upper part a smooth articular surface for articulation with the femur. Elsewhere, its surface is rough for the attachment of tendon fibers and the entrance of blood vessels. The patella is the largest sesamoid bone in the body. It so interrupts the quadriceps tendon, in which it lies, that the part of the tendon between it and the tibia is known as the *patellar ligament.*

FUNCTIONAL/CLINICAL NOTE 16-1

By holding the tendon of the quadriceps farther forward, the patella adds a great deal to the effectiveness of the quadriceps in extending the leg. In the absence of the patella, about 30% more force is required to extend the leg completely.

Knee Joint

The joint capsule of the knee joint is somewhat complex and, unlike that of most joints, does not form a complete covering around the joint. Anteriorly, it is replaced by the insertion of the quadriceps muscle on the patella, the patella itself, and the patellar ligament. The synovial membrane (lining) of the joint rests directly against parts of these structures. On either side of the quadriceps tendon, between the patella and the femoral and tibial condyles, the joint capsule is formed by fibers from the fascia lata (the deep fascia of the thigh) and expansions from the quadriceps tendon; these parts are called the *medial* and *lateral patellar retinacula.* Posteriorly, the joint capsule consists of interlacing fibers that are reinforced by a strong attachment from the semimembranosus tendon (Fig. 16-1). The band derived from this tendon runs obliquely upward and laterally as the *oblique popliteal ligament.*

Closely related to the posterolateral aspect of the joint is the tendon of the popliteus muscle at the knee. This tendon lies deep to the lateral part of the joint capsule. It is separated from the joint cavity only by a fold of synovial membrane but is attached to both the capsule and the lateral meniscus. The popliteus muscle exits through a hole in the posterior part of the capsule. The upper edge of this opening is strengthened by some arching fibers that constitute the *arcuate popliteal ligament.*

Sensory innervation to the knee joint is provided by branches from the femoral nerve, obturator nerve, and sciatic nerve (both tibial and common fibular components).

Collateral ligaments

Hinge joints typically have special medial and lateral ligaments, and the knee joint is no exception to this. The medial ligament of the knee, the *tibial collateral ligament,* is a broad band that is fused posteriorly with the capsule of the knee joint, passing from the medial epicondyle of the femur to the medial surface of the proximal end of the tibia. The cordlike lateral ligament of the knee, the *fibular collateral ligament,* runs from the lateral epicondyle of the femur

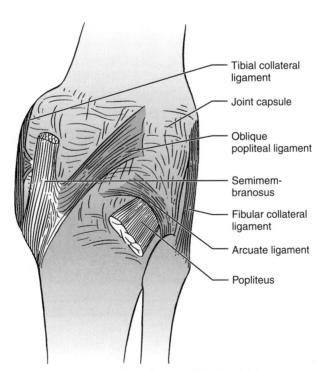

Tibial collateral ligament

Joint capsule

Oblique popliteal ligament

Semimembranosus

Fibular collateral ligament

Arcuate ligament

Popliteus

Figure 16-1 Posterior view of the knee joint.

to the head of the fibula. In contrast to the tibial collateral ligament, the fibular collateral ligament has no attachment to the joint capsule but lies just lateral to it.

FUNCTIONAL/CLINICAL NOTE 16-2

The fibular collateral ligament and the posterior part of the tibial collateral ligament are made taut by extension of the knee and relaxed by flexion. The anterior part of the tibial collateral ligament, however, remains tense in all positions of the knee. The two ligaments together restrain rotation and lateral movement at the knee, especially in the extended position, and the tibial collateral ligament is an important stabilizer of the knee in all positions. Tearing of this ligament as a result of a forcible blow to the outside of the knee is a common injury in football players.

Joint cavity

The cavity of the knee joint is extensive. It passes some distance proximally anterior to the femur, between the femur and the overlying quadriceps muscle. The cavity is usually continuous with the *suprapatellar bursa,* although the bursa may be separate. The *articularis genus muscle* inserts into the posterior surface of the superior reflection of the synovial membrane. Below the patella and between the femur and tibia, the cavity is subdivided by structures lying within the capsule of the joint. A fold of synovial membrane, the *infrapatellar synovial fold,* sweeps downward and posteriorly from the posterior surface of the patella and, becoming wider as it does so, attaches to the inner border of the articular surfaces of both the femoral and tibial condyles. The *infrapatellar fat pad* lies between the patellar ligament and the synovial membrane. In consequence, the cavity of the knee joint between the femur and tibia is divided into medial and lateral parts that communicate only anteriorly and are separated from each other by the structures extending between the intercondylar fossa of the femur and the intercondylar areas of the tibia, primarily, the cruciate ligaments.

Associated with the anterior region of the knee are two subcutaneous bursae. The *prepatellar bursa* lies between the skin and the lower part of the patella and the patellar ligament, and the *subcutaneous infrapatellar bursa* is positioned between the skin and the tibial tuberosity. These bursae can become inflamed and painful when subjected to trauma such as that associated with frequent kneeling on a floor or with repeated contact of an athlete's knee on a hard surface. Neither bursa is connected to the synovial cavity or to the deep bursae of the knee joint.

Menisci

The medial and lateral parts of the cavity are, in turn, partly subdivided by semilunar cartilages, the *medial* and *lateral menisci* (Fig. 16-2). These crescentic cartilages are wedge-shaped in cross-section, with the thinnest part on the inner edge. Around this free inner border, the part of the synovial cavity between a femoral condyle and a meniscus is continuous with that between the meniscus and the corresponding tibial condyle. On their outer border, both menisci are attached to the synovial and fibrous layers of the joint capsule. Although the medial meniscus is also anchored firmly to the strong tibial collateral ligament, the lateral meniscus has only slight attachments to the weak lateral portion of the capsule, from which it is partially separated by the tendon of the popliteus muscle. The lateral meniscus has no attachment to the fibular collateral ligament.

FUNCTIONAL/CLINICAL NOTE 16-3

This marked difference in the relationship of the menisci to the collateral ligaments may be one of the reasons why the medial cartilage is more often torn, in conjunction with tearing of ligaments at the knee, than is the lateral cartilage; the concept is that the medial cartilage is less mobile and more likely to be caught and torn as the femur moves it back and forth, or rotates it, on the tibia.

Both menisci are anchored to the tibia by strong fibrous bands continuous with the ends of the cartilages, and these also limit their movement.

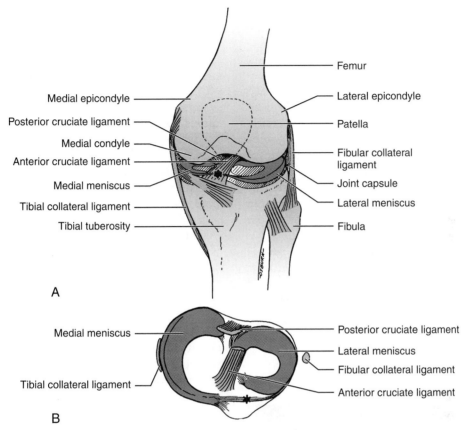

Medial epicondyle

Posterior cruciate ligament

Medial condyle

Anterior cruciate ligament

Medial meniscus

Tibial collateral ligament

Tibial tuberosity

Femur

Lateral epicondyle

Patella

Fibular collateral ligament

Joint capsule

Lateral meniscus

Fibula

A

Medial meniscus

Tibial collateral ligament

Posterior cruciate ligament

Lateral meniscus

Fibular collateral ligament

Anterior cruciate ligament

B

Figure 16-2 The principal structures of the interior of the knee joint. **A**, Anterior view. **B**, Superior view with the femur omitted. Menisci are shown in *dark color;* ligaments are in *light color.* (A transverse ligament, marked with an *asterisk,* may be present, attaching to both the medial and lateral menisci.)

The menisci serve in small part to deepen the articular surfaces on the upper end of the tibia, allow better adaptation of these surfaces to the femoral condyles, and apparently facilitate rotation at the knee.

FUNCTIONAL/CLINICAL NOTE 16-4

The menisci are most likely to be torn by rotation of the femur on the supporting tibia when the knee is flexed: for instance, when a runner suddenly changes direction, rotating the body and therefore the femur on the tibia while that limb is supporting weight. The torn part of a meniscus usually rolls up and locks the joint. This is accompanied by pain and swelling at the knee.

Menisci have also been thought to be particularly important in maintaining an even film of synovial fluid and aiding in lubrication of the joint. If the cartilages are torn by violence, they can be removed; however, the weight-bearing areas on the femur and tibia have been shown to be decreased by almost 50% by such removal. This concentration of the weight on a smaller area, and perhaps a poorer lubrication, may account for the finding that in time the articular cartilages of both the femur and tibia may manifest early degenerative arthritic changes.

Cruciate ligaments

The anterior cruciate (crossed) ligament and the posterior cruciate ligament are especially important ligaments of the knee joint, lying within the joint capsule but covered anteriorly and on both sides by reflections of the synovial membrane. The *anterior cruciate ligament* ascends from the anterior area between the tibial condyles and runs proximally, posteriorly, and somewhat laterally to attach toward the back of the medial surface of the lateral femoral condyle. The *posterior cruciate ligament* arises from the posterior intercondylar area and extends proximally and somewhat anteriorly and medially to attach to the lateral side of the medial femoral condyle. Both ligaments seem to be fairly tense in all positions, but particularly so in extreme extension and extreme flexion. The cruciate ligaments apparently contribute significantly to the stability of the knee joint in all positions, preventing anteroposterior displacement of the tibia and limiting rotation of the femur upon the tibia. They are, however, apparently not as important in limiting rotation as are the collateral ligaments.

FUNCTIONAL/CLINICAL NOTE 16-5

Rupture of the anterior cruciate ligament alone has been reported as a result from a hard blow (such as a block or a tackle in football) on the anterolateral side of the limb while the foot bearing all the weight was in slight medial rotation. This differs little from the mechanism of rupture of the tibial collateral ligament. A common severe athletic injury to the knee results in tearing of the tibial collateral and anterior cruciate ligaments (and often of the medial meniscus). The resulting instability makes it difficult or impossible for a runner to suddenly change course, and surgical repair or replacement of the torn ligament or ligaments is necessary. The large muscle on the front of the thigh that extends the knee, the quadriceps femoris, must always be strengthened in such cases, because it rapidly loses strength in any disability of the knee. In the nonathlete with less severe injury, development of the quadriceps may be all that is necessary to restore adequate stability.

Rupture of the posterior cruciate ligament alone can result from an automobile accident in which the tibia of an occupant comes in violent contact with the dashboard, forcing the tibia posteriorly. The usual test for a ruptured cruciate ligament consists of trying to displace the tibia anteriorly or posteriorly on the femur with the leg flexed. Rupture of the anterior cruciate ligament allows abnormal anterior displacement, the *anterior drawer sign*, whereas rupture of the posterior ligament permits abnormal posterior displacement, the *posterior drawer sign*.

Tibiofibular Joint

The **tibiofibular joint** is of the plane type. A capsule with no particular distinguishing features surrounds the small cavity. On occasion, it communicates with the knee joint.

Surface Anatomy

Numerous bony landmarks can be palpated in the anterior and lateral parts of the thigh and at the knee. The **iliac crest,** palpable laterally, marks the superior border of the bony pelvis. It can be followed anteriorly where it ends at the **anterior superior iliac spine** (origin for the sartorius muscle). The **pubis** can be felt anteriorly, near the midline, and if it is followed laterally, the **pubic tubercle** can normally be palpated. On the femur, the **greater trochanter** is easily located laterally on the thigh, several inches distal to the iliac crest. Most of the femur is surrounded by muscles, but distally, the **medial** and **lateral condyles and epicondyles** can be identified. In the same region, anteriorly, the **patella** is quite obvious. With flexion and extension of the leg, the articulation between the femur and tibia is palpable. Just distal to the knee joint, the **condyles of the tibia** can be felt medially and laterally, and the sharp anterior border indicates the position of the **tibial tuberosity.** Just below the lateral tibial condyle, the **head of the fibula** is palpable subcutaneously.

FASCIA AND SUPERFICIAL NERVES AND VESSELS OF THE THIGH

Fascia

The superficial fascia of the thigh contains superficial nerves and vessels, the important superficial inguinal lymph nodes, and a varying amount of fat, but it otherwise has no particular distinguishing features. The deep fascia of the thigh is the **fascia lata** (meaning "broad fascia"); it resembles the fascia of the arm and forearm in that it is a tough layer that completely surrounds the musculature of the thigh. Laterally, it is thickened and strengthened by additional longitudinal fibers to form the **iliotibial tract.** This important band has three origins: anteriorly, from the attachment of the tensor fasciae latae muscle; posteriorly, from much of the insertion of the gluteus maximus; and in between, from the crest of the ilium through the fascia covering the gluteus medius. The fascia lata is attached to the femur for much of its length by the lateral intermuscular septum; distally, it reinforces the capsule of the knee joint and attaches anterolaterally to the lateral tibial condyle.

Posterolaterally, the fascia lata extends over the gluteus medius. It also continues on both sides of the tensor fasciae latae and the gluteus maximus and attaches to the iliac crest, the sacrotuberous ligament, and the ischial tuberosity. Anteromedially, it is attached to the inguinal ligament and the pubis. It sends **medial and lateral intermuscular septa** to the femur in the lower part of the thigh and is attached around the knee to various bony prominences to help form the medial and lateral patellar retinacula.

Nerves

The **lateral cutaneous nerve of the thigh** (lateral femoral cutaneous nerve), a branch of the lumbar plexus that penetrates the fascia lata a little below the anterior superior iliac spine, innervates the skin of the anterolateral aspect of the thigh. Branches of the **femoral nerve** innervate most of the anterior and anteromedial surfaces of the thigh. These branches pierce the fascia lata at various levels to branch in the superficial fascia. A small area of skin on the medial surface of the thigh is usually innervated by a branch of

the **obturator nerve,** while the posterior aspect of the thigh is innervated by the **posterior cutaneous nerve of the thigh** (posterior femoral cutaneous nerve).

Vessels

Many small veins form a network in the superficial fascia of the thigh, but the prominent vein here is the **great saphenous** (saphenous means "obvious," probably a reference to the usual involvement of this vein in varicose veins of the lower limb). The great saphenous vein ascends from the medial side of the leg to the medial side of the thigh. It runs slightly forward to reach the anterior surface of the thigh, where, a little below the inguinal ligament, it penetrates the fascia lata and ends in the femoral vein. The gap in the fascia lata that it passes through is the *saphenous hiatus.* Just before the great saphenous vein goes through the hiatus, it usually receives veins from the lower abdominal and pudendal regions.

LUMBAR PLEXUS

The lumbar plexus (Fig. 16-3) innervates the muscles and the skin on the anterior and medial sides of the thigh and the skin on the medial side of the leg and

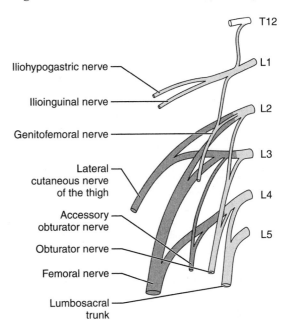

Figure 16-3 Diagram of the lumbar plexus. The posterior portions of the plexus are *shaded.*

foot. Although it arises deep within the abdomen, its pattern of formation and branching are best studied at this time to understand the nerves in the thigh. Similarly, the sacral plexus supplies posterior skin and muscles of the thigh, as well as muscles of the gluteal region. Because the lumbar and sacral plexuses are connected, and because both innervate primarily the lower limb, they are frequently described together as the *lumbosacral plexus* (Fig. 16-4). The sacral part of the lumbosacral plexus is described in Chapter 17.

The origin of the **lumbar plexus** is from the *anterior rami of spinal nerves L1 to L3 and a variable part of L4, with usually a small communication from T12*. Because it is formed at the lumbar level of the

vertebral column, the plexus itself lies on the inner surface of the posterior abdominal wall; during dissection, it must be approached from the abdominal cavity. At its origin, it is embedded in the psoas major muscle. The definitive peripheral nerves arising from the plexus exit from the psoas muscle and pass into the lower part of the anterior abdominal wall or into the thigh.

The plexus is usually arranged as follows: L1, having received a communication from T12, divides into two branches. The upper one of these gives rise to the *iliohypogastric* and *ilioinguinal nerves* to the lowermost part of the abdominal wall. The other branch joins a small branch from L2 to form the *genitofemoral*

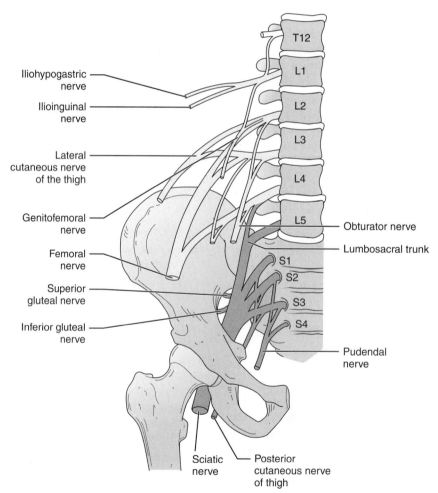

Figure 16-4 Diagram of the lumbosacral plexus. The lumbar plexus is in *light shading;* the sacral plexus is in *dark shading.* Only the major branches of the sacral plexus are depicted. See Figure 17-1 for a more detailed diagram of the sacral plexus.

nerve to the scrotum or labia majora and some of the skin of the upper anterior surface of the thigh. Small anterior branches from L2 to L4 join to form the *obturator nerve.* Branches from L3 and L4 form an *accessory obturator nerve* in up to 10% of plexuses.

Contributions from the larger, posterior portions of the anterior rami of L2 and L3 form the *lateral cutaneous nerve of the thigh.* The remainder of the posterior portions of these two rami joins a part of L4 to form the largest branch of the plexus, the *femoral nerve.* Typically, L4 divides into two parts, one part going into the lumbar plexus to help form the obturator and femoral nerves, and the remainder passing downward to join the sacral plexus. There is considerable variation in the relative sizes of the contributions of L4 to the two plexuses. If L4 fails to participate in the lumbar plexus but goes entirely to the sacral plexus, the plexus is known as a *prefixed* one. If all of L4, and perhaps even some of L5, go into the lumbar plexus, this plexus is known as a *postfixed* one.

In the brachial plexus, a division between anterior and posterior parts of the plexus is obvious; the anterior part, as exemplified by medial and lateral cords and their branches, innervates the anterior, or flexor, muscles of the limb, while the posterior part, consisting of the posterior cord and its branches, innervates the posterior, or extensor, muscles. A similar division and distribution also exists in both lumbar and sacral plexuses, although they are somewhat less obvious than in the upper limb because of the extensive rotation that the lower limb has undergone during development. The anterior portion of the lumbar plexus is distributed to the anterior abdominal wall or its derivatives (through the iliohypogastric, ilioinguinal, and genitofemoral nerves) and to the adductor or anteromedial surface of the thigh (through the obturator nerve). This part of the thigh represents the cephalic part of the original flexor surface of the limb. Similarly, the lateral cutaneous nerve of the thigh and femoral nerve, the posterior elements of the lumbar plexus, are distributed to the original posterior or extensor surface of the thigh. In the sacral plexus, the gluteal nerves and the common fibular nerve, the larger parts of the posterior division of this plexus, are distributed also to original posterior (extensor) muscles of the gluteal region and of the

leg. The tibial nerve and its derivatives innervate the more caudal muscles of the original flexor surface of the thigh and the flexor (original anterior) muscles in the leg and foot.

MUSCLES
Anterior Muscles of the Thigh

Sartorius
The anterior muscles of the thigh are depicted in Figure 16-5 and Figure 16-6; origins and insertions of muscles are depicted in Figure 16-7 and listed in Table 16-1. The most superficial muscle on the anterior aspect of the thigh is the **sartorius** ("tailor" muscle). This long ribbon-like muscle winds across the anterior and medial surfaces of the thigh. Its *origin* is from the anterior superior iliac spine, and its *insertion* is on the medial surface of the shaft of the tibia below the tuberosity. At its insertion, its tendon is closely associated with the tendons of two other muscles, the gracilis (medially) and the semitendinosus (posteriorly). Because it crosses anterior to the hip joint, the *action* of the sartorius is as a flexor there; because it usually crosses posterior to the axis of motion of the knee joint, it participates in flexion of the knee. Moreover, it is an abductor of the thigh (although a very weak one), and because of its lateral origin and its medial position at the knee, it is also a lateral rotator of the thigh. These four actions of the muscle together produce the once common cross-legged sitting position used in the past by tailors; hence the name. (None of these actions of the sartorius is a strong one. In order to assume this position, other muscles, which produce one or two of the necessary movements, must also be used. Abduction by the sartorius is especially weak.) The sartorius receives *innervation* from branches of the femoral nerve.

The sartorius muscle forms the lateral boundary of the **femoral triangle,** which is situated in the upper part of the thigh (Fig. 16-8, *A*). The floor and the medial wall are composed of other muscles of the thigh, and the femoral nerve and vessels enter the thigh deep to the inguinal ligament (see Fig. 16-8, *B*), the upper border of the triangle. The nerve breaks up into branches in the triangle, and the femoral

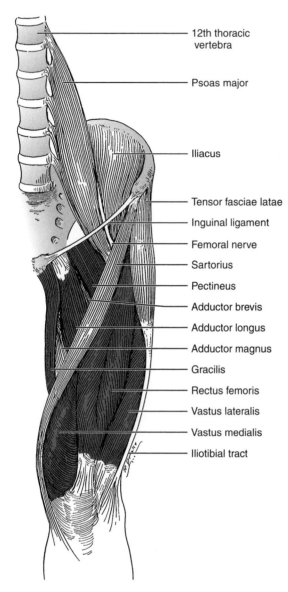

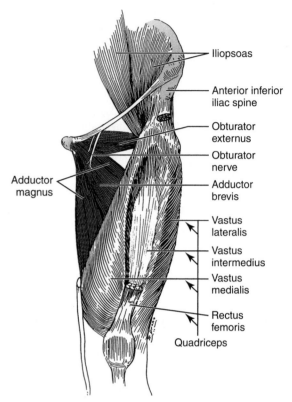

Figure 16-6 Deeper muscles of the anterior and medial *(highlighted in color)* aspects of the thigh; the more superficial muscles are omitted.

Figure 16-5 Some of the more superficial muscles of the anterior aspect of the thigh *(highlighted in color)*. The space between the pectineus and the adductor longus is exaggerated so that the position of the adductor brevis can be shown. (Note that the sartorius and tensor fasciae latae muscles are also superficial but are not shown in color.)

artery gives off its chief branch, the deep artery of the thigh (profunda femoris or deep femoral artery) before continuing distally in the thigh deep to the sartorius muscle, separated from it by a heavy layer of fascia.

Tensor fasciae latae

The **tensor fasciae latae** takes *origin* from the iliac crest just posterior to the anterior superior iliac spine. It is a short, straplike muscle enclosed between two layers of the fascia lata as they attach to the iliac crest. This muscle runs distally and slightly posteriorly to an *insertion* onto the iliotibial tract. Although anteriorly placed, it is actually a muscle of the gluteal region. It receives its *innervation* from the superior gluteal nerve. Its *action* is to assist in flexion of the thigh at the hip joint. Because of its oblique posterior direction, it medially rotates as it flexes. It also works with the gluteus medius and gluteus minimus muscles in abduction of the thigh, or at least in preventing undue sagging of the opposite side of the pelvis when the weight is supported on one limb. However, the tensor fasciae latae can contribute very little to the latter action.

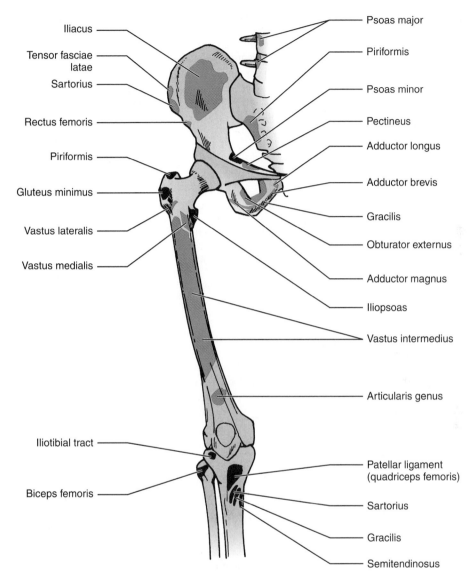

Figure 16-7 Anterior view of the bones of the pelvis, thigh, and knee region, depicting origins *(color)* and insertions *(black)* of the anterior and adductor muscles of the thigh (and posterior muscles that can be observed in this view). The attachment of the quadriceps femoris to the patella is not depicted. However, the insertion of the muscle onto the tibial tuberosity by way of the patellar ligament is shown.

Quadriceps femoris

The **quadriceps femoris** is the large muscle mass covering the anterior, medial, and lateral aspects of the femur. It is divisible into four parts, as its name indicates. The **rectus femoris** is the rounded, more anterior, head of the quadriceps, appearing as a separate muscle except at its insertion. Its *origin* is from

the anterior inferior iliac spine and, by a posteriorly arching part of its tendon of origin, from the ilium just above the acetabulum. It combines with the other members of the quadriceps group in an *insertion* upon the patella and through the patellar ligament upon the tibial tuberosity; therefore, it shares with these others the *action* of extension of the leg at the knee. It is

Table 16-1   ANTERIOR MUSCLES OF THE THIGH

Muscle	Origin (Proximal Attachment)	Insertion (Distal Attachment)	Action	Innervation
Sartorius	Anterior superior iliac spine	Medial surface of proximal end of tibia just distal to tibial tuberosity	Flexion, abduction, and lateral rotation of thigh; flexion of leg	Femoral nerve
Tensor fasciae latae	Iliac crest posterior to anterior superior iliac spine	Iliotibial tract	Flexion, medial rotation, and abduction of thigh	Superior gluteal nerve
Quadriceps femoris				
1. Rectus femoris	Anterior inferior iliac spine; ilium above acetabulum	Patella and through patellar ligament to tibial tuberosity	Extension of leg; flexion of thigh	Femoral nerve
2. Vastus medialis	Medial lip of linea aspera; lower part of intertrochanteric line	Patella and through patellar ligament to tibial tuberosity	Extension of leg	Femoral nerve
3. Vastus lateralis	Lateral lip of linea aspera of femur; limited origin from intertrochanteric line	Patella and through patellar ligament to tibial tuberosity	Extension of leg	Femoral nerve
4. Vastus intermedius	Anterior and lateral surfaces of femur	Patella and through patellar ligament to tibial tuberosity	Extension of leg	Femoral nerve
Articularis genus	Distal part of anterior surface of femur	Synovial membrane of knee joint	Pulls synovial membrane of knee proximally during extension of leg	Femoral nerve (nerve to vastus intermedius)
Iliopsoas				
1. Psoas major	Bodies and transverse processes of all lumbar vertebrae (and possibly last thoracic vertebra)	Lesser trochanter of femur	Flexion of thigh; slight adduction of thigh of free limb	Second to fourth lumbar nerves
2. Iliacus	Iliac fossa	Lesser trochanter of femur (with psoas major)	Flexion of thigh; slight adduction of thigh of free limb	Femoral nerve
Psoas minor	Twelfth thoracic and first lumbar vertebrae	Superior ramus of pubis	Upward rotation of pelvis	First or second lumbar nerve (or both)
Pectineus	Superior ramus of pubis	Femur just distal to lesser trochanter	Flexion and adduction of thigh	Femoral nerve; possibly obturator and/or accessory obturator nerve

the only member of the quadriceps group that passes across the hip joint, and it is a flexor at this joint.

The other three heads of the quadriceps femoris muscle are the *vastus medialis,* the *vastus lateralis,* and the *vastus intermedius.* They are difficult to distinguish individually throughout much of their course

because both the vastus medialis and vastus lateralis arise in part from septa that they share with the intermedius. The **vastus medialis** seems to cover much of the medial surface of the femur, but it is actually kept away from contact with the femur's surface by the vastus intermedius. The vastus medialis has an *origin*

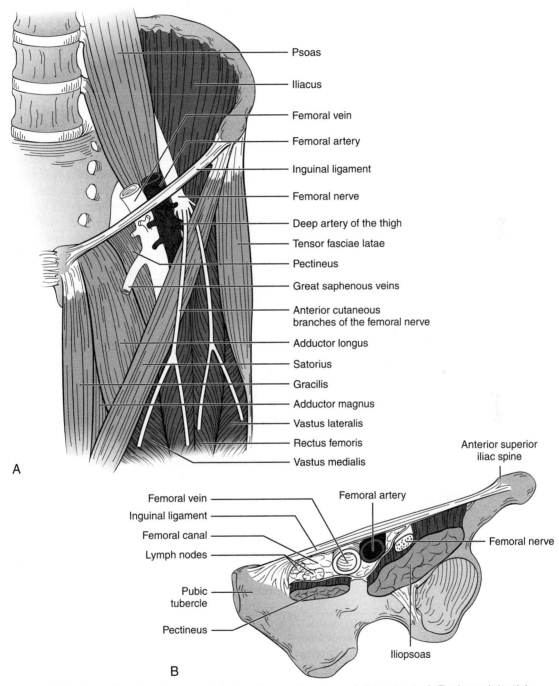

Psoas

Iliacus

Femoral vein

Femoral artery

Inguinal ligament

Femoral nerve

Deep artery of the thigh

Tensor fasciae latae

Pectineus

Great saphenous veins

Anterior cutaneous
branches of the femoral nerve

Adductor longus

Satorius

Gracilis

Adductor magnus

Vastus lateralis

Rectus femoris

Vastus medialis

A

Femoral vein

Inguinal ligament

Femoral canal

Lymph nodes

Pubic
tubercle

Pectineus

Femoral artery

Anterior superior
iliac spine

Femoral nerve

Iliopsoas

B

Figure 16-8 The femoral triangle and a view of a section through the upper end of the triangle. **A,** The femoral sheath is omitted, to expose the femoral nerve and vessels. **B,** The positions of the femoral nerve, vessels, and canal can be seen deep to the inguinal ligament.

chiefly from the medial lip of the linea aspera—that is, from the posterior aspect of the femur—but has some origin anteriorly from the lower part of the intertrochanteric line. The **vastus lateralis** has a slight attachment on the anterior surface of the femur (intertrochanteric line) above the origin of the vastus intermedius, but it too has an *origin* primarily from the posterior aspect of the femur, along the lateral lip of the linea aspera. The **vastus intermedius** has its *origin* from the anterior and lateral surfaces of the shaft of the femur.

All three vastus muscles unite with the rectus femoris and have their *insertion* on the patella, through which their pull is transferred to the patellar ligament and then to the tibia.

FUNCTIONAL/CLINICAL NOTE 16-6

The patella not only provides an enduring surface to withstand the friction that would otherwise affect the quadriceps tendon at the knee joint but also provides additional leverage for the quadriceps by holding the tendon away from the axis of motion. As mentioned previously, the quadriceps must develop as much as 30% more power in order to extend the knee after patellectomy. Although exercise of the quadriceps is important after any injury to the knee, it may not significantly increase the muscle's strength in some individuals. Therefore, methods have been developed to repair the tendon after patellectomy so that the additional strength needed is minimal.

The *action* of the four heads of the quadriceps is to extend the leg, and the muscle as a whole forms the chief extensor at the knee. The last 15 degrees of extension are brought about by the three vastus muscles. Each head of the muscle receives *innervation* from one or more branches of the femoral nerve.

Articularis genus

Under cover of the lower part of the vastus intermedius, the **articularis genus** muscle has an *origin* from the distal part of the anterior surface of the femur,

and its *insertion* is on the upper part of the synovial membrane of the knee joint. *Innervation* to the muscle is provided by the nerve to the vastus intermedius. Its *action* is to draw the synovial membrane upward as the leg is extended.

Iliopsoas

The **iliopsoas** muscle actually consists of two muscles, the psoas major and the iliacus. These muscles blend as they go to a common insertion and have a common action. The **psoas major** has its *origin* within the abdomen from the anterolateral aspect of the lumbar vertebral bodies and from their transverse processes (and possibly from the lower border of the twelfth thoracic vertebra). At its origin, the roots and branches of the lumbar plexus are embedded in it. The muscle descends, simultaneously passing somewhat laterally, and leaves the abdomen deep to the inguinal ligament to reach the anterior aspect of the thigh. As it does so, it is joined by the iliacus. The conjoined muscles run posteriorly around the medial aspect of the thigh to an *insertion* on and below the lesser trochanter. The iliopsoas passes across the anterior aspect of the hip joint, and in this position, a bursa (iliopectineal) usually intervenes between the muscle and the capsule of the hip. The bursa may communicate with the hip joint. The psoas major receives *innervation* from the anterior rami of the second to the fourth lumbar spinal nerves.

The **iliacus** muscle, like the psoas major, has its *origin* from within the abdomen, but from the inner surface of the ilium (iliac fossa) rather than from the vertebral column. The muscle makes its exit deep to the inguinal ligament in close association with the psoas major and runs with this to an *insertion* on the lesser trochanter. The iliacus receives *innervation* from branches of the femoral nerve. The psoas major and iliacus muscles form a part of the floor of the femoral triangle, and the femoral nerve enters the thigh in the groove formed at the junction of the two muscles. The femoral vessels lie more medially, separated from the nerve by fascia that covers the muscles.

The *action* of the iliopsoas muscle is as a powerful flexor at the hip. In infants, it is apparently a very strong lateral rotator, but in adults, it has minimal, if any, rotatory function.

Taking their fixed points from below, the two iliopsoas muscles flex the trunk on the hip, as in sitting up in bed, and are essential to this movement. In so doing, their pull on the anterior portion of the lumbar vertebral column results first in an increase in the normal lumbar curvature, producing lordosis or extension in the lumbar region. In the erect posture, the pull of the iliopsoas muscles on the lumbar column can aid in flexion of the trunk against resistance.

Psoas minor

Associated with the psoas major, lying on its anterior surface, there may be a small muscle known as the **psoas minor.** The psoas minor has its *origin* from the anterolateral surfaces of only two or three vertebrae, usually the twelfth thoracic and the first lumbar. It ends as a long, flat tendon that has its *insertion* on the superior ramus of the pubis. Its *action* is to assist in upward rotation of the pelvis. Its *innervation* is variable, but it is usually supplied by a branch of the lumbar plexus (often L1 or L2, or both). This muscle is, of course, not really a muscle of the thigh.

Pectineus

Medial to the iliopsoas is the **pectineus** muscle, sometimes regarded as a member of the anterior group and sometimes as one of the adductor group. Its *origin* is from the superior ramus of the pubis,

and its *insertion* is on the femur just below the lesser trochanter. The *action* of the pectineus is to flex and adduct the thigh. Although it usually receives *innervation* from the femoral nerve (as do the other anterior muscles), it may be innervated by the obturator nerve and is rather regularly innervated in part by the accessory obturator nerve, when that is present.

Adductor Group of Muscles

The adductor muscles form an anteromedial group and are primarily adductors, flexors, and rotators at the hip joint (Table 16-2; see Figs. 16-5, 16-6, and 16-7). As just noted, the pectineus is sometimes included with this group because it lies somewhat between the anterior and anteromedial groups and is sometimes supplied by the obturator nerve, the nerve of the adductor group. The more superficial adductor muscles are the adductor longus and the gracilis; the deeper ones are the adductor brevis, the adductor magnus, and the obturator externus.

Adductor longus

The **adductor longus** muscle takes *origin* from the pubic tubercle and has its *insertion* on the medial lip of the linea aspera between the attachments of the

Table 16-2 ADDUCTOR GROUP OF MUSCLES				
Muscle	**Origin (Proximal Attachment)**	**Insertion (Distal Attachment)**	**Action**	**Innervation**
Adductor longus	Pubic tubercle	Medial lip of linea aspera of femur	Adduction and flexion of thigh	Obturator nerve
Gracilis	Inferior ramus of pubis; ramus of ischium	Medial surface of proximal end of tibia just distal to medial condyle	Adduction of thigh; flexion of leg; medial rotation of flexed leg	Obturator nerve
Adductor brevis	Body and inferior ramus of pubis	Pectineal line; proximal part of linea aspera of femur	Adduction and flexion of thigh	Obturator nerve
Adductor magnus	Inferior ramus of pubis; ramus of ischium; ischial tuberosity	Linea aspera (anterior fibers); adductor tubercle of femur (posterior fibers)	Adduction of thigh; flexion of thigh (anterior fibers); extension of thigh (posterior fibers)	Obturator nerve (anterior fibers); sciatic nerve (posterior fibers)
Obturator externus	Obturator membrane; bone around obturator foramen on external surface of pelvis	Trochanteric fossa of femur	Lateral rotation of thigh	Obturator nerve

vastus medialis and the adductor magnus to this line. Its *action* is as an adductor and a flexor of the thigh. It receives *innervation* from the anterior branch of the obturator nerve.

Heavy fascia between the adductor muscles and the vastus medialis forms a canal deep to the sartorius muscle and anterior to all the adductor muscles. This is called the **adductor canal.** The femoral vessels and some branches of the femoral nerve pass through this canal, across the adductor longus close to its insertion. They continue distally from a similar position on the pectineus and adductor brevis, and thereafter they lie on the adductor magnus (Fig. 16-9). The deep artery of the thigh (from the femoral artery), accompanied by a corresponding vein, passes downward behind the adductor longus and is separated from the femoral artery by this muscle.

Gracilis

The **gracilis** is a thin, straplike muscle on the medial surface of the thigh. It has its *origin* from the inferior ramus of the pubis and the ramus of the ischium, and its *insertion* is on the medial surface of the proximal end of the tibia close to the insertion of the sartorius and that of a posterior muscle of the thigh, the semitendinosus. Its *action* is to adduct the thigh and to flex the leg. It also helps rotate the flexed leg medially. If the leg is kept extended, the muscle helps flex the thigh at the hip. Like the preceding muscle, its *innervation* is by the anterior branch of the obturator nerve.

Adductor brevis

The **adductor brevis** muscle lies under cover of the pectineus and adductor longus. The *origin* of the muscle is from the body and the inferior ramus of the pubis, and its *insertion* is on the lower part of the line between the lesser trochanter and the linea aspera (pectineal line) and the upper portion of the linea aspera. The *action* of the adductor brevis is to flex and adduct the thigh. The anterior branch of the obturator nerve runs anterior to the muscle, and the posterior branch runs posterior to it. Either branch may supply *innervation* to the muscle. Both the femoral and the deep femoral vessels (deep artery of the thigh and profunda femoris vein) run anterior to the muscle.

Adductor magnus

The **adductor magnus** muscle is by far the largest muscle of the adductor group, with an *origin* from the inferior ramus of the pubis, the ramus of the ischium, and the ischial tuberosity. Its upper anterior fibers run almost horizontally to an *insertion* on the linea aspera; its lower, most posterior fibers run almost straight downward from the ischial tuberosity to insert on the adductor tubercle at the distal medial end of the linea aspera. The intervening fibers spread out in a fan-shaped manner to insert between the upper and lower fibers along almost the whole length of the linea aspera. The adductor magnus has a double *innervation:* the anterior and more oblique fibers are innervated by the posterior branch of the obturator nerve, while the straighter, more posterior fibers are innervated by the sciatic nerve. The *action* of the entire muscle is to adduct the thigh. The fibers innervated by the obturator nerve assist the other adductors in flexion of the thigh, while the fibers running from the ischial tuberosity to the adductor tubercle, and innervated by the sciatic nerve, work with the hamstrings in extension of the thigh. In action and in innervation, therefore, the adductor magnus is composed of two elements: an adductor, flexor, or obturator portion and a hamstring, extensor, or sciatic portion. (The adductor magnus, as well as the adductor longus, has also been described as a medial rotator of the thigh.)

A little above the adductor tubercle, the adductor magnus has in its tendon a gap called the **adductor hiatus.** Through this hiatus, the femoral vessels, lying on the muscle's anterior surface, pass to the back of the thigh and leg, where they are then called popliteal vessels.

Obturator externus

The **obturator externus** lies deeply in the thigh, behind the pectineus and the upper ends of the three adductor (longus, brevis, and magnus) muscles. Its *origin* is from the outer surface of the pelvis, around the obturator foramen, and from the obturator membrane that almost fills that foramen. From this circular origin, the muscle tapers and runs laterally and posteriorly, so that it has somewhat the form of a misshapen ice cream cone. It passes just below and then upward, posterior to the

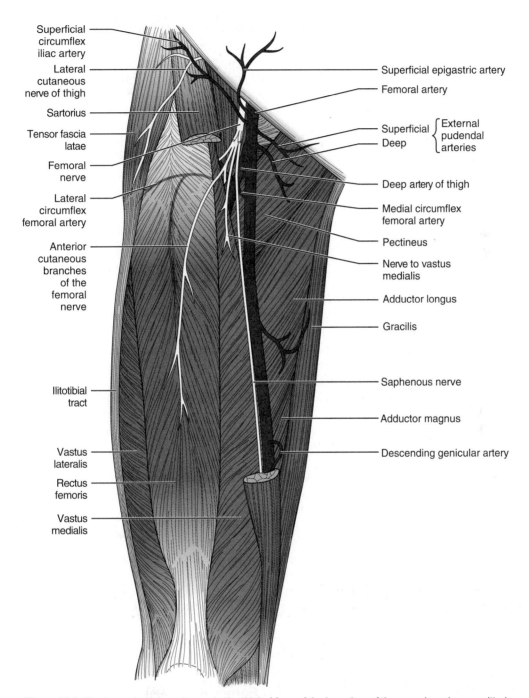

Superficial circumflex iliac artery

Lateral cutaneous nerve of thigh

Sartorius

Tensor fascia latae

Femoral nerve

Lateral circumflex femoral artery

Anterior cutaneous branches of the femoral nerve

Ilitotibial tract

Vastus lateralis

Rectus femoris

Vastus medialis

Superficial epigastric artery

Femoral artery

Superficial $\left.\begin{array}{l}\\\\\end{array}\right\}$ External pudendal arteries

Deep

Deep artery of thigh

Medial circumflex femoral artery

Pectineus

Nerve to vastus medialis

Adductor longus

Gracilis

Saphenous nerve

Adductor magnus

Descending genicular artery

Figure 16-9 The femoral artery and nerve in the thigh. Many of the branches of the nerve have been omitted.

hip joint, to an *insertion* into a small pit (the trochanteric fossa) on the medial side of the greater trochanter. The *action* of the muscle is to laterally rotate the thigh. Its *innervation* is by a branch of the obturator nerve given off before this nerve enters the thigh. The anterior branch of the obturator nerve usually runs anterior to the muscle as the nerve emerges from the obturator canal by which it leaves the pelvis. The posterior branch runs through the muscle. The obturator artery largely ends in the muscle.

Surface Anatomy

Of the muscles, the **quadriceps** as a whole is easily identified on the front of the thigh, and its tendon can be traced to the patella. The **patellar ligament** can also be traced between the patella and the tibial tuberosity. The distal ends of the **vastus lateralis** and the more bulky **vastus medialis** can easily be identified close to their insertions on the patella. The proximal end of the **rectus femoris** can be traced upward, if the thigh and leg are raised, with the leg extended, while in a sitting position. The sharp upper border of the **sartorius** can also be identified and followed toward the anterior superior iliac spine; this is easiest if, from a sitting position, the thigh is sharply flexed, so as to lift the foot from the floor, and at the same time laterally rotated.

The adductor muscles can be felt to contract when the thighs are forcefully adducted. The most easily identified member of this group is the **adductor longus,** whose strong tendon of origin can be traced to the pubis. The **gracilis** is difficult to recognize close to its insertion because its flat tendon is closely applied on the medial side of the knee to the tendon of a posterior muscle (semimembranosus) of the thigh. When the gracilis is contracted, however, its sharp posterior border can be palpated in about the middle of the thigh.

ANTEROMEDIAL NERVES AND VESSELS

The **femoral nerve, artery, and vein,** in that order from lateral to medial sides, pass deep to the inguinal ligament to lie in the femoral triangle (see Fig. 16-8, *B*). The femoral nerve enters the thigh on the anterior surface of the iliopsoas muscle, in the same fascial compartment with that muscle. The femoral artery and vein enter in a separate, more medial compartment, bringing with them a funnel-shaped continuation of the fascia lining the abdomen. This fascia surrounding the vessels is the **femoral sheath.** It contains three compartments: a lateral one for the artery, a middle one for the vein, and a medial one, the **femoral canal,** empty except for a little loose connective tissue and a lymph node or two. Because the femoral canal represents a part of the diverticulum from the abdominal fascia, it is open above, and peritoneum and viscera may descend into it and enter the thigh as a *femoral hernia.*

The distributions of the femoral and obturator nerves are diagrammed in Figures 16-10 and 16-11.

Femoral Nerve

A short distance below the inguinal ligament, the **femoral nerve** divides (see Figs. 16-8, *A* and 16-9) into muscular and cutaneous branches that are distributed to the quadriceps, sartorius, and pectineus muscles and to the skin of the anterior surface of the thigh. One long cutaneous branch, the *saphenous nerve,* runs deeply in the thigh (with the femoral vessels in the adductor canal) but becomes subcutaneous just above the knee. It is distributed to skin of the medial surface of the knee and leg and to the medial border of the foot as far as the base of the big toe.

FUNCTIONAL/CLINICAL NOTE 16-7

Interruption of the femoral nerve abolishes active extension of the knee because the quadriceps is the sole muscle that can do this. The extended knee, however, does support the body as long as the center of gravity is kept anterior to the axis of the knee joint.

Femoral Artery

Just below the inguinal ligament, the **femoral artery** (Fig. 16-12) gives off small branches to the lower part of the abdomen and perineal region (*superficial epigastric, superficial circumflex iliac, superficial external*

FEMORAL NERVE

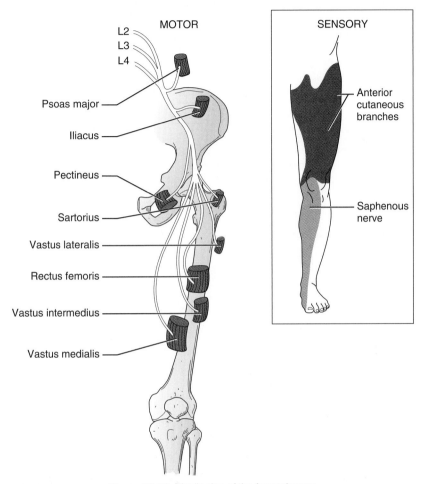

MOTOR

L2
L3
L4

Psoas major

Iliacus

Pectineus

Sartorius

Vastus lateralis

Rectus femoris

Vastus intermedius

Vastus medialis

SENSORY

Anterior
cutaneous
branches

Saphenous
nerve

Figure 16-10 Distribution of the femoral nerve.

pudendal, and *deep external pudendal arteries*), and then at least one large branch, the *deep artery of the thigh* (profunda femoris or deep femoral artery) (see Figs. 16-9 and 16-12). Close to its origin, the deep artery of the thigh usually gives off two branches, the *medial* and *lateral circumflex femoral arteries,* which encircle the limb to anastomose with each other and with other vessels in the upper posterior part of the thigh. (Either or both of the circumflex arteries may arise from the femoral artery above the deep artery instead of from the latter vessel.) The deep artery of the thigh runs distally, anterior to the pectineus, adductor brevis, and adductor magnus muscles

(in that order), and posterior to the adductor longus. It gives off a series of *perforating arteries* (usually four) that go through the tendons of the adductors brevis and magnus close to the femur and supply the musculature on the back of the thigh.

After giving off the deep artery of the thigh, the femoral artery continues down the anteromedial aspect of the thigh between the quadriceps and adductor group of muscles, lying in the adductor canal formed by these muscles and fascia between them, and provides branches to muscles within the thigh. At the distal end of the adductor canal, the femoral artery gives off a *descending genicular*

OBTURATOR NERVE

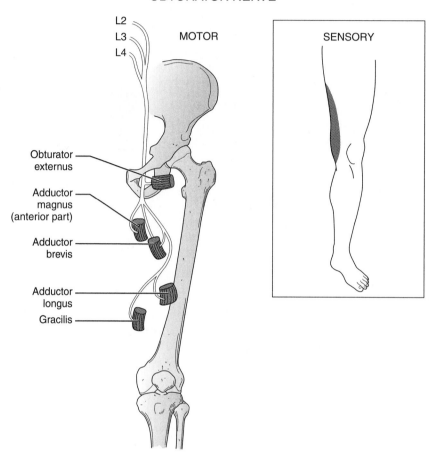

L2
L3
L4

MOTOR

SENSORY

Obturator externus

Adductor magnus (anterior part)

Adductor brevis

Adductor longus

Gracilis

Figure 16-11 Distribution of the obturator nerve.

artery. It then passes through the adductor hiatus in the insertion of the adductor magnus, and in that manner reaches the posterior aspect of the lower part of the thigh. Here it is known as the *popliteal artery.*

The tributaries of the femoral vein and their names correspond to the branches of the femoral artery. The one exception is the great saphenous vein, to which there is no corresponding artery.

Popliteal Artery

The **popliteal artery** passes through the popliteal fossa, deep (anterior) to the popliteal vein. It provides branches to the knee joint and surrounding tissues and ends by dividing into the *anterior and posterior tibial arteries* that continue through the leg. The

popliteal provides a *middle genicular artery* that supplies the cruciate ligaments and synovial membrane of the joint and numerous branches that form anastomoses around the knee (Fig. 16-13). These branches are the *superior lateral and medial genicular arteries* and the *inferior lateral and medial genicular arteries.* Also entering into the anastomoses are the *descending branch of the lateral circumflex femoral artery,* the *descending genicular artery* from the femoral artery, the *anterior and posterior* (an inconstant branch) *tibial recurrent arteries* from the anterior tibial artery, and the *circumflex fibular artery* from the posterior tibial artery.

Even with this large number of vessels forming anastomoses at the knee, their total diameters are so small, in comparison with that of the popliteal artery, that they cannot furnish an adequate blood supply

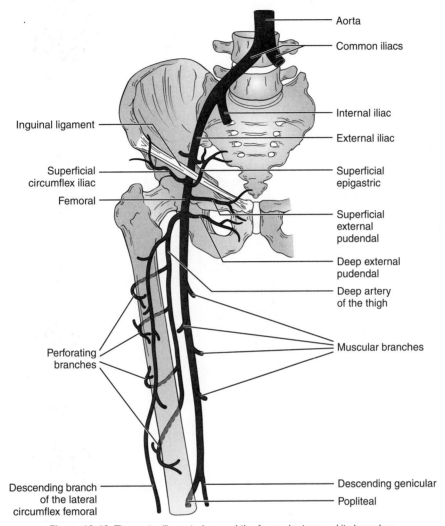

Aorta

Common iliacs

Internal iliac

External iliac

Superficial
epigastric

Superficial
external
pudendal

Deep external
pudendal

Deep artery
of the thigh

Muscular branches

Descending genicular

Popliteal

Inguinal ligament

Superficial
circumflex iliac

Femoral

Perforating
branches

Descending branch
of the lateral
circumflex femoral

Figure 16-12 The aorta, iliac arteries, and the femoral artery and its branches.

to the leg and foot if the popliteal artery is suddenly occluded.

Obturator Nerve

The **obturator nerve,** a branch of the lumbar plexus, passes through the obturator foramen and appears deeply within the adductor group of muscles (see Fig. 16-6). As it enters the thigh, it divides into *anterior* and *posterior branches.* These branches supply the muscles of the adductor group, with the exception of the posterior portion of the adductor magnus. The nerve also supplies a limited amount

of skin on the medial aspect of the thigh, gives off one or more *branches to the hip joint,* and continues along the femoral artery to give off *branches to the knee joint.*

A lesion of the anterior branch of the obturator nerve would not seriously affect adduction, because the adductor magnus is innervated both by the posterior branch of the obturator nerve and by the sciatic nerve. In fact, this branch has been intentionally sectioned as part of an operation to relieve adduction contraction resulting from spastic cerebral palsy. However, a lesion of the entire obturator nerve, which would have to be above (proximal to) the

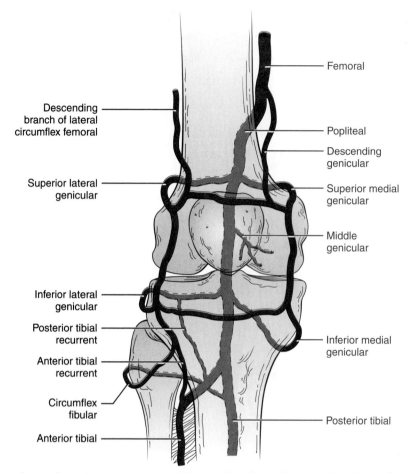

Figure 16-13 The major arteries and anastomoses around the knee joint. Posteriorly placed arteries are illustrated with *dotted outline* and *lighter color.* The patellar and collateral ligaments are not included on the illustration.

inguinal ligament, would leave the limb so abducted that walking would not be possible.

Obturator Artery

The **obturator artery** (which arises from the internal iliac artery), with its accompanying vein, emerges through the foramen with the obturator nerve but supplies blood chiefly to structures immediately around the obturator membrane, primarily the obturator externus muscle and the bone adjacent to the foramen. It also gives off a branch that enters the acetabulum to supply tissue there and continues through the ligament of the head of the femur to help supply blood to the femoral head.

Surface Anatomy

Of the vessels, the pulse of the **femoral artery** can be felt in the femoral triangle a little below the inguinal ligament. Parts of the **greater saphenous vein** may be visible through the skin on the medial side of the thigh. The deep artery of the thigh and most of the femoral artery lie too deeply to be recognizable. The fact that the femoral artery lies in the adductor canal, however, should facilitate visualizing its course.

Neither of the two large anterior **nerves** of the thigh is distinctly palpable because the femoral nerve breaks up into branches in the upper part of the femoral triangle, and the obturator lies too deep (Table 16-3).

Table 16-3	ANTEROMEDIAL NERVES OF THE THIGH		
	Muscle		
Nerve and Origin	**Name**	**Segmental Innervation***	**Chief Action(s)**
Branches of lumbar plexus (psoas major) and femoral nerve (iliacus) L2–L4	Iliopsoas	L2–L4	Flexion at hip
Femoral L2–L4	Sartorius	L2, L3	Flexion and rotation at hip and knee
	Quadriceps	L2–L4	Extension at knee
	Articularis genus	L3, L4	Pulling synovial membrane of knee joint upward
	Pectineus	L2, L3	Flexion and adduction at hip
Obturator L2–L4	Pectineus (sometimes)	L2, L3	Flexion and adduction at hip
	Adductor longus	L2, L3	Adduction and flexion at hip
	Gracilis	L2, L3	Adduction at hip, flexion at knee
	Adductor brevis	L3, L4	Adduction and flexion at hip
	Adductor magnus (ant. part)	L3, L4	Adduction and flexion at hip
	Obturator externus	L3, L4	Lateral rotation at hip

*A common segmental origin or innervation. The composition of both the chief nerves and their muscular branches varies somewhat among persons. Note: The tensor fasciae latae is included in Table 17-3.

REVIEW QUESTIONS

1   What is the function or purpose of the patella?

2   Describe in detail the anatomy of the knee joint. What types of movements are possible at this joint? What are the functions of the anterior and posterior cruciate ligaments? How would their structural integrity be tested?

3   Sensory innervation to the skin on the anterior and anteromedial aspects of the thigh is provided by which nerve? Which nerve provides sensory innervation to the skin on the anterolateral aspect of the thigh?

4   What is the relationship of the structures lying deep to the inguinal ligament as they enter the thigh?

5   Describe the anatomy of the iliopsoas muscle.

6   Describe the origin, insertion, action, and innervation of the adductor magnus muscle. What is the adductor hiatus? What passes through the hiatus?

7   What is the origin of the obturator artery? How does it gain access to the thigh?

8 Describe the course of the femoral artery in the thigh. What are its branches?

9 Describe the arterial anastomoses around the knee.

10 A lesion of the femoral nerve as it enters the thigh would have what effect on movements of the leg at the knee?

EXERCISES

1 On a skeleton, demonstrate the anatomy of the distal half of the femur. Do the same exercise for the proximal end of the tibia.

2 Draw a schematic for the lumbar plexus showing anterior rami that contribute fibers, the pattern of fiber mixing, and the branches of the plexus.

3 By palpation, locate the following:
   a iliac crest
   b anterior superior iliac spine
   c greater trochanter
   d lateral condyle of the femur
   e tibial tuberosity
   f patellar ligament

17 GLUTEAL REGION AND POSTERIOR THIGH

CHAPTER CONTENTS

Sacral Plexus

Fascia and Superficial Nerves and Vessels of the Gluteal Region

Muscles

Nerves and Vessels

Movements of the Bony Pelvis

SACRAL PLEXUS

The sacral plexus supplies the musculature of the gluteal region (buttocks) and gives rise to the large sciatic nerve that runs through the gluteal region to supply the posterior muscles of the thigh and all the muscles below the knee. The plexus lies deeply, partly within and partly outside the pelvis, and as it is taking form, the plexus passes through the greater sciatic foramen. Its method of formation can be seen from within the pelvis, where the nerve trunks contributing to it lie on the anterior surface of the sacrum. An even better concept of the plexus and its branches can be obtained by approaching it from the posterior aspect, removing a lateral portion of the sacrum and the adjacent portion of the ilium after the dissection of the gluteal region is completed. A diagram of the sacral plexus is shown in Figure 17-1; it and the lumbar plexus together are illustrated in Figure 16-4.

The **sacral plexus** is typically formed *by the union of part of the anterior ramus of spinal nerve L4 with all of the anterior ramus of L5 to form a lumbosacral trunk, and by the union of this trunk with the anterior rami of S1 to S3 or of S1 to S4.* Anterior branches from almost all these anterior rami—that is, L4, L5, S1, S2, and S3—usually unite to form the tibial nerve, the anterior component of the sciatic nerve. Posterior branches of the lumbosacral trunk, S1 and S2, unite to form the posterior component of the sciatic, the common fibular nerve. These two parts of the sciatic nerve regularly lie in a common connective tissue sheath in the thigh. The tibial nerve lies more medially, and the common fibular nerve more laterally. Together, they form a single large nerve until they separate from each other just proximal to the knee. On occasion, they are separate at their origin from the plexus.

Other branches from the posterior part of the sacral plexus include the *superior gluteal nerve,* derived from the lumbosacral trunk and S1; the *inferior gluteal nerve,* derived from the lumbosacral trunk, S1, and S2; one or more *branches to the piriformis muscle;* and a part of the *posterior cutaneous nerve of the thigh* (posterior femoral cutaneous nerve). Branches from the anterior part of the plexus also contribute to the posterior cutaneous nerve of the thigh. This nerve, derived from S1, S2, and S3, lies at the boundary between original posterior and anterior surfaces of the thigh (which in the adult, because of the twisting that the limb has undergone during development, is the posterior midline of the thigh; the original posterior surface is lateral to this, and the original anterior one is medial). The anterior parts of the lumbosacral trunk and of S1 and S2 also give rise to the *nerve to the quadratus femoris* and the *nerve to the obturator internus.* These two nerves supply innervation to the four small external rotator muscles of the gluteal region. The nerve to the quadratus femoris innervates the quadratus femoris and inferior gemellus, and the nerve to the obturator internus provides innervation to the obturator internus and the superior gemellus. Finally, anterior portions of S2 and S3 unite with a part of S4 to form the *pudendal nerve,* the lowest branch of the sacral plexus. This is distributed to the area (pudendal region) between the thighs—that is, to the anal and genital regions. If a very large continuation from L4 enters the sacral plexus, the contribution of S4 to the pudendal nerve is often reduced or lacking; in other cases, a part of S4 may contribute to the tibial nerve.

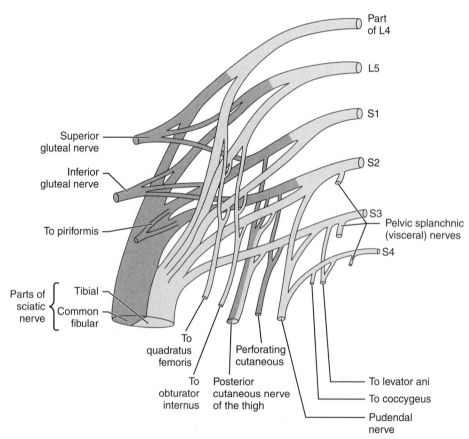

Figure 17-1 Diagram of the sacral plexus. The posterior parts of the plexus have *dark shading.*

FASCIA AND SUPERFICIAL NERVES AND VESSELS OF THE GLUTEAL REGION

The subcutaneous tissue of the gluteal region is thick, for it is a favored area for the deposition of fat. The gluteus maximus, the most superficial muscle of the gluteal region, is enclosed in a strong fascia that is well developed on the deep surface of the muscle. It is continuous with the heavy deep fascia of the thigh, the *fascia lata,* and much of the gluteus maximus is inserted into this fascia. The anterior part of the gluteus medius, where it is not covered by the gluteus maximus, is provided with a tendinous fascia from which some of the muscle fibers take origin; this also is continuous with the fascia lata. The tensor fasciae latae muscle is also enclosed in the fascia lata and inserts entirely into a special part of that fascia, the *iliotibial tract.*

Posterior rami of the first three lumbar nerves pierce the fascia close together, just above the posterior part of the iliac crest, to run downward over the gluteal region and help innervate skin of this area. Smaller *posterior rami of the first three sacral nerves* appear closer to the midline over the sacrum and spread laterally. The *posterior cutaneous nerve of the thigh,* as it runs down the posterior aspect of the thigh, gives off recurrent branches that turn upward to innervate skin of the gluteal region. There are no superficial blood vessels of any importance.

MUSCLES
Muscles of the Gluteal Region

Gluteus maximus
The musculature of the gluteal region and the origins and insertions of the muscles are diagrammed in Figures 17-2 and 17-3 and listed in Table 17-1. The **gluteus maximus,** the most superficial muscle, covers the other muscles of this region. It is a large, coarse, quadrangular muscle that has its *origin* from the sacrum, the posterior sacroiliac ligaments, a small area of the ilium in the region of the posterior superior iliac spine (behind the posterior gluteal line), and the sacrotuberous ligament. The upper half of the muscle has its *insertion* entirely into the strong lateral portion of the fascia lata, the iliotibial tract. The fibers

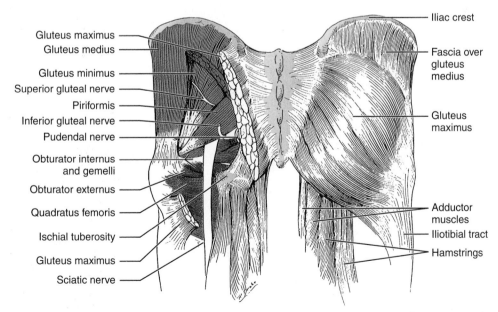

Figure 17-2 The musculature of the gluteal region. The deeper muscles are highlighted with *color.* On the left side, the space between the inferior gemellus and quadratus femoris is exaggerated so that the insertion of the obturator externus can be shown.

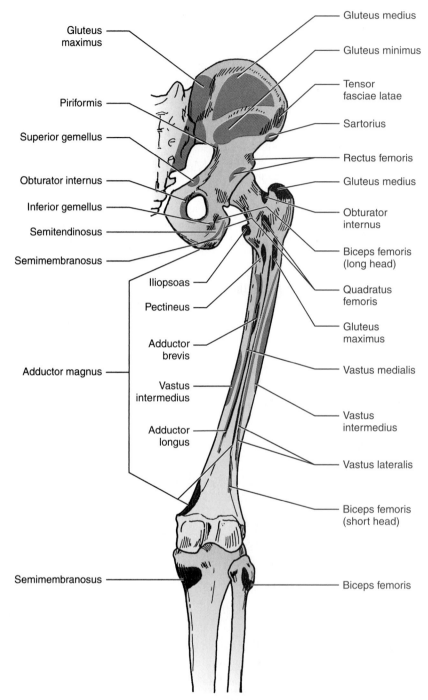

Figure 17-3 Posterior view of the bones of the pelvis, thigh, and knee region, illustrating origins *(color)* and insertions *(black)* of the anterior, adductor, and posterior muscles of the thigh.

Table 17-1	MUSCLES OF THE GLUTEAL REGION			
Muscle	Origin (Proximal Attachment)	Insertion (Distal Attachment)	Action	Innervation
Gluteus maximus	Lateral surface of ilium behind posterior gluteal line; posterior sacroiliac and sacrotuberous ligaments; posterior surface of sacrum	Iliotibial tract; gluteal tuberosity of femur	Extension, lateral rotation, abduction (upper fibers), and adduction (lower fibers) of thigh	Inferior gluteal nerve
Gluteus medius	Lateral surface of ilium between anterior and posterior gluteal lines	Greater trochanter of femur	Abduction of thigh; medial rotation and flexion (anterior fibers) and lateral rotation and extension (posterior fibers) of thigh	Superior gluteal nerve
Gluteus minimus	Lateral surface of ilium between anterior and inferior gluteal lines	Greater trochanter of femur	Abduction of thigh; medial rotation and flexion of thigh	Superior gluteal nerve
Piriformis	Sacrum (anterior surface)	Greater trochanter of femur	Lateral rotation of thigh; abduction of thigh when thigh is flexed	S1 and S2
Obturator internus	Obturator membrane; bone around obturator foramen on internal surface of pelvis	Medial surface of greater trochanter above trochanteric fossa of femur	Lateral rotation of thigh; abduction of thigh when thigh is flexed	Nerve to obturator internus
Superior gemellus	Ischial spine	Superior border of obturator internus tendon	Lateral rotation of thigh; abduction of thigh when thigh is flexed	Nerve to obturator internus
Inferior gemellus	Ischial tuberosity	Inferior border of obturator internus tendon	Lateral rotation of thigh; abduction of thigh when thigh is flexed	Nerve to quadratus femoris
Quadratus femoris	Ischial tuberosity	Posterior surface of femur between greater and lesser trochanters	Lateral rotation and adduction of thigh	Nerve to quadratus femoris

of the lower half of the muscle divide at their *insertion*, approximately half of them inserting into the iliotibial tract and the remaining, deeper ones on the upper lateral extension from the linea aspera, the gluteal tuberosity. Where the tendon of the muscle passes over the greater trochanter, there is a bursa between the two.

The gluteus maximus receives *innervation* from the inferior gluteal nerve, a branch of the sacral plexus. This nerve leaves the pelvis inferior to the piriformis muscle and close to the lateral edge of the sacrotuberous ligament, where it is accompanied by

the inferior gluteal artery and vein (Fig. 17-4). Nerve and vessels penetrate the heavy fascia on the deep surface of the muscle before spreading out between the two, so that it is impossible to reflect the muscle to its origin without severing them.

The *action* of the gluteus maximus is to extend the thigh, the muscle being used especially in straightening up from a bending position, in walking up stairs, and in other movements that require powerful extension at the hip joint. It is also a lateral rotator, an abductor (upper fibers), and an adductor (lower fibers) of the thigh. Because of its extensive insertion

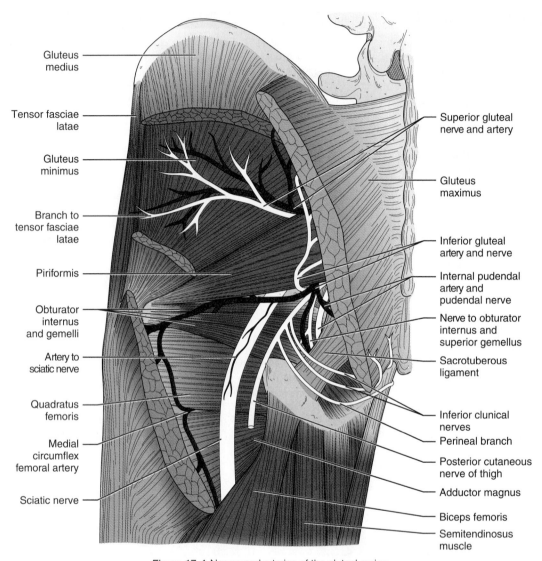

Figure 17-4 Nerves and arteries of the gluteal region.

Labels on figure:
- Gluteus medius
- Tensor fasciae latae
- Gluteus minimus
- Branch to tensor fasciae latae
- Piriformis
- Obturator internus and gemelli
- Artery to sciatic nerve
- Quadratus femoris
- Medial circumflex femoral artery
- Sciatic nerve
- Superior gluteal nerve and artery
- Gluteus maximus
- Inferior gluteal artery and nerve
- Internal pudendal artery and pudendal nerve
- Nerve to obturator internus and superior gemellus
- Sacrotuberous ligament
- Inferior clunical nerves
- Perineal branch
- Posterior cutaneous nerve of thigh
- Adductor magnus
- Biceps femoris
- Semitendinosus muscle

into the iliotibial tract and the attachment of the iliotibial tract to the femur by an intermuscular septum, the gluteus maximus attains much greater leverage than can be obtained through its insertion on the gluteal tuberosity.

Gluteus medius and gluteus minimus

After the gluteus maximus is reflected, most of the muscles of the gluteal region and the nerves and vessels to or passing through the region can be seen. The posterior part of the **gluteus medius** lies under cover of the gluteus maximus, but the anterior part projects in front of it. The *origin* of the gluteus medius is from a major part of the upper lateral surface of the wing of the ilium (between the anterior and posterior gluteal lines), and the anterior part also arises from its covering fascia. Because of the convexity of the ilium, parts of the muscle lie in front of and behind the hip joint, as well as lateral to it. The *insertion* of the muscle is on the greater trochanter. It receives *innervation* from the superior gluteal nerve and blood supply from the superior gluteal vessels. Both nerve and vessels leave the pelvis above the upper border of the piriformis muscle and turn upward and laterally to run deep to the gluteus medius.

Under cover of the gluteus medius is the **gluteus minimus,** which has its *origin* from the lower part of the lateral surface of the wing of the ilium (between the anterior and inferior gluteal lines) and its *insertion* on the greater trochanter. Like the gluteus medius, this muscle also receives *innervation* from the superior gluteal nerve and blood supply from the superior gluteal vessels. The nerve and vessels run between the gluteus minimus and the overlying gluteus medius. One branch of the superior gluteal nerve passes forward to supply the **tensor fasciae latae,** a medial rotator and flexor of the hip that is a member of the gluteal group but is best studied on the anterior part of the thigh (see Chapter 16).

The gluteus medius and the gluteus minimus not only have the same nerve and blood supply but also have a similar *action,* which is to strongly abduct the thigh. When the weight is supported on one limb, the other side of the pelvis tends to sag, a movement equivalent to adduction of the supporting limb. Because the glutei medius and minimus are abductors, they oppose this movement. In walking, therefore, the muscles of the two sides have to contract alternately, as the weight is shifted from side to side.

Although the major function of both muscles is abduction of the thigh, the muscles have been reported to be involved variably in other movements. The anterior fibers of the gluteus medius take part in medial rotation and flexion of the thigh, while the posterior fibers act in lateral rotation and extension. The gluteus minimus medially rotates the thigh and may assist in flexion.

Piriformis

Below the posteroinferior edge of the gluteus medius is a series of small muscles. The upper one of these, the **piriformis** (meaning "pear-shaped") muscle, has its *origin* from the anterior surface of the sacrum and passes to an *insertion* on the inner surface of the upper part of the greater trochanter. The muscle largely fills the greater sciatic foramen as it passes from origin to insertion. Above and below this muscle emerge the important branches of the sacral plexus and the branches of the internal iliac artery (the artery to the pelvis) that leave the pelvis through the greater

sciatic foramen. The piriformis receives *innervation* from one or two small branches from the anterior rami of either the second or the first and second sacral nerves, which enter its pelvic surface and are not visible from the gluteal region. Its *action* is to laterally rotate the thigh, but when the thigh is flexed, it becomes an abductor.

Obturator internus and the superior and inferior gemelli

Below the piriformis is the tendon of the **obturator internus,** which is associated with two small muscles on its upper and lower borders, the superior and inferior gemelli. The obturator internus has its *origin* from the inner surface of the pelvis, both from the obturator membrane and the edges of the obturator foramen. The muscle passes posteriorly through the lesser sciatic notch, turning sharply laterally as it does so; it largely fills the lesser sciatic foramen. It becomes tendinous on its deep surface and is provided with a bursa to allow free movement over the bone of the notch. The tendon receives the attachments of the two gemelli and passes to an *insertion* onto the medial surface of the greater trochanter just above the trochanteric fossa.

The superior and inferior gemelli are small muscles accessory to the obturator internus, and one or both may be absent. The **superior gemellus** has its *origin* from the ischial spine, and its *insertion* is on the upper border of the obturator internus tendon. The **inferior gemellus** takes *origin* from the ischial tuberosity and has its *insertion* on the lower border of the obturator internus tendon. The superior gemellus and obturator internus receive their *innervation* from the same nerve, the nerve to the obturator internus, a branch of the sacral plexus (see Fig. 17-1). It runs across the superficial surface of the superior gemellus and lateral to the pudendal nerve and vessels, and like these, it disappears into the lesser sciatic foramen on the surface of the obturator internus. The inferior gemellus muscle receives *innervation* from the nerve to the quadratus femoris and from the sacral plexus. The nerve runs deep to all the small muscles below the piriformis, against the posterior surface of the capsule of the hip joint. The *action* of the obturator internus is to laterally rotate the thigh; when the thigh is flexed, it, like the piriformis, may act as an abductor. The gemelli have similar actions.

Quadratus femoris

The **quadratus femoris** is a small quadrangular muscle with its *origin* from the ischial tuberosity. It extends transversely to an *insertion* on the posterior surface of the femur about midway between the lesser and greater trochanters. Its *innervation* is in common with that of the inferior gemellus. Its *action* is to laterally rotate the thigh and also, because of its position below the head of the femur, to adduct the thigh.

Obturator externus

The **obturator externus** is an anteromedial muscle of the thigh and is described in Chapter 16 with other muscles of its group. Its insertion, however, is visible only from the gluteal region and can be reviewed here. It passes posteriorly just below the hip joint and then upward and laterally across the posterior aspect of the joint, deep to the quadratus femoris, to an *insertion* into a pit, termed the *trochanteric fossa*, immediately below the insertion of the obturator internus.

Posterior Muscles of the Thigh

The three muscles of the posterior aspect of the thigh are known as the *hamstring muscles* (or posterior hamstrings when the sartorius and gracilis are also called hamstrings) and include the semitendinosus, semimembranosus, and biceps femoris (Fig. 17-5 and Table 17-2). The more vertical portion of the adductor magnus, running from the ischial tuberosity to the adductor tubercle, functions with these hamstrings (see Chapter 16) and has been regarded as the remains of a muscle that once continued across the knee joint.

Semitendinosus

The **semitendinosus** muscle has its *origin* from the ischial tuberosity, where it is intimately blended with the long head of the biceps femoris. Diverging from this, it passes down on the medial side of the posterior aspect of the thigh. Posterior to the knee joint, it curves anteriorly and has its *insertion* on the tibia medial and a little inferior to the tibial tuberosity, where it is closely associated with the insertions of the gracilis and sartorius muscles. A bursa intervenes between the tendons of insertion of the semitendinosus and gracilis muscles and the overlying tendon

of insertion of the sartorius. This bursa also extends (or there is a separate bursa) between the tendons of the semitendinosus and gracilis and the tibial collateral ligament. The associated tendons of insertion of these three muscles are sometimes referred to as the *pes anserinus* ("goose's foot"), and the bursa is accordingly named the *anserine bursa.*

Semimembranosus

The **semimembranosus** takes *origin* from the lateral aspect of the ischial tuberosity and crosses deep (anterior) to the semitendinosus and long head of the biceps femoris. The long, wide tendon of origin of the semimembranosus, from which the muscle derives its name, gives rise to a muscular "belly," which at the knee is succeeded by a thick, rounded tendon that passes on the posteromedial side of the knee. The *insertion* is on the posteromedial aspect of the medial tibial condyle. At the knee, the semimembranosus tendon has a bursa between it and the joint capsule. The tendon of insertion of the semimembranosus gives off the **oblique popliteal ligament,** a heavy band that runs obliquely upward and laterally and blends with the posterior capsule of the knee joint.

Biceps femoris

The **biceps femoris** arises by two heads. The *origin* of the *long head* is from the ischial tuberosity, in common with the semitendinosus, and is joined above the knee by the *short head,* which arises from the linea aspera on the posterior aspect of the femur and from the lateral intermuscular septum. The tendon derived from the union of the two heads runs on the posterolateral aspect of the knee joint to an *insertion* on the head of the fibula. The biceps femoris forms the upper lateral border of the somewhat diamond-shaped popliteal fossa, and the semitendinosus and semimembranosus form the upper medial border. The two heads of the most superficial muscle of the calf, the gastrocnemius, form the lower borders.

Actions and innervation of the hamstring muscles

At the knee, all three hamstring muscles give off expansions to the fascia of the leg. Also, all three have similar *actions* as good extensors and very weak adductors of the thigh and as good flexors of the leg.

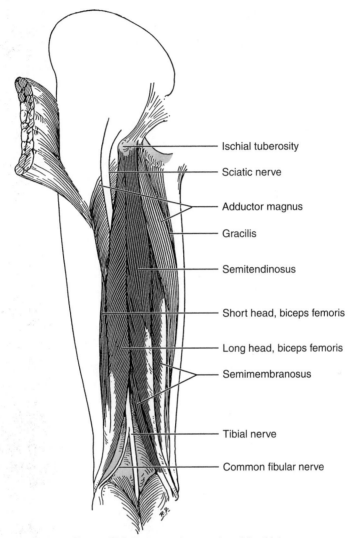

Ischial tuberosity

Sciatic nerve

Adductor magnus

Gracilis

Semitendinosus

Short head, biceps femoris

Long head, biceps femoris

Semimembranosus

Tibial nerve

Common fibular nerve

Figure 17-5 The posterior muscles of the thigh.

Their lengths are such that they can with difficulty be stretched over both joints during combined flexion at the hip and extension at the knee. They act passively to check such movements as high kicking or bending over to touch the floor with the legs extended. The short head of the biceps femoris does not participate in extension of the thigh because it does not cross the hip joint. In addition to these actions, the semitendinosus and semimembranosus serve as weak medial rotators of the thigh and medial rotators of the leg at the knee when the leg is flexed. The long head of the biceps femoris may act as a lateral rotator of the thigh; both heads laterally rotate the leg when it is flexed, and both help to flex the leg. The long head, however, is said to participate in only the early part of flexion and to relax as the leg becomes semiflexed.

FUNCTIONAL/CLINICAL NOTE 17-1

The hamstring muscles and the posterior part of the adductor magnus work with the gluteus maximus in extending the thigh (in such movements as straightening up from a

Continued

Table 17-2 POSTERIOR MUSCLES OF THE THIGH				
Muscle	**Origin (Proximal Attachment)**	**Insertion (Distal Attachment)**	**Action**	**Innervation**
Semitendinosus	Ischial tuberosity	Medial surface of proximal end of tibia	Extension of thigh; flexion of leg; medial rotation of flexed leg	Sciatic nerve: tibial part
Semimembranosus	Ischial tuberosity	Medial condyle of tibia	Extension of thigh; flexion of leg; medial rotation of flexed leg	Sciatic nerve: tibial part
Biceps femoris	Long head: ischial tuberosity Short head: linea aspera of femur and lateral intermuscular septum	Head of fibula	Extension of thigh (long head); flexion of leg; lateral rotation of flexed leg	Sciatic nerve: tibial part to long head; common fibular part to short head

bending position). It has been reported that they contribute 31% to 48% of the strength of this movement, their greatest contribution occurring when the hip is flexed to 90 degrees. However, they cannot contribute much to rising from a sitting position, because this involves simultaneous extension at both hip and knee, and they are flexors at the knee.

Each of these three muscles is *innervated* by branches (usually multiple branches) of the sciatic nerve. When, as sometimes occurs, the sciatic nerve is divided into its tibial and common fibular components at a level higher than normal, it is evident that the semitendinosus and semimembranosus and the long head of the biceps femoris are innervated by the tibial portion of the sciatic nerve, while the short head of the biceps femoris is innervated by the common fibular portion. Most of the branches of the sciatic nerve in the thigh arise from the medial, or tibial, portion of the sciatic nerve and course medially. The surgeon takes advantage of this fact in an operative approach to the posterior aspect of the thigh, knowing that the lateral side of the sciatic nerve is the side of relative safety.

As has already been noted, the adductor magnus can be considered as two muscles from the standpoint of actions and innervations. The obliquely running portion of the adductor magnus is innervated by the obturator nerve and belongs functionally with the adductor group of muscles. The more vertical postero-medial portion of the adductor magnus arises from the ischial tuberosity, as do the hamstrings proper, and is innervated from the tibial portion of the sciatic nerve, as are these muscles. Although this portion of the adductor magnus cannot flex the knee, it functions with the hamstrings in extension at the hip.

Surface Anatomy

The most superior of the bony landmarks in the gluteal region is the **iliac crest.** It is easily palpable because it is subcutaneous and the abdominal muscles above it yield readily to pressure. It can be traced anteriorly to the **anterior superior iliac spine** and posteriorly to the **posterior superior iliac spine.** The iliac crest extends to its highest point posteriorly, which is at the *level of the fourth lumbar vertebra.* The posterior superior iliac spine, although it may not be clearly palpable, is indicated by the permanent dimple of the skin over the region where the crest meets the sacrum (at the *level of the second sacral vertebra*). The **posterior inferior iliac spine** lies slightly inferior and anterior to it. The **sacrum** can be identified between the two hip bones. The **greater trochanter** is identifiable on the lateral side of the thigh, somewhat more than a hand's breadth below the iliac crest. The **ischial tuberosity** is most clearly felt in a sitting position; in an erect position (thigh extended), it is covered by the gluteus maximus muscle. As described in Chapter 16, the condyles and epicondyles of the femur, the joint region, and condyles of the tibia are all easily palpated.

Of the muscles, the **gluteus maximus** and **gluteus medius** are the only two that can be reliably identified in the gluteal region. The gluteus maximus can be felt when it contracts as a person straightens up from bending over. The gluteus medius of one thigh is felt as all the weight of the body is shifted onto that limb.

In the thigh, the hamstrings can be felt as a unit as they arise from the ischial tuberosity, and at the borders of the **popliteal fossa,** some of their tendons can be identified. The tendon on the lateral side of the popliteal fossa is that of the **biceps femoris.** The first (most lateral) tendon on the medial side, and the most prominent tendon, when the knee is forcefully flexed, is the **semitendinosus.** Medial to it is the broader tendon of the **semimembranosus,** which does not project so much on flexion. Closely applied to the medial side of this tendon, and distinguishable from it only with difficulty, is the thin flat tendon of the **gracilis.**

NERVES AND VESSELS
Nerves and Vessels of the Gluteal Region

The nerves (Table 17-3) and vessels in the gluteal region all emerge through the greater sciatic foramen, which is in close contact with the piriformis muscle (see Fig. 17-4). Only the superior gluteal nerve and vessels normally pass superior to the piriformis. The others, whether they end in the gluteal region or merely pass through it, typically first appear at the lower border of the piriformis.

The **inferior gluteal nerve** emerges through the greater sciatic foramen inferior to the piriformis muscle, in company with the inferior gluteal vessels, and passes directly into the gluteus maximus. The larger branches of the inferior gluteal vessels are distributed to the gluteus maximus. Smaller branches are provided to the adjacent small muscles of the gluteal region, to the upper ends of the posterior muscles of the thigh, and to the posterior surface of the sciatic nerve.

The **superior gluteal nerve** emerges through the greater sciatic foramen superior to the piriformis muscle (in company with the superior gluteal vessels). It runs laterally between the glutei medius and minimus, supplying both, and continues beyond these muscles to enter the deep surface of the tensor

fasciae latae. The superior gluteal vessels are largely distributed with the nerve, but the artery sends a superficial branch between the piriformis and the gluteus medius to the upper part of the gluteus maximus.

The **nerve to the piriformis** enters the pelvic surface of the muscle and is difficult to demonstrate in a posterior dissection.

The **nerve to the obturator internus** (which also innervates the superior gemellus) emerges from the greater sciatic foramen inferior to the piriformis muscle close to the ischial spine and turns around this spine to supply a branch to the superior gemellus. It then enters the lesser sciatic foramen to run on the perineal (internal) surface of the obturator internus. Medial to the nerve to the obturator internus, and also passing around the ischial spine from the greater sciatic foramen into the lesser sciatic foramen, is the pudendal nerve to the perineal region (the region of the anus and of the external genitals). The internal pudendal vessels lie medial to the pudendal nerve. The nerve and vessels have no distribution to the gluteal region but simply pass through it.

The **nerve to the quadratus femoris** (which also innervates the inferior gemellus) usually arises from the sacral plexus as the main elements converge to form the sciatic nerve. It runs deep to the two gemelli and the obturator internus to enter the deep surface of the quadratus femoris, having previously given off a branch to the inferior gemellus. This nerve also supplies the posterior aspect of the hip joint.

The two remaining nerves appearing in the gluteal region are the posterior cutaneous nerve of the thigh and the sciatic. The large **sciatic nerve** makes its exit through the greater sciatic foramen, appearing inferior to the lower edge of the piriformis muscle, and runs down the thigh. It gives off no branches to the gluteal region.

FUNCTIONAL/CLINICAL NOTE 17-2

On occasion, the sciatic nerve is split at this level into its two component parts, the tibial nerve and the common fibular nerve. Sometimes, when this occurs, the common

Continued

Table 17-3	NERVES OF GLUTEAL REGION AND POSTERIOR PART OF THIGH		
	Muscle		
Nerve and Origin*	**Name**	**Segmental Innervation***	**Chief Action(s)**
Superior gluteal L4–S1	Gluteus medius	L4–S1	Abduction and lateral and medial rotation at hip
	Gluteus minimus	L4–S1	Abduction and medial rotation at hip
	Tensor fasciae latae	L4–S1	Flexion, medial rotation, and abduction at hip
Inferior gluteal L5–S2	Gluteus maximus	L5–S2	Extension and adduction at hip
Nerve to piriformis S1 and S2	Piriformis	S1, S2	Lateral rotation at hip
Nerve to obturator internus L5–S2	Obturator internus	L5–S2	Lateral rotation at hip
	Superior gemellus	L5–S2	Lateral rotation at hip
Nerve to quadratus femoris L4–S1	Quadratus femoris	L4–S1	Lateral rotation at hip
	Inferior gemellus	L4–S1	Lateral rotation at hip
Tibial nerve, from L4–S3	Semitendinosus	L5–S2	Extension at hip, flexion at knee
	Semimembranosus	L5–S2	Extension at hip, flexion at knee
	Biceps, long head	L5–S2	Extension at hip, flexion at knee
	Adductor magnus, posterior part	L4, L5	Extension and adduction at hip
Common fibular L4–S2	Biceps, short head	L5, S1	Flexion at knee

*A common segmental origin or innervation.

fibular portion of the nerve may emerge through the piriformis instead of below it. In rare instances, the entire nerve passes through the piriformis. The abnormal relation of the nerve to the piriformis muscle has been held responsible for some cases of sciatic pain; the concept is that a spastic piriformis muscle may so squeeze the nerve as to produce pain over its distribution (piriformis syndrome).

The small **posterior cutaneous nerve of the thigh** runs almost exactly in the posterior midline, behind the sciatic nerve, and gives off recurrent branches to the skin of the gluteal region. It then passes down the posterior surface of the thigh, just deep to the fascia lata, giving off a series of branches that pierce the fascia lata to supply the overlying skin. It continues a variable distance down the leg.

Nerves and Vessels of the Posterior Thigh

The **sciatic nerve** is the sole posteriorly placed deep nerve of the thigh, although the posterior cutaneous nerve of the thigh runs for much of its course deep to the fascia lata. The sciatic nerve enters the thigh by passing just lateral to the ischial tuberosity, and it runs straight downward in about the midline to its division into **common fibular and tibial branches** in the popliteal fossa (Fig. 17-6; see Table 17-3). Besides its terminal branches, its branches in the thigh

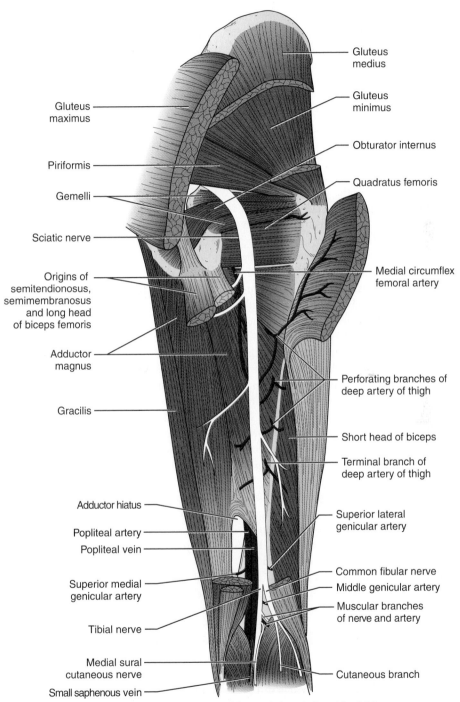

Gluteus medius

Gluteus minimus

Obturator internus

Quadratus femoris

Medial circumflex femoral artery

Perforating branches of deep artery of thigh

Short head of biceps

Terminal branch of deep artery of thigh

Superior lateral genicular artery

Common fibular nerve

Middle genicular artery

Muscular branches of nerve and artery

Cutaneous branch

Gluteus maximus

Piriformis

Gemelli

Sciatic nerve

Origins of semitendionosus, semimembranosus and long head of biceps femoris

Adductor magnus

Gracilis

Adductor hiatus

Popliteal artery

Popliteal vein

Superior medial genicular artery

Tibial nerve

Medial sural cutaneous nerve

Small saphenous vein

Figure 17-6 The sciatic nerve and the posterior arteries of the thigh.

are to the hamstring muscles. These branches arise in variable patterns, but the tibial side of the nerve gives off one or more branches into the long head of the biceps femoris and into the semimembranosus and semitendinosus and the posterior part of the adductor magnus. The common fibular side gives rise only to the nerve to the short head of the biceps femoris. To explain this distribution, it has already been noted that the posterior midline of the thigh represents the junction of original anterior and posterior parts of the limb: the anterior part lying medially and the posterior part lying laterally. Therefore, the anterior or tibial component of the sciatic supplies muscles arising medial to the posterior midline, and the common fibular component supplies the sole muscle arising laterally.

After they separate, the tibial nerve continues the downward course of the sciatic nerve and disappears deep to the muscles of the calf. The common fibular nerve diverges to the lateral side of the leg. Both nerves give off cutaneous branches to the leg as they leave the thigh.

Because there is no longitudinal artery in the posterior side of the thigh above the popliteal fossa, the blood supply to the muscles comes largely from the **perforating branches of the deep artery of the thigh** that come through the adductor magnus. In addition, there are *twigs from the inferior gluteal artery and from branches of the two circumflex femoral arteries to the upper ends of the muscles, and from the femoral and popliteal arteries to their lower ends.*

The **popliteal vessels,** the continuations of the femoral vessels below the adductor hiatus, appear only briefly in the thigh. The popliteal vein is more superficial than the artery in the popliteal fossa. Immediately distal to the fossa, both the vessels and the tibial nerve lie deep to the muscles of the calf. The branches of the popliteal artery and the anastomoses at the knee are discussed in Chapter 16.

Surface Anatomy

Of the vessels and nerves, none of those in the gluteal region can be palpated, and the only one in the posterior aspect of the thigh that can be palpated is the **popliteal artery.** The pulse of even this large artery may be difficult to obtain because of the depth at which the vessel lies.

Although none of the nerves can be clearly palpated, the courses of the sciatic nerve and its tibial continuation, and that of the posterior cutaneous nerve of the thigh, can be fairly easily visualized. The **sciatic nerve** runs just lateral to the ischial tuberosity and then straight down the midline of the thigh. Injections into the gluteal region, when needed, are given in the upper lateral region to prevent injury to the sciatic nerve. The **tibial nerve** lies in the middle of the popliteal space. The **posterior cutaneous nerve of the thigh** lies posterior to the sciatic and tibial nerves; therefore, it is also in the posterior midline of the thigh.

Because the sciatic nerve has a much greater distribution in the leg and foot than it does to the thigh, its distribution is illustrated later (see Chapter 19).

MOVEMENTS OF THE BONY PELVIS

The muscles that rotate and tilt the bony pelvis form a heterogeneous group; none of them are, strictly speaking, muscles of the pelvis. **Downward rotation** of the pelvis is assisted especially by the anterior thigh muscles attaching to the front of the pelvis, and it is a concomitant of any increase in the lumbar curvature. The latter can be brought about by the psoas muscles that, taking their fixed points from below, can pull on the front of the lumbar portion of the vertebral column. More commonly, it is brought about by gravity and by relaxation of the anterolateral abdominal muscles. **Upward rotation** of the pelvis is brought about especially by the upward pull on the pubis of the anterolateral abdominal muscles, probably assisted by the downward pull of the hamstring muscles on the ischial tuberosity. **Lateral rotation** of the pelvis and trunk as a whole on one femoral head, as occurs in walking, is brought about mostly by certain rotators of the thigh, assisted also by the anterolateral abdominal muscles.

Lateral tilting of the pelvis tends to occur when the weight is put on one leg. It is opposed by the passive checking action of the fascia lata, particularly the iliotibial tract, and, as already noted, by the active contraction of the glutei medius and minimus, probably assisted slightly by the tensor fasciae latae.

REVIEW QUESTIONS

1 Which anterior rami contribute to the sacral plexus? What are the branches of the plexus?

2 Which muscles form the upper borders of the popliteal fossa?

3 What is the course of the sciatic nerve in the gluteal region and posterior thigh? Where should injections into the gluteal region be given to avoid injuring the nerve?

4 What are the functions of each of the following muscles?
a piriformis
b quadratus femoris
c semitendinosus
d obturator internus

5 Describe the anatomy of the biceps femoris muscle.

6 A patient with noticeable atrophy of the gluteal region of one side complains of difficulty in climbing stairs normally. What muscle might be atrophied? If a nerve lesion is suspected, what nerve might be involved?

EXERCISES

1 On an articulated skeleton or a figure of the same, demonstrate the areas of origin of the gluteus maximus, medius, and minimus muscles. What is the motor innervation to each muscle? What is the segmental innervation of each muscle?

2 By palpation, locate the following:
a ischial tuberosity
b sacrum
c posterior inferior iliac spine
d tendons of the biceps femoris, semitendinosus, and semimembranosus muscles

18 MOVEMENTS OF THE THIGH AND LEG

CHAPTER CONTENTS

Movements at the Hip Joint

Movements at the Knee Joint

Maintenance of Stability at the Hip and Knee Joints

Analyses of Activities and Associated Movements

MOVEMENTS AT THE HIP JOINT

Extension of the Thigh

The muscles producing **extension of the thigh** at the hip joint lie in the gluteal region and the posterior aspect of the thigh (Fig. 18-1). The large *gluteus maximus,* extending as it does from the sacrum, sacrotuberous ligament, and posterior wing of the ilium to the fascia lata and femur, is a particularly strong extensor at the hip. In this action, it is assisted by the part of the *adductor magnus,* which arises from the ischial tuberosity and is innervated by the tibial portion of the sciatic nerve. Because the posterior hamstring muscles, the *semimembranosus, semitendinosus,* and *biceps femoris,* attach proximally to the ischial tuberosity, they are also extensors of the thigh. However, because they are likewise flexors of the leg, they cannot contribute strongly to extension of the thigh unless the knee is kept from flexing. They become active in any forward bending at the hips and act as antigravity or postural muscles.

In the movement of bending over to touch the floor with the fingers, the extensors of the thigh must contract and then slowly relax (an eccentric contraction) in order to control the movement. The hamstrings are active throughout the movement of bending over and straightening up, but the gluteus maximus contracts most toward the end of flexion and the beginning of extension. The *posterior fibers of the gluteus medius* aid in extension. Although the piriformis has also been thought to contribute to extension, and the obturator internus may contribute

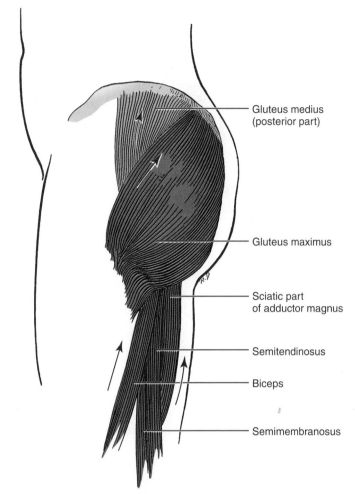

Figure 18-1 Extensors of the thigh. The chief extensors are illustrated in *dark color*.

if the movement starts from a sharply flexed position, neither is of any real importance in this movement. Because they pass across the hip and knee joints, the hamstrings are subject to stretching when the leg is kept extended as the thigh is flexed. Therefore, pain is felt behind the knee with floor-touching or high-kicking exercises.

Abduction of the Thigh

In **abduction of the thigh,** the chief function of the muscles is to keep the pelvis approximately horizontal when all the weight is put on one limb (Fig. 18-2). Normally, they contract enough to raise the unsupported side of the pelvis slightly above the horizontal position. If the abductor muscles of the supporting limb are weak, however, there is marked sagging of the pelvis on the opposite, unsupported side. This is known as *Trendelenburg's sign.* To compensate for these weak abductors and to balance the weight on one limb, the hip will be protruded laterally, and the trunk will be flexed laterally toward the supporting limb side.

From the standpoint of supporting the pelvis, there are only two really good abductors of the thigh: the *gluteus medius* and *gluteus minimus.* When these muscles are weakened, the gait is much disturbed by the constant tilting of the pelvis and the consequent

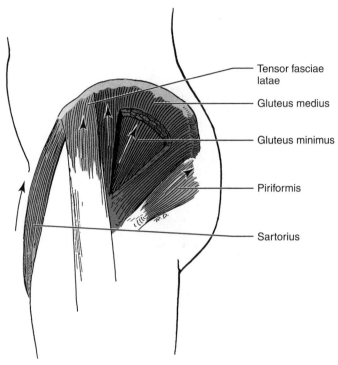

Tensor fasciae latae

Gluteus medius

Gluteus minimus

Piriformis

Sartorius

Figure 18-2 The abductors of the thigh. The most important abductors of the thigh are illustrated in *dark color.*

side-to-side sway of the trunk. Other muscles that may assist in abduction of the thigh are the *tensor fasciae latae, sartorius,* and, to even a lesser extent, the *piriformis, obturator internus,* and *upper fibers of the gluteus maximus.* Although these muscles may assist in abducting the limb when the foot is free from weight bearing, they are by no means capable of replacing the gluteus medius and minimus in the important weight-bearing function of the abductors. The tensor fasciae latae comes closest to doing that, but it has been estimated that it can exert no more than one fifth of the combined pull of the two glutei, and it contributes almost nothing to abduction of the free limb. Only if the thigh is flexed to a right angle does the gluteus maximus help abduct the limb; in other positions, this muscle is an adductor.

Lateral and Medial Rotation of the Thigh

Various interpretations are available concerning which muscles produce lateral rotation of the thigh and which produce medial rotation. The action

of muscles as rotators is often incidental to other movements in which the muscle is involved and can be dependent on the position of the thigh at the time of muscle activity. Because of such factors, accounts of rotation may vary. One interpretation of muscles producing rotation of the thigh is presented here.

Numerous muscles are involved in **lateral rotation of the thigh** (Fig. 18-3). Of the posterior muscles, the lateral direction of the fibers of the *gluteus maximus* makes this a powerful lateral rotator. All the short muscles in the gluteal region—that is, *both obturators* and the *piriformis, quadratus femoris,* and *gemelli*—are positioned so that they can assist in lateral rotation. The *posterior fibers of the gluteus medius* produce lateral rotation as they extend the thigh. The *long head of the biceps femoris* exerts a very weak lateral rotatory action and the *sartorius* produces some lateral rotation as it flexes and abducts the thigh and flexes the leg. (The involvement of the sartorius provides an example of rotation being coupled with other actions of a muscle.) As presented in Chapter 16, the

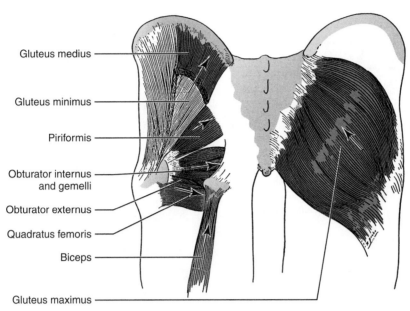

Figure 18-3 The posteriorly placed lateral rotators of the thigh. Only the posterior fibers of the gluteus medius are involved in lateral rotation. The gluteus minimus is considered a medial rotator.

Labels: Gluteus medius; Gluteus minimus; Piriformis; Obturator internus and gemelli; Obturator externus; Quadratus femoris; Biceps; Gluteus maximus

iliopsoas is a strong lateral rotator in the infant, but in the adult, its function as a rotator is negligible.

Many muscles have been given credit for being involved in **medial rotation of the thigh,** but this movement is produced mainly by the *gluteus minimus, tensor fasciae latae,* and *anterior fibers of the gluteus medius* (Fig. 18-4). The *semitendinosus* and *semimembranosus* may assist in medial rotation, but their action is weak.

In summary, many of the rotators of the thigh rotate only incidentally as they flex, extend, abduct, or adduct the thigh, although the small posteriorly placed rotators do little except rotate. The gluteus maximus is the most important lateral rotator; the gluteus minimus, tensor fasciae latae, and anterior fibers of the gluteus medius are the more important medial rotators.

Flexion of the Thigh

Flexion of the thigh is produced by muscles lying mostly on the anterior or anteromedial surface of the hip region (Fig. 18-5). The only head of the quadriceps that crosses the hip joint, the *rectus femoris,* is also a flexor of the thigh; however, it can exert little power

in flexion until other muscles have started this movement. The strongest action of the *sartorius* is in flexion of the thigh, and the *tensor fasciae latae* apparently participates regularly in this movement. The *iliopsoas,* crossing the front of the joint, is a powerful flexor, the strongest of the group, but it is not used unless a strong movement is needed. The *pectineus, adductor longus, adductor brevis,* and the more *anterior portion of the adductor magnus* assist in flexion. The *anterior fibers of the gluteus medius,* as well as the *gluteus minimus,* have also been regarded as flexors of the thigh.

The *adductor magnus* has been included with both the flexors and the extensors of the thigh. This is because the muscle actually consists of two parts that, although blended well anatomically, have fairly distinct functions. The portion arising from the pubis and the ramus of the ischium, sweeping obliquely across to insert on the linea aspera and innervated by the obturator nerve, acts with other members of the adductor group in *flexing and adducting the thigh.* The second part of the adductor magnus arises from the ischial tuberosity, running downward to insert on and a little above the adductor tubercle. It is innervated by the tibial portion of the sciatic nerve. It is an *adductor,* but it acts with the hamstrings as an *extensor of the thigh.*

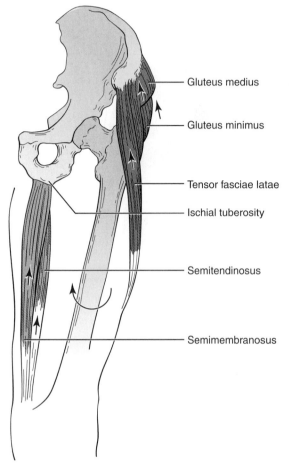

- Gluteus medius
- Gluteus minimus
- Tensor fasciae latae
- Ischial tuberosity
- Semitendinosus
- Semimembranosus

Figure 18-4 Medial rotators of the thigh. The tensor fasciae latae, gluteus minimus, and anterior fibers of the gluteus medius *(dark color)* are considered the main medial rotators of the thigh. The semitendinosus and semimembranosus *(light color)* are weak medial rotators.

Adduction of the Thigh

The **adductors of the thigh** (Fig. 18-6) include the *pectineus,* the *adductors longus* and *brevis,* and the *obturator portion of the magnus.* These muscles are also flexors, and, in general, the more posteriorly they arise, the more important they are as adductors (and the less important as flexors). Other adductors of the thigh include the *gluteus maximus* (particularly the lower fibers), *quadratus femoris,* and *obturator externus;* the *hamstrings,* including the sciatic part of the adductor magnus, and the *gracilis;* and with the thigh flexed, the *iliopsoas.*

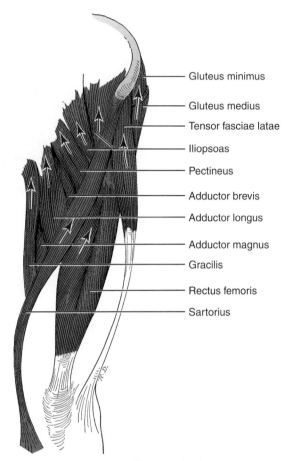

- Gluteus minimus
- Gluteus medius
- Tensor fasciae latae
- Iliopsoas
- Pectineus
- Adductor brevis
- Adductor longus
- Adductor magnus
- Gracilis
- Rectus femoris
- Sartorius

Figure 18-5 Flexors of the thigh.

Innervation

The same nerve, the superior gluteal, innervates the chief abductors, the gluteus medius, the gluteus minimus, and the tensor fasciae latae. Injury to this single nerve markedly affects stability of the pelvis, abduction of the femur, and, to some slight extent (because the gluteus minimus, anterior fibers of the gluteus medius, and tensor fasciae are also medial rotators), medial rotation of the thigh.

The chief *extensors,* the gluteus maximus and hamstrings, are innervated from the sacral plexus but by separate nerves. The gluteus maximus is supplied by the inferior gluteal nerve, while the hamstrings are supplied by the sciatic nerve.

The *adductor group* of muscles is innervated by the obturator nerve (except for the posterior part of the

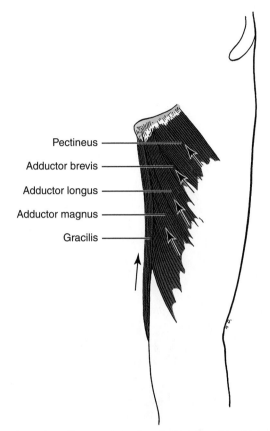

Figure 18-6 The anteriorly placed adductors of the thigh.

Pectineus

Adductor brevis

Adductor longus

Adductor magnus

Gracilis

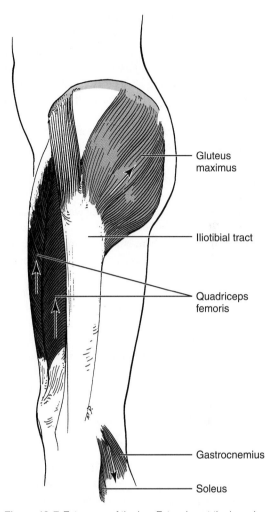

Gluteus maximus

Iliotibial tract

Quadriceps femoris

Gastrocnemius

Soleus

Figure 18-7 Extensors of the leg. Extension at the knee is produced primarily by the quadriceps muscle *(dark color)*. The gluteus maximus, gastrocnemius, and soleus also contribute in this movement *(light color)*.

adductor magnus). Injury to this single nerve may diminish the power of adduction, although muscles innervated through the sacral plexus may still carry out the movement.

The *lateral rotators* in the gluteal region are innervated by a number of branches from the sacral plexus. Therefore, marked disturbance of lateral rotation by an isolated nerve injury is impossible. The same is true for the *flexors* of the thigh that are innervated by the femoral, obturator, and superior gluteal nerves. The main *medial rotators* are innervated by the superior gluteal nerve.

The segmental innervation of the various muscle groups is so diverse that limited lesions of the lumbar or sacral plexuses affect no one movement in particular. More extensive lesions of the lumbar plexus involves the muscles supplied by the obturator and femoral nerves, therefore especially affecting flexion and adduction of the thigh. Similar lesions of the sacral plexus involve the gluteal and hamstring muscles and particularly affect the movements of extension and abduction.

MOVEMENTS AT THE KNEE JOINT

Extension of the Leg

Extension of the leg (Fig. 18-7) is produced mainly by the *quadriceps* muscle. The four heads of the muscle insert on the patella and are continued from this to the tibial tuberosity by the patellar ligament, which is, in actuality, the tendon of insertion of the quadriceps muscle. Because the femoral nerve innervates all four heads of the quadriceps, injury to this nerve prevents active extension at the knee against gravity. In walking slowly on level ground, however, the gait with a paralyzed quadriceps may be approximately normal. As long as the forward swing of the affected limb is not great enough to produce flexion of the leg, the limb is stable because the weight-bearing extended knee stays extended through the action of other muscles. These other muscles would appear to have little to do with extension of the leg. In the weight-bearing limb, however, with the foot fixed, flexion at the knee can occur only when there is also flexion at the hip and dorsiflexion at the ankle. The *gluteus*, in extending the weight-bearing limb, also helps extend the leg or keep it extended, and the *gastrocnemius* and *soleus*, muscles of the leg that produce plantar flexion of the foot, have a similar action as they resist dorsiflexion or promote plantar flexion of the foot.

The main part of the iliotibial tract passes just in front of the center of the knee joint on the lateral side of the knee, and therefore both the tensor fasciae latae and gluteus maximus have been reported to exert an effect on the knee through this tract. Although the tensor fasciae latae apparently contracts during extension of the leg, stimulation of either it or the gluteus maximus, or pulling on the iliotibial tract (which is anchored to the femur by the lateral intermuscular septum) does not produce extension. It seems that neither muscle should be described as acting directly at the knee through the tract, although the tensor fasciae latae may be contracting during extension to help stabilize the joint.

Flexion of the Leg

Flexion of the leg (Fig. 18-8) is brought about largely by the *semitendinosus, semimembranosus, biceps femoris, gracilis*, and *sartorius*. The *long head of the biceps femoris* is said to function as a flexor only until the knee is semiflexed, becoming relaxed as flexion is carried further. In addition to these muscles of the thigh, there are also muscles of the calf of the leg that extend across the knee joint and have a flexor action here. These are the *gastrocnemius, plantaris*, and especially

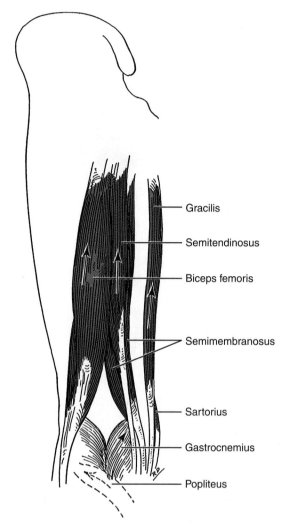

Figure 18-8 The flexors of the leg. The most important flexors are illustrated with *color.*

the *popliteus muscles*. The plantaris is so tiny that it can be disregarded. The gastrocnemius is primarily a plantar flexor at the ankle, and as already noted, it helps extend the leg when the leg is supporting weight. When the leg is free, the gastrocnemius helps flex it. The popliteus is a weak flexor. Although it contracts at the beginning of flexion, its real contribution is that of rotation of the leg at the knee in preparation for flexion. The popliteus also helps stabilize the knee (when standing with the knee bent) by resisting forward movement of the femur on the tibia.

Medial and Lateral Rotation of the Leg

The rotators of the leg are, for the most part, the same muscles that have just been described as flexors (Figs. 18-9 and 18-10; see also Fig. 18-8). **Medial rotation of the leg** is produced by the *sartorius, gracilis, semitendinosus,* and *semimembranosus,* all of which pass across the medial side of the knee joint to insert on the tibia. The *popliteus,* passing distally and medially across the posterior aspect of the knee joint, is also a medial rotator. **Lateral rotation of the leg** is produced by only one muscle, the *biceps femoris,* which passes laterally to insert on the fibula (see Fig. 18-10).

Rotation of the leg is most free with the leg flexed, in which position the total range of movement, from full lateral to full medial rotation, may amount to about 40 degrees, on average. Most of the muscles concerned with rotation are at a mechanical disadvantage for this movement when the leg is extended, and even passive rotation in the extended position is very much limited by the tautness of the ligaments of the knee. However, during the last phase of this movement, with complete extension of the leg and with the foot planted on the ground, the medial femoral condyle slides slightly posteriorly on the corresponding tibial condyle. This results in a slight medial rotation of the femur with further

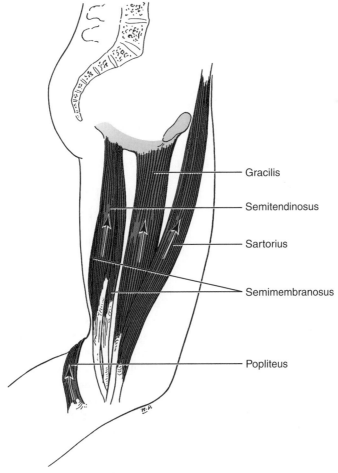

Gracilis

Semitendinosus

Sartorius

Semimembranosus

Popliteus

Figure 18-9 Medial rotators of the leg.

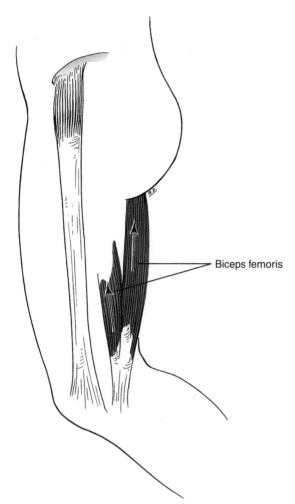

Figure 18-10 The biceps femoris is the only lateral rotator of the leg. The iliotibial tract, also shown, stabilizes the knee joint but apparently does not contribute to movement of the joint.

tightening of the collateral ligaments. If the foot is free, the leg is correspondingly rotated laterally during the last phase of extension. It is in reversing this terminal lateral rotation of the leg or, in the weight-bearing limb, the terminal medial rotation of the femur that the popliteus has its chief function during flexion. At its fixed point from below, when the foot is firmly on the floor, it laterally rotates the femur on the fixed leg and therefore prepares the knee joint for flexion.

Innervation

The hamstring flexors are innervated by the sciatic nerve; the sartorius, by the femoral nerve; the gracilis, by the obturator nerve; and the gastrocnemius, plantaris, and popliteus, by the tibial nerve. As mentioned earlier, injury to the femoral nerve affects extension of the leg. Similarly, severe injury to the sciatic nerve as a whole interferes with maintenance of extension of the thigh, because the hamstrings, rather than the stronger gluteus maximus, normally perform this. Such an injury abolishes flexion and rotation of the leg (and paralyzes muscles of the leg and foot), resulting in a flail-like extremity. Both heads of the biceps femoris apparently participate in lateral rotation of the leg. Because separate nerves arise from the tibial nerve and common fibular portions of the sciatic nerve to supply the two heads, a single nerve lesion can paralyze the muscle as a whole only when it affects the entire sciatic nerve. Other movements of the knee are carried out by several muscles acting together. The diversity of their nerve supply, both segmental and peripheral (see Tables 16-1 to 16-3 and Tables 17-2 and 17-3), is such that limited lesions of either the sacral plexus or peripheral nerves have no marked effect on movements at the knee.

MAINTENANCE OF STABILITY AT THE HIP AND KNEE JOINTS

The actions of the muscles across the hip and knee have now been considered, and reference has also been made, in the sections on these joints, to the parts played by some of the ligaments. Although the following discussion must repeat at least some of this information, the importance of the lower limb in supporting the body is such that the mechanics of the static limb merit a summary here.

The entire weight of the body in standing is transmitted from the pelvis onto the heads of one or both femurs. Because the line of gravity of the erect body is posterior to the center of movement of the head of the femur (see Fig. 1-5), the weight of the body tends to force the hip joint into extension. The strong iliofemoral ligament in particular, and the pubofemoral and ischiofemoral ligaments to a lesser extent, resist extension of the thigh. The hip can therefore be maintained in the extended weight-bearing position with little or no muscular effort.

When the weight is supported on one limb only, the center of gravity of the body lies to the medial side of the head of the supporting femur. This tends to force the unsupported side of the pelvis downward, a movement equivalent to adduction of the limb. The abductors then resist this movement, normally raising the unsupported side slightly above the horizontal position. The iliotibial tract exerts a passive checking action on any significant drooping of the unsupported side.

With the weight on both limbs, the bracing action of the two femora and the ligamentous checking of extension allow complete relaxation of the muscles around the hip, except for occasional slight contractions of the hamstrings and the iliopsoas that may be necessary to keep the body properly balanced. The hip is equipped to support the weight of the body with little expenditure of energy.

At the knee, somewhat the same fundamental conditions hold true. The line of gravity is anterior to the center of movement through the knee, so that the weight of the body also tends to keep this joint in extension, once it has been completely extended by the quadriceps. The role that the gluteus maximus and the muscles of the calf may play in extension when the limb is supporting weight has already

been mentioned. The gluteus maximus is relaxed during quiet standing. Because the line of gravity lies anterior to the ankle joint, the calf muscles are partly contracted in order to prevent dorsiflexion of the foot. They also tend to keep the leg extended. Extension of the leg results in a tightening of the collateral ligaments with further stabilization of this joint. When the weight is placed on only one leg, the leg is usually extended slightly further. This terminal extension involves a medial rotation of the femur on the tibial condyles with consequent further tightening of the collateral ligaments and so-called "locking" of the joint. Although this "locking" or "screwing home" of the knee in extension is often described as if it were an inevitable factor of weight-supporting extension, most persons, standing with the weight equally distributed between the two legs, do not actually extend the knee joints completely. Rather, they stand with the legs very slightly flexed, avoiding the final locking of the joint, but with the weight so distributed on the condyles of the femur that the leg is easily maintained in this almost completely extended position.

In patients with torn collateral or cruciate ligaments, or both, the stability of the knee joint depends largely on muscles. Under these circumstances, it is especially important that the quadriceps be of good strength, and therapeutic exercises to achieve this end are often prescribed for such patients.

ANALYSES OF ACTIVITIES AND ASSOCIATED MOVEMENTS

Activity: *Crossing the Legs.* The individual movements of the thigh at the hip joint and of the leg at the knee joint have just been described. These movements are often combined to accomplish specific activities. Complicated activities such as walking, running, and climbing stairs require the combination of many movements, numerous muscles, and more joints in addition to the hip and knee. Even seemingly simple activities may be more complex than they initially appear. Consider the movements at the hip and knee joints involved in "crossing the legs": that is, causing one thigh and

leg to overlap the other, with the posterior surface of the knee of the limb in motion coming to rest on the anterior surface of the other knee. In initiating the activity from a sitting position with either the right or left leg, the thigh must be flexed to raise the leg and foot from the floor. As flexion of the thigh takes place, the leg is extended so that the moving limb clears the stationary limb. The thigh is adducted (to cross the limbs) and then extended as it comes to rest on the other limb. The leg then relaxes into a position of flexion at the knee. The stationary limb is also active. Before the moving limb can be raised, the stationary limb must be planted firmly on the floor; the muscle activity in the thigh of the latter can be verified, with one hand placed on the posteromedial surface of the thigh and the other placed just distal to the ischial tuberosity, as the other limb is raised. In addition, when the moving limb is placed on the stationary limb, the thigh of the latter adducts, bringing the knee of the stationary limb closer to the body's midline.

The movements that take place to allow one limb to be placed over the other are not isolated events but occur in a coordinated manner. Each, however, can be analyzed individually to determine which muscles are involved. Reference can be made to the previous sections and the diagrams of specific movements. The major muscles that are used in flexion of the thigh include the tensor fasciae latae, sartorius, iliopsoas, and rectus femoris. Extension of the leg is produced by the quadriceps, and adduction of the thigh involves the pectineus, the adductors longus and brevis, and the obturator part of the adductor magnus. As the moving limb is placed over the other limb, gravity is involved, but muscle activity is necessary to control the placement. In the stationary limb, the hamstrings and adductor magnus (and possibly the gluteus maximus) contract in an attempt to extend the thigh, resulting in firmly fixing the foot of the stationary limb on the floor, providing stability for movement of the other limb.

This activity can be modified. If the legs are crossed in such a manner as to allow the ankle of the moving limb to come to rest on the opposite knee, the thigh of the moving limb must (in addition to some of the movements discussed previously) be abducted and laterally rotated.

With any analysis of an activity, consideration should be given to the effect of nerve lesions on the ability to perform the activity. For example, a lesion of the obturator nerve weakens the movement of adduction of the thigh as the moving limb is crossed over the stationary limb. Although weakened, the movement may still be possible as a result of the action of muscles innervated by other nerves.

Activity: *Pedaling a Bicycle.* Riding and maintaining balance on a bicycle involves numerous joints throughout the body. In pedaling the bicycle, the predominant movements at the hip and knee joints are flexion and extension. The limb that is producing downward force on the pedal starts the movement from a flexed position at both the knee and hip joints. As the thigh and leg are extended, the pedal is pushed downward to its lowest point. As this part of the sequence occurs, the opposite limb changes from an extended position to a position in which both the thigh and leg are flexed. The sequence then alternates between the limbs.

Most of the muscle action in this activity occurs during extension; flexion is typically the more passive movement produced by the upward push of the pedal. Powerful extension at the hip joint is produced mainly by the gluteus maximus and the part of the adductor magnus that arises from the ischial tuberosity, while extension of the leg at the knee is produced mainly by the quadriceps femoris. Flexion can be more active if the toes of the foot that is moving upward are held in place with a toe clip or a clipless pedal in which the shoe is attached to the pedal. With this arrangement, muscles producing flexion can then pull upward on the pedal, rather than having the pedal push the foot upward. Muscles capable of producing flexion of the thigh would be the sartorius, the tensor fasciae latae, muscles on the anterior and anteromedial aspects of the thigh (including the pectineus, the adductors longus and brevis, and the anterior part of the adductor magnus), the gluteus minimus, and anterior fibers of the gluteus medius. The iliopsoas can also flex the thigh, but it is used only when power is needed. Flexion of the leg is produced by the semitendinosus, semimembranosus, biceps femoris, gracilis, and sartorius. Movements of the foot at the ankle, specifically plantar flexion and dorsiflexion, also occur with this activity. These movements are discussed in Chapter 19.

ANALYSES OF ACTIVITIES AND ASSOCIATED MOVEMENTS—cont'd

Activity: *Digging a Hole with a Shovel.* The lower limb provides the force to dig a hole with a shovel. With the shovel held firmly by the upper limbs, one foot is placed on the top of the shovel blade. To accomplish this, the thigh and leg are flexed, and the foot is dorsiflexed (the front of the foot is raised upward). To raise the limb off the ground, the opposite limb must support the weight of the body, which requires stabilizing or raising the pelvis slightly on the unsupported side. The leg is then extended to position the foot on the top of the blade of the shovel. Once the foot is positioned, the body weight is again supported by both limbs. To drive the shovel blade into the ground, the leg and thigh are extended with force, while the foot is held in a fixed position.

Muscles involved in flexion of the thigh include the sartorius and the tensor fasciae latae. The iliopsoas and the rectus femoris, the only part of the quadriceps that crosses the hip joint, can also aid in flexion. Flexion of the leg at the knee can be produced by gravity as the thigh is flexed. However, because the sartorius crosses both the hip and knee joints, it flexes the thigh and leg. Contraction of the hamstrings and gracilis, if they are needed, would also produce flexion of the leg. Dorsiflexion of the foot is the result of the action of several muscles (tibialis anterior, extensor digitorum longus, and fibularis tertius) described in Chapter 19. To support the weight of the body as the limb is being lifted, the gluteus medius and gluteus minimus on the supporting side must contract. These muscles produce abduction of the thigh, an action that, because the limb is fixed on the ground, causes the pelvis to be raised slightly above the horizontal position on the unsupported side.

Extension of the leg to position the foot on the shovel and to begin forcing the blade downward is produced by the quadriceps femoris. The gluteus maximus and the part of the adductor magnus that is innervated by the tibial nerve provide forceful extension of the thigh.

REVIEW QUESTIONS

1 If when standing on one leg the pelvis sags or drops on the unsupported side, which muscles are probably weak or unable to contract?

2 Which muscles contribute to adduction of the thigh?

3 When the leg is approaching maximum extension at the knee joint and the foot is fixed on the ground, what type of movement is the femur undergoing? Which muscle "undoes" this terminal movement of the femur to prepare the knee joint for flexion?

4 Is the short head of the biceps femoris muscle capable of producing any movement at the hip joint? Why?

5 Which muscles of the thigh, due to their origin and insertion, are capable of producing movement at both the hip and knee joints?

6 What is the position of the line of gravity in relation to the hip and knee joints? What effect does this have on these joints?

7 Injury to the superior gluteal nerve at its origin from the sacral plexus could affect which muscles and what movements? What effect would loss of the obturator nerve have on movements of the thigh?

8 What movements take place at the hip and/or knee joint, and what muscles are involved at these joints in performing the following activities?
a holding a box of popcorn between the legs
b stepping onto a bus
c squatting to lift a heavy box

EXERCISES

1 In a sitting position with the foot resting on a stool, palpate the quadriceps femoris muscle, its tendon of insertion on the patella, and the patellar ligament. Palpate the same structures as the leg is extended.

2 While climbing stairs and palpating the gluteal region, anterior thigh, and posterior thigh, attempt to identify the muscles as they contract.

19 THE LEG

CHAPTER CONTENTS

General Considerations

Bones

Fascia and Superficial Nerves and Vessels

Muscles

Nerves and Vessels

Movements of the Foot

*Analyses of Activities and Associated
    Movements*

GENERAL CONSIDERATIONS

In the leg, three muscles cross the knee joint. One of these crosses only the knee joint, and the other two cross both the knee and the ankle (talocrural) joints. The other muscles of the leg originate distal to the knee and act at the ankle or both at the ankle and at a more distal part of the foot, including the toes.

The movements of the leg at the knee joint are discussed in Chapter 18. Those at the **ankle joint** are almost entirely limited to flexion and extension. Because of the rotation of the lower limb during development and the adult position attained by the foot, the foot can be regarded as normally being in a position of hyperextension. To avoid any confusion created by this position and the usual definitions of flexion and extension (see Chapter 1 and Glossary), it is preferable to avoid the terms "flexion" and "extension" in trying to describe movements at the ankle. The sole of the foot is usually referred to as the plantar surface, and the top of the foot is the dorsum. By use of these terms, it is possible to qualify the terms of direction so that there can be no misunderstanding concerning what movement at the ankle is being described. The movement of moving the distal end of the foot (the toes) downward in a sagittal plane (rising up on the toes) is **plantar flexion of the foot.** Moving the distal end of the foot upward in a sagittal plane toward the anterior surface of the leg (standing upon the heels) is **dorsiflexion of the foot.**

Just as movement of the hand is not restricted to movement at the radiocarpal joint but occurs also among the carpals, movement of the foot is not restricted to the ankle joint but occurs also among the tarsals. Through certain joints among the tarsals, the sole of the foot can be turned inward, as if to appose

307

it to the sole of the opposite side. This movement, occurring distal to the ankle joint, is known as **inversion.** The movement in the opposite direction, turning the sole of the foot outward, occurs at the same joints and is known as **eversion.** Inversion is normally accompanied by **adduction** (a medial flexion of the anterior part of the foot on the posterior part), and eversion by **abduction** (lateral flexion). These combined movements are frequently referred to, particularly by clinicians, as **supination** and **pronation,** respectively. (The terms *varus* and *valgus,* already defined as indicating inward and outward bending, respectively, are used to describe position, not movement. Therefore, a pronated or everted foot is in the valgus position, or is a pes valgus.)

In contrast to the confusion in terminology regarding flexion and extension at the ankle, there is none in regard to these movements of the toes. **Flexion of the toes** always means plantar flexion, and **extension of the toes** means straightening or dorsiflexing them. As is true of the fingers, **abduction of the toes** is the act of spreading the toes apart, and **adduction** is the act of bringing them together. In the foot, however, the reference for abduction-adduction is the *second digit* rather than the third digit.

BONES

Tibia and Fibula

The tibia and fibula, the bones of the leg, have been studied partly in connection with the thigh and knee (Fig. 19-1). At its proximal end, the slender **fibula** has a *head* (with a pointed *apex*) that bears an articular surface for the synovial joint between it and the tibia. Most of the *shaft* is so marked by the attachments of muscles that its surfaces and borders are difficult to follow, but a sharp edge that is directed medially is its *interosseous border.* At its distal end, the fibula enlarges to form the *lateral malleolus,* which has an articular surface that forms the lateral side of the ankle joint.

The proximal end of the **tibia,** the much heavier medial bone of the leg, has been described in Chapter 16. In summary, the *medial and lateral condyles* have articular surfaces for the femoral condyles. These articular surfaces are separated from each other by the nonarticular intercondylar areas and *intercondylar*

eminence. On the posteroinferior aspect of the lateral condyle is an articular surface for the fibula. The *shaft* of the tibia is somewhat triangular. Its anterior border, marked above by the *tibial tuberosity* for the attachment of the patellar ligament, is subcutaneous, as is its medial surface. Its *interosseous border* faces laterally, toward the interosseous border of the fibula. Close to the distal end, the tibia expands to form the *medial malleolus.* On the lateral surface of the downward-projecting malleolus is an articular surface that forms the medial side of the ankle joint. This is continuous with the inferior articular surface of the tibia, on the distal end of that bone, through which weight is transmitted from the leg to the foot.

The tibia and fibula are united proximally by the **tibiofibular joint** and are united throughout most of their length by a heavy interosseous membrane that stretches between their interosseous borders. At their distal ends, there is a **tibiofibular syndesmosis** (nonsynovial joint) provided with special ligaments. Sometimes a part of the synovial cavity of the ankle joint extends upward between the distal ends of the two bones to convert the joint into a synovial one.

FUNCTIONAL/CLINICAL NOTE 19-1

The tibia transmits most of the weight (about five sixths) from the femur to the foot because the fibula does not reach the knee joint and articulates on the side of the ankle joint. The fibula is important, however, because it gives rise to many muscles, and its presence is necessary to stabilize the ankle joint. The uppermost bone at the ankle, the talus, is normally gripped firmly between the medial and lateral malleoli, and this is the reason that only dorsiflexion and plantar flexion are possible at the ankle joint. When the lateral malleolus is fractured, or the lower end of the fibula is missing, the foot may be badly twisted at the ankle.

Bones of the Ankle and Foot

Because many muscles of the leg insert on the foot, the bones of the ankle and foot are identified now (more detailed coverage is presented in Chapter 20). There

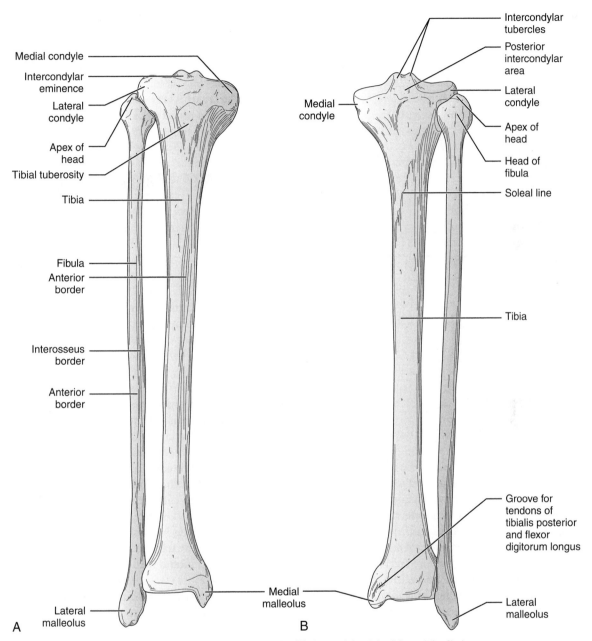

Figure 19-1 Anterior **(A)** and posterior **(B)** views of the right tibia and the fibula.

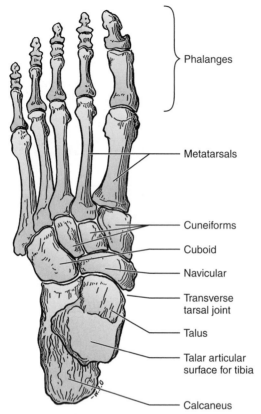

Phalanges

Metatarsals

Cuneiforms

Cuboid

Navicular

Transverse
tarsal joint

Talus

Talar articular
surface for tibia

Calcaneus

Figure 19-2 The bones of the left ankle and foot *(dorsal view).*

are seven **tarsal bones** (Fig. 19-2). Of these, the **talus** alone enters into the articulation with the bones of the leg. It rests on the **calcaneus;** the posteriorly projecting part of the calcaneus gives the plantar flexors inserting into it much better leverage than the other plantar flexors have. The posterior end of the calcaneus receives all the weight on the heel. Its anterior end, and that of the talus, are higher and normally not in contact with the ground, because they are lateral and medial parts of the arch of the foot. Between the talus and the calcaneus is the important **subtalar joint,** and between the anterior ends of both bones and the more distal tarsals is the important **transverse tarsal joint** (see Fig. 20-6). These joints are discussed in Chapter 20 but are mentioned here because they allow inversion and adduction (supination), and eversion and abduction (pronation). The transverse tarsal joint also allows additional plantar flexion and dorsiflexion.

Distal to the calcaneus is the **cuboid bone.** Immediately distal to the talus is the **navicular bone,** and distal to that are three **cuneiforms,** *medial, intermediate, and lateral.* The cuboid and the cuneiforms articulate with the **metatarsals,** essentially similar to the metacarpals. These in turn articulate with the proximal **phalanges** of the toes. Except in size, the phalanges of the toes are similar to those of the fingers and thumb.

FUNCTIONAL/CLINICAL NOTE 19-2

Because of the arch of the foot, in a standing position the weight of the body is normally transmitted to the ground only through the posterior end of the calcaneus and the heads (distal ends) of the metatarsals. The toes, especially the big toe, participate in the thrust in walking when the weight is shifted forward onto the ball of the foot.

Surface Anatomy

Several bony landmarks can be palpated in the leg. A part of the **tibia** is subcutaneous throughout its entire course in the leg and can be traced without difficulty from the **condyles** and **tuberosity** above to the **medial malleolus** on the medial side of the ankle. The **head of the fibula** is also subcutaneous and can easily be palpated just below the knee. More distally, the fibula is covered by muscles and can be felt only indistinctly. Above the ankle, it again becomes subcutaneous and can then be palpated down to the prominent **lateral malleolus.**

FASCIA AND SUPERFICIAL NERVES AND VESSELS

Fascia

The **deep fascia of the leg** (crural fascia) resembles the deep fascia found elsewhere on the limbs. It is a tough, fibrous layer the upper part of which gives origin to some of the musculature. It blends with the periosteum of the subcutaneous part of the tibia throughout most of the length of the leg and laterally sends two septa to the fibula. The *anterior intermuscular septum* separates the anterior from the lateral muscles of the leg, and the *posterior intermuscular septum* separates the lateral muscles from the posterior muscles. Each of the three groups of muscles lies in its own compartment. In addition, the fascia of the calf gives rise to the *transverse crural septum,* or *deep transverse crural fascia,* that passes across the calf and separates a superficial group of calf muscles from a deep group.

FUNCTIONAL/CLINICAL NOTE 19-3

Both the anterior and the deep posterior groups of muscles lie in such tight compartments that any trauma to them that produces swelling interferes very quickly with their circulation, which can lead to their rapid degeneration.

Close to the ankle, the crural fascia is thickened by more or less transverse fibers to form retinacula, similar to those at the wrist, that hold the tendons of the muscles of the leg close to the bones as they cross the ankle. Because there are three sets of muscles of the leg, there are three sets of retinacula. The **flexor retinaculum** lies posteromedially and extends between the medial malleolus and the calcaneus (see Figs. 19-4 and 19-6). The tendons of the deep muscles of the calf pass deep to it, as do also the nerve and vessels that continue from the calf into the sole of the foot. There are two lateral or **fibular** (peroneal) **retinacula.** The *superior fibular retinaculum* passes between the lateral malleolus and the calcaneus, and the *inferior fibular retinaculum* is attached at both its ends to the calcaneus (see Fig. 19-8). The tendons of the two lateral muscles of the leg (fibular muscles) pass deep to these retinacula. There are also two anterior or **extensor retinacula** (see Figs. 19-8 and 19-9). The *superior extensor retinaculum* is a transverse thickening that passes between the tibia and fibula above the malleoli. The *inferior extensor retinaculum,* once called the "cruciate ligament," resembles a Y lying on its side. The stem of the Y is attached to the lateral and dorsal surfaces of the calcaneus. As it is traced medially, across the dorsum of the foot, its two limbs diverge. The upper one goes to the medial malleolus, and the lower one blends with the fascia of the medial side of the foot. The tendons of the anterior muscles of the leg pass deep to the superior and through the inferior retinaculum.

As the posterior tendons pass through the flexor retinaculum, and as the anterior tendons pass through the inferior extensor retinaculum, most of them lie in separate compartments, each lined with a synovial membrane. These membranes form synovial sheaths that extend for varying distances above and below the retinacula. The two lateral muscles pass together through a single compartment and have a common synovial sheath deep to the superior fibular retinaculum, but the sheath divides into a part around each tendon, separated by a septum, deep to the inferior retinaculum.

Nerves

Posteriorly, the skin of the leg is supplied by branches from both the tibial and common fibular nerves. These branches, the medial sural cutaneous nerve from the tibial nerve and the sural communicating branch from the common fibular nerve, unite to form the **sural nerve,** which continues to the lateral side of the foot. Medially, the **saphenous nerve,** a branch of the femoral nerve, supplies the leg and continues into the foot. Anterolaterally, the upper part of the leg is supplied by a branch of the common fibular nerve that may arise either with or separate from the branch that joins the sural nerve; the lower part of the leg is supplied by the **superficial fibular nerve,** which also continues into the foot.

Vessels

Two large superficial veins are located in the leg. The **great saphenous vein** (see Fig. 14-4), beginning on the medial border of the foot, runs along the medial side of the leg, then into the thigh, where its course has already been described. The **small saphenous vein** begins on the lateral border of the foot and runs proximally on the posterior surface of the leg, communicating with the great saphenous vein and sometimes joining that vein in the thigh. It usually ends by penetrating the deep fascia in the hollow behind the knee (popliteal fossa) and joins the popliteal vein.

MUSCLES

The muscles of the leg are conveniently categorized into three groups: *posterior muscles,* or *muscles of the calf; anterior muscles;* and *lateral muscles.* The posterior muscles are primarily plantar flexors of the foot at the ankle and flexors of the toes. The anterior muscles are dorsiflexors at the ankle and extensors of the toes, whereas the lateral muscles are evertors of the foot. (Certain anterior

and posterior muscles invert the foot.) All three groups of muscles are innervated by major branches of the sciatic nerve. The *posterior muscles are innervated by the tibial nerve.* The *lateral and anterior muscles are innervated by the superficial and deep fibular nerves, respectively.* The two fibular nerves are branches of the common fibular nerve; both the common fibular and tibial nerves are terminal branches of the sciatic nerve.

The muscles of the calf can be categorized into a superficial and a deep group, each lying in its own fascial compartment. (The origins and insertions of the muscles are illustrated in Fig. 19-3.) The muscles

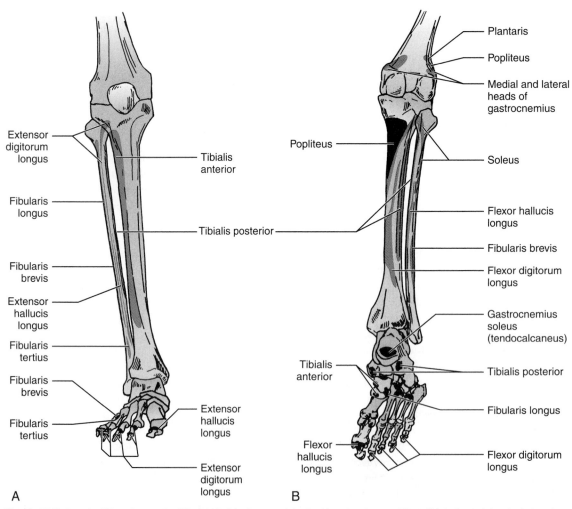

Figure 19-3 Anterior **(A)** and posterior **(B)** views of the bones of the knee region, leg, and foot, illustrating origins *(color)* and insertions *(black)* of the anterior, lateral, and posterior muscles of the leg.

of the superficial group are the *gastrocnemius, soleus,* and *plantaris.* They all insert on the posterior end of the calcaneus, and the gastrocnemius and soleus share the same tendon of insertion. In addition to having individual names, the two heads of the gastrocnemius and the soleus are grouped together and called the **triceps surae.**

Superficial Muscles of the Calf

Gastrocnemius

The **gastrocnemius,** the superficial member of the triceps surae group and the most superficial muscle of the calf, has medial and lateral heads, which have *origins* from the posterior surface of the femur just proximal to the corresponding condyles (Fig. 19-4 and Table 19-1).

These two heads quickly unite to form the bulk of the muscle. Approximately halfway down the calf, the gastrocnemius ends in a flat tendon that receives on its deep (anterior) surface the attachment of the next underlying muscle, the soleus. The tendon becomes more rounded and proceeds downward as the calcaneal tendon (tendo calcaneus, or Achilles tendon). Its *insertion* is on the lower part of the projecting posterior portion of the calcaneus. There is usually a bursa between the tendon and the upper region of the calcaneus. The *action* of the gastrocnemius is as a powerful plantar flexor of the foot, and it can help flex the leg when the leg is not supporting

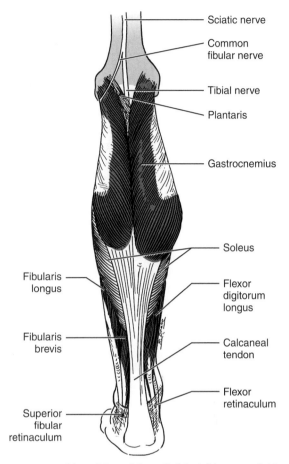

Figure 19-4 Musculature of the calf of the left leg, superficial view.

Table 19-1	SUPERFICIAL MUSCLES OF THE CALF			
Muscle	**Origin (Proximal Attachment)**	**Insertion (Distal Attachment)**	**Action**	**Innervation**
Gastrocnemius	Posterior surface of femur just proximal to medial and lateral condyles	Calcaneus, through calcaneal tendon	Plantar flexion of foot: flexion of leg of free limb	Tibial nerve
Soleus	Soleal (or popliteal) line; posterior surface of upper third and medial border of middle third of tibia; proximal third of posterior surface of fibula	Calcaneus through calcaneal tendon	Plantar flexion of foot	Tibial nerve
Plantaris	Lateral epicondyle of femur	Calcaneus, anteromedial to calcaneal tendon	Weak plantar flexion of foot; weak flexion of leg	Tibial nerve

weight. With the foot fixed in weight bearing, however, its posterior position at the ankle allows it to resist dorsiflexion at that joint. Because flexion of the weight-bearing limb at the knee cannot occur without accompanying dorsiflexion at the ankle, the gastrocnemius helps maintain extension of the leg. It receives *innervation* from the tibial nerve, which passes between its two heads to a deeper position in the calf in company with the large vessels (popliteal vessels) that run from the thigh to the leg.

Soleus

The **soleus muscle** lies immediately deep to the gastrocnemius and also has two heads (Fig. 19-5). One has its *origin* from the soleal line across the upper third of the posterior surface of the tibia and from the middle third of the medial border. The *origin* of the other head is from the proximal third of the posterior surface of the fibula. As the two heads unite to form a flattened muscle mass, the tibial nerve and the popliteal vessels pass deeply to lie adjacent to the anterior surface of the muscle. The *insertion* of the soleus is on the calcaneus through its attachment to the deep (anterior) surface of the calcaneal tendon. Because it has no attachment across the knee joint, it does not share the function of flexion of the knee with the gastrocnemius. The *action* of the soleus is to work with the gastrocnemius in plantar flexion of the foot and in complete plantar flexion when the knee is flexed and the gastrocnemius is at a disadvantage. Taking its fixed point from below, the soleus, like the gastrocnemius, prevents dorsiflexion at the ankle and therefore flexion at the knee. It is usually the soleus rather than the gastrocnemius that does this during quiet standing. It typically receives *innervation* from two branches of the tibial nerve, one into its superficial surface and one into its deep surface.

Plantaris

The small **plantaris muscle** (see Fig. 19-5) has its *origin* from the lateral epicondyle of the femur just above the attachment of the lateral head of the gastrocnemius. Its muscular "belly" is approximately 2 to 4 inches (51 to 102 mm) long, but its slender tendon is very long. The tendon passes distally between the gastrocnemius and soleus to an *insertion* on the calcaneus, anteromedial to the calcaneal tendon;

it sometimes fuses with the calcaneal tendon or the flexor retinaculum. (In some animals, the plantaris is a powerful muscle whose tendon extends over the heel onto the plantar surface of the foot, becoming continuous there with the heavy plantar aponeurosis. In these animals, the plantaris is the equivalent of the palmaris longus of the forearm and hand.) Because of its anatomical arrangement, it is capable of two *actions:* flexion of the leg and plantar flexion of the foot. Both actions, however, are weak. The plantaris receives *innervation* from a branch of the tibial nerve.

Deep Muscles of the Calf

The deep muscles of the calf are the *popliteus* (a muscle behind the knee) and three muscles that arise from the tibia and fibula and continue deep to the flexor retinaculum into the foot: the *flexor hallucis longus, flexor digitorum longus,* and *tibialis posterior* (Fig. 19-6 and Table 19-2). These muscles are separated from the superficial group by a fascial septum that extends across the leg from the deep fascia and is reinforced in its upper part by a slip from the semimembranosus tendon. Below the popliteus, this fascia helps give origin to the deep muscles, but lower in the leg, it covers them more loosely. This layer of fascia is thickened at the ankle to form the flexor retinaculum and is pierced in the upper part of the leg by the tibial nerve and popliteal vessels, the continuations of which lie deep to the fascia and among the deep muscles.

Popliteus

The **popliteus muscle** forms part of the floor of the popliteal fossa (Fig. 19-7; see Fig. 19-6). Its tendon, variably described as its tendon of *origin* or insertion, attaches within the joint capsule of the knee joint to the lateral condyle of the femur and runs posteriorly and medially between the fibrous and synovial layers of the joint capsule. The muscle also has attachments to the lateral meniscus and to the arcuate popliteal ligament. It emerges through a gap in the posterior part of the capsule below the arcuate ligament and runs obliquely across the posterior aspect of the knee joint to an *insertion* on the proximal third of the posterior surface of the tibia, proximal and medial to the tibial origin of the soleus. The *action* of the

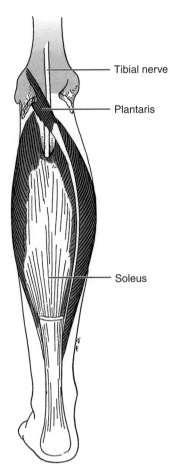

Figure 19-5 Musculature of the calf. The gastrocnemius is omitted in order to illustrate the deeper lying muscles of the superficial group.

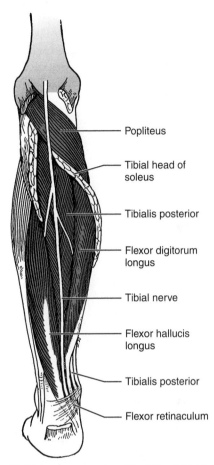

Figure 19-6 The deep muscles of the left calf *(highlighted in color).*

Table 19-2	DEEP MUSCLES OF THE CALF			
Muscle	**Origin (Proximal Attachment)**	**Insertion (Distal Attachment)**	**Action**	**Innervation**
Popliteus	Lateral condyle of femur	Proximal third of posterior aspect of tibia (proximal to soleal line)	Medial rotation of leg on femur; lateral rotation of femur on leg	Tibial nerve
Flexor hallucis longus	Middle half of posterior surface of fibula	Distal phalanx of big toe	Flexion of big toe; weak plantar flexion of foot	Tibial nerve
Flexor digitorum longus	Middle third of posterior surface of tibia	Distal phalanges of lateral four toes	Flexion of distal phalanges of lateral four toes; weak plantar flexion and inversion of foot	Tibial nerve
Tibialis posterior	Proximal two-thirds of posterior surface of tibia; proximal two-thirds of fibula; interosseous membrane	Navicular; cuneiforms; cuboid; bases of second to fourth metatarsals	Adduct front of foot; inversion and plantar flexion of foot	Tibial nerve

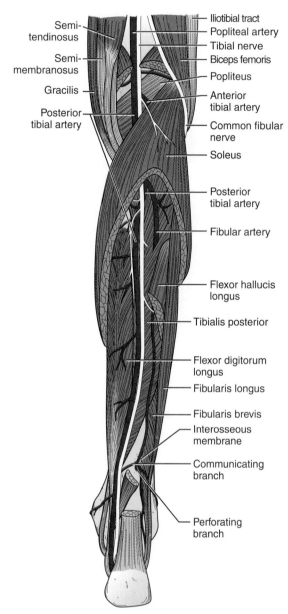

Semi-
tendinosus

Semi-
membranosus

Gracilis

Posterior
tibial artery

Iliotibial tract

Popliteal artery

Tibial nerve

Biceps femoris

Popliteus

Anterior
tibial artery

Common fibular
nerve

Soleus

Posterior
tibial artery

Fibular artery

Flexor hallucis
longus

Tibialis posterior

Flexor digitorum
longus

Fibularis longus

Fibularis brevis

Interosseous
membrane

Communicating
branch

Perforating
branch

Figure 19-7 Nerves, arteries and muscles of the right calf.

popliteus is to medially rotate the leg on the femur or laterally rotate the femur on the leg. It is an unimportant flexor at the knee. However, in standing with the knee partly flexed, it contracts to help prevent forward displacement of the femur on the tibia. *Innervation* is provided by a branch of the tibial nerve that typically passes around the lower edge of the muscle to penetrate the muscle on its deep (anterior) surface.

Flexor hallucis longus

The three remaining muscles of the calf cover the posterior aspect of the tibia, fibula, and interosseous membrane. The **flexor hallucis longus,** the most lateral, has its *origin* from the lateral side of about the middle half of the posterior aspect of the fibula. Its tendon of insertion begins just above the ankle and passes obliquely downward, medially, and forward to enter the foot deep to the flexor retinaculum. The tendon of the flexor hallucis longus is the most posterolateral of the three tendons posterior to the medial malleolus. In the foot, it runs forward to an *insertion* on the distal phalanx of the big toe. The *action* of the muscle is primarily as a flexor of the big toe, as its name implies. It is a very weak plantar flexor of the ankle. *Innervation* to the flexor hallucis longus is provided by the tibial nerve.

Flexor digitorum longus

The most medial of the three muscles is the **flexor digitorum longus,** that has its *origin* from about the middle third of the posterior aspect of the tibia. As this muscle passes distally, it is crossed on its anterior surface by the tibialis posterior, and at the ankle, the tendon of the flexor digitorum longus lies between those of the tibialis posterior and flexor hallucis longus. The tendon of the flexor digitorum longus begins somewhat higher above the ankle than does that of the flexor hallucis. It passes through the flexor retinaculum and, therefore, posterior to the medial malleolus. In the sole of the foot, it spreads out to its *insertion* on the distal phalanges of the four lateral digits. In the foot, these tendons are associated with the origins of the lumbrical muscles and pass through the divided tendons of the flexor digitorum brevis (an intrinsic muscle of the foot). The flexor digitorum longus of the leg corresponds to the flexor digitorum profundus of the forearm. The *action* of the flexor digitorum longus is to flex the distal phalanges of the four lateral toes. It is also a weak plantar flexor and can assist in inversion and adduction (supination) of the foot. The flexor digitorum longus receives *innervation* from the tibial nerve.

Tibialis posterior

The third muscle of the group, the **tibialis posterior,** has its *origin* from the proximal two thirds of the lateral side of the posterior surface of the shaft of the tibia, approximately the corresponding part of the medial portion of the posterior surface of the fibula, and from the posterior aspect of the interosseous membrane between these two bones. It lies between the flexor hallucis longus and the flexor digitorum longus. Distally, it becomes tendinous and runs medially and forward so that its tendon passes deep to the tendon of the flexor digitorum longus. In this way, it assumes an anterior, rather than an intermediate, position posterior to the medial malleolus. The tendon of the tibialis posterior passes through the flexor retinaculum in its own compartment, grooving the back of the medial malleolus as it does so, and then passes to the medial side of the plantar surface of the foot. Its *insertion* is primarily onto the navicular bone, but it also extends to attach, with some variation, to all the other tarsals except the talus and to the bases of the second, third, and fourth metatarsals. The *action* of this muscle is to adduct the front of the foot and to aid in inversion and plantar flexion. *Innervation* is provided by the tibial nerve.

Lateral Muscles of the Leg

Fibularis longus

The **fibularis longus** (Fig. 19-8 and Table 19-3; see Figs. 19-3 and 19-7, *C*) has its *origin* from the proximal two thirds of the lateral surface of the fibula and the surrounding fascia and intermuscular septa. It is more superficial than the fibularis brevis. The fibularis longus shares a common synovial sheath with the fibularis brevis above the ankle and passes posterior to the lateral malleolus and deep to the two fibular retinacula onto the lateral border of the foot.

Its tendon rounds the lateral border of the foot to run in a deep position across the sole of the foot to an *insertion* on the base of the first metatarsal and the adjacent medial cuneiform bone. It receives *innervation* from the superficial fibular nerve and often receives a branch from either the common or the deep fibular nerve. The *action* of the fibularis longus is as a good evertor of the foot and a weak plantar flexor. The common fibular nerve, or the superficial and deep fibular nerves together, pass deep to the upper part of the fibularis longus, between it and the fibula. The deep fibular continues forward into the anterior muscles, but the superficial fibular nerve runs distally between the two fibular muscles to become subcutaneous in the distal third of the leg.

Fibularis brevis

The **fibularis brevis** (see Figs. 19-3, 19-7, and 19-8) takes *origin* from much of the distal two thirds of the lateral surface of the fibula and the adjacent intermuscular septa. Its tendon passes through a common synovial sheath with that of the fibularis longus and then posterior to the lateral malleolus to an *insertion* on the dorsal part of the base of the fifth metatarsal bone. The fibularis brevis receives its *innervation* from branches of the superficial fibular nerve. Its *action* is to evert the foot; it also is a weak plantar flexor.

Anterior Muscles of the Leg

Extensor digitorum and fibularis tertius

Of the anterior muscles of the leg, the **extensor digitorum longus** is the most lateral (Fig. 19-9 and Table 19-4). Its *origin* is from a small portion of the lateral condyle of the tibia and from about the proximal three fourths of the anterior surface of the fibula, and it also has some attachment to the interosseous membrane and the covering crural fascia. The muscle becomes tendinous above the ankle, and its tendon then divides into four tendons that insert on the four lateral toes. The insertion of the extensor digitorum longus is similar to that of the extensor digitorum in the hand. The tendons reinforce the thin dorsal capsules of the metatarsophalangeal and interphalangeal joints. Each tendon divides into a central slip that has an *insertion* on the middle phalanx and two

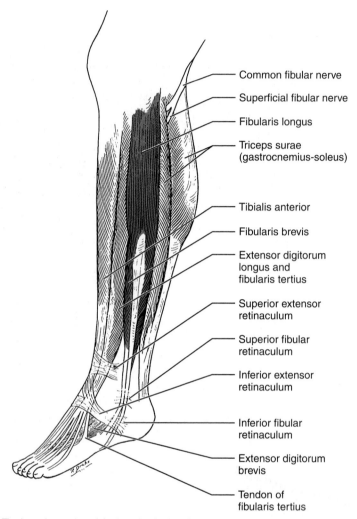

Common fibular nerve

Superficial fibular nerve

Fibularis longus

Triceps surae
(gastrocnemius-soleus)

Tibialis anterior

Fibularis brevis

Extensor digitorum
longus and
fibularis tertius

Superior extensor
retinaculum

Superior fibular
retinaculum

Inferior extensor
retinaculum

Inferior fibular
retinaculum

Extensor digitorum
brevis

Tendon of
fibularis tertius

Figure 19-8 The lateral muscles of the leg, the fibularis longus and the fibularis brevis *(highlighted in color).*

Table 19-3	LATERAL MUSCLES OF THE LEG			
Muscle	**Origin (Proximal Attachment)**	**Insertion (Distal Attachment)**	**Action**	**Innervation**
Fibularis longus	Proximal two thirds of lateral surface of fibula; adjacent fascia and intermuscular septa	Base of first metatarsal; medial cuneiform	Eversion and weak plantar flexion of foot	Superficial fibular nerve (and often a branch from common or deep fibular nerve)
Fibularis brevis	Distal two thirds of lateral surface of fibula; adjacent intermuscular septa	Dorsal surface of base of fifth metatarsal	Eversion and weak plantar flexion of foot	Superficial fibular nerve

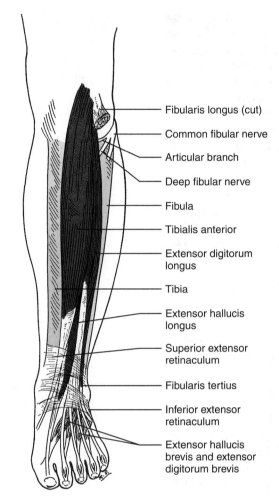

Fibularis longus (cut)

Common fibular nerve

Articular branch

Deep fibular nerve

Fibula

Tibialis anterior

Extensor digitorum longus

Tibia

Extensor hallucis longus

Superior extensor retinaculum

Fibularis tertius

Inferior extensor retinaculum

Extensor hallucis brevis and extensor digitorum brevis

Figure 19-9 The anterior muscles of the left leg *(highlighted in color)*.

lateral slips that are continued onto the distal phalanx. As the tendons to the second, third, and fourth toes expand on the metatarsophalangeal joints, they are joined by the three tendons of the extensor digitorum brevis, a muscle of the foot that has no counterpart in the normal hand.

Closely associated with the extensor digitorum longus, and continuous at its origin from the fibula with the lower fibers of origin of the longus, is the **fibularis tertius.** The fibers of this muscle end in a tendon that seems to be a fifth, most lateral, tendon of the extensor digitorum longus on the dorsum of the foot. Instead of passing to the toes, however, it has an *insertion* on the dorsal surface of the base of

the fifth metatarsal. The muscle varies considerably in size and is sometimes absent.

The *action* of the extensor digitorum longus is to extend the toes. It is also a dorsiflexor and weak evertor of the foot. The fibularis tertius also acts in dorsiflexion and eversion, but it is a better evertor than it is a dorsiflexor. Both muscles receive *innervation* from the deep fibular nerve (as do the other anterior muscles). This nerve passes deep to the extensor digitorum longus before running distally in the leg.

Extensor hallucis longus

The **extensor hallucis longus** is, at its origin, covered by the extensor digitorum longus and a more medial muscle, the tibialis anterior. Its *origin* is from approximately the middle third of the anterior surface of the fibula and the adjacent interosseous membrane. The muscle appears between the extensor digitorum longus and the tibialis anterior muscles somewhat above the ankle. It runs deep to the superior extensor retinaculum and through the inferior extensor retinaculum and goes to an *insertion* on the distal phalanx of the big toe. The *action* of the extensor hallucis longus is to extend the big toe. It is also a weak dorsiflexor at the ankle and invertor of the foot. *Innervation* is provided by the deep fibular nerve, which courses with the anterior tibial vessels between the extensor hallucis longus and tibialis anterior muscles. The nerve and vessels pass deep to the extensor hallucis longus near the ankle and lie lateral to its tendon on the dorsum of the foot.

Tibialis anterior

The **tibialis anterior** has its *origin* from the lateral condyle and the proximal two thirds of the lateral surface of the tibia, the deep fascia of the leg, and the interosseous membrane. After passing deep to the superior and through the inferior extensor retinaculum, the tendon of this muscle goes to the medial side of the foot to an *insertion* on the medial cuneiform bone and the base of the first metatarsal, almost over onto the sole of the foot. The *action* of the tibialis anterior is to strongly invert and dorsiflex the foot. It receives *innervation* from several branches of the deep fibular nerve.

	Table 19-4	ANTERIOR MUSCLES OF THE LEG			
Muscle	**Origin (Proximal Attachment)**	**Insertion (Distal Attachment)**	**Action**	**Innervation**	
Extensor digitorum longus	Lateral condyle of tibia; proximal three fourths of anterior surface of fibula; interosseous membrane and crural fascia	Middle and distal phalanges of lateral four toes	Extension of lateral four toes; dorsiflexion and eversion of foot	Deep fibular nerve	
Fibularis tertius	Fibula in common with lower fibers of extensor digitorum longus	Dorsal surface of base of fifth metatarsal	Dorsiflexion and eversion of foot	Deep fibular nerve	
Extensor hallucis longus	Middle third of anterior surface of fibula; interosseous membrane	Distal phalanx of big toe	Extension of big toe; dorsiflexion and inversion of foot	Deep fibular nerve	
Tibialis anterior	Lateral condyle of tibia; proximal two thirds of lateral surface of tibia; interosseous membrane; and deep fascia of leg	Medial cuneiform; base of first metatarsal	Inversion and dorsiflexion of foot	Deep fibular nerve	

Surface Anatomy

The muscles of the calf are largely covered by the gastrocnemius. Therefore, only this muscle is identifiable in the upper part of the calf. The level at which its muscular part gives way to the calcaneal tendon is plainly visible. The **calcaneal tendon** can be followed without difficulty to the posterior end of the calcaneus, and below the gastrocnemius, the **soleus** can be palpated deep to and on the sides of the wider upper part of the tendon. Both the soleus and gastrocnemius are more easily palpated if the foot is brought into plantar flexion, as in standing on the toes. The long deep muscles of the calf are not easily identified individually, although their tendons can be identified as a group just posterior to the medial malleolus, particularly if the foot is inverted or the toes are flexed.

The **fibularis longus and brevis** can be felt to contract when the foot is everted, and their tendons can be felt together as they emerge from posterior to the lateral malleolus and pass anteriorly below it. The **tendon of the fibularis brevis** can be palpated as it inserts on the base of the fifth metatarsal.

The anterior muscles of the leg can be palpated on the lateral side of the tibia, and at the ankle, some of their tendons can be recognized. As the foot is inverted and dorsiflexed, the heavy **tendon of the tibialis anterior** can be visualized and felt as it runs across the medial side of the anterior surface of the ankle and dorsum of the foot. If the big toe is dorsiflexed, the sharper **tendon of the extensor hallucis longus** can be palpated just lateral to the tendon of the tibialis anterior. As the remaining toes are dorsiflexed, the **tendon of the extensor digitorum longus** can be felt lateral to the extensor of the big toe, and some of the tendons can be visualized and felt as they diverge toward the various digits. The **tendon of the fibularis tertius** may be palpable lateral to these tendons. It is best visualized during dorsiflexion and eversion of the foot.

NERVES AND VESSELS
Nerves and Vessels of the Calf

The **tibial nerve** leaves the sciatic nerve as its larger and medial terminal branch in the popliteal fossa. It is, in direction and size, the more direct continuation of the sciatic nerve. The tibial nerve leaves the popliteal fossa by passing between the two heads of the gastrocnemius. Almost immediately, it passes deep to the soleus to lie between it and the tibialis posterior, deep to the fascia covering the deep group of muscles of the leg. It runs distally on the tibialis posterior in company with the posterior tibial vessels (see Fig. 19-7); at the ankle, it lies between the tendons of the flexor hallucis longus and flexor digitorum longus. The tibial nerve innervates all the muscles in the calf of the leg. As it passes through the flexor retinaculum to reach the plantar surface of the foot, it divides into *medial* and *lateral plantar nerves.*

The direct continuation of the femoral artery is known as the **popliteal artery** as it passes from the anteromedial to the posterior aspect of the thigh through the gap in the adductor magnus tendon. The popliteal artery (see Fig. 16-13), in addition to muscular branches including the *sural arteries* to the soleus and gastrocnemius, gives off paired *superior* and *inferior genicular branches* that anastomose with each other around the knee and an unpaired *middle genicular artery* that enters the knee joint. The popliteal artery then divides, usually on the posterior surface of the popliteus muscle, into *anterior* and *posterior tibial arteries.*

The **anterior tibial artery** passes anteriorly between the tibia and fibula through a gap at the proximal end of the interosseous membrane to reach the anterolateral aspect of the leg. Its course there is described later. The **posterior tibial artery** takes the same course in the calf as does the tibial nerve. It gives off muscular branches in the calf, and as it passes through the flexor retinaculum in the same compartment as the nerve, it divides, as the nerve does, into *medial* and *lateral plantar branches.* In addition to its *muscular branches* and the *nutrient artery* to the tibia, the posterior tibial artery gives off one large branch in the leg, the **fibular (peroneal) artery.** This artery arises high, from the proximal end of the posterior tibial artery. On the lateral side of the leg, it runs deep to or in the flexor hallucis longus, lying close to the interosseous membrane and the fibula. At the ankle, the fibular artery communicates with the posterior tibial artery, supplies branches around the ankle, and gives rise to a *perforating branch* that passes forward between the tibia and the fibula to reach the dorsum of the foot.

The tibial and fibular arteries are usually each accompanied by two correspondingly named veins, which unite in a variable pattern to form a single **popliteal vein.** Usually, the popliteal vein receives the **small saphenous vein.** Before the popliteal vein passes through the adductor hiatus to continue as the femoral vein, there is frequently a communication with perforating branches of the profunda femoris vein (deep vein of the thigh).

Nerves and Vessels of the Anterolateral Aspect of the Leg

The **common fibular nerve,** the lateral terminal branch of the sciatic nerve in the popliteal fossa, runs laterally across the lateral head of the gastrocnemius muscle. It is subcutaneous just distal to the head of the fibula, a position in which it is easily damaged. As it passes between the fibula and the fibularis longus muscle, it divides into two branches or, sometimes, three. These branches include the superficial and deep fibular nerves and an articular branch to the knee joint that usually arises from the deep fibular but may arise as a terminal branch of the common fibular. The **superficial fibular nerve** lies between the fibularis muscles, supplying both, and becomes subcutaneous by emerging at the anterior border of these muscles near the middle of the leg. Its distribution in the foot is described later.

The **deep fibular nerve** passes anteriorly, deep to the fibularis longus, into the anterior muscles of the leg. It gives off branches to all these muscles and courses close to the interosseous membrane, in company with the anterior tibial artery, to be continued onto the dorsum of the foot (Fig. 19-10).

After the **anterior tibial artery** passes between the tibia and fibula above the superior edge of the interosseous membrane to reach the anterior surface of this membrane, it gives off an *anterior tibial recurrent branch* to the knee (see Fig. 19-10). As it runs distally with the deep fibular nerve (which crosses from its lateral to its medial side), it supplies the four anterior muscles, and after giving off branches around the ankle, it continues onto the dorsum of the foot as the *dorsalis pedis artery.*

Surface Anatomy

Of the two major nerves, the tibial and common fibular, the tibial nerve cannot be satisfactorily located by palpation. The **common fibular nerve,** however,

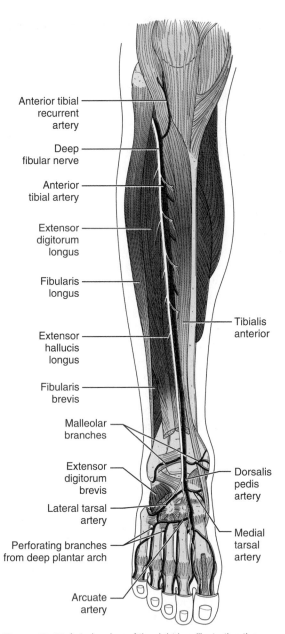

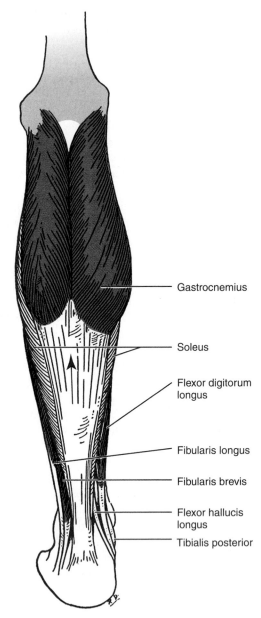

Figure 19-10 Anterior view of the right leg, illustrating the deep fibular nerve and the anterior tibial artery.

Figure 19-11 The plantar flexors of the left foot. All the potential plantar flexors are shown, although some (see text) may contribute little or nothing to plantar flexion. Note: The soleus is not shown in color.

can usually be palpated as it passes laterally around the fibula. The courses of both nerves can be visualized without difficulty. The **tibial nerve** continues the course of the sciatic nerve through the popliteal fossa and runs distally between the superficial and deep muscles of the calf. It diverges just enough medially to pass posterior to the medial malleolus with the posterior tibial artery. The common fibular nerve runs laterally and distally, leaving the popliteal fossa to cross the fibula just distal to its head. Its superficial branch then runs between the fibularis muscles. Its deep branch continues farther anteriorly and then turns down in company with the anterior tibial artery.

Of the vessels, parts of the **great and small saphenous veins** are frequently visible through the skin. The arteries are, for the most part, so deep that they cannot be palpated, but it is common practice for the pulse to be obtained from the **posterior tibial artery,** posterior to the medial malleolus. The fibular artery lies entirely deep. The anterior tibial artery also lies deep, but its pulse can be felt in its continuation, the **dorsalis pedis artery,** which passes onto the dorsum of the foot. This artery lies between the tendons of the extensor hallucis longus and extensor digitorum longus muscles, just below the ankle joint. In about 12% of limbs, however, the anterior tibial artery ends largely in the leg, so that the dorsalis pedis artery is not palpable, and in others, the dorsalis pedis has an abnormal course or origin and is largely covered by tendons on the foot.

MOVEMENTS OF THE FOOT

Plantar Flexion

Plantar flexion is caused primarily by the actions of the powerful *gastrocnemius* and *soleus* muscles (triceps surae) on the calcaneus (Fig. 19-11). The other three muscles in the calf that send their tendons posteriorly around the medial malleolus (*flexor hallucis longus, flexor digitorum longus,* and *tibialis posterior*) have usually been described as playing a very important role in assisting in plantar flexion. Similarly, the *fibularis longus* and *fibularis brevis* can be plantar flexors.

FUNCTIONAL/CLINICAL NOTE 19-4

All these muscles have much poorer leverage, however, than does the triceps surae, for the latter uses the posterior part of the calcaneus as its lever arm, while the other muscles pass close to the malleoli. As a result, even the best of the muscles have only about one-fifth the efficiency of the triceps surae. Because of the shortness of the lever arm of the triceps surae, it must exert a pull of about 200 lb (91 kg) in order to achieve plantar flexion of the foot against a weight of 100 pounds. Therefore, even it is at a disadvantage. Furthermore, the other muscles combined have much less strength than the triceps surae, and calculations, taking into account both their relative strength and their efficiency, indicate that these other muscles can produce a pull of only about 5% to perhaps 15% of that of the triceps surae.

With loss of the action of the triceps surae, walking becomes less smooth because of the lack of propulsion during "push-off." In addition, it has been shown that in many individuals, the fibularis longus and fibularis brevis are not normally used to produce plantar flexion of the foot. If the tibial nerve is destroyed, all potential plantar flexors at the ankle except the fibularis longus and fibularis brevis are paralyzed; among such cases, in fewer than half has plantar flexion of the unopposed foot been possible at all. Because the fibularis muscles were used when the patients were asked to evert their feet, there was obviously no weakness or disability of these muscles. It seems that some persons are accustomed to using the fibularis longus and fibularis brevis primarily as evertors of the foot, and they may not have learned to use them as plantar flexors. This can be learned, however. In irreparable paralysis of the triceps surae, the fibularis longus is sometimes attached to the calcaneus to give it better leverage for plantar flexion.

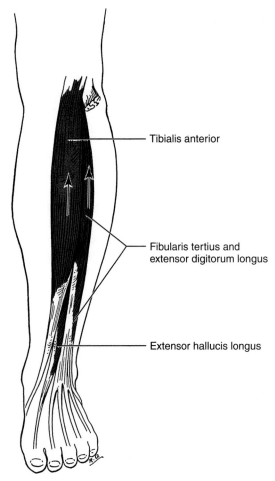

Figure 19-12 The dorsiflexors of the foot.

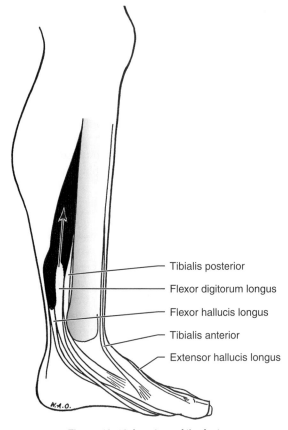

Figure 19-13 Invertors of the foot.

Dorsiflexion

Dorsiflexion is produced by the actions of all the muscles crossing the front of the ankle (Fig. 19-12). The *tibialis anterior* is the most important muscle involved in this action, but the *extensor digitorum longus* and its associated *fibularis tertius* assist, and the *extensor hallucis longus* can contribute weakly. When the tibialis anterior is paralyzed, the other muscles contract more strongly to dorsiflex the foot, and the extensor hallucis longus dorsiflexes the big toe. The extensor digitorum longus may dorsiflex the other toes, but this is not as noticeable because its action is primarily on the proximal phalanges, and these are usually maintained in dorsiflexion anyway.

Dorsiflexion with paralysis of the tibialis anterior may be accompanied by eversion of the foot because the fibularis tertius and the extensor digitorum longus, especially the former, may evert more strongly than the extensor hallucis longus inverts.

Inversion and Eversion

Inversion and eversion of the foot involve little movement at the hingelike ankle joint; almost all of this movement occurs at the subtalar and transverse tarsal joints. **Inversion** is brought about by all the muscles passing to or around the medial border of the foot (Fig. 19-13). Therefore, posteriorly, the *tibialis posterior, flexor hallucis longus,* and *flexor digitorum longus* all invert the foot. Anteriorly, the *tibialis anterior* is a strong invertor of the foot—the strongest of all—and the *extensor hallucis longus* is a weak one.

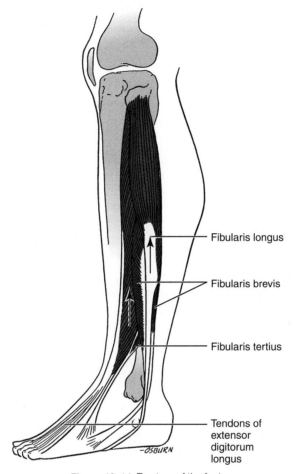

Figure 19-14 Evertors of the foot.

Eversion of the foot is brought about by all *three fibularis muscles* and the *extensor digitorum longus,* particularly its lateral part (Fig. 19-14).

Movement Dysfunction

The muscles of the calf are all innervated by the tibial nerve (Fig. 19-15 and Table 19-5). Therefore, injuries to this nerve may not only markedly interfere with "push-off" in walking (for the fibularis muscles are the only plantar flexors not supplied by the tibial nerve) but may make it impossible for the limb to bear weight unless an ankle brace is worn. The line of gravity of the body lies anterior to the ankle joint. Therefore, the activity of plantar flexors is necessary to prevent the foot from going into dorsiflexion, with a resultant forward shift of the weight of the body. The tibial nerve receives fibers from almost all the elements entering into the sacral plexus. The fibers distributed through it to the muscles of the calf are mostly from spinal nerves L5, S1, and S2.

The anterolateral muscles of the leg, all innervated by branches of the common fibular nerve, may be paralyzed by injury to this nerve (Fig. 19-16; see Table 19-5). Because of its subcutaneous position against the proximal end of the fibula, the common fibular nerve is one of the more commonly injured nerves in the body. The outstanding symptom of its injury is an inability to dorsiflex the foot, resulting in

TIBIAL NERVE

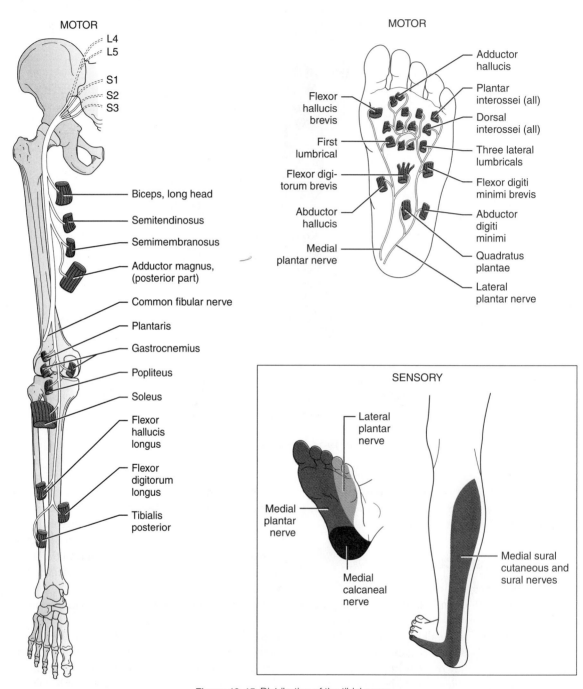

Figure 19-15 Distribution of the tibial nerve.

Table 19-5	NERVES			
	Muscle			
Nerve and Origin*	**Name**	**Segmental Innervation***	**Chief Action(s)**	
Tibial	Gastrocnemius	S1, S2	Plantar flexion at ankle	
L4–S3	Soleus	S1, S2	Plantar flexion at ankle	
	Plantaris	L4–S1	Plantar flexion at ankle	
	Popliteus	L5, S1	Rotation and flexion at knee	
	Tibialis posterior	L5, S1	Adduction and inversion of foot	
	Flexor digitorum longus	L5, S1	Flexion of lateral four toes	
	Flexor hallucis longus	L5–S2	Flexion of big toe	
Superficial fibular	Fibularis longus	L4–S1	Eversion of foot	
L4–S1	Fibularis brevis	L4–S1	Eversion of foot	
Deep fibular	Tibialis anterior	L4–S1	Inversion and dorsiflexion of foot	
L4–S2	Extensor digitorum longus	L4–S1	Extension of four lateral toes; dorsiflexion of foot	
	Fibularis tertius	L4–S1	Eversion and dorsiflexion of foot	
	Extensor hallucis longus	L4–S1	Extension of big toe	

*A common segmental origin or innervation.

footdrop when the lower limb is raised from contact with the ground. When a person with this condition attempts to walk, the foot must be raised far enough from the ground to provide clearance for the toes. Because it is impossible to make the heel strike first, as a result of the inability to dorsiflex the foot, the foot is simply flopped down. The common fibular nerve is composed primarily of fibers from L4, L5, S1, and S2. Most of the anterolateral muscles of the leg receive fibers from L4, L5, and S1.

Because the muscles of the leg, rather than those of the foot, move the foot, underdevelopment, contracture, fibrosis, or imbalance of the muscles of the leg can markedly distort the foot. There are numerous grades and directions of distortion. The general name of **clubfoot** (talipes) can be given to any of these distortions but is usually applied more specifically to the congenital deformity known also as *talipes equinovarus*. In this deformity, the foot is in plantar flexion and is adducted, and inverted, much of which is caused by contracture or underdevelopment of the triceps surae muscle group. Because the foot is in plantar flexion and the heel is turned inward and cannot bear the weight of the body, the weight is shifted to the lateral side of the front of the foot.

Correction of deformities is largely a matter of correcting the relations of the bones of the foot to each other and of restoring muscle balance. These corrections can sometimes be made, especially in congenital conditions, by applying a succession of casts or by performing surgery to realign the bones and to lengthen or transplant tendons.

COMMON FIBULAR NERVE

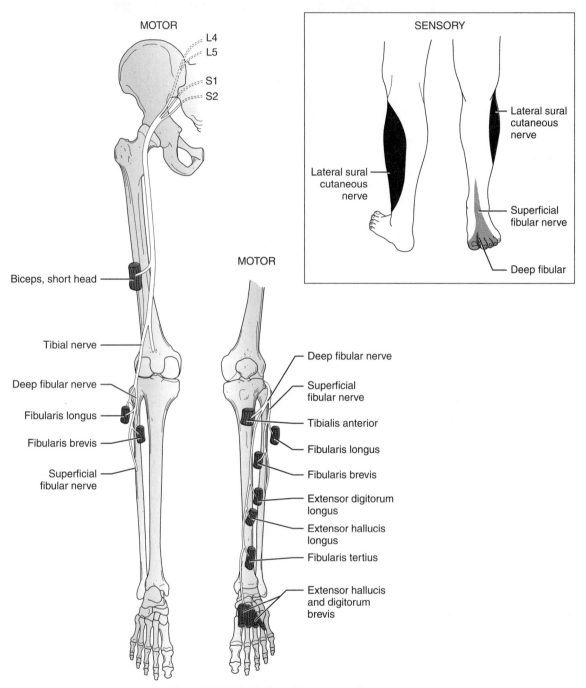

Figure 19-16 Distribution of the common fibular nerve.

ANALYSES OF ACTIVITIES AND ASSOCIATED MOVEMENTS

Activity: *Operating the Gas Pedal of a Car* The information just presented on movements of the foot and the muscles that produce them can be used to analyze everyday activities. Consider the movements the foot undergoes in depressing and releasing the gas pedal of a car. If the heel is held in a stationary position and is used as a pivot point, the pedal can be depressed by plantar flexion and released (raised) by dorsiflexion of the foot. Plantar flexion is produced mainly by the action of the soleus and gastrocnemius, but the deeper muscles of the calf can assist in the movement. The primary muscle producing dorsiflexion is the tibialis anterior; the other anterior muscles (extensor hallucis longus, extensor digitorum longus, and fibularis tertius) can all contribute to the movement but are weaker dorsiflexors. Depending on the layout of the gas and brake pedals of the car and the position of the foot, if the heel remains in contact with the floor, the same foot can be inverted and plantar flexed to apply light pressure to the side of the brake pedal. Inversion is the result of contraction of the tibialis anterior, as well as the deeper muscles of the calf (flexor hallucis longus, flexor digitorum longus, and tibialis posterior).

Nerve injuries have been discussed in this chapter, but it is appropriate to discuss a lesion that could affect the activity just described. The effect of nerve lesions on movements depends on the extent of the injury. If only the branches to an individual muscle are involved, other muscles having the same function could produce the movement. If, however, a major nerve is injured, the movement could be greatly weakened or abolished. A lesion of the tibial nerve before it reaches the musculature of the posterior leg would eliminate innervation to all of the calf muscles. The ability to perform plantar flexion would be greatly impaired or possibly lost. The only muscles capable of producing plantar flexion that would be spared by such a lesion are the fibularis longus and fibularis brevis; their action, however, is very weak. The individual with a lesion of the tibial nerve would not be able to depress the gas pedal effectively through plantar flexion of the foot.

Activity: *Walking with an Injured Foot* Walking with an injured foot often requires redistribution of the weight of the body to avoid pain or additional trauma to the injured area. For example, if the big toe is injured, the foot can be turned to distribute the weight in that limb to the lateral side of the foot to avoid the normal contact of the big toe on the ground. To accomplish this, the foot is inverted and adducted. Muscles capable of producing these combined movements are the tibialis anterior, tibialis posterior, flexor hallucis longus, and the flexor digitorum longus.

If the injury is on the lateral side of the foot, the foot can be everted and abducted to redistribute weight to the medial side of the heel, ball of the foot, and big toe. Contraction of the fibularis muscles (longus, brevis, and tertius) and the extensor digitorum longus provides the desired movements of eversion and abduction of the foot.

Activity: *Inspecting the Plantar Surface of the Foot* For a person to look at a blister on the sole of his or her own foot, the foot must be raised and inverted to observe its plantar surface. Such placement requires movement of the foot at the ankle and intertarsal joints but also movement at the hip and knee joints. If the activity is started from a sitting position, the thigh is flexed at the hip and the leg is flexed at the knee (see Chapter 18 for muscles involved) to place the foot on the thigh of the opposite limb. To observe the plantar surface of the foot, the foot is plantar flexed at the ankle and inverted. Muscles responsible for plantar flexion are primarily the gastrocnemius and soleus. The tibialis posterior, flexor hallucis longus, and flexor digitorum longus can all assist with plantar flexion and also produce inversion of the foot because their tendons pass around the medial malleolus. The tibialis anterior can produce inversion while dorsiflexing the

Continued

foot; therefore, it does not contribute to movements in this activity. This can be verified by palpation of the muscle and tendon of the tibialis anterior while performing plantar flexion and inverting the foot.

REVIEW QUESTIONS

1 Define the following sets of opposing movements of the foot:
   a inversion-eversion
   b adduction-abduction
   c supination-pronation

2 What is the course of the small saphenous vein?

3 The triceps surae consists of which muscles?

4 Describe the arterial supply of the leg.

5 Which muscles insert on the calcaneus by way of the calcaneal tendon?

6 What is the origin of the extensor digitorum longus muscle? Describe in detail the insertion of the muscle.

7 What is the order of the structures (in relation to the medial malleolus) that pass deep to the flexor retinaculum at the ankle?

8 Describe the course of the tibial nerve in the leg, and include in the discussion its relationship to muscles and vessels in the area.

9 What are the primary muscles involved in plantar flexion? What muscles can assist in this movement?

10 What movement would best accentuate the following muscles and/or their tendons for palpation?
   a extensor digitorum longus
   b fibularis brevis
   c tibialis anterior

11 A pedestrian is hit by a car and suffers a severe injury to the lateral side of the leg at the knee joint. It is suspected that, among other problems, the common fibular nerve has been crushed. If this is true, what sensory deficits would be expected?

12 What is footdrop? Explain the anatomy of this condition.

13 What movements of the foot take place, and what muscles described in this chapter are involved, in the following activities?
   a standing on the toes to reach something on a shelf and then bringing the heel to the floor again
   b kicking a soccer ball with the medial surface of the foot
   c putting on a shoe

1 By palpation, while moving the foot, identify the tendons and indicate the movements performed to accentuate the tendons of the following muscles:

    a extensor hallucis longus

    b fibularis brevis

    c tibialis anterior

    d extensor digitorum longus

2 Demonstrate plantar flexion and dorsiflexion of the foot. These movements take place between which bones?

20 THE FOOT

CHAPTER CONTENTS

General Considerations

Bones and Joints

Superficial Nerves and Vessels

Fascia and the Plantar Aponeurosis

Plantar Muscles

Plantar Nerves and Vessels

Dorsum of the Foot

Movements of the Toes

The Ankle and Foot in Supporting Weight

Gait

GENERAL CONSIDERATIONS

The foot (pes) has been described in part in connection with the leg. The surfaces of the foot are referred to as *plantar* and *dorsal surfaces,* and its borders are referred to as *medial* or *tibial* and as *lateral* or *fibular.* The big (great) toe is the *hallux* and the little toe is the *digitus minimus* (littlest toe). The toes are numbered, beginning with the big toe.

BONES AND JOINTS

The individual bones of the foot have already been identified but should be reviewed, and their articulations should be studied, in preparation for the study of the soft tissues of the foot (Fig. 20-1; see also Fig. 19-2).

Bones

Calcaneus

The **calcaneus** (which forms the heel) projects posteriorly behind the ankle, providing leverage for the triceps surae, which inserts on its posterior end. The lower projecting surface of the posterior end, the *calcaneal tuberosity,* has rounded *medial and lateral processes* that support the weight transmitted to the heel. The upper surface has articular facets for the talus, the largest surface being on the *sustentaculum tali,* a medially projecting ledge of the calcaneus. The anterior end articulates with the cuboid bone.

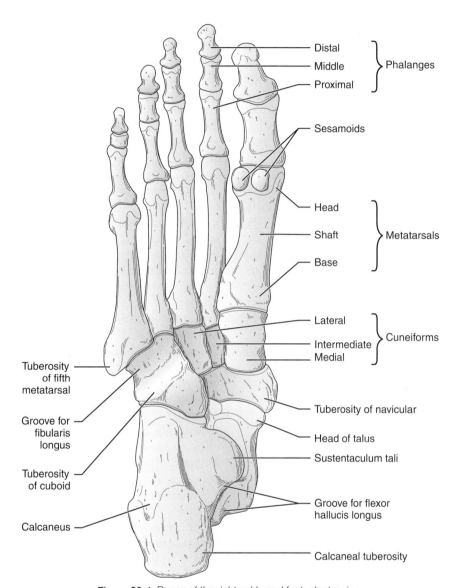

Figure 20-1 Bones of the right ankle and foot, plantar view.

Talus

The **talus** rests on the superior surface of the calcaneus. The superior, posterior part of the talus is called the *trochlea* (pulley), which is shaped somewhat like a short, transversely placed segment of a rod and is provided above and on its medial and lateral ends with an articular surface. The upper part of the articular surface articulates with the end of the tibia; the medial part, with the medial malleolus of the tibia; and the lateral part, with the lateral malleolus of the fibula. The anterior end of the talus is called the *head.* It articulates anteriorly with the navicular bone and inferiorly with the calcaneus and a ligament that stretches between the calcaneus and the navicular. The chief articulations between the talus and calcaneus are posterior to the head.

Navicular, cuneiforms, and cuboid

The remaining bones of the foot are smaller and less complex. The **navicular** lies anterior to the talus on the medial side of the foot. It has a concave proximal articular surface for the head of the talus and a convex distal articular surface with three impressions for the three cuneiform bones. Its lateral surface is attached to the cuboid by a heavy ligament.

The three **cuneiforms,** *medial, intermediate,* and *lateral,* lie anterior to the navicular. Their proximal ends articulate with the navicular through a synovial joint, and they also articulate with each other. The lateral cuneiform articulates with the cuboid, but the articular surfaces on their sides are small because the articulations are only in part through synovial joints. Heavy ligaments unite the rough parts of the adjacent surfaces. The distal ends are, however, largely smooth for articulation with the bases (proximal ends) of the metatarsals.

The **cuboid** has a proximal articular surface for the calcaneus, a distal one for the two lateral metatarsals, and a small medial one for the lateral cuneiform, to which it is also bound by a heavy ligament.

Metatarsals and phalanges

The **metatarsals** resemble the metacarpals of the hand. Each consists of a *base,* a *shaft,* and a *head.* Each **phalanx** also has a *base, shaft,* and *head,* although the middle and distal phalanges are such short bones that each of these parts is not very distinct. The bases of the metatarsals articulate with each other and with the cuneiform and cuboid bones; their heads articulate with the bases of the proximal phalanges, whose heads in turn articulate with the bases of the middle phalanges, and so forth. The distal phalanges, of course, end freely. There are often two **sesamoid bones** at the metatarsophalangeal joint of the big toe.

The arches and the transmission of weight in the foot

Ligaments hold the bones of the foot together so that in a normal foot, none of the parts between the posterior end of the calcaneus and the heads of the metatarsal bones transmits weight to the ground. Therefore, all the weight transmitted to the talus by the leg is in turn transmitted posteriorly and inferiorly to the posterior end of the calcaneus or anteriorly and inferiorly to the heads of the metatarsals (ball of the foot). In normal standing, the weight is divided approximately equally between the calcaneus and the ball of the foot. The curvatures of the plantar surface between these points form the two **arches** of the foot, a longitudinal arch and a transverse arch.

The **longitudinal arch** is obviously higher on its medial side than on its lateral side, and because of this, it is described as consisting of two parts (Fig. 20-2). Its *medial part* starts posteriorly with the calcaneus and proceeds through the talus, the navicular, and the three cuneiforms to the heads of the three medial metatarsals. The *lateral part* also starts with the calcaneus but proceeds through the cuboid to the heads of the two lateral metatarsals.

The **transverse arch** is more difficult to describe. The head of the talus and the navicular bone form the highest part of the arch on the medial side. The adjacent ends of the calcaneus and cuboid form the highest part on the lateral side. Anteriorly, the transverse arch gradually flattens out, and the heads of the metatarsals are all on the same plane and therefore all share in weight bearing. Posteriorly, the arch is directed not only laterally and inferiorly but also posteriorly and inferiorly, so that this part of the arch resembles a segment of a dome. When the two feet are together, the posterior ends of the two transverse arches form approximately a half-dome.

Studies of the way in which weight is transmitted through the foot indicate that this description is at best an anatomical one and that, functionally, the foot has a single, although admittedly complex, arch. Stresses on the arch are apparently not proportioned according to a medial, lateral, and transverse part; instead, they spread out in all directions through the foot. The stress at any particular point is proportional to its height on the curve, not to which curve it lies upon. This is similar to the pattern of stress placed on an arch built of stone or concrete.

Ankle Joint

The distal ends of the tibia and fibula have already been described in Chapter 19, as has the articular surface of the talus. It has been noted that the malleoli so grip the trochlea tali between them that the

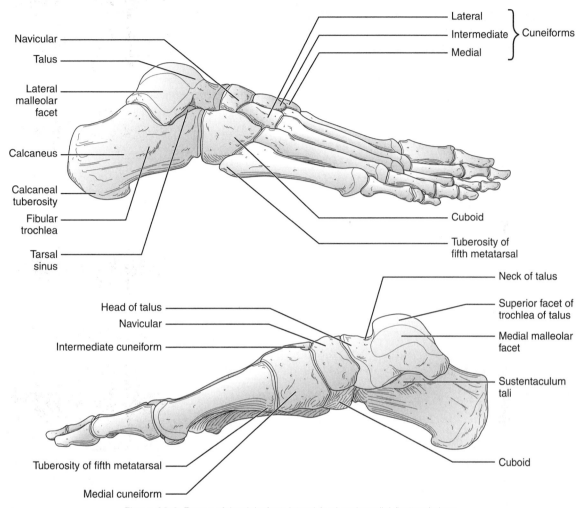

Navicular

Talus

Lateral
malleolar
facet

Calcaneus

Calcaneal
tuberosity

Fibular
trochlea

Tarsal
sinus

Lateral
Intermediate } Cuneiforms
Medial

Cuboid

Tuberosity of
fifth metatarsal

Head of talus

Navicular

Intermediate cuneiform

Neck of talus

Superior facet of
trochlea of talus

Medial malleolar
facet

Sustentaculum
tali

Tuberosity of fifth metatarsal

Medial cuneiform

Cuboid

Figure 20-2 Bones of the right foot, lateral *(top)* and medial *(bottom)* views.

ankle (talocrural) **joint** is primarily a hinge-type joint (Fig. 20-3). The joint is tightened still further when the foot is dorsiflexed, because the trochlea tali is slightly wider in front than it is behind.

Medial (deltoid) ligament
As is typical of hinge joints, the capsule of the ankle joint is thin anteriorly and posteriorly, but it is reinforced on its sides by special ligaments. The ligament on the medial side is called the *medial (deltoid) ligament* because of the way it fans out from the medial malleolus of the tibia (Fig. 20-4). It is composed of four parts: *anterior and posterior tibiotalar, tibiocalcaneal,* and *tibionavicular.* This important ligament

resists eversion of the foot. Weakness of the ligament, allowing eversion and throwing a greater weight than usual on the medial side of the arch, has been thought to be a predisposing cause of flatfoot.

Lateral ligament and ligament injury
The **lateral ligament** of the ankle joint consists of three parts that fan out from their attachments on the lateral malleolus: the *anterior talofibular ligament, posterior talofibular ligament,* and *calcaneofibular ligament.* These ligaments check inversion of the foot. They and the parts of the medial ligament are also so arranged that they check anteroposterior movement at the ankle joint.

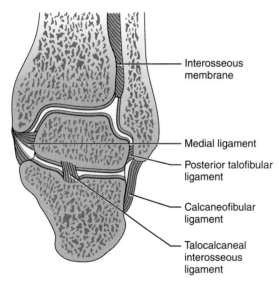

Interosseous membrane

Medial ligament

Posterior talofibular ligament

Calcaneofibular ligament

Talocalcaneal interosseous ligament

Figure 20-3 Frontal section through the ankle and subtalar joints. Ligaments, the interosseous membrane, and articular cartilages are highlighted in *color.*

Joints of the Foot

Ligaments

The tarsal bones are united by three sets of ligaments. Those on the dorsal surface of the foot are collectively called the *dorsal tarsal ligaments.* The ligaments on the plantar surface are the *plantar tarsal ligaments.* Those that stretch between adjacent surfaces of the bones and interrupt the synovial cavities are the *interosseous tarsal ligaments.*

The numerous individual ligaments are usually named according to the bones that they connect. There are dorsal and plantar cuboideonavicular ligaments, dorsal and plantar intercuneiform ligaments, and so forth. The dorsal ligaments, because they are on the top of the bony arch, are generally thin; the plantar ligaments, lying below the arch, and therefore acting as tie rods that support it, are much heavier.

Two of the plantar ligaments are particularly important and merit special comment. One of these, the *plantar calcaneonavicular ligament,* passes from the inferior surface of the calcaneus to the inferior surface of the navicular bone and, in so doing, forms a sling on which the lower surface of the head of the talus rests (Fig. 20-5; see Fig. 20-4). This ligament, by resisting downward movement of the head of the talus, helps support the highest part of the arch. Because it has been credited for some of the elasticity of the arch, it is frequently called the "spring ligament." The other, the *long plantar ligament,* lies more laterally, stretching between the calcaneus posteriorly and the cuboid and lateral three metatarsals anteriorly (see Fig. 20-5). This ligament extends for most of the length of the lateral part of the arch and is the chief support of this side.

Of the interosseous ligaments, the *talocalcaneal interosseous ligament* is particularly strong. One part of it partially fills the grooves on the adjacent surfaces of the talus and calcaneus and divides the joint between these two bones into two synovial cavities, one posterior to the ligament and one anterior to it (Fig. 20-6). There are also interosseous ligaments between the cuboid and navicular, the cuboid and lateral cuneiform, and the three cuneiforms.

Intertarsal joints

The **intertarsal joints** are the *subtalar, talocalcaneonavicular, calcaneocuboid, transverse tarsal,* and *cuneonavicular.* The slight gliding movements between the various tarsals are greatest at the complex subtalar and transverse tarsal joints.

The **subtalar joint,** between the talus and the calcaneus, has a synovial cavity both posterior and anterior to the *talocalcaneal interosseous ligament* (see Fig. 20-6); the anterior cavity is also part of the **talocalcaneonavicular joint.** The latter joint, the highest

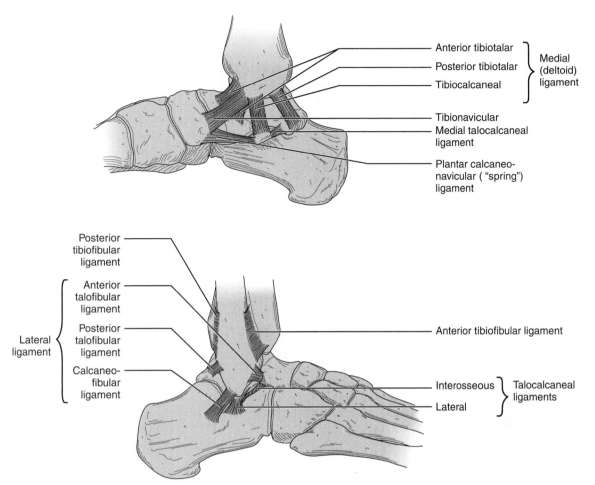

Figure 20-4 Ligaments of the ankle and subtalar joints, medial and lateral views.

in the foot, is closed inferiorly by the *plantar calcaneonavicular* ("spring") *ligament.* Lateral to it is the **calcaneocuboid joint.** The **transverse tarsal joint** is a name for the combined calcaneocuboid joint and the talonavicular part of the talocalcaneonavicular joint. Stretching across the foot almost transversely, these two joints work together (with the subtalar joint) in allowing the foot to move in inversion and eversion. The transverse tarsal joint also allows flexion and extension of the forepart of the foot, increasing or decreasing the height of the arch. The **cuneonavicular joint** lies, as its name implies, between the navicular and the cuneiforms, and it extends slightly between the cuneiforms and between the cuboid and the lateral cuneiform.

Tarsometatarsal and intermetatarsal joints

The **tarsometatarsal joint** of the big toe is a separate cavity. The corresponding joints of the second and third toes have a shared articular cavity. Likewise, the tarsometatarsal joints between the fourth and fifth toes and the cuboid bone also have a combined, single synovial cavity. Ligaments of the tarsometatarsal joints are the *dorsal* and *plantar tarsometatarsal ligaments* and the *cuneometatarsal interosseous ligaments.*

The **intermetatarsal joints** are small extensions from the tarsometatarsal joints. There is typically none between the first and second toes. *Dorsal* and *plantar metatarsal ligaments* and the *metatarsal interosseous ligaments* bind the metatarsals together.

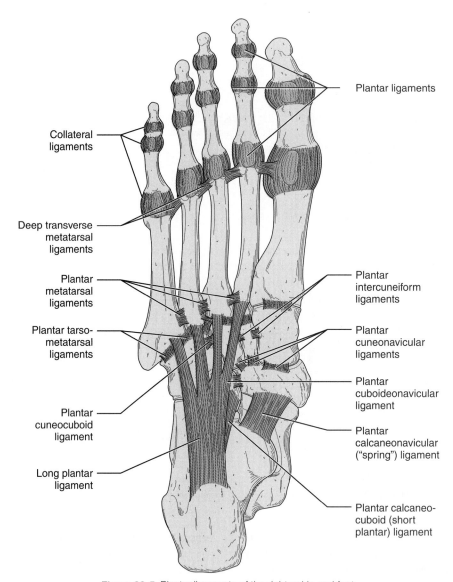

Collateral ligaments

Plantar ligaments

Deep transverse metatarsal ligaments

Plantar metatarsal ligaments

Plantar intercuneiform ligaments

Plantar tarso-metatarsal ligaments

Plantar cuneonavicular ligaments

Plantar cuboideonavicular ligament

Plantar cuneocuboid ligament

Plantar calcaneonavicular ("spring") ligament

Long plantar ligament

Plantar calcaneo-cuboid (short plantar) ligament

Figure 20-5 Plantar ligaments of the right ankle and foot.

Metatarsophalangeal joints

The **metatarsophalangeal joints** are condylar ones, usually maintained in a variable degree of dorsiflexion that varies with the height of the heel of the shoe. *Collateral ligaments,* similar to those found in the corresponding joints of the hand, are situated laterally. Dorsally, the extensor tendon reinforces the joint capsule. On the plantar surface are heavy *plantar ligaments* that complete the joint capsules and serve as gliding surfaces for the flexor tendons (see Fig. 20-5). The foot's plantar ligaments and metatarsal heads are connected to adjacent ligaments and heads by *deep transverse metatarsal ligaments,* corresponding to the similar ligaments of the hand. In the hand, there is no transverse ligament between the thumb and

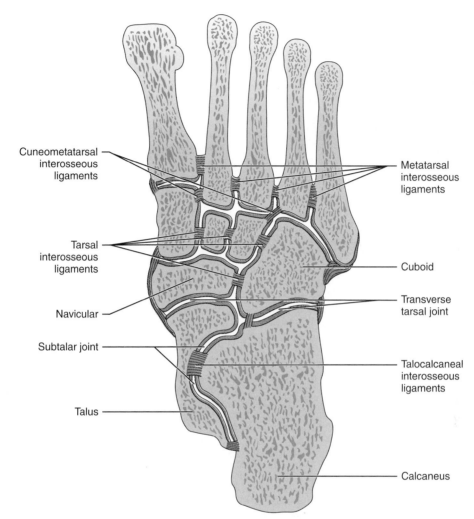

Figure 20-6 Section of the right foot, illustrating intertarsal joints, ligaments, and articular cartilages.

forefinger, which allows for greater mobility of the thumb. However, in the foot, the big toe, like the other toes, is connected to the second toe by such a ligament.

Interphalangeal joints

The **interphalangeal joints** are similar to corresponding joints in the hand. Each has *collateral ligaments* at the sides and a *plantar ligament* on the flexor surface, and the dorsal portion of the capsule is completed by the extensor tendon. The interphalangeal joints are hinge joints.

Innervation of the joints

The intertarsal and tarsometatarsal joints are innervated on their plantar aspects by branches of the medial and lateral plantar nerves. Branches of the deep fibular nerve supply their dorsal aspects. The more distal joints are innervated by the digital nerves.

Surface Anatomy

Of the bones and bony features of the ankle region and foot, the **medial and lateral malleoli** are useful landmarks and can easily be palpated. The posterior end of the **calcaneus** and the insertion of the **calcaneal tendon** can be palpated with no difficulty. Inferior and anterior to the medial malleolus, the **talus** and the **sustentaculum tali** can be felt on the medial border of the foot. Medially, the **navicular bone** can be palpated, but the **medial cuneiform** is difficult to identify distinctly. The **metatarsals** are palpable on the dorsum of the foot, especially toward their heads. The medial border of the **first metatarsal** can be easily followed distally to its head. The **base of the fifth metatarsal** is prominent on the lateral side of the foot; the **cuboid bone** lies just posteriorly but is difficult to palpate. The **phalanges** are palpable distally.

SUPERFICIAL NERVES AND VESSELS

The cutaneous innervation of the sole of the foot is through branches of the medial and lateral plantar nerves, the two terminal divisions of the tibial nerve. The **medial plantar nerve** is distributed in the foot in a manner similar to the distribution of the median nerve in the hand. It gives off branches to the medial side of the sole of the foot and breaks up into digital branches that supply approximately three and a half toes. The **lateral plantar nerve** corresponds in its distribution to the ulnar nerve in the hand, except that it has no dorsal cutaneous branch. The cutaneous distribution of the lateral plantar nerve is to the lateral side of the plantar surface of the foot and to the lateral one and a half toes. Frequently, a communication exists between the digital branches of the medial and lateral plantar nerves so that the nerve to the adjacent sides of the third and fourth toes is formed from both. This nerve and its branches are particularly subject to a painful tumor (neuroma) that necessitates resection of the portion of the nerve involved.

The skin on the medial side of the foot is innervated by the **saphenous nerve,** which continues to about the level of the metatarsophalangeal joint. Similarly, the skin on the lateral border of the foot is supplied by the **sural nerve.** The skin of the dorsum of the foot is innervated by both branches of the common fibular nerve, but the **superficial fibular nerve** innervates most of the area. This nerve innervates all the skin on the dorsum of the foot and toes except for a variable lateral part innervated by the sural nerve,

and the adjacent sides of the first and second toes, which are innervated by the **deep fibular nerve.**

Because superficial veins in the sole of the foot would be constantly subjected to so much pressure that they would be unable to function adequately, there is no large venous network on this aspect of the foot. Rather, the venous drainage passes quickly into the deep veins or around the borders of the foot and between the toes into the dorsal venous network. The veins on the dorsum of the foot are usually fairly obvious, and in addition to the network here, they form a venous arch on the distal part of the foot. This arch is continued along the medial border of the foot as the **great saphenous vein** and along the lateral margin of the foot as the **small saphenous.** The larger veins of the dorsal network unite the two saphenous veins on the foot or drain upward to end in either vein but primarily in the great saphenous vein.

FASCIA AND THE PLANTAR APONEUROSIS

The fascia of the dorsum of the foot is thin and merits no particular description. The plantar fascia resembles the palmar fascia of the hand but is even stronger and better developed. The **plantar aponeurosis** is essentially a strong, superficially placed ligament that extends in the middle part of the foot from the calcaneus to the toes. It plays an important part in supporting the arch of the foot. Like the palmar aponeurosis, the plantar aponeurosis sends slips to the digits. These slips help to reinforce the flexor digital synovial sheaths and attach around the tendons to the distal ends of the metatarsals and the bases of the proximal phalanges. The plantar aponeurosis blends laterally and medially with the thinner fascia over the short muscles of the big and little toes, and at these points, it sends a *medial* and a *lateral intermuscular septum* toward the first and fifth metatarsals, respectively.

The aponeurosis and its septa form a central compartment in the foot more complicated than, but somewhat comparable with, that in the hand. The compartment contains the flexor digitorum tendons and lumbrical muscles, as does that of the hand. Most of the muscles of the big and little toes lie similarly in medial and lateral compartments, as do those of the thumb and little finger.

PLANTAR MUSCLES

The muscles of the foot can be more easily described and dissected in layers than by compartments. The muscles and the long tendons of the toes form four layers.

Superficial Layer

The superficial layer is composed, medially to laterally, of the *abductor hallucis, flexor digitorum brevis,* and *abductor digiti minimi* (Figs. 20-7 and 20-8 and Table 20-1).

Abductor hallucis
The **abductor hallucis** has its *origin* from the medial process of the calcaneal tuberosity, the flexor retinaculum, and the medial intermuscular septum. Its *insertion* is on the tibial side of the flexor surface of the proximal phalanx of the first (big or great) toe. The medial and lateral plantar nerves and vessels, the continuations of the tibial nerve and posterior tibial vessels into the foot, pass deep to the posterior end of this muscle as they enter the foot. The abductor hallucis receives its *innervation* from the medial plantar nerve. Its *action* is to flex and abduct at the metatarsophalangeal joint. It usually functions better as a flexor.

Flexor digitorum brevis
The **flexor digitorum brevis** is the central muscle of the superficial layer. This muscle, the equivalent of the flexor digitorum superficialis in the upper limb, has its *origin* from the medial process of the calcaneal tuberosity and both intermuscular septa and gives rise to four tendons that run forward to the four lateral toes. (The tendon to the little toe is frequently missing; when it is present, it often arises from a separate muscular slip attached to the tendon of the flexor digitorum longus.) Each of the four tendons divides to allow a tendon of the flexor

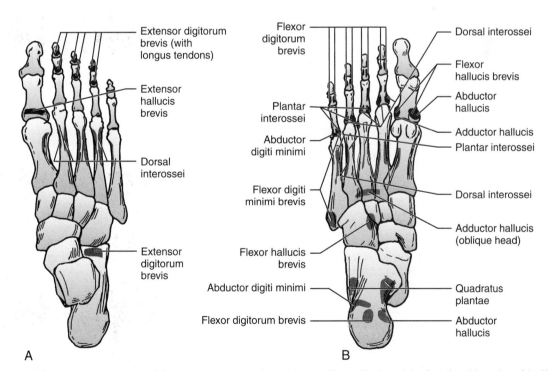

Figure 20-7 Dorsal **(A)** and plantar **(B)** views of the bones of the right foot, illustrating the origins *(color)* and insertions *(black)* of the muscles.

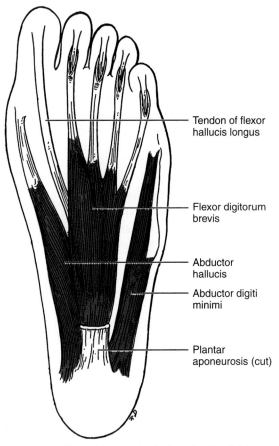

Tendon of flexor hallucis longus

Flexor digitorum brevis

Abductor hallucis

Abductor digiti minimi

Plantar aponeurosis (cut)

Figure 20-8 Superficial muscles in the sole of the left foot.

digitorum longus to pass through it, and each then unites again to go to an *insertion* on the middle phalanx of their respective toe. The tendons of the flexor digitorum brevis lie in digital synovial sheaths with those of the flexor digitorum longus. In contrast to those of the hand, none of these sheaths usually join the flexor synovial sheath situated at the ankle. The lateral plantar nerves and vessels run deep to the muscle toward the lateral part of the foot (above it if the person is in a standing position), but it receives its *innervation* from the medial plantar nerve. Its *action* is to flex the middle phalanges of the four lateral toes.

Abductor digiti minimi

The third muscle of the superficial group, the **abductor digiti minimi,** has its *origin* from the lateral process of the calcaneal tuberosity, the bone between the two processes, and a small part of the medial process, and also from the adjacent fascia. Its *insertion* is on the lateral side of the proximal phalanx of the little toe. The abductor digiti minimi may send a slip to the extensor tendon of the toe. On occasion, a portion of the muscle also attaches to the tuberosity of the fifth metatarsal to form an abductor of this bone (abductor ossis metatarsi quinti). The abductor digiti minimi receives its *innervation* from a branch of the lateral plantar nerve. Its *action* is to both flex and abduct the little toe.

Table 20-1	PLANTAR MUSCLES: SUPERFICIAL LAYER			
Muscle	**Origin (Proximal Attachment)**	**Insertion (Distal Attachment)**	**Action**	**Innervation**
Abductor hallucis	Medial process of calcaneal tuberosity; flexor retinaculum; medial intermuscular septum	Proximal phalanx of big toe (tibial side of flexor surface)	Flexion and abduction of big toe at metatarsophalangeal joint	Medial plantar nerve
Flexor digitorum brevis	Medial process of calcaneal tuberosity; medial and lateral intermuscular septa	Middle phalanges of lateral four toes	Flexion of middle phalanges of lateral four toes	Medial plantar nerve
Abductor digiti minimi	Lateral process of calcaneal tuberosity; medial process (small area); intervening surface of calcaneus; adjacent fascia	Proximal phalanx of little toe (lateral side)	Flexion and abduction of little toe	Lateral plantar nerve

Second Layer

The second layer in the foot consists partly of the *tendons of the long flexors of the toes, the flexor hallucis longus* and *the flexor digitorum longus*, and partly of the *quadratus plantae*, and *four lumbricals*, both of which are closely associated with the flexor digitorum longus tendon (Fig. 20-9 and Table 20-2).

Tendon of the flexor hallucis longus

The **tendon of the flexor hallucis longus** (see Chapter 19 for a complete description of this muscle) enters the foot posterior to the medial malleolus, lying in a synovial sheath that it loses at about the point at which it crosses above the tendon of the flexor digitorum longus. It usually gives off a tendinous

slip that joins the flexor digitorum and then runs anteriorly on the inferior surface of the flexor hallucis brevis muscle of the big toe. As it reaches the level of the metatarsophalangeal joint, it acquires a digital synovial sheath essentially similar to those of the other toes and to those of the fingers. Within this sheath, it goes to its *insertion* on the distal phalanx of the big toe.

Tendon of the flexor digitorum longus

The **tendon of the flexor digitorum longus** (see Chapter 19 for a complete description of this muscle) also enters the foot by passing deep to the flexor retinaculum and posterior to the medial malleolus, and it usually loses its synovial sheath in the proximal part of the foot. It passes superficial to the tendon of

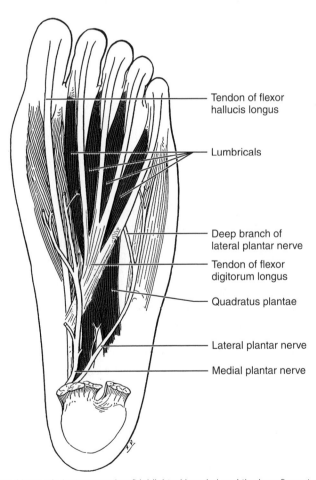

Tendon of flexor
hallucis longus

Lumbricals

Deep branch of
lateral plantar nerve

Tendon of flexor
digitorum longus

Quadratus plantae

Lateral plantar nerve

Medial plantar nerve

Figure 20-9 The second layer of plantar muscles *(highlighted in color)* and the long flexor tendons in the left foot.

Table 20-2	PLANTAR MUSCLES: SECOND LAYER			
Muscle	**Origin (Proximal Attachment)**	**Insertion (Distal Attachment)**	**Action**	**Innervation**
Quadratus plantae	Medial and lateral sides of plantar surface of calcaneus (distal to calcaneal tuberosity)	Lateral and posterior margin of flexor digitorum longus tendon	Aids in flexion of lateral four toes by modifying pull of flexor digitorum longus tendon	Lateral plantar nerve
Lumbricals	Flexor digitorum longus tendons	Expansions of extensor tendons of lateral four toes	Flexion of metatarsophalangeal joints; possible extension of interphalangeal joints	Medial plantar nerve to first lumbrical; lateral plantar nerve to second, third, and fourth lumbricals

the flexor hallucis longus and, as it nears the center of the foot, receives on its lateral border the insertion of the quadratus plantae muscle. As the tendon divides to go to the four lateral toes, the lumbrical muscles have *origins* from the tendons, just as corresponding muscles in the hand take origin from the flexor digitorum profundus tendon. On the toes, the tendons of the flexor digitorum longus enter digital synovial sheaths with the flexor digitorum brevis and pass through the split tendons of the brevis. The *insertion* of the tendons is on the distal phalanges of the toes.

Quadratus plantae

The **quadratus plantae** is a muscle that has no counterpart in the hand. Its *origin* is by two heads from the medial and lateral sides of the plantar surface of the calcaneus, distal to the calcaneal tuberosity, and its *insertion* is on the lateral and posterior margin of the flexor digitorum longus tendon just before this divides into its four terminal slips. Its *action* is to aid the flexor digitorum longus in flexing the four lateral toes, helping convert the pull of its tendon from a posteromedial one to a more directly posterior one. Unlike that of the flexor digitorum longus, its action is not affected by the degree of plantar flexion or dorsiflexion of the foot. *Innervation* is provided by the lateral plantar nerve as this crosses its lower surface.

Lumbricals

The four **lumbrical muscles** are essentially like those in the hand. They have *origins* from the flexor digitorum longus tendons and pass across the tibial side of the metatarsophalangeal joints of the lateral four toes

to *insertions* on the expansions of the extensor tendons on the dorsum of these toes. The *action* of the muscle is to aid in flexion of the metatarsophalangeal joints and, at least theoretically, in extension of the interphalangeal ones. The first lumbrical usually receives *innervation* from the medial plantar nerve, and the other three by the deep branch of the lateral plantar nerve.

Third Layer

The third layer of the plantar muscles is composed of the *flexor hallucis brevis, adductor hallucis,* and *flexor digiti minimi brevis* (see Fig. 20-10 and Table 20-3; see Fig. 20-7).

Flexor hallucis brevis

The **flexor hallucis brevis** has its *origin* from the cuboid bone, the lateral cuneiform bone, and the tendon of the tibialis posterior muscle. It divides into two "bellies." The *insertion* of one is on the medial side of the flexor surface of the proximal phalanx of the big toe, and that of the other is onto the lateral side of this phalanx. The medial part, at its insertion, fuses with the abductor hallucis; the combined tendons of insertion of the two muscles also attach to the medial sesamoid bone of the metatarsophalangeal joint of the big toe. The lateral part unites with the adductor hallucis, and the combined tendon of insertion has some attachment to the lateral sesamoid bone of the metatarsophalangeal joint. The *action* of the flexor hallucis brevis is to flex the proximal phalanx of the big toe. Its *innervation* is from the medial plantar nerve.

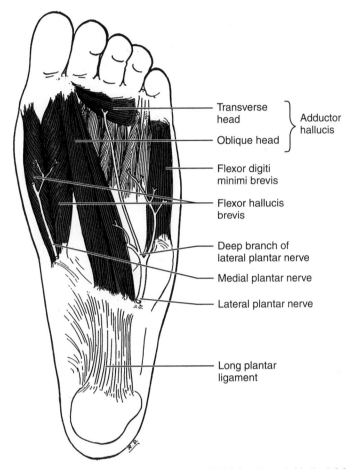

Figure 20-10 The third layer of plantar muscles *(highlighted in color)* in the left foot.

Adductor hallucis

The **adductor hallucis** resembles the adductor of the thumb, in that it has an oblique head and a transverse head. The oblique head, the larger of the two, has its *origin* from the bases of the second to the fourth metatarsals and the sheath of the fibularis longus tendon. The small transverse head arises from the capsules of the third, fourth, and fifth metatarsophalangeal joints and the intervening deep transverse metatarsal ligaments. The two heads unite and join the lateral head of the flexor hallucis brevis to have an *insertion* on the base of the proximal phalanx of the big toe. The muscle receives *innervation* from the deep branch of the lateral plantar nerve. Its *action* is to aid in flexion and adduction of the big toe. Like other short muscles of the big toe, the adductor

hallucis may send an expansion to the extensor tendon, helping in extending the distal phalanx.

Flexor digiti minimi brevis

The **flexor digiti minimi brevis** takes *origin* from the base of the fifth metatarsal. Its tendon blends with that of the abductor digiti minimi, and its *insertion* is on the plantar aspect of the base of the proximal phalanx of the little toe. Its *action* is to flex that proximal phalanx. *Innervation* is provided by the lateral plantar nerve.

Deep Layer

The fourth or deepest layer of plantar muscles consists of *seven interossei: three plantar* and *four dorsal* (Fig. 20-11 and Table 20-4; see Fig. 20-7). The

Table 20-3	PLANTAR MUSCLES: THIRD LAYER			
Muscle	**Origin (Proximal Attachment)**	**Insertion (Distal Attachment)**	**Action**	**Innervation**
Flexor hallucis brevis	Cuboid bone; lateral cuneiform bone; tendon of tibialis posterior muscle	Medial and lateral sides of proximal phalanx of big toe	Flexion of proximal phalanx of big toe	Medial plantar nerve
Adductor hallucis	Oblique head: bases of second to fourth metatarsals; sheath of fibularis longus tendon Transverse head: capsules of third to fifth metatarsophalangeal joints; associated deep transverse metatarsal ligaments	Base of proximal phalanx of big toe	Adduction and flexion of big toe	Lateral plantar nerve
Flexor digiti minimi brevis	Base of fifth metatarsal	Base of proximal phalanx of little toe (plantar surface)	Flexion of proximal phalanx of little toe	Lateral plantar nerve

interossei of the foot are essentially similar to the corresponding muscles in the hand but vary in two ways. First, they are arranged so as to abduct or adduct around the second rather than the middle toe; therefore, the midline of the foot passes through the second digit, rather than the third digit as in the hand. Second, all the interossei attach primarily to the proximal phalanges, rather than having strong insertions into the extensor tendons as do most of those of the hand.

Plantar interossei

The three **plantar interossei** have *origins* from the medial side of the third, fourth, and fifth metatarsals, respectively, and have their *insertions* on the medial side of the proximal phalanges of the corresponding digits. The *action* of the plantar interossei is to adduct the digits. *Innervation* is provided by the lateral plantar nerve.

Dorsal interossei

The four **dorsal interossei** each have two heads of origin. The first of these muscles has its *origin* from the adjacent surfaces of the first and second metatarsals and has an *insertion* on the medial side of the proximal phalanx of the second toe. The second takes *origin* from the second and third metatarsals and has its *insertion* on the lateral side of the

proximal phalanx of the second toe. The third has its *origin* from the third and fourth metatarsals, and the fourth takes *origin* from the fourth and fifth metatarsals; their *insertions* are on the lateral side of the proximal phalanges of the third and fourth toes, respectively. As in the hand, the *action* of the dorsal interossei is to abduct the digits. The muscles receive their *innervation* from branches of the lateral plantar nerve.

Surface Anatomy

Most of the muscles on the plantar surface are difficult to palpate because they lie deep to the skin, plantar aponeurosis, and heavy padding on that surface of the foot. The **abductor hallucis** and the **abductor digiti minimi** can be palpated on the medial and lateral sides of the plantar surface of the foot, respectively, as the big and little toes are abducted.

On the lateral aspect of the foot, the **tendons of the fibularis longus and brevis** can be felt when the foot is everted as they pass anteriorly from their position posterior to the lateral malleolus. The **tendon of the fibularis tertius** can be felt as it inserts on the base of the fifth metatarsal.

The surface anatomy of the dorsum of the foot is considered later in this chapter.

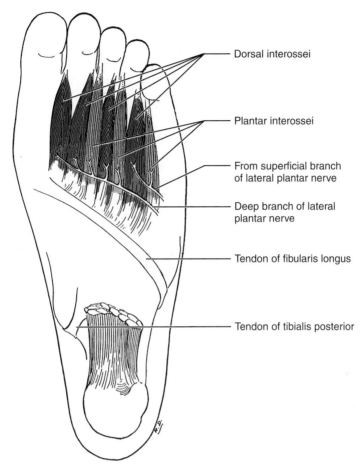

Figure 20-11 The deep layer of plantar muscles in the left foot. Dorsal interossei are illustrated in *dark color.* Plantar interossei are illustrated in *light color.*

Labels in figure:
- Dorsal interossei
- Plantar interossei
- From superficial branch of lateral plantar nerve
- Deep branch of lateral plantar nerve
- Tendon of fibularis longus
- Tendon of tibialis posterior

PLANTAR NERVES AND VESSELS

Nerves

As the tibial nerve passes through the flexor retinaculum at the ankle with the posterior tibial artery, lying between the compartments of the flexor hallucis longus and the flexor digitorum longus, it divides into medial and lateral plantar branches. These branches pass deep to the origin of the abductor hallucis to enter the foot and are distributed in the same manner as the median and ulnar nerves are in the hand (see Figs. 20-9 to 20-11).

The **medial plantar nerve,** comparable with the median nerve of the hand, innervates *skin of about three and a half digits* and also innervates the *flexor digitorum brevis,* the *abductor hallucis,* the *flexor hallucis brevis,* and the *first lumbrical* (see Fig. 19-15). In the hand, the median nerve supplies the equivalent flexor digitorum superficialis, abductor pollicis brevis, and flexor pollicis brevis (but the first two lumbricals instead of only one).

The **lateral plantar nerve,** comparable to the ulnar nerve, runs laterally deep to the flexor digitorum brevis, turns anteriorly, between this and the abductor digiti minimi, and divides into superficial and deep branches. In its course, this nerve innervates the *quadratus plantae* (not represented in the hand) and the *musculature of the little toe,* just as the ulnar nerve innervates the musculature of the little finger (see Fig. 19-15). The *superficial branch* of the nerve innervates

	Table 20-4	PLANTAR MUSCLES: DEEP LAYER			
Muscle	**Origin (Proximal Attachment)**	**Insertion (Distal Attachment)**	**Action**	**Innervation**
Plantar interossei	Medial side of third through fifth metatarsals	Medial side of proximal phalanges of same toes	Adduction of toes	Lateral plantar nerve
Dorsal interossei	Adjacent sides of metatarsals	Proximal phalanges: First interosseus muscle, to medial side of second toe; Second through fourth, to lateral side of correspondingly numbered toes	Abduction of toes	Lateral plantar nerve

approximately one and a half or more digits and may give off the muscular branches to the third plantar and fourth dorsal interosseous muscles. The *deep branch* runs transversely from the lateral to the medial side of the foot in close association with the plantar arterial arch. It innervates the *two or three lateral lumbricals, all the interossei not supplied by the superficial* branch, and *both heads of the adductor hallucis.* It corresponds very closely to the deep branch of the ulnar nerve in the hand, in that it innervates lumbricals and interossei and the plantar equivalent of the adductor pollicis. The minor differences are only that some interossei may be supplied by the nerve's superficial branch and that the nerve usually supplies three lumbricals.

Vessels

The posterior tibial artery also divides into medial and lateral plantar branches deep to the flexor retinaculum. The **medial plantar artery** is small and is distributed largely to the muscles of the big toe. Its superficial branch, however, helps supply blood to the skin of the medial side of the sole and sends tiny twigs distally along the digital branches of the medial plantar nerve, toward the toes. These join the metatarsal branches of the plantar arch but contribute little to the circulation of the toes.

The **lateral plantar artery** accompanies the nerve of the same name. It runs laterally and anteriorly at first deep to the abductor hallucis and then deep to the flexor digitorum brevis. It gives off a branch to the lateral side of the little toe and may also give off a twig that joins the metatarsal artery between this and the fourth toe. It then arches medially across

the foot, with the deep branch of the lateral plantar nerve, as the **deep plantar arch** (Fig. 20-12). The plantar arch is completed on the medial side of the foot by the deep plantar artery, a branch of the dorsalis pedis artery (see the following section) that reaches the plantar surface by passing between the two heads of the first dorsal interosseous muscle (as the radial artery does in the hand).

From the plantar arch, four *plantar metatarsal arteries* are given off. These run anteriorly and, after they receive small superficial branches from the medial and lateral plantar arteries, continue as *common plantar digital arteries,* short arteries, which are not labeled in Figure 20-12. Each common plantar digital artery divides into two *proper plantar digital arteries* (also termed *plantar digital arteries proper*) that supply blood to the toes. Between the heads of the interossei, the plantar arch is connected by *perforating branches* to the dorsal metatarsal arteries. Other perforating branches pass from the plantar to the dorsal vessels between the heads of the metatarsals or in the webs of the toes.

Surface Anatomy

The vessels and nerves of the plantar surface of the foot cannot be palpated, but the pattern of cutaneous innervation can be reviewed. The distribution of the **medial and lateral plantar nerves** can be recalled more easily by remembering that the medial plantar nerve has a distribution almost exactly comparable with that of the median nerve in the hand, and the lateral plantar nerve has a distribution comparable with that of the palmar portion of the ulnar nerve (see Fig. 19-15).

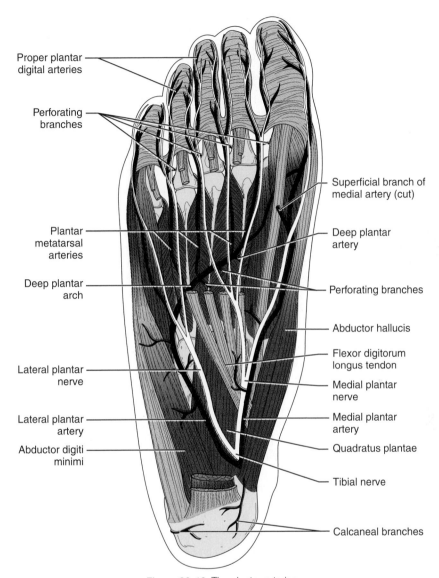

Proper plantar digital arteries

Perforating branches

Superficial branch of medial artery (cut)

Plantar metatarsal arteries

Deep plantar artery

Deep plantar arch

Perforating branches

Lateral plantar nerve

Abductor hallucis

Flexor digitorum longus tendon

Medial plantar nerve

Lateral plantar artery

Medial plantar artery

Abductor digiti minimi

Quadratus plantae

Tibial nerve

Calcaneal branches

Figure 20-12 The plantar arteries.

DORSUM OF THE FOOT

Muscles

In contrast to the hand, the dorsum of the foot contains only two muscles. They are closely associated at their origin. The lateral and larger one, the **extensor digitorum brevis** (Table 20-5), takes *origin* laterally from the superior (dorsal) surface of the calcaneus and divides into three tendons that run toward the second,

third, and fourth toes (see Figs. 19-8 and 19-9). Near the distal ends of the metatarsals, these short extensor tendons unite with the long extensor tendons of the corresponding toes. Sometimes there is also a tendon to the fifth toe. The *insertion* of the extensor digitorum brevis is with the tendons of the long extensor onto the middle phalanges (by the middle band) and distal phalanges (by the lateral bands). The second muscle, the **extensor hallucis brevis,** may seem to be simply a larger medial part of the extensor digitorum

Table 20-5	DORSAL MUSCLES			
Muscle	**Origin (Proximal Attachment)**	**Insertion (Distal Attachment)**	**Action**	**Innervation**
Extensor digitorum brevis	Calcaneus (dorsal surface)	With extensor digitorum longus tendons to middle and distal phalanges of second to fourth toes	Extension of second to fourth toes	Deep fibular nerve
Extensor hallucis brevis (often considered medial part of extensor digitorum brevis)	Calcaneus (dorsal surface)	Base of proximal phalanx of big toe	Extension of big toe	Deep fibular nerve

brevis and has been described as such. Its single tendon has an *insertion* on the base of the proximal phalanx of the big toe. It may send a slip to the tendon of the long extensor. The *action* of the extensor digitorum brevis (including the extensor hallucis) is to assist the long extensors in extension of the toes. Its *innervation* is from the deep fibular nerve.

Nerves and Arteries

The **deep fibular nerve,** after innervating muscles of the leg, passes onto the dorsum of the foot, where it innervates the *short extensors,* sends branches to the *intertarsal joints,* and ends as the cutaneous branch, already mentioned, to the *adjacent surfaces of the big and second toes.*

The **anterior tibial artery,** which gives off branches around the ankle, is continued onto the foot as the **dorsalis pedis artery** (see Figs. 19-10 and 14-3). This artery supplies small branches to the region of the tarsus, gives off the arcuate artery running transversely across the foot, and then ends by dividing into the deep plantar and the first dorsal metatarsal arteries. The *deep plantar artery* passes between the two heads of the first dorsal interosseous muscle to form, with the lateral plantar artery, the plantar arch. The *first dorsal metatarsal artery* divides into branches that supply both sides of the big toe and the medial side of the second toe. The *arcuate artery,* as it runs across the foot, gives off three more dorsal metatarsal branches that run forward to supply the skin of the digits. The *dorsal metatarsal arteries* are connected to the plantar arch and to the plantar metatarsal arteries by *perforating branches.*

The arcuate artery is often very small, and the perforating branches may be the chief source of blood to the dorsal metatarsal arteries. In about 3.5% of feet, the dorsalis pedis artery is not the continuation of the anterior tibial artery but is formed by the perforating branch of the fibular artery.

Surface Anatomy

On the dorsum of the foot, the short extensors lie deep to the long tendons of the muscles of the anterior compartment of the leg. The **tendons of the extensor digitorum longus** can be easily observed and palpated as the lateral four toes are extended. The **extensor digitorum brevis** can be palpated anterior to the lateral malleolus, just lateral to the tendons of the longus; it can be felt contracting when the toes are extended. If the foot is inverted and dorsiflexed, the **tendon of the tibialis anterior** can be felt as it courses to its insertion on the medial cuneiform and base of the first metatarsal. With extension of the big toe, the **tendon of the extensor hallucis longus** can be palpated lateral to the tendon of the tibialis anterior and then followed to its insertion.

Only a few of the vessels of the dorsum of the foot can be observed or palpated, but none of the nerves is identifiable. The **dorsal venous plexus** may be visible. This plexus connects with the **great saphenous vein,** which passes anterior to the medial malleolus, and the **small saphenous vein** lying posterior to the lateral malleolus (see Fig. 14-4). The pattern of superficial veins on the dorsum may be visible, and when the **dorsalis pedis artery** is in its proper position and of normal size, it can be palpated on the foot, where it lies between the long extensor of the big toe and that of the other digits.

MOVEMENTS OF THE TOES

Extension

Extension of the distal phalanx of the big toe is brought about by the *extensor hallucis longus,* and extension of the proximal phalanx, by the *extensor hallucis brevis.* The short muscles that sometimes attach in part to the tendon of the extensor hallucis longus—the extensor hallucis brevis, for instance—can help extend the distal phalanx when they attach in this way. Extension of the other toes is carried out by the *extensor digitorum longus* and the parts of the *extensor digitorum brevis* associated with each of these, except the little toe. These muscles, although they insert on the middle and distal phalanges, act primarily at the metatarsophalangeal joints, which are normally hyperextended and can be hyperextended still more. The distal phalanges are usually kept flexed by the pull of the flexors. Because the interossei of the foot, in contrast to those of the hand, have little insertion on the extensor tendons, they are largely ineffective in extension of the interphalangeal joints. Although the lumbricals do insert into the extensor tendons, they also have little effect.

Flexion

Flexion of the big toe is carried out by the *flexor hallucis brevis, flexor hallucis longus, abductor hallucis,* and *adductor hallucis.* Flexion of the remaining toes is carried out by the *flexor digitorum longus* and *flexor digitorum brevis,* assisted by the *lumbricals,* both sets of *interossei,* and the *quadratus plantae.* The fifth digit is also flexed by the *flexor digiti minimi brevis* and *abductor digiti minimi.* All these muscles act at the metatarsophalangeal joints, directly or indirectly. The interphalangeal joint of the big toe is flexed by the flexor hallucis longus. The *flexor digitorum brevis* acts on the proximal interphalangeal joints of the remaining toes, and the *flexor digitorum longus,* assisted by the *quadratus plantae,* is the flexor of the distal phalanges.

Abduction and Adduction

Abduction of the toes is brought about by the *dorsal interossei* and the *abductor hallucis* and *abductor digiti minimi.* **Adduction** is brought about by the *plantar interossei* and the *adductor hallucis.*

Innervation

Because the tibial nerve innervates all the muscles in the sole of the foot, tibial nerve injury may result in paralysis of them all. Their segmental innervation is from L5, S1, and S2. The extensor digitorum brevis, innervated by the deep fibular nerve, probably receives fibers from L5 and S1, just as do most of the anterolateral muscles of the leg (Table 20-6).

THE ANKLE AND FOOT IN SUPPORTING WEIGHT

The line of gravity of the body passes posterior to the hip joint and anterior to the knee joint, so that the weight borne on the extended limb helps keep these joints extended. Because hyperextension is resisted by ligaments, no sustained muscular effort is required to hold the pelvis, thigh, and leg together as a supporting pillar.

The situation is different at the ankle, however, where the line of gravity passes anterior to the normally dorsiflexed joint, so that the weight of the body tends to dorsiflex it even farther. Therefore, even quiet standing requires contraction of the plantar flexors of the foot, a function that the soleus normally performs. If there is any difficulty in keeping the balance, as there is in standing on one foot, practically all the muscles of the leg contract in order to stabilize the intertarsal and ankle joints and to prevent any inversion or eversion of the foot.

Because all weight is transmitted to the rest of the foot through the talus, the position of this bone on the arch of the foot is important. For one thing, the talus is not centered over the longitudinal midline of the foot but is somewhat to the medial side of this line. This means that weight is first transmitted to the medial side of the arch, which is also the highest side. Indeed, although weight thereafter spreads out in all directions through the arch, measurements

Table 20-6	NERVES OF THE FOOT		
	Muscle		
Nerve and Origin*	**Name**	**Segmental Innervation***	**Chief Action(s)**
Medial plantar L5 and S1	Abductor hallucis	L5, S1	Abduction-flexion of big toe
	Flexor hallucis brevis	L5, S1	Flexion of big toe
	Flexor digitorum brevis	L5, S1	Flexion of four lateral toes
	First lumbrical	L5, S1	Flexion of second toe
Lateral plantar S1 and S2	Three lateral lumbricals	S1, S2	Flexion of lateral three toes
	Quadratus plantae	S1, S2	Assists flexion of four lateral toes
	Flexor digiti minimi brevis	S1, S2	Flexion of little toe
	Abductor digiti minimi	S1, S2	Abduction of little toe
	Adductor hallucis	S1, S2	Adduction of big toe
	Plantar interossei	S1, S2	Adduction and flexion of three lateral toes
	Dorsal interossei	S1, S2	Abduction and flexion of second, third, and fourth toes
Deep fibular L4–S2	Extensor digitorum and hallucis brevis	L5, S1	Extension of toes

*A common segmental origin or innervation.

indicate that the medial side of the anterior end of the arch, represented by the head of the first metatarsal, bears approximately twice the weight that any of the other metatarsals bears. Furthermore, the medial position of the talus means that weight bearing produces a tendency toward eversion (pronation) of the foot, which results in placing greater weight than normal on the medial side and possibly in some flattening of the medial side of the arch. If eversion does occur, it can set up a vicious cycle. The subtalar joint is normally tilted slightly downward and anteriorly so that there is a tendency for the talus to slip in this direction. Eversion both increases the weight on the medial side of the foot and increases the tendency of the talus to be displaced medially and downward. This, in turn, distributes more weight to the medial side and encourages more eversion and flattening.

The fact that the talus is situated posterior to the middle of the longitudinal arch of the foot has less obvious consequences but does increase the strain placed on the arch. Because of the position of the talus, it would normally transmit to the calcaneus, through the shorter posterior end of the arch, 80% of the weight it bears and only 20% anteriorly to the heads of the five metatarsals. Even in quiet standing, however, the contraction of the posterior leg muscles pulls upward on the calcaneus (sufficiently

to redistribute the weight equally, rather than in an 80:20 ratio, between the calcaneus and the metatarsals). The arch is subject not only to the weight bearing on it but also to the pull exerted by the posterior muscles. This pull obviously becomes much greater when all the weight is shifted forward onto the ball of the foot and the heel is lifted from the ground. In fact, because of the short lever arm on which the triceps surae has to work, the pull must be sufficient to support twice the weight that is on the ball of the foot. Therefore, the strain on the arch of a weight-bearing foot in plantar flexion is very great, approximately three times the actual weight that the foot is bearing.

In view of the considerations just discussed, it is obvious that an arch that remains normal must be very strongly constructed. A fundamental consideration is the bony conformation: whether, for instance, the subtalar joint is slanted slightly more inferiorly and medially than usual. There have been varied opinions as to which soft tissues contribute to the support of the arch and to what degree. Extreme opinions have been (1) that the heavy plantar ligaments normally contribute no support whatsoever and (2) that they are the primary support of the arch.

Numerous experiments have shown that the plantar ligaments are indeed the primary support of

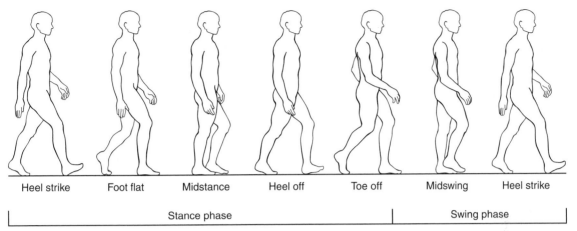

Heel strike   Foot flat   Midstance   Heel off   Toe off   Midswing   Heel strike

| Stance phase | Swing phase |

Figure 20-13 The gait cycle.

the arch. In quiet standing, the normal foot needs no other support, for the muscles of the leg and foot show only slight intermittent activity associated with small shifts in balance. When additional support is needed, as in standing on the toes or in walking, the short muscles of the foot become active. The support of the arch, therefore, comes from the plantar ligaments and, when necessary, the plantar muscles, which stretch along the arch like tie rods.

The long muscles seem to contribute to the preservation or destruction of the arch only in that they are responsible for keeping the foot properly balanced between eversion and inversion, for the normal distribution of weight over the arch. If the long muscles fail to do this, excess weight is placed on either the medial or the lateral side of the arch, which may be more than the ligaments can withstand without stretching, even with the aid of the short muscles. Although imbalance of the long muscles may lead to deformation of and pain from a normal arch, strengthening them by exercise cannot be expected to increase the support of the arch.

GAIT

Gait is the manner of walking. It involves not only movements of the lower limbs but also accompanying activities such as the usual rhythmic swinging of the upper limbs and the movements of the trunk. Only the involvement of the lower limbs is considered here.

Gait can be divided into a stance phase and a swing phase, each of which is initiated by a particular momentary activity. The **stance phase** begins with "heel-strike" and ends with "toe-off" and, therefore, is the time when the *limb is supporting weight.* The **swing phase** is initiated by "toe-off" and lasts until "heel-strike" and, therefore, is the time when the *limb is not supporting weight.* A **gait cycle** (Fig. 20-13) is the activity that takes place from heel-strike of one limb to the next heel-strike of the *same* limb. The stance phase occupies about 60% of this cycle; the swing phase, about 40%. In normal walking, the cycle is such that as one heel is making contact with the ground (heel-strike), the other heel is lifting off the ground (heel-off). During this brief period of time, both feet are in contact with the ground. This is called a period of *double support* (which occurs twice during each cycle). At all other times in the gait cycle, only one limb supports the weight of the body. As the pace of walking increases, the period of double support decreases, and in running there is no period of double support.

Stance Phase

The **stance phase** can be subdivided into different parts: *heel-strike, foot-flat, midstance, heel-off,* and *toe-off* (see Fig. 20-13). (Heel-off and toe-off are sometimes combined and together may be termed *push-off.*) For the most part, these terms provide an indication of the sequence of positions the foot goes through during the stance phase. Midstance, as would be expected, is in the middle of the phase when the weight of the body is over the supporting foot. The following account considers the stance phase of a limb that has just completed the swing phase. Keep in mind that as the stance phase is beginning in this limb, the other limb is initiating the swing phase.

At *heel-strike*, the thigh is partially flexed, the leg is slightly flexed at the knee (apparently in part to help absorb the shock of contact of the limb with the ground), and the foot is in a midposition (or neutral position) between dorsiflexion and plantar flexion. To avoid rapid plantar flexion of the foot during heel-strike, the muscles of the anterior compartment of the leg, particularly the tibialis anterior, contract. As the heel is beginning to make contact, the short muscles of the foot contract to help support the arches of the foot. As the stance phase proceeds toward the position of *foot-flat*, the weight is redistributed from the heel to the lateral side and ball of the foot. Just before heel-strike, the gluteus maximus contracts to promote extension of the thigh. (A person with a weak gluteus maximus may lurch backward at heel-strike to stop the forward movement of the trunk and produce a passive extension at the hip.) The quadriceps contracts to extend the leg after the foot makes contact. The hamstrings also contract, but this is usually interpreted as being primarily to prevent hyperextension of the leg. (If the hamstrings are paralyzed, a hyperextension deformity develops at the knee.)

As the cycle is proceeding to *midstance*, the anterior leg muscles cease contracting, and passive dorsiflexion of the foot then occurs as the weight of the body is shifted forward over the foot. The plantar flexors (primarily the gastrocnemius and soleus) contract to control this dorsiflexion and to initiate toe-off of the next cycle. During the midstance, the weight of the body is over the supporting limb, and the other foot is clear of the ground in swing phase. At this time, the gluteus medius and gluteus minimus of the supporting limb contract to prevent drooping of the unsupported side of the pelvis to keep the pelvis basically horizontal. If the gluteus medius and gluteus minimus are weak on the supporting side, lurching to the supporting side occurs, putting the weight more over the joint.

As the limb continues through midstance, the leg is maintained in extension, and the thigh begins to

hyperextend. Continued contraction of the triceps surae lifts the heel off the ground *heel-off*, and *toe-off* follows. If the triceps surae is paralyzed, or if the calcaneal tendon has been severed, toe-off can be accomplished to a lesser extent by extension of the hip produced by the gluteus maximus and the posterior hamstrings. (Initiation of toe-off can be passive. As the body leans forward, producing dorsiflexion of the foot, the posterior leg muscles can act primarily to check the forward movement of the body.)

Swing Phase

The limb involved in the swing phase is not supporting weight; therefore, the foot is off the ground. The swing phase begins at toe-off, and in this phase there is a period of *acceleration,* then *midswing,* and finally a period of *deceleration* in preparation for heel-strike.

Immediately after toe-off, the beginning of the swing phase involves almost simultaneous flexion of the thigh and leg, followed by dorsiflexion of the foot. These movements are necessary to enable the limb to clear the ground. Flexion of the thigh is produced by the tensor fasciae latae, pectineus, sartorius, and probably the iliopsoas; flexion of the leg is produced by the hamstrings (which may simply produce passive pull) and gravity. Dorsiflexion is mainly the result of contraction of the tibialis anterior. At this time, the limb is in the *acceleration period.* At *midswing,* the limb is "shortened" as much as possible by flexion at the hip and knee and dorsiflexion at the ankle to ensure clearance of the ground. After midswing, a period of *deceleration* follows to prepare the limb for heel-strike. The thigh (through contraction of the gluteus maximus) and knee (by contraction of the quadriceps) begin to extend. Much of the extension of the leg is passive, brought about by the forward swing of the limb. Therefore, if a person walks on level ground at an appropriate speed, the limb can be extended at heel-strike, even if the quadriceps is paralyzed. Under such circumstances, as the weight is shifted forward during the stance phase, the knee stays extended as long as the weight is centered anterior to the knee joint.

The foot is again maintained in a neutral position by the anterior leg muscles. Heel-strike then follows, and the stance phase of this limb is then initiated.

Running

In running, extension at the hip and knee is very powerful, and the triceps surae contracts strongly before the foot touches the ground, preventing heel-strike by transferring all the weight onto the ball of the foot (and in consequence, subjecting the arch to enormous stress). As mentioned previously, in running there is no period of double support, and, in fact, there are periods of no support in which neither foot is in contact with the ground.

REVIEW QUESTIONS

1 Describe the lateral ligament of the ankle joint. Which could potentially injure this ligament: forced eversion or forced inversion? Why?

2 What muscles make up the superficial layer of muscles on the plantar surface of the foot?

3 What is the action of the quadratus plantae muscle?

4 Describe the arrangement of the interossei in the foot. Which toe is used to define the midline or axis of movement within the foot?

5 The function of which muscles of the foot would be lost with a complete lesion of the tibial nerve just proximal to the ankle? Which muscles would be affected with a lesion of the deep fibular nerve?

6 Compare and contrast the innervation provided by the medial plantar nerve of the foot and the median nerve of the hand.

7 In a standing position where does the line of gravity lie in relation to the ankle joint and what effect does this have on the joint? What overcomes this effect?

8 What would be the effect on an individual's gait at the midstance phase if the gluteus medius and gluteus minimus muscles of the supporting limb were not able to contract? How might an individual compensate for this weakness or loss?

EXERCISES

1 On an articulated skeleton, identify the bones of the foot and the major bony landmarks and areas on each bone.

2 Demonstrate the pattern of sensory innervation to the skin of the foot.

SECTION 5 The Head, Neck, and Trunk

21 THE HEAD AND NECK

CHAPTER CONTENTS

Skull

Meninges and Brain

Facial Muscles

Orbit

Muscles of Mastication and the
Temporomandibular Joint

Muscles of the Tongue

Muscles of the Neck

Pharynx, Larynx, Trachea, and Esophagus

Nerves and Vessels

Surface Anatomy

SKULL

The bones of the skull can be divided into two groups, the *cranium* (cranial skeleton), which supports, surrounds, and protects the brain, and the *facial skeleton* (Fig. 21-1), which includes the mandible (lower jaw). The bones of the cranium are held together tightly by joints termed *sutures*. At these joints, there is virtually no movement. With the exception of the mandible, the facial bones are similarly united by sutures with each other and with the cranial bones. The mandible articulates with the skull by synovial joints.

Cranium

The roof of the skull (calvaria) is formed anteriorly by the unpaired **frontal bone** (see Fig. 21-1). The paired **parietal bones** are posterior to the frontal bone, and the unpaired **occipital bone** forms the most posterior portion of the skull (Figs. 21-2 and 21-3). The occipital bone surrounds the large *foramen magnum*, through which the lower part of the brain stem joins the spinal cord. The floor of the cranial cavity is formed in part by the occipital bone; the unpaired **sphenoid,** which lies anterior to the occipital bone; and a horizontal portion of the frontal bone that also forms the roof of the orbit (the cavity that contains the eyeball and its associated muscles, nerves, and

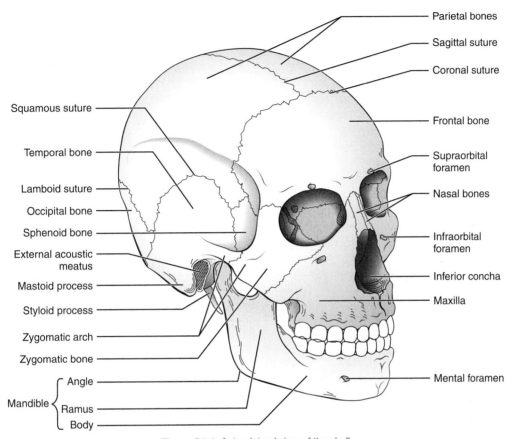

Figure 21-1 Anterolateral view of the skull.

vessels). The **ethmoid bone** forms a small portion of the floor of the skull anteriorly along the midline. Finally, a part of the **temporal bone,** its petrous part, forms a lateral part of the floor between the occipital and sphenoid bones.

Most of the bones of the floor and roof of the cranial cavity also extend laterally to form its lateral walls. The temporal bone, appearing on the side of the skull in the region of the external ear, contains the *middle ear cavity*. The part of the temporal bone behind the external acoustic meatus, the *mastoid process*, contains mastoid air cells that communicate with the middle ear cavity. The *petrous part* of the temporal bone contains the complex *inner ear*.

The ethmoid is an unpaired bone that forms part of the medial wall of each orbit and part of the lateral walls of the nasal cavity, and it helps form the septum

that separates the two nasal passages from each other. The part of the ethmoid bone forming the roof of the nasal cavity transmits the nerves concerned with olfaction (the sense of smell) to the cranial cavity. The ethmoid bone is a fragile bone containing large cavities, the *ethmoidal cells* or ethmoidal sinuses, which are filled with air. Other *paranasal sinuses* lie in the frontal, sphenoid, and maxillary bones and receive their names from these bones. All of the paranasal sinuses communicate with the nasal cavity and are subject to infection from this cavity.

Facial Skeleton

The paired facial bones include the **zygomatic** (cheek) **bones** that form the prominence of the cheek. Each has a projecting process that unites with a similar process of the temporal bone to form the *zygomatic*

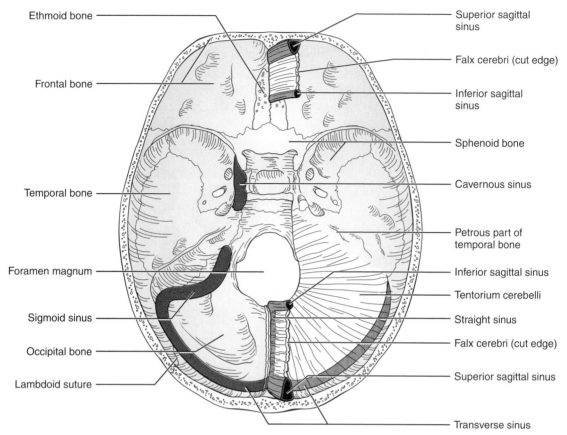

Figure 21-2 View of the interior of the base of the skull. All dura mater is omitted except for the anterior and posterior parts of the falx cerebri and the tentorium cerebelli on the *right.* The position of the transverse, sigmoid, and cavernous venous sinuses are shown on the *left,* and the transverse and straight sinuses are illustrated within the tentorium. The sagittal sinuses are evident at the cut edges of the falx cerebri. Note: There are numerous other venous sinuses in the cranium that are not illustrated.

arch. The zygomatic arch is also contributed to by the **maxilla,** the tooth-bearing bone of the upper jaw. The **nasal bones** form the bridge of the nose. A horizontal process from the maxilla of each side contributes to the *hard palate,* which separates the anterior part of the nasal cavity from the corresponding part of the oral cavity. The **lacrimal bones** are located in the medial wall of the orbit. Other bones of the facial skeleton include the **inferior nasal conchae** and the unpaired **vomer,** located within the nasal cavity, and the **palatine bones,** which contribute to the framework of the nasal cavity and form the posterior part of the hard palate.

The **mandible** is the unpaired bone of the lower jaw. It consists of paired *rami,* the vertically oriented

parts of the bone, and a heavy, tooth-bearing *body.* Each ramus is continuous with the body at the *angle* of the mandible. On the upper end of each ramus, two processes are present: a *coronoid process,* to which the temporalis muscle attaches, and a *condylar process,* which articulates with the temporal bone to form the *temporomandibular joint.*

Sutures

As noted previously, the majority of the bones of the skull articulate at sutures. Sutures are fibrous joints in which the surfaces of the bones entering the joint are united by fibrous connective tissue. At most sutures, the bones have irregular surfaces that interlock with

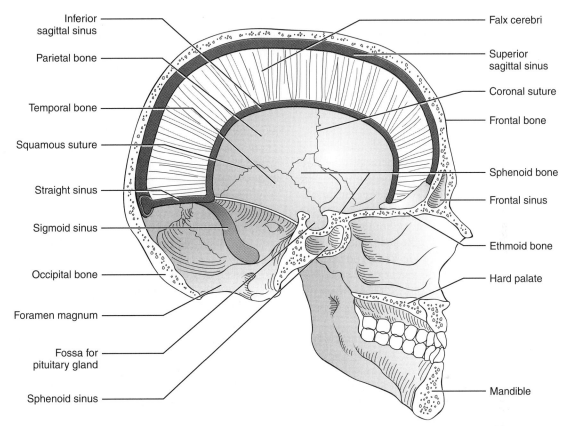

Inferior sagittal sinus

Parietal bone

Temporal bone

Squamous suture

Straight sinus

Sigmoid sinus

Occipital bone

Foramen magnum

Fossa for pituitary gland

Sphenoid sinus

Falx cerebri

Superior sagittal sinus

Coronal suture

Frontal bone

Sphenoid bone

Frontal sinus

Ethmoid bone

Hard palate

Mandible

Figure 21-3 Medial view of a skull sectioned parallel to the median plane. The falx cerebri is shown with the superior and inferior sagittal venous sinuses within its outer and inner edges, respectively; the straight sinus connects them posteriorly. The position of the sigmoid sinus is shown in the posterior part of the cranium as it passes downward to exit the skull as the internal jugular vein. (The tentorium cerebelli and the transverse sinus, with which the sigmoid sinus is continuous, are not illustrated.)

each other. The major sutures of the cranial bones are the: *sagittal, coronal, squamous,* and *lambdoid.* The **sagittal suture** is located in the midline, running in an anteroposterior direction between the parietal bones. The **coronal suture** marks the juncture between the parietal bones and frontal bone. Its plane of orientation is at a right angle to that of the sagittal suture. The **squamous suture** is apparent laterally between the temporal and parietal bones, and posteriorly the **lambdoid suture** lies between the parietal and occipital bones.

Fontanelles

In the newborn, the bones of the cranium, instead of being tightly joined by sutures, are united by membranes that are gradually converted into bone.

The membranes allow for considerable deformation of the infant's head during birth. In locations where more than two bones come together, the membranes are particularly extensive and constitute **fontanelles** (of which there are six), or "soft spots," in the baby's head. The largest is the *anterior fontanelle,* which is located where the originally paired frontal bones and the two parietal bones approach each other in the midline and is easily palpated. The *posterior fontanelle,* between the two parietal bones and the occipital bone, is also palpable but for a much shorter time because it closes earlier than the anterior fontanelle. In addition, there are two fontanelles on each lateral aspect of the skull: the *anterolateral fontanelle,* at the juncture of the parietal, frontal, sphenoid, and temporal bones, and the *posterolateral fontanelle,* located where the temporal, occipital, and parietal bones meet. All of the fontanelles are typically closed by around the end of the second year of life.

MENINGES AND BRAIN

Meninges

The brain lies within the cranial cavity and, like the spinal cord, is supplied with three meninges: the *dura mater, arachnoid mater*, and *pia mater*. An outer part of the **dura mater** is in contact with the skull and is actually the periosteum of the inner surface of the cranium (Fig. 21-4). Folds of the inner part of the dura mater also pass between the two cerebral hemispheres as the *falx cerebri* (see Fig. 21-3) and between cerebral hemispheres and the cerebellum as the *tentorium cerebelli* (see Fig. 21-2). In addition, there are several other smaller reflections of dura mater present within the cranial cavity.

In certain locations, the dura mater contains **cranial venous sinuses** that receive the blood from the brain (see Figs. 21-2 and 21-3). The unpaired *superior sagittal sinus* is situated in the midline against the skull (see Fig. 21-4) in the outer edge of the falx cerebri (where in the infant a needle can be easily inserted into it through the anterior fontanelle). The smaller *inferior sagittal sinus* lies in the free edge of the falx. These two sagittal sinuses are connected posteriorly by the *straight sinus.* Running laterally from the straight sinus, the paired *transverse sinuses* are continuous with the *sigmoid sinuses.* The sigmoid sinuses curve downward to leave the skull as the *internal jugular veins.* The paired *cavernous sinuses* are situated near the floor of the skull, on the sides of the body (central portion) of the sphenoid bone.

The superior sagittal sinus receives veins from the brain; it also receives the drainage of the cerebrospinal fluid from the arachnoid villi that project into this sinus. The transverse sinuses receive the blood from the superior sagittal sinus and also veins from much of the rest of the brain. The transverse sinuses and their continuations, the sigmoid sinuses, form the chief venous pathways leaving the skull. Although the cavernous sinuses are smaller than the other sinuses, they are significant because of their anatomical relationships with other structures. They lie adjacent to a very important part of the brain, the *hypothalamus.* In addition, the internal carotid artery and several cranial nerves pass through the cavernous sinuses.

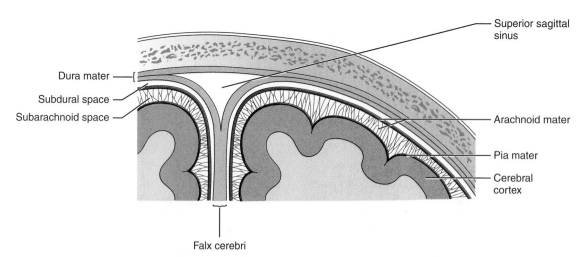

Dura mater

Subdural space

Subarachnoid space

Superior sagittal sinus

Arachnoid mater

Pia mater

Cerebral cortex

Falx cerebri

Figure 21-4 Coronal section through the cranial cavity, demonstrating the cranial meninges close to the midline of the roof of the skull. The two layers of the dura mater (dura) are illustrated. The subdural space is a potential space only, created by separation of the closely adherent arachnoid mater and dura mater (as by a subdural hemorrhage). The arachnoid mater (arachnoid) consists of a condensed layer adjacent to the dura mater and a trabeculated layer within the subarachnoid space.

The dura mater of the brain resembles that of the spinal cord in being a tough, fibrous membrane. Where venous sinuses are located, the walls of these sinuses consist largely of the dura mater and an endothelial lining. The dura mater and arachnoid mater are separated from each other by a potential space containing a film of fluid.

The **arachnoid mater** is more closely applied to the dura mater than to the brain (see Fig. 21-4), and it runs smoothly from one high point to another; therefore, it fails to dip into the folds of the cerebral hemispheres or to dip in any farther than the dura mater between the cerebral hemispheres and between those and the cerebellum. The **pia mater,** in contrast, follows exactly the outer surface of the brain, dipping in at every fold of this organ. Therefore, a considerable amount of space is left between the arachnoid mater and pia mater. This *subarachnoid space* is occupied by the cerebrospinal fluid, which helps cushion the brain and at the same time takes the place of the lymphatic system, which is lacking in the brain. In some locations, such as around certain parts of the base of the brain, the subarachnoid space is particularly large, and considerable accumulations of cerebrospinal fluid exist. These larger subarachnoid spaces are known as *cisterns.* The largest of these, the *cisterna magna* or *cerebellomedullary cistern,* lies between the lower surface of the cerebellum and the posterior surface of the medulla.

FUNCTIONAL/CLINICAL NOTE 21-1

It is possible to insert needles into the cisterna magna, for the purpose of obtaining cerebrospinal fluid or to measure the pressure of this fluid, without injuring delicate nerve structures that lie immediately adjacent to it.

Brain

The brain consists of several parts. The **cerebral hemispheres** fill a large part of the cranial cavity. Their surfaces are arranged in numerous convolutions, or *gyri.* The smaller **cerebellum,** which also has numerous but smaller folds of its outer layers, lies in the posteroinferior part of the cranial cavity. More centrally placed are the **diencephalon** and the **brainstem** (Fig. 21-5). The latter is continuous with the spinal cord through the foramen magnum. The cerebral hemispheres and the cerebellum, instead of having all their nerve cell bodies buried close to their centers, also have layers of cell bodies, *gray matter,* on their surfaces. This outer layer of gray matter is termed the *cerebral cortex* (meaning "bark") or *pallium* (meaning "cloak"). In the brainstem, however, the arrangement of cells and fibers is essentially like that in the spinal cord: The outside is composed of *white matter,* which is made up mainly of nerve fibers, and the gray matter lies deeper.

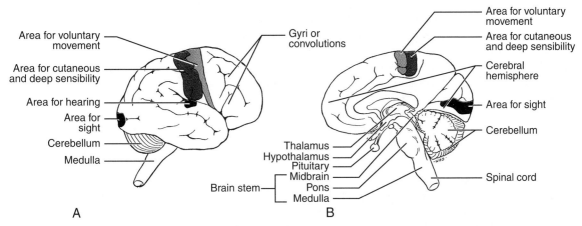

Figure 21-5 Illustrations of a brain sectioned on a median plane, showing its major structures and cortical areas. **A,** Lateral view. **B,** Medial view.

Because the brain is derived from a hollow tube, its various parts contain cavities within them. The largest cavities lie within the cerebral hemispheres and are known as the *lateral ventricles* of the brain. Vascular folds, called *choroid plexuses,* project into the lateral ventricles and are the chief source of cerebrospinal fluid. This fluid circulates downward through other cavities or ventricles to escape into the subarachnoid space at about the junction of the brain and spinal cord.

Cerebral hemispheres

The **cerebral hemispheres** are the parts of the brain concerned with recognition of sensations, initiation of voluntary movements, and the intricate mental processes involved in memory, judgment, and interpretation. The nerve cells have an almost infinite number of connections with lower centers, with the other cerebral cortex, and with both their close and distant neighbors in the same cortex. Different parts of the cortex have different functions. The locations of the parts having the functions of initiating voluntary movement (motor cortex) or appreciating sensations of several kinds are shown in Figure 21-5. Injuries to the cortex may or may not involve one or more of these cortical areas. Furthermore, because the areas are relatively large, injuries may involve only a part of one area, producing, for instance, paralysis or loss of sensation of a limited part of the body or partial loss of sight.

Certain masses of gray matter that lie deeper within the cerebral hemispheres are sometimes categorized together as the basal ganglia. These include, among other structures, the *caudate nucleus, putamen,* and *globus pallidus.* (*Corpus striatum* has been used as a term that includes all three of these structures.) The putamen and globus pallidus can be categorized together as the *lentiform nucleus.* These structures are important parts of the extrapyramidal motor system (see Chapter 13). Although they do not send fibers directly into the spinal cord, they send nerve impulses to various centers in the brain stem that do give rise to extrapyramidal fibers, and they also send impulses to the cerebral cortex. They play a role in helping to govern voluntary movements.

FUNCTIONAL/CLINICAL NOTE 21-2

Lesions of the basal ganglia, or of other extrapyramidal centers with which it is closely connected, are typically associated with an increased contraction of all muscles (rigidity), which makes movements difficult, and with some type of abnormal, unwilled movement. *Parkinsonism* (*Parkinson disease* or *paralysis agitans*), in which muscular rigidity and rhythmic involuntary movements are combined, is one of the better known syndromes associated with disease of the extrapyramidal system.

On the inner surface of the lentiform nucleus, separating this nucleus posteriorly from the thalamus and anteriorly from the caudate nucleus, is a very heavy bundle of fibers known as the *internal capsule.* The internal capsule contains almost all the fibers that are either going to the cerebral cortex or leaving it, except those that go from one cortex to the other through the *corpus callosum* (a heavy bundle of fibers connecting the cerebral hemispheres).

FUNCTIONAL/CLINICAL NOTE 21-3

Because sensory and motor fibers of the corpus callosum are so closely packed together in the internal capsule, a lesion of corpus callosum unlike one of the cortex, is likely to cause both paralysis and loss of sensation over one entire side of the body.

Cerebellum

The **cerebellum,** lying dorsal to the pons and an upper portion of the medulla of the brain stem (see next section), is concerned primarily with helping control voluntary movement. It receives impulses from many sources but chiefly from muscles and from the cerebral cortex. Unlike the cerebral cortex, the cerebellar cortex has nothing to do with sensation. The cerebellum helps to control voluntary movement both through impulses that it sends back to the cerebral cortex and through others that it sends to extrapyramidal centers in the brain stem.

FUNCTIONAL/CLINICAL NOTE 21-4

Damage to the cerebellum may affect primarily the ability to keep the trunk balanced, but more often, it affects movements of the limbs. Without the influence of the cerebellum, the muscles of the limb lack the coordination in sequence and strength of contraction necessary to produce a smooth movement, so that there is tremor on attempting to move the limb; difficulty in carrying out precise movements, such as touching the tip of the nose with a finger; and difficulty in carrying out rapid movements that involve alternating use of two different muscle groups (e.g., pronation and supination). Lesions of the cerebellum affect the same side of the body, instead of the opposite side, as cerebral cortical lesions do.

Diencephalon

The **diencephalon** consists of several parts, two of which are the *thalamus* and *hypothalamus*. The large paired *thalami* receive incoming sensory impulses, integrate the impulses in complex patterns, and forward them to the cerebral hemispheres. The *hypothalamus*, an important center of reflex action, is especially concerned with reflexes involving the autonomic nervous system and correlations between the autonomic and the voluntary nervous system, such as the maintenance of body temperature. The hypothalamus also governs the release of hormones from the pituitary gland (hypophysis).

Brainstem

The **brainstem** is made up of the midbrain, pons, and myelencephalon (medulla oblongata). The *midbrain* serves as a center for reflexes involving the eye and ear, but much of it consists of fibers passing to or from higher centers. The *pons* is the segment of brainstem below the midbrain. It gets its name, which means "bridge," from the heavy bundle of transverse fibers on its ventral surface that go to the cerebellum and therefore seem to connect the two sides of the cerebellum (they are really a connection from the cerebral cortex to the cerebellum). Both the pons and the *myelencephalon (medulla oblongata),* which lies inferior to the pons, transmit large ascending and descending tracts and contain the nuclei of various cranial nerves. They are also important sources of extrapyramidal fibers to the spinal cord. The various centers giving rise to these latter fibers (reticulospinal, vestibulospinal) are in turn under the influence of higher, extrapyramidal centers. Besides those features just mentioned, the myelencephalon contains various cell groups or combinations of groups, usually called *centers*, that are concerned with the control of certain vital functions such as blood pressure, cardiac rate, and respiration. On each side of the ventral midline of the myelencephalon, the corticospinal fibers form a prominent projection known as a *pyramid*. This accounts for the alternative name, the *pyramidal tracts,* to the corticospinal tracts and is the anatomical basis for distinguishing between pyramidal and extrapyramidal motor fibers.

Blood Supply of the Brain

The brain receives its blood supply from the paired vertebral and internal carotid arteries (Fig. 21-6). The **vertebral arteries,** branches of the subclavian arteries at the base of the neck, run up in a deep position in the neck, through the transverse foramina in the transverse processes of the upper six cervical vertebrae. They penetrate the posterior atlanto-occipital membrane to enter the vertebral canal, pass upward through the foramen magnum, and unite on the anterior surface of the medulla to form the **basilar artery.** From the vertebral and basilar arteries, vessels are given off to the cerebellum, myelencephalon, and spinal cord and to the pontine region of the brain. The basilar artery ends by dividing into two *posterior cerebral arteries.* These arteries are distributed to the lower part of the medial surfaces of the cerebral hemispheres and to the inferior surfaces of the hemispheres. Close to its origin from the basilar artery, each vessel receives a posterior communicating branch that unites it to the internal carotid arteries.

The **internal carotid arteries** enter the cranial cavity through foramina in the cranial floor and pass

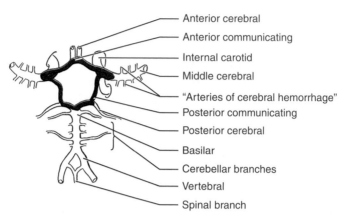

- Anterior cerebral
- Anterior communicating
- Internal carotid
- Middle cerebral
- "Arteries of cerebral hemorrhage"
- Posterior communicating
- Posterior cerebral
- Basilar
- Cerebellar branches
- Vertebral
- Spinal branch

Figure 21-6 The cerebral arterial circle *(highlighted in color)* and other arteries at the base of the brain.

through the cavernous sinuses. They give off large *middle cerebral arteries* that are distributed to most of the lateral surfaces of the cerebral hemispheres. Smaller *anterior cerebral arteries* also arise from the internal carotids and are distributed to the upper portions of the medial surfaces of the hemispheres. The internal carotid arteries are connected by the *posterior communicating arteries* to the posterior cerebral arteries and, therefore, to the basilar artery. An anterior communicating artery connects the anterior cerebral arteries to each other. A complete "circle" of arteries (really a hexagon), called the **cerebral arterial circle (circle of Willis),** is formed at the base of the brain. A knowledge of the detailed distribution of the various vessels just mentioned, and of other small but important branches, is of great importance to neurologists and neurosurgeons.

FUNCTIONAL/CLINICAL NOTE 21-5

Certain small branches from the middle cerebral artery and the arterial circle supply the internal capsule with its ascending and descending tracts connecting to the cerebral hemispheres. These vessels have no free anastomoses with other vessels, and therefore their occlusion leads to damage to the function of some or most of these pathways, resulting in the more common type of "stroke." Because of the relative frequency with which these arteries are involved when vascular accidents occur in the brain, these vessels are known as the *arteries of cerebral hemorrhage*. This should not be interpreted, however, to mean that all cerebral hemorrhages or all strokes result from damage to these specific vessels.

The venous drainage of the brain is by numerous, mostly unnamed, veins that in general run into the nearest cranial venous sinuses. The veins from the convexity of the cerebral hemispheres pass into the superior sagittal sinus, those from posterior parts of the inferior surfaces of the hemispheres and from the upper surface of the cerebellum pass into the transverse sinuses, and so forth.

FACIAL MUSCLES

The facial muscles differ from most muscles in that, instead of moving one bone on another, they move primarily skin. Although many have some attachment to the bones of the face, their insertions are chiefly into the skin. Because of their effects on facial expression, they are sometimes known as the **muscles of facial expression** or **mimetic muscles.**

The facial muscles may be divided into four groups: one group around the mouth, a second around the nose, a third around the eye and forehead, and a fourth around the ear (Fig. 21-7). A single muscle, the platysma, forms a fifth group, which, although it lies chiefly in the neck rather than in the face, really belongs to the facial group.

The paired muscles around the mouth include the **depressor anguli oris** and the **depressor labii inferioris,** which pull the corner of the mouth and lower lip downward, respectively; the **risorius** and the two **zygomaticus muscles,** which pull the corners of the mouth laterally (for the risorius) and laterally and upward (for the zygomaticus muscles); and the **levator labii superioris** and the **levator anguli oris,** which elevate the upper lip and corner of the mouth,

respectively. The **orbicularis oris** encircles the mouth and closes it or puckers the lips, as for a kiss.

The **buccinator** muscle forms the muscular part of the cheek. By contracting, it prevents food from collecting in the space between the cheeks and the teeth. The buccinator is used in such actions as swallowing and blowing wind instruments.

The muscles connected with the nose are primarily compressors, depressors, or dilators of the nares (external openings of the nose). They are small and vary considerably in their development.

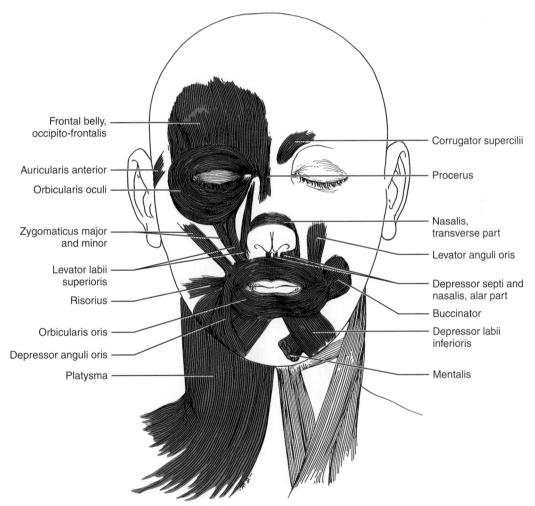

Frontal belly, occipito-frontalis
Corrugator supercilii
Auricularis anterior
Procerus
Orbicularis oculi
Nasalis, transverse part
Zygomaticus major and minor
Levator anguli oris
Levator labii superioris
Depressor septi and nasalis, alar part
Risorius
Buccinator
Orbicularis oris
Depressor labii inferioris
Depressor anguli oris
Mentalis
Platysma

Figure 21-7 Muscles of facial expression. The more superficial ones are shown on the right side of the face, the deeper ones on the left. The medial muscle of the two labeled *levator labii superioris* is also a levator of part of the nose; the muscles together are called the *levator labii superioris alaeque nasi*. The platysma is included on this figure because, like the facial muscles, it is innervated by the facial nerve and because it blends with the facial muscles around the mandible.

The **orbicularis oculi,** a broad muscle that surrounds the orbit and extends into both upper and lower eyelids, is responsible for closing the eyelids. The upper eyelid is raised by a muscle lying within the orbit the levator palpebrae superioris (see the following "Orbit" section).

One of the muscles of the forehead is the **frontalis** (the frontal belly of the occipitofrontalis), which runs downward from the scalp to the skin above the orbit. When it contracts, it wrinkles the forehead transversely. Another muscle, the **corrugator supercilii,** produces the small vertical folds between the eyebrows that are associated with a "worried look." Because the frontalis muscle attaches to the scalp, it and a corresponding scalp muscle in the occipital region, the **occipitalis** (the occipital belly of the occipitofrontalis), can move the scalp posteriorly and anteriorly.

There are several small muscles connected with the ears, so placed that they may move the ears anteriorly, upward, or posteriorly such as in "wiggling the ears." These muscles are rudimentary in humans and are not typically subject to voluntary control in most individuals.

The **platysma** muscle lies in the superficial fascia of the neck, extending from the upper part of the thorax to the mandible, where its fibers interlace with the musculature around the mouth. This muscle draws the corners of the mouth and lower lip downward and laterally, as in an expression of horror. Taking its fixed point from above, it tightens the superficial fascia of the neck. Because the platysma lies just under the skin, its vertically oriented fibers can easily be visualized when the muscle contracts.

The entire group of facial muscles, including the platysma, receives *innervation* from branches of the facial nerve (cranial nerve VII). The **facial nerve** rounds the posterior aspect of the ramus of the mandible, passes through the parotid gland, and branches out to reach all the muscles of the face. Interruption of this nerve as a whole produces a unilateral facial paralysis, or *Bell palsy* (see "Cranial Nerves" section later in this chapter).

ORBIT

The eyeball is moved by a number of muscles, all of which lie within the orbit (Fig. 21-8). They are divided into four rectus (meaning straight) muscles and two oblique muscles according to the way in which they insert on the eyeball. The **superior, inferior, medial,** and **lateral recti** direct the pupil upward, downward, medially, and laterally, respectively. The **superior oblique** directs the pupil downward and laterally, and the **inferior oblique** directs it upward and laterally; the two muscles together tend to overcome the slight medial pull exerted by the superior and inferior recti. All these muscles, with the exception of the inferior oblique, arise from or close to a tendinous ring placed at the apex (posterior end) of the orbit. The inferior oblique arises more anteriorly, from the floor of the orbit.

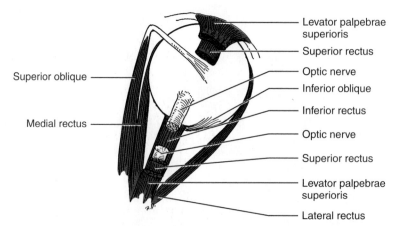

Superior oblique

Medial rectus

Levator palpebrae superioris

Superior rectus

Optic nerve

Inferior oblique

Inferior rectus

Optic nerve

Superior rectus

Levator palpebrae superioris

Lateral rectus

Figure 21-8 Muscles of the orbit. Parts of the levator palpebrae superioris, superior rectus, and optic nerve are omitted. The back of the eyeball with its attached portion of optic nerve has been rotated up and forward.

In addition to these muscles, the orbit contains the **levator palpebrae superioris,** levator of the upper eyelid. This muscle works in conjunction with the superior rectus, so that as the pupil is turned upward, the eyelid is raised further. It is attached to the upper eyelid both through tendinous fibers and through a smooth muscle that, by its contraction, which is controlled by sympathetic innervation, can open the eyelid even further than by the action produced by the levator.

Three cranial nerves supply the voluntary muscles of the orbit. *Innervation* to the superior oblique muscle is provided by the trochlear nerve (cranial nerve IV). The lateral rectus is innervated by the abducens nerve (cranial nerve VI), and the remaining muscles of the orbit are innervated by the oculomotor nerve (cranial nerve III). The oculomotor nerve also brings into the orbit parasympathetic nerve fibers that synapse in the *ciliary ganglion.* (The ganglion is about the size of the head of a pin and is located between the optic nerve and the lateral rectus muscle.) The postganglionic fibers given off by the ciliary ganglion produce constriction of the pupil of the eye and accommodation of the lens for near vision. Sympathetic fibers derived from the plexus on the internal carotid artery also innervate the eye, to produce dilation of the pupil.

In addition to the three nerves supplying ocular muscles, the *optic nerve,* which is the large nerve of sight, occupies a prominent position in the orbit. The branches of the ophthalmic division of the trigeminal nerve (cranial nerve V) pass through the orbit in their course toward the face, and the maxillary division of the trigeminal nerve runs for some distance in the floor of the orbit.

MUSCLES OF MASTICATION AND THE TEMPOROMANDIBULAR JOINT

Muscles

There are four major muscles involved with the process of chewing food or mastication. Of these muscles, the *masseter* and *temporalis* are largely superficial, while the *lateral pterygoid* and *medial pterygoid* lie deep to the mandible (Figs. 21-9 and 21-10 and Table 21-1); all of the muscles insert onto the mandible.

The **masseter** has its *origin* from the zygomatic arch and lies superficial to the ramus of the mandible. Fibers of its superficial head are inclined downward and slightly posteriorly, while those of its deep head are oriented more vertically (see Fig. 21-9). The *insertion* is onto the ramus and angle of the mandible.

The **temporalis** takes *origin* from much of the lateral aspect of the skull in front of and above the external ear. Its anterior fibers are vertically oriented, whereas its posterior fibers are horizontally oriented. The muscle fibers pass deep to the zygomatic arch and converge to a tendon that has its *insertion* onto the coronoid process, the anterior of the two projections on the superior border of the ramus of the mandible, and the medial surface of the anterior part of the ramus of the mandible.

The **lateral pterygoid** has two heads: a small superior head and a much larger inferior head. The superior head has its *origin* from the greater wing of the sphenoid bone at the base of the skull; the inferior head takes *origin* from the lateral surface of the lateral pterygoid plate of the sphenoid bone. Fibers of both heads are directed posterolaterally and lie predominantly in a horizontal plane. The fibers converge toward the neck of the condyle of the mandible. The fibers of the superior head have an *insertion* primarily into the joint capsule and disc of the temporomandibular joint. The fibers of the inferior head insert onto the neck of the mandible (area just below the condyle).

The **medial pterygoid** has its *origin* mostly from the medial surface of the lateral pterygoid plate and partly from the maxilla just behind the last molar (maxillary tuberosity). Its *insertion* is on the medial surface of the ramus and angle of the mandible.

Muscle Action and Innervation

Muscles acting on the mandible can produce several movements. *Elevation* is an upward movement of the mandible resulting in closure of the mouth. *Depression* is a downward movement of the mandible that results in opening the mouth. In *protrusion* (protraction), the mandible moves anteriorly; during *retrusion* (retraction), it moves posteriorly. *Lateral excursion* is movement to the side.

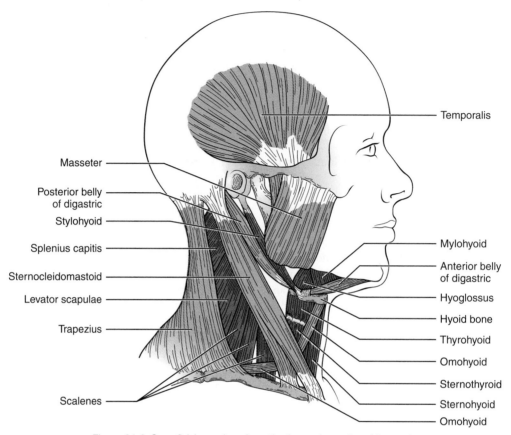

Masseter

Posterior belly
of digastric

Stylohyoid

Splenius capitis

Sternocleidomastoid

Levator scapulae

Trapezius

Scalenes

Temporalis

Mylohyoid

Anterior belly
of digastric

Hyoglossus

Hyoid bone

Thyrohyoid

Omohyoid

Sternothyroid

Sternohyoid

Omohyoid

Figure 21-9 Superficial muscles of mastication and muscles of the neck.

The major *action* of the masseter, temporalis, and medial pterygoid is to elevate the mandible. The posterior (horizontal) fibers of the temporalis produce retrusion. The action of the inferior head of the lateral pterygoid is to draw its side of the mandible forward; both sides working together cause protrusion of the mandible, a movement necessary for complete opening of the mouth. The superficial head of the masseter, as a result of its muscle fiber orientation, can possibly aid in protrusion of the mandible. The superior head of the lateral pterygoid does not contract in protrusion but does contract during retrusion (although it does not produce retrusion) to stabilize the capsule and disc complex. All of the muscles are involved in lateral excursion, which can be used to produce the side-to-side movement used in chewing. Lateral movement to one side involves the two superficial muscles of that side, the temporalis and masseter, and

the deeper lateral and medial pterygoid muscles of the opposite side. Depression of the mandible can be produced by muscles inferior to the mandible such as the digastric, mylohyoid, and geniohyoid (described later) and also by gravity.

All of the muscles of mastication receive their *innervation* from the third, or mandibular, branch of the trigeminal nerve (cranial nerve V).

Temporomandibular Joint

The temporomandibular joint is a synovial joint between the condyle of the mandible and the temporal bone of the skull (see Fig. 21-10). Because the two temporomandibular joints are connected by way of a bony arch, the mandible, it is a functionally complex joint. Movement of one joint will in some way affect the other joint.

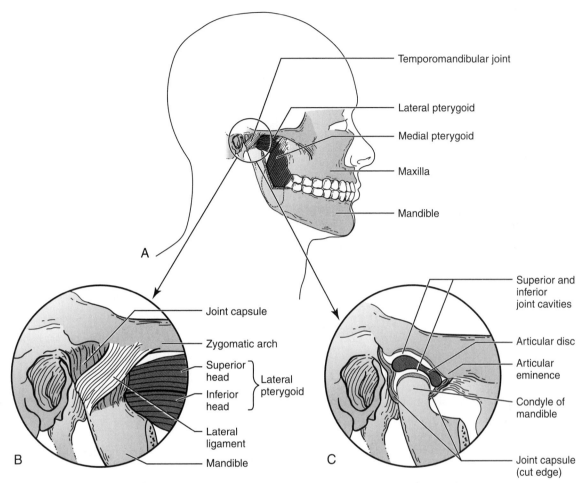

Figure 21-10 Temporomandibular joint and associated structures. **A,** Lateral view with par of the mandible omitted to expose the lateral and medial pterygoid muscles. **B,** Enlargement of the temporomandibular joint, showing the joint capsule, the lateral ligament, and the lateral pterygoid muscle. **C,** With the capsule and ligament omitted, the articular disc and articular cavities can be seen (the lateral pterygoid muscle is not depicted).

The joint is surrounded by a joint capsule that attaches above to the temporal bone and below to the neck of the condyle of the mandible. The capsule is strengthened laterally by the *lateral (temporomandibular) ligament*. Most of the fibers of the ligament are directed postero-inferiorly. This fiber orientation prevents the mandible from moving posteriorly and inferiorly. Movement at the joint is primarily in a forward direction or a forward and downward direction. Other smaller ligaments are also present at the joint to aid in its stability.

The articular areas of the bones at the temporo-mandibular joint are the anterosuperior surface of the condyle of the mandible and the posterior and inferior surfaces of the articular eminence of the temporal bone. (On a skeletal preparation, it appears that the condyle articulates in the mandibular fossa; however, no direct articulation occurs there.) The articular surfaces are covered by *fibrous connective tissue* rather than the hyaline cartilage that is found in most other synovial joints. The fibrous connective tissue is better suited to the forces that occur at the joint, especially shear forces. A fibrous *articular disc* is situated between the condyle and temporal bone. The disc is thicker anteriorly and posteriorly than in its midregion. Because of the presence of the disc, the articular cavity is divided into two parts: a superior

Table 21-1 MUSCLES OF MASTICATION				
Muscle	**Origin**	**Insertion**	**Action**	**Innervation**
Masseter	Zygomatic arch	Ramus and angle of mandible (lateral surface)	Elevation of mandible; may aid in protrusion of mandible (superficial head)	Trigeminal nerve: mandibular division
Temporalis	Lateral surface of skull (temporal fossa)	Coronoid process and anterior part of ramus of mandible (medial surface)	Elevation of mandible; retrusion of mandible (posterior fibers)	Trigeminal nerve: mandibular division
Lateral pterygoid	Inferior head: lateral surface of lateral pterygoid plate of sphenoid bone; Superior head: sphenoid bone (greater wing)	Inferior head: neck of mandible Superior head: capsule and disc of temporomandibular joint	Protrusion of mandible	Trigeminal nerve: mandibular division
Medial pterygoid	Medial surface of lateral pterygoid plate of sphenoid bone; maxillary tuberosity	Ramus and angle of mandible (medial surface)	Elevation of mandible	Trigeminal nerve: mandibular division

cavity and an inferior cavity. The disc is held more firmly to the condyle of the mandible by the joint capsule than to the temporal bone. Therefore, the condyle and disc act as a functional unit. The condyle can rotate on the undersurface of the disc, and the condyle and disc complex can move downward and forward on the articular eminence as a unit.

Two types of movement occur at the temporomandibular joint. If the mandible is depressed to open the mouth, the initial movement that occurs at the joint is a *rotation (hinge) movement*, in which the condyle rotates around its medial-lateral axis. The rotary movement occurs between the condyle and the undersurface of the disc. The extent of the rotary movement at the temporomandibular joint is limited, in part, by contact of the mandible with soft tissue as the angle and ramus move posteriorly during depression. To continue depression of the mandible, a *gliding movement* must take place to allow the condyle and disc complex to move forward on the articular eminence of the temporal bone. This gliding movement produces protrusion of the mandible. When coupled with continued rotation of the condyle on the disc, gliding enables the mouth to be fully opened.

Two ligaments, *stylomandibular* and *sphenomandibular ligaments,* attach to the inner surface of the mandible. These have been described as accessory ligaments of the joint, but their specific role in the function of the joint has been variably interpreted. The capsule of the temporomandibular joint is innervated by branches of the mandibular part (division) of the trigeminal nerve.

MUSCLES OF THE TONGUE

The tongue itself is composed of interlacing skeletal muscle fibers arranged longitudinally, horizontally, and transversely (Fig. 21-11 and Table 21-2). There are four pairs of extrinsic muscles of the tongue: the *hyoglossus, styloglossus, genioglossus,* and *palatoglossus;* there are also several *intrinsic muscles.*

The **hyoglossus** has its *origin* from the hyoid bone, and its *insertion* is on the sides of the tongue. Its *action* is to depress the tongue by pulling its sides downward toward the floor of the oral cavity.

The **styloglossus** takes *origin* from the styloid process. It passes downward and anteriorly to its *insertion* on the sides of the tongue, where it blends with the fibers of the hyoglossus. The *action* of the styloglossus is to pull the tongue upward and posteriorly, and as it does this, it creates a trough on the surface of the tongue.

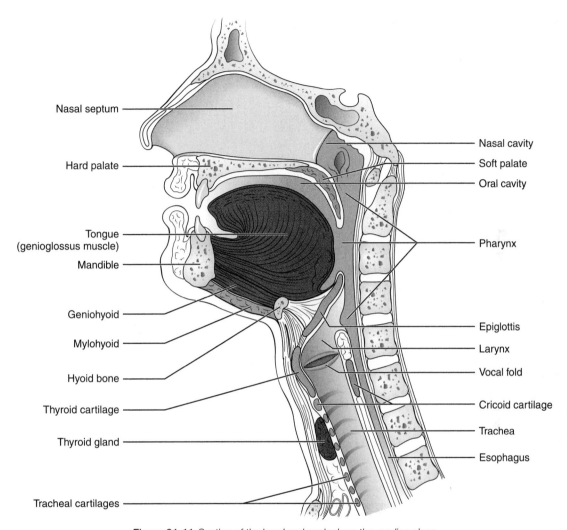

Figure 21-11 Section of the head and neck along the median plane.

The **genioglossus** has its *origin* from the inner surface of the anterior part of the mandible from small bony processes, the superior mental spines, on each side of the midline. Its fibers pass posteriorly and also upward and have an *insertion* into the body and dorsum of the tongue. A few of its inferior fibers insert into the hyoid bone. The major *action* of the genioglossus is to produce protrusion of the tip of the tongue out of the oral cavity. The more vertical fibers can help depress the central part of the tongue.

The remaining extrinsic muscle, the **palatoglossus,** is a small muscle that takes *origin* from the soft palate and passes to an *insertion* on the sides and dorsal surface of the tongue. Its *action* is to elevate (raise) the back of the tongue and, therefore, assist in moving material from the oral cavity into the oropharynx. By this action the muscle approximates the posterior part of the tongue to the soft palate to help close the opening between the oral cavity and oropharynx.

The intrinsic muscles, which have both their origin and insertion in the tongue, are responsible for changing the shape of the tongue. Both the extrinsic and intrinsic muscles are used in speaking, mastication, and

Table 21-2	MUSCLES OF THE TONGUE			
Muscle	**Origin**	**Insertion**	**Action**	**Innervation**
Hyoglossus	Hyoid bone	Sides of tongue	Depression of tongue (pulls sides of tongue downward toward floor of oral cavity)	Hypoglossal nerve
Styloglossus	Styloid process	Sides of tongue	Pulls tongue upward and posteriorly, forming trough on tongue surface	Hypoglossal nerve
Genioglossus	Inner surface of anterior part of mandible on each side of midline (superior mental spines)	Body and dorsum of tongue; some fibers to hyoid bone	Protrusion of tongue	Hypoglossal nerve
Palatoglossus	Soft palate	Sides and dorsal surface of tongue	Elevation of posterior part of tongue	Vagus nerve

swallowing. All of the muscles of the tongue, except for the palatoglossus, receive their *innervation* from the hypoglossal nerve (cranial nerve XII); the palatoglossus is innervated by the vagus nerve (cranial nerve X). If an individual has a lesion of the hypoglossal nerve on one side and is asked to "stick out" (protrude) the tongue, the tongue deviates (points to) the side of the lesion.

MUSCLES OF THE NECK

Suprahyoid Muscles

The **mylohyoid** forms the sloping floor of the oral cavity (Table 21-3). The muscle fibers of each pass downward from an *origin* on the medial surface of the mandible (mylohyoid line) on each side to an *insertion* on the hyoid bone and along the midline with the muscle of the other side. The mylohyoid muscles receive *innervation* from a branch of the mandibular division of the trigeminal nerve of each side. Their *action* is to raise the floor of the mouth and the base of the tongue. Because they are attached to the hyoid bone, they may also assist the digastric in opening the mouth when the hyoid bone is fixed in place.

The **geniohyoid** has its *origin* on the inner surface of the mandible near the midline (inferior mental spines), just inferior to the origin of the genioglossus, and its *insertion* is on the hyoid bone. It lies just superior to the mylohyoid. The *action* of the geniohyoid is to help pull the hyoid bone upward and forward or

depress the mandible if the hyoid bone is fixed in place. Its *innervation* is from a branch of spinal nerve C1.

The **digastric** (meaning "two-bellied") takes *origin* from an area on the base of the skull (digastric notch) just medial to the mastoid process. It has an *insertion* on the inner surface of the anterior part of the mandible (behind the chin) adjacent to the midline (digastric fossa). The tendon connecting the two "bellies" of the muscle is attached by a sling of fascia to the hyoid bone. The *action* of the muscle is to raise the hyoid bone or aid in opening the mouth. Its posterior belly receives *innervation* from the facial nerve, and its anterior belly, by a branch from the mandibular division of the trigeminal nerve.

Because all three of the muscles just described have an attachment to the hyoid bone and the mandible, they can depress the mandible (open the mouth) if the hyoid bone is fixed in place by contraction of the muscles attaching to it from below.

The **stylohyoid** has its *origin* from the styloid process. It passes forward and downward to an *insertion* on the hyoid bone. Its tendon of insertion typically surrounds the tendon connecting the two bellies of the digastric muscle. The *action* of the stylohyoid is to pull the hyoid bone upward and posteriorly. *Innervation* is provided by fibers from the facial nerve.

The suprahyoid muscles can raise the hyoid bone, or they can cooperate with the infrahyoid muscles (described in the next section) to stabilize or move the hyoid bone during swallowing and speech production.

Table 21-3	SUPRAHYOID MUSCLES			
Muscle	**Origin**	**Insertion**	**Action**	**Innervation**
Mylohyoid	Medial surface of mandible (mylohyoid line)	Hyoid bone; along midline with muscle of other side	Elevates floor of oral cavity; depresses mandible when hyoid bone is fixed	Trigeminal nerve: mandibular division
Geniohyoid	Inner surface of anterior part of mandible on each side of midline (inferior mental spines)	Hyoid bone	Pulls hyoid bone upward and anteriorly; depresses mandible when hyoid bone is fixed	Branch form anterior ramus of C1
Digastric	Medial to mastoid process (digastric notch)	Inner surface of mandible adjacent to midline (digastric fossa); intermediate tendon held to hyoid bone by fascia	Pulls hyoid bone upward and anteriorly; depresses mandible when hyoid bone is fixed	Anterior belly: trigeminal nerve: mandibular division Posterior belly: facial nerve
Stylohyoid	Styloid process	Hyoid bone	Pulls hyoid bone upward and posteriorly	Facial nerve

Sternocleidomastoid

The heaviest musculature in the neck is the upward continuation of the muscles of the back. In addition to these and the trapezius, the **sternocleidomastoid** (Fig. 21-12 and Table 21-4; see Fig. 21-9) is a prominent component of the muscles of the neck. This muscle takes *origin* by a tendinous head from the manubrium of the sternum and by fleshy fibers from the medial third of the clavicle. Its *insertion* is on the mastoid process behind the ear (see Fig. 21-9). *Motor innervation* is provided by the accessory nerve (cranial nerve XI), but *sensory innervation* is from fibers of the upper cervical spinal nerves, usually C2 and sometimes C3. The *action* of the sternocleidomastoids (acting together) is to powerfully flex the head and neck. Contraction of the muscle of one side laterally flexes the head and neck toward the same side and turns the face upward and toward the opposite side.

The anatomy of the neck is so complicated that it is often convenient to divide the anterolateral part into subsidiary regions on the basis of muscular landmarks. The sternocleidomastoid is the most prominent of these landmarks and, for descriptive purposes, is used to divide the neck into two major triangles. The *posterior triangle* lies posterior to the muscle, between it and the trapezius, and the *anterior triangle* lies anterior and medial to the muscle and extends to the midline.

FUNCTIONAL/CLINICAL NOTE 21-6

An abnormal position of the head and neck (*torticollis* or *wryneck*) may be maintained by various muscles of the neck. In the simplest type, the sternocleidomastoid is responsible, but in other types, there seems to be a contraction of many muscles: the large muscles, such as the sternocleidomastoid, trapezius, scalene, and vertebral muscles; the short muscles associated with the skull; and even the hyoid musculature.

Infrahyoid Muscles

There are several thin muscles in the front of the neck that lie inferior to the level of the hyoid bone (see Table 21-4). They are known collectively as the **infrahyoid muscles** or as the **strap muscles of the neck.** These muscles include the sternohyoid, sternothyroid, thyrohyoid, and omohyoid. The **sternohyoid** and **sternothyroid** muscles have *origins* from the sternum and have *insertions* on the hyoid bone and thyroid cartilage, respectively. The sternohyoid is positioned superficial to the sternothyroid. The two muscles cover the anterior and lateral surfaces of the thyroid gland. The **thyrohyoid**

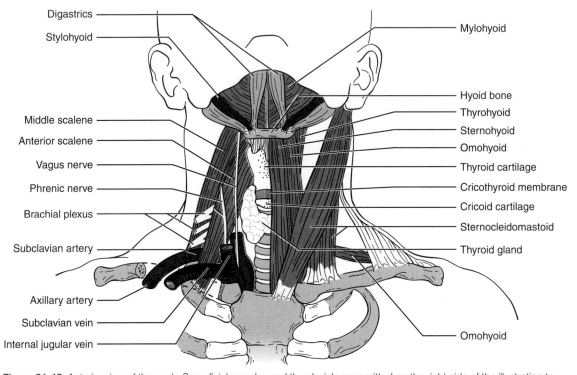

Figure 21-12 Anterior view of the neck. Superficial muscles and the clavicle are omitted on the right side of the illustration to reveal deeper structures. Branches of the subclavian and axillary arteries are not illustrated.

has its *origin* from the thyroid cartilage, and its *insertion* is on the hyoid bone. It seems to be an upward continuation of the sternothyroid muscle. The **omohyoid** muscle has its *origin* from the scapula, hence the prefix *omo-* ("shoulder"), and its *insertion* is on the hyoid bone. It consists of two bellies, one superior and one inferior, united by a tendon that is anchored to the clavicle by a sling of fascia. The superior belly of the omohyoid muscle runs almost parallel but lateral to the sternohyoid. The inferior belly runs almost transversely across the base of the neck from its attachment on the shoulder.

All the infrahyoid muscles except the thyrohyoid receive *innervation* from a nerve loop, the *ansa cervicalis*, derived usually from branches of spinal nerves C1 to C3. The thyrohyoid muscle receives *innervation* from C1 fibers that travel with the hypoglossal nerve (cranial nerve XII). The *action* of the infrahyoid muscles is to pull the hyoid bone and thyroid cartilage downward.

FUNCTIONAL/CLINICAL NOTE 21-7

As noted earlier, cooperation between the infrahyoid and suprahyoid muscles enables the hyoid bone and thyroid cartilage to be moved up and down, as in swallowing or singing up or down a scale. These muscles also help to stabilize the hyoid bone to provide a firm base on which the hyoglossus can contract to pull the sides of the tongue downward or the mylohyoid, digastric, and geniohyoid can contract to depress the mandible.

Scalene Muscles

Most of the muscles connected with the vertebral column in the neck have already been described in connection with the back muscles. Anterolaterally in the neck, however, there are three scalene (scalenus)

Table 21-4	MUSCLES OF THE NECK			
Muscle	**Origin**	**Insertion**	**Action**	**Innervation**
Sternocleido-mastoid	Sternum and medial third of clavicle	Mastoid process of temporal bone	Both muscles: flexion of head and neck. One muscle: lateral flexion (turns face to opposite side)	Accessory nerve (motor); spinal nerves C2 and C3 (sensory)
Sternohyoid	Sternum (posterior surface)	Hyoid bone	Depression and/or fixation of hyoid bone	Anterior rami of first three cervical spinal nerves through ansa cervicalis
Sternothyroid	Sternum (posterior surface)	Thyroid cartilage	Depression and/or fixation of thyroid cartilage	Anterior rami of first three cervical spinal nerves through ansa cervicalis
Thyrohyoid	Thyroid cartilage	Hyoid bone	Depression and/or stabilization of hyoid bone; if hyoid bone is fixed, elevation of thyroid cartilage	Anterior ramus of C1 by way of hypoglossal nerve
Omohyoid	Superior border of scapula	Hyoid bone	Depression and/or fixation of hyoid bone	Anterior rami of first three cervical spinal nerves through ansa cervicalis
Anterior scalene	Transverse processes of third to sixth cervical vertebrae	First rib	Fixation or elevation of first rib during inhalation. With rib fixed: lateral flexion of neck	Anterior rami of cervical spinal nerves at origin of muscle
Middle scalene	Transverse processes of lower five or six cervical vertebrae (possibly the atlas)	First rib	Fixation or elevation of first rib during inhalation. With rib fixed: lateral flexion of neck	Anterior rami of cervical spinal nerves at origin of muscle
Posterior scalene	Transverse processes of fourth to sixth cervical vertebrae	Second rib	Fixation or elevation of second rib. With rib fixed: lateral flexion of neck	Anterior rami of cervical spinal nerves at origin of muscle

muscles arising from the vertebral column and inserting on the ribs: anterior, middle, and posterior (Fig. 21-13; see Figs. 21-9 and 21-12).

The **anterior scalene** (scalenus anterior) muscle takes *origin* from the anterior tubercles of the transverse processes of approximately the third to sixth cervical vertebrae, and its *insertion* is on the upper surface of the first rib toward its sternal attachment. The subclavian vein and phrenic nerve (nerve to the diaphragm) lie anterior to this muscle.

The **middle scalene** (scalenus medius) has a similar *origin* from the lower five or six or all the cervical vertebrae and *insertion* onto the first rib. The anterior and middle scalenes are separated from each other by the roots of the brachial plexus and the subclavian artery (see Fig. 21-12).

The **posterior scalene** (scalenus posterior) lies behind the middle scalene and has its *origin* from the transverse processes of the fourth through the sixth cervical vertebrae. It passes inferiorly to an *insertion* on the second rib.

The scalene muscles receive *innervation* from short branches of the anterior rami of the cervical nerves corresponding to the levels of their origins. Taking their fixed points below, their *action* is to flex the neck laterally or turn it slightly toward the opposite side. Taking their fixed points above, they are respiratory muscles, serving to fix the first two ribs in quiet inspiration and to raise these ribs in forced inspiration.

Because of its position between the anterior and middle scalenes, the brachial plexus is subject to pressure from the contraction of these muscles or to being stretched over the first rib raised by their spastic contraction. Spasm of the anterior scalene, in particular, has been thought to be responsible for certain cases of injury to the plexus at the base of the neck, and the operation of scalenotomy, or section of the anterior scalene, has been reported to relieve selected cases. The *scalenus anticus syndrome,* like other signs of compression of the brachial plexus, is often precipitated or exaggerated by a lower position of the shoulder and is often amenable to physical therapy.

Longus Colli and Longus Capitis

The longus colli and longus capitis (see Fig. 21-13) are discussed with the back but are reviewed briefly here (see Chapter 13 and Table 13-6 for more detailed information). The muscles lie on the anterior surface of the upper region of the vertebral column. The **longus colli** has its *origin* as three groups of muscle fibers from the upper thoracic and lower and middle cervical vertebrae; the **longus capitis** takes *origin* from the middle cervical vertebrae. The *insertion* of the longus colli is onto the cervical vertebrae, and its *action* is to flex the vertebral column. The longus capitis has its *insertion* on the occipital bone, and its *action* is to flex the head and vertebral column. *Innervation* to both muscles is provided by the anterior rami of the upper cervical nerves.

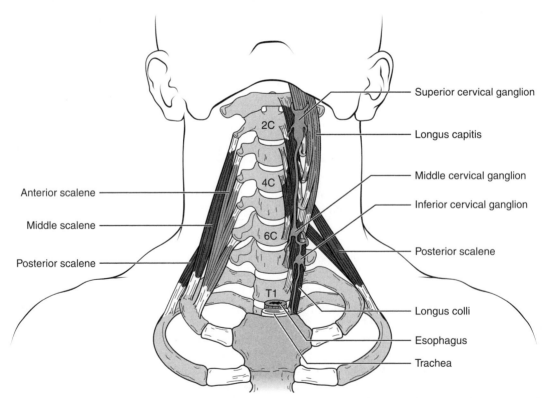

Figure 21-13 Deep muscles of the neck. The scalene muscles are illustrated on the right side of the figure. The longus capitis and longus colli, the sympathetic trunk and ganglia, and the posterior scalene are included on the left.

PHARYNX, LARYNX, TRACHEA, AND ESOPHAGUS

The essential anatomy of these structures is diagrammed in Figure 21-11. The pharynx is formed by the union of nasal and oral cavities, posterior and inferior to the soft palate. The pharynx, therefore, is the common chamber in the head and upper part of the neck for the respiratory and digestive systems. At the level of the thyroid cartilage, the pharynx is continuous with the larynx of the respiratory system anteriorly and with the esophagus of the digestive system posteriorly.

Pharynx

The soft palate extends downward and posteriorly from the back of the hard palate. It is essentially a muscular partition that, during swallowing, separates the nasopharynx from the oropharynx so that liquid and food pass downward toward the esophagus and do not enter the nasal cavity. The most important muscles here are those that lift or tense the soft palate, the *levator veli palatini* and *tensor veli palatini;* these attach to the skull. Other muscles extend from the soft palate to the walls of the pharynx (the *palatopharyngeus*) or to the tongue (the *palatoglossus*). Movements of the soft palate are essential for proper phonation and for swallowing.

FUNCTIONAL/CLINICAL NOTE 21-9

Defects in the soft palate, especially cleft palate but also those involved in paralysis of the musculature of the palate, lead to difficulty in swallowing and sometimes result in the outflow of liquids through the nose.

Also essential to swallowing is the action of the muscles in the walls of the pharynx. These muscles are arranged to compress the pharynx and are termed the **constrictors of the pharynx.** The *superior, middle,* and *inferior pharyngeal constrictors* overlap each other so that by their contraction, which begins superiorly, they pass food or liquids down into the esophagus. Their malfunction, therefore, leads to difficulty in swallowing. The pharyngeal constrictors and most of the muscles of the soft palate receive *innervation* from pharyngeal branches of the vagus nerves. The sensory supply to the posterior wall of the pharynx is partly through the glossopharyngeal nerve (cranial nerve IX) and partly through the vagus nerve (cranial nerve X).

Larynx and trachea

The pharynx is a common chamber for the respiratory and digestive systems. From the pharynx, the respiratory tract continues anteriorly and then inferiorly as the larynx and trachea, and the digestive tract continues inferiorly as the esophagus. At the upper end of the larynx is the *epiglottis,* a cartilaginous plate that is covered by mucosa (see in Fig. 21-11). It projects posterosuperiorly and is important during swallowing to help keep food and liquids out of the respiratory tract (see later "Swallowing" section). The walls of the respiratory tract are held open by the *thyroid* and *cricoid cartilages* in the region of the larynx, and by a series of C-shaped *cartilaginous rings in the trachea* (see Figs. 21-11 and 21-12). The opening into the larynx can, however, be closed, as in holding the breath, by the action of muscles acting on the folds in the laryngeal walls. One pair of these folds is termed the **vocal folds,** or **vocal cords,** which not only can be brought together in the midline but also can be lengthened or shortened. These folds are thrown into vibration by the passage of air between them to produce sound, and the pitch of the voice is altered by changes in the length and tenseness of the vibrating portions of the cords. Within the thorax the trachea divides into the two *main bronchi* that enter the lungs.

The musculature of the larynx is complex and is not described in this text. Most of the laryngeal musculature receives its *innervation* from the recurrent laryngeal branch of the vagus nerve, which leaves the main vagus stem in the lower part of the neck or in the thorax (differing on the two sides) and ascends alongside the trachea and esophagus to reach the level of the larynx.

The recurrent nerve is subject to injury during operations on the thyroid gland, and such injury, if bilateral, may have serious consequences. Paralysis of the musculature of the larynx may lead to gradual closure of the airway, so that breathing becomes increasingly difficult. If an artificial opening into the airway is needed, a *tracheotomy* or *tracheostomy* can be performed by creating a hole in the upper tracheal rings. This is best done in a controlled surgical environment, because of the complex anatomy of the area. In true emergency situations, a *cricothyroidotomy* (also known as *coniotomy* or *cricothyrotomy*) can be performed by making an opening in the anterior midline through the skin and underlying cricothyroid membrane that occupies the space between the thyroid and cricoid cartilages (see Fig. 21-12).

Esophagus

The **esophagus,** the more direct continuation of the pharynx, is a muscular tube that lies between the trachea and the vertebral column. The part of it in the neck has skeletal muscle in its walls, but before the esophagus reaches the stomach, this muscle has been replaced by smooth muscle. Except when it is distended by the passage of food or liquids, the walls of the esophagus are collapsed.

Swallowing

The initial phase of swallowing (deglutition) is voluntary. The liquid or the masticated material, which is formed into a mass called a *bolus,* is forced upward and posteriorly toward the hard palate by the tongue (Fig. 21-14). When the material to be swallowed reaches the junction of the oral cavity and pharynx, the process becomes involuntary. The soft palate is tensed and raised to close off the upper part of the pharynx and nasal cavity. As the laryngeal opening constricts, the larynx is elevated toward the epiglottis. The epiglottis is pulled downward to meet the rising larynx, and their contact helps close off the laryngeal opening. (The upward movement of the larynx can be verified by palpating the thyroid cartilage during swallowing.) Sequential contraction of the pharyngeal constrictors (from above, downward) causes the swallowed material to move toward the esophagus.

It is apparent that numerous muscles and nerves are involved in the complex procedure of swallowing. Movements of the tongue rely on input mainly from the hypoglossal nerve and those of the soft palate, the vagus nerve, and the trigeminal nerve. The movements of the larynx and pharynx involve predominantly input from the vagus nerve, but the glossopharyngeal nerve also innervates a muscle of the pharynx, the stylopharyngeus.

NERVES AND VESSELS

Cranial Nerves

The cranial nerves consist of 12 pairs of nerves that can be identified by name or by Roman numerals. They largely arise from various parts of the brain and must make their exit through the skull to reach the periphery. Some of these nerves are widely distributed; others have a very limited distribution (Fig. 21-15 and Table 21-5). With the exception of the first two cranial nerves, the sensory fibers of the cranial nerves arise from ganglia similar to those of the posterior root ganglia of spinal nerves. The motor fibers originate from cell groups in the brain stem known as *motor nuclei,* the equivalent of the anterior horn cells in the spinal cord, except that instead of being a continuous mass, most of the motor nuclei supply fibers to only one cranial nerve. The incoming sensory fibers also end largely in a discrete collection of nerve cells, so that there are both motor and sensory nuclei for the cranial nerves. The nerves that contain parasympathetic preganglionic fibers, cranial nerves III, VII, IX, and X, also have nuclei composed of the cell bodies of these fibers.

The **olfactory nerve** (cranial nerve I) is a purely sensory nerve associated with the sense of smell. The fibers of the olfactory nerves originate from cells that lie in the nasal mucosa on the roof of the nasal cavity. Their fibers pass upward through the ethmoid bone into the cranial cavity. They then pass into the

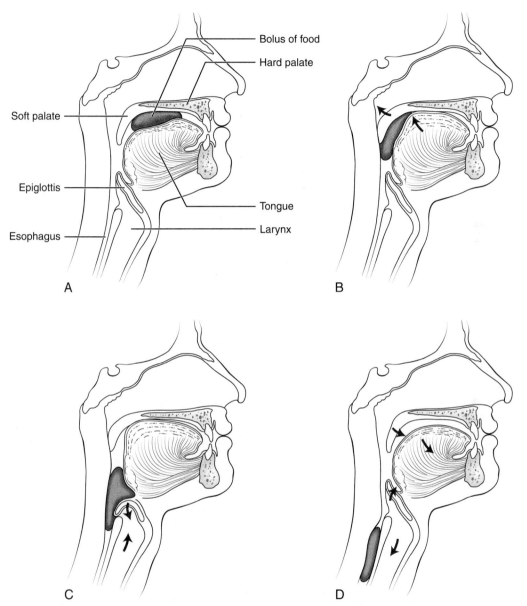

Figure 21-14 Sequence of swallowing. **A,** The bolus of food (highlighted with color) is pushed to the back of the oral cavity by the tongue. **B,** The tongue moves up and back, and the soft palate elevates to close off the upper part of the pharynx. The bolus moves into the pharynx. **C,** The larynx moves upward, and its opening is narrowed by muscle action. The epiglottis is bent downward to seal off the opening of the larynx. The bolus moves toward the esophagus by the contraction of the pharyngeal constrictors. **D,** By continued action of the constrictors, the bolus moves downward through the esophagus, and the structures return to their normal positions.

olfactory bulbs that lie on the under surface of the cerebral hemispheres. The olfactory bulbs and olfactory tracts (which connect to the brain) are really parts of the brain (the telencephalon).

The **optic nerve** (cranial nerve II) is the sensory nerve associated with sight. Its fibers originate from cells in the retina of the eyeball, course posteriorly through the orbit, and then enter the cranial cavity.

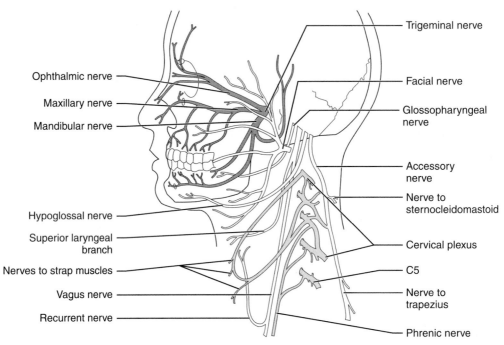

Figure 21-15 The cervical plexus and selected cranial nerves. The outlines of the mandible and other osteological features are included for orientation only; some of the nerves lie deep to or within the bones illustrated. The cervical nerves have *light color,* and the trigeminal nerve and branches have *dark color.*

Table 21-5	CHIEF FUNCTIONS AND DISTRIBUTIONS OF THE CRANIAL NERVES	
Nerve	**Afferent Innervation**	**Efferent Innervation**
I. Olfactory	Smell: nose	—
II. Optic	Sight: eye	—
III. Oculomotor	—	Motor to skeletal muscle: levator palpebrae superioris; superior, medial, and inferior recti; and inferior oblique of eyeball Parasympathetic: smooth muscle of eyeball
IV. Trochlear	—	Motor to skeletal muscle: superior oblique of eyeball
V. Trigeminal	Touch, pain: skin of face, mucous membranes of nasal cavity, sinuses, oral cavity, anterior two thirds of tongue	Motor to skeletal muscle: muscles of mastication; anterior belly of digastric; mylohyoid, tensor veli palatine, and tensor tympani
VI. Abducens	—	Motor to skeletal muscle: lateral rectus of eyeball
VII. Facial	Taste: anterior two thirds of tongue	Motor to skeletal muscle: facial muscles, stylohyoid, and posterior belly of digastric Parasympathetic: lacrimal gland, submandibular and sublingual salivary glands, glands of nasal mucosa
VIII. Vestibulocochlear	Hearing: ear Balance: ear	—

Table 21-5	CHIEF FUNCTIONS AND DISTRIBUTIONS OF THE CRANIAL NERVES—cont'd	
Nerve	**Afferent Innervation**	**Efferent Innervation**
IX. Glossopharyngeal	Visceral sensory*: posterior one third of tongue, pharynx Taste: posterior one third of tongue	Motor to skeletal muscle: stylopharyngeus Parasympathetic: parotid gland
X. Vagus	Visceral sensory: pharynx, larynx, respiratory tract, digestive tract to transverse colon Taste: epiglottis	Motor to skeletal muscle: palatoglossus, muscles of palate (except tensor veli palatine), muscles of pharynx (except stylopharyngeus), and muscles of larynx Parasympathetic: thoracic and abdominal viscera
XI. Accessory	—	Motor to skeletal muscle: sternocleidomastoid and trapezius
XII. Hypoglossal	—	Motor to skeletal muscle: hyoglossus, styloglossus, and genioglossus; intrinsic muscles of tongue

Note: In addition to innervation from cranial nerve V and branches of the cervical plexus, the skin of the external ear and associated canal receives general sensory innervation variably from cranial nerves VII, IX, and X.
*Sensory innervation associated with visceral structures such as internal organs and blood vessels.

The fibers meet those from the other eye at the optic chiasm (chiasma) and continue through the optic tracts to the diencephalon.

The **oculomotor nerve** (cranial nerve III) emerges from the midbrain and contains motor fibers, which innervate some of the muscles within the orbit, and parasympathetic nerve fibers. The oculomotor nerve innervates the levator palpebrae superioris muscle of the upper eyelid and the superior rectus, inferior rectus, medial rectus, and inferior oblique muscles of the eye. The parasympathetic fibers synapse in the *ciliary ganglion,* and the postganglionic fibers innervate smooth muscle that produces constriction of the pupil and accommodation of the lens for near vision. (See the earlier "Orbit" section.)

The **trochlear nerve** (cranial nerve IV) arises from the midbrain and is the only nerve to leave the brain dorsally. The trochlear innervates only one muscle of the eye, the superior oblique.

The **trigeminal nerve** (cranial nerve V) has three branches or divisions: the ophthalmic (V_1) nerve, maxillary (V_2) nerve, and mandibular (V_3) nerve. Each passes through different openings in the skull. All three contain sensory fibers, but only the mandibular nerve contains both sensory and motor fibers.

The *ophthalmic nerve* is distributed to the skin of the forehead and much of the scalp as far back as the ears (supraorbital and supratrochlear nerves), the upper eyelid, and the bridge of the nose (Fig. 21-16). It also innervates some of the paranasal sinuses.

The *maxillary nerve* innervates skin over the prominence of the cheek, the side of the nose, and the upper lip (infraorbital nerve). It also innervates much of the mucosa in the nasal cavity and most of the paranasal sinuses, the roof of the mouth (nasopalatine and greater palatine nerves), and the teeth of the maxilla (superior alveolar nerves). To perform dental work on the teeth of the maxilla, branches of the superior alveolar nerve are anesthetized.

The sensory part of the *mandibular nerve* innervates the mandibular teeth (inferior alveolar nerve); anterior two thirds of the tongue (lingual nerve); floor of the oral cavity (lingual nerve); inner surface of the cheek (buccal nerve); and skin (see Fig. 21-16) of the cheek (buccal nerve), over the mandible (buccal and mental nerves) and of the temporal region in front of the ear (auriculotemporal nerve). The innervation to the anterior two thirds of the tongue provided by nerve fibers from the mandibular nerve is general sensory innervation, not taste. The motor component of the mandibular nerve innervates the muscles of mastication (temporalis, masseter, and medial and lateral pterygoids), anterior belly of the digastric, mylohyoid, tensor veli palatini of the soft palate, and tensor tympani of the middle ear.

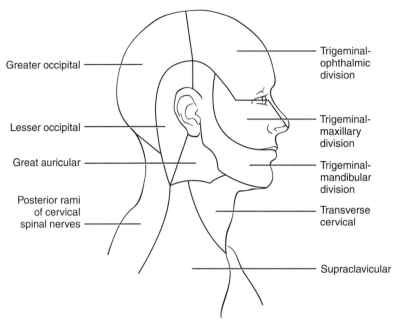

Figure 21-16 Cutaneous innervation of the head and neck.

The cutaneous branches of these three parts of the trigeminal nerve produce a relatively specific pattern of innervation to the skin of the face. The main branch of the ophthalmic nerve (supraorbital nerve) becomes subcutaneous by passing through the supraorbital foramen in the upper border of the orbit, not far from the bridge of the nose, and innervates the skin of the forehead. Other branches of the ophthalmic nerve to the skin of the face are those to the skin around the eye (lacrimal, supratrochlear and infratrochlear nerves) and one to the tip of the nose (external nasal nerve). The chief cutaneous branch of the maxillary nerve (infraorbital nerve) to the skin of the lower eyelid, lateral side of the nose and the upper lip passes through the infraorbital foramen. Other branches of the maxillary nerve provide innervation to the skin posterior to the eye (zygomaticotemporal nerve) and skin over the prominence of the cheek (zygomaticofacial nerve). The cutaneous branches of the mandibular nerve are rather widely separated as they approach the skin, one appearing just anterior to the ear (auriculotemporal nerve), one in the cheek (buccal nerve), and one on the chin through the mental foramen (mental nerve).

FUNCTIONAL/CLINICAL NOTE 21-11

The trigeminal nerve joins the brain stem at the pontine level. Its long sensory root between the trigeminal ganglion and the brainstem is sometimes surgically cut in order to alleviate attacks of severe pain in the face known as *trigeminal neuralgia.*

The **abducens nerve** (cranial nerve VI) emerges from the pontomedullary junction of the brainstem. It provides innervation to the lateral rectus muscle of the eye.

The **facial nerve** (cranial nerve VII) also emerges at the pontomedullary junction of the brainstem. It is a mixed nerve with several types of fibers. It has motor fibers that are distributed to all of the muscles of facial expression and to several other muscles (stapedius and stylohyoid and posterior belly of the digastric). In addition, it provides taste fibers to the anterior two thirds of the tongue and parasympathetic motor fibers to the submandibular, sublingual and minor salivary glands, lacrimal gland, and glands within the mucous membrane of the nasal cavity. The parasympathetic fibers reach synapse in either the submandibular or pterygopalatine ganglion.

The **vestibulocochlear nerve** (cranial nerve VIII) is distributed to the inner (internal) ear that lies within the temporal bone. It conveys impulses from the parts of the inner ear that are concerned with hearing (cochlea) and balance (utricle, semicircular ducts, and saccule). This nerve does not leave the skull because the inner ear is entirely enclosed within the temporal bone. Its fibers are connected to the pontomedullary junction of the brainstem.

The **glossopharyngeal nerve** (cranial nerve IX) is a mixed nerve containing both motor and sensory fibers. Its fibers emerge from the medulla. It passes through a foramen of the skull (jugular foramen) with the vagus nerve (cranial nerve X) and accessory nerve (cranial nerve XI). The foramen is the same one through which the sigmoid venous sinus of the cranial cavity is continuous with the internal jugular vein. The motor fibers are distributed to the stylopharyngeus muscle of the pharynx. The sensory fibers are distributed to the middle ear cavity, pharyngotympanic (auditory or eustachian) tube, pharynx, and posterior third of the tongue (both taste and general sensation). The nerve is responsible for the gag reflex associated with the posterior part of the oral cavity and the related region of the pharynx. The glossopharyngeal nerve also contains parasympathetic fibers that synapse in the otic ganglion and innervate the parotid salivary gland.

The **vagus nerve** (cranial nerve X) contains both motor (including parasympathetic) and sensory fibers. (The wide distribution of this nerve is the reason for the name *vagus*, meaning "wanderer.") It emerges from the medulla. The vagus nerve runs downward through the neck, just posterior to the internal and common carotid arteries. It sends motor fibers to the palatoglossus of the tongue and muscles of the soft palate (except the tensor veli palatini, which is innervated by the mandibular branch of the trigeminal nerve), the pharynx (except for the stylopharyngeus but including the constrictors of the pharynx), and the larynx. The sensory fibers of the vagus nerve provide innervation to the pharynx, larynx, trachea, thoracic viscera, and many of the abdominal viscera. The vagus nerve provides innervation to taste buds located on the epiglottis. Its parasympathetic fibers innervate the musculature of the lower part of the esophagus and the thoracic and abdominal viscera.

Some specific branches of the vagus nerve within the head and neck are of interest. The *superior laryngeal nerve* provides sensory innervation to the upper region of the larynx. The cough reflex, an important protective reflex of the respiratory system, is associated with this vagal innervation. The superior laryngeal nerve also provides motor innervation to one muscle of the larynx, the cricothyroid. The recurrent laryngeal branch of the vagus nerve innervates the rest of the muscles of the larynx and provides sensory innervation to the lower part of the larynx. The right recurrent laryngeal nerve arises from the right vagus nerve as it passes anterior to the subclavian artery. It then turns upward, posterior to this artery, and ascends to the larynx (see Fig. 22-8). The left recurrent laryngeal nerve leaves the vagus nerve in the thorax, rather than in the neck, and passes inferior and then posterior to the arch of the aorta before ascending to the larynx.

The **accessory nerve** (cranial nerve XI) arises in part by rootlets from the medulla that are in line with those of cranial nerves IX and X and in part by rootlets that arise from the upper four or five segments of the spinal cord. The latter run upward through the foramen magnum in the base of the skull to join the medullary rootlets. As the accessory nerve passes through the jugular foramen with the glossopharyngeal and vagus nerves, the fibers in the cranial rootlets of the accessory join the vagus nerve and are distributed with it. The fibers of the spinal rootlets alone form the accessory nerve that is typically described in gross anatomy. It carries motor fibers to the sternocleidomastoid and trapezius muscles. The accessory nerve contains no sensory fibers; sensory fibers to the sternocleidomastoid and trapezius are provided by branches of spinal nerves C2 and C3.

The **hypoglossal nerve** (cranial nerve XII) emerges from the medulla. It provides motor innervation to all intrinsic muscles of the tongue and most of the extrinsic muscles (the styloglossus, hyoglossus, and genioglossus).

Cervical Plexus

In the neck, the upper cervical nerves, with the frequent exception of the first, enter into the formation of the **cervical plexus** (see Fig. 21-15). The plexus is formed chiefly by the union of the *anterior rami of spinal nerves C1 to C4.* Like other plexuses of the spinal nerves, it contains both sensory and motor fibers. From this plexus, there arise a number of cutaneous (sensory) nerves that innervate skin of the neck and of the posterior part of the head. Motor fibers are provided to adjacent muscles, including the longus colli, longus capitis, and levator scapulae.

The *ansa cervicalis,* the major nerve supply to the infrahyoid muscles, is formed by the junction of C1 fibers that travel for a short distance with the hypoglossal nerve and fibers of C2 and C3 directly off the cervical plexus. The ansa cervicalis innervates the sternohyoid, sternothyroid, and omohyoid. The

thyrohyoid receives innervation from the C1 fibers traveling with the hypoglossal nerve.

The **phrenic nerve,** the nerve to the diaphragm, is also derived largely from the cervical plexus because it usually contains fibers from the anterior rami of C3, C4, and C5. The phrenic nerve passes through the lower part of the neck almost vertically, where it lies on the anterior surface of the anterior scalene muscle. After passing through the neck, it runs the length of the thorax to provide all of the motor and most of the sensory innervation to the diaphragm. Intercostal nerves can provide some sensory innervation to the very periphery of the diaphragm.

Sympathetic Trunks

Within the cervical region, the **sympathetic trunks** (see Fig. 21-13) lie deeply, anterior to the longus colli and longus capitis muscles. Each is an upward continuation of the thoracic part of the sympathetic trunk (see Chapter 3 for a summary of the sympathetic nervous system). Like the thoracic part, the cervical part of the sympathetic trunk is composed of ganglia and nerve fibers that connect the ganglia. In the cervical region, instead of the expected eight ganglia to correspond with the eight cervical nerves, there are typically only three cervical ganglia in each of the sympathetic trunks. A *superior cervical ganglion* is located high in the neck at about the level of the second cervical vertebra, and a small *middle cervical ganglion* lies at the level of the sixth cervical vertebra. At the base of the neck, near the seventh cervical vertebra and first rib, is the *inferior cervical ganglion.* The latter ganglion may be fused with the first ganglion of the thoracic part of the trunk to form the *cervicothoracic* (stellate) *ganglion.*

All of the fibers given off from the sympathetic trunk in the cervical region are postganglionic fibers, having already synapsed in the cervical ganglia. These ganglia give off fibers, gray rami communicantes, to all the cervical nerves (the inferior or cervicothoracic nerve being the chief sympathetic supply to the blood vessels and sweat glands of the upper limb). They also give rise to descending nerves that help innervate the heart, increasing the rate and strength of the heartbeat. Finally, the superior cervical ganglion sends a great number of fibers upward along the external and, in particular, the internal carotid arteries. These fibers supply blood vessels, sweat glands, and other structures of the face and head, including a muscle that dilates the pupil of the eye. Because all the preganglionic fibers to the cervical sympathetic ganglia come from thoracic nerves (cervical nerves have no white rami communicantes), interruption of the cervical sympathetic trunk eliminates the sympathetic innervation to the face and head.

Arteries

At the base of the neck on the right side, the **brachiocephalic trunk,** the first large branch from the aorta, divides into **right subclavian and right common carotid arteries** (Fig. 21-17). On the left side, the **left common carotid and left subclavian arteries** appear as separate branches from the aorta (see Fig. 22-8). The **subclavian arteries** arch across the base of the neck to enter the axillae, and the **common carotid arteries** run upward, lateral to the trachea and esophagus. The pulse of the latter vessels can easily be felt in the neck. At about the level of the upper border of the thyroid cartilage, the common carotid arteries branch into external and internal carotids. The **internal carotid arteries** continue upward and end by supplying blood to the brain. The **external carotid arteries** branch to supply numerous vessels to structures in the head and neck.

The pharynx, larynx, and upper parts of the trachea and esophagus receive their blood supplies from numerous branches derived ultimately from either the external carotid or subclavian arteries. The thyroid gland is supplied by the *superior thyroid arteries,* the first branch of the external carotid artery on each side, and the *inferior thyroid arteries,* indirect branches of the subclavian arteries.

Except for the brain, the blood supply of which has already been described as being derived from the internal carotid and vertebral arteries, most of

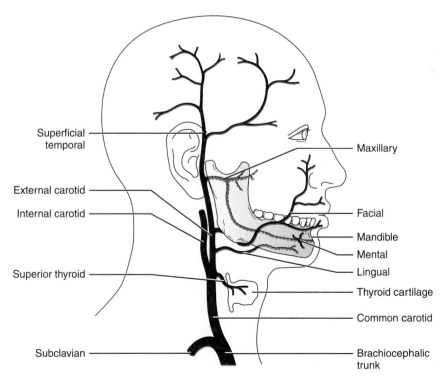

Figure 21-17 Diagram of the carotid arteries on the right side of the body. The common carotid artery divides into the internal and external carotid arteries at or near the upper border of the thyroid cartilage. The internal carotid artery enters the cranial cavity through the base of the skull. Some of the branches of the external carotid artery are illustrated.

the structures of the head are supplied by various branches of the **external carotid artery** (see Fig. 21-17). The *lingual artery* supplies the tongue and oral cavity. The *facial artery* crosses the inferior edge of the mandible just anterior to the attachment of the masseter muscle and runs toward the angle between the nose and eye (as the angular artery), giving off branches to the face in its course. The *superficial temporal artery*, from which the pulse is sometimes taken, ascends anterior to the ear and superficial to the zygomatic arch to supply blood to the region of the head over the temporalis muscle. The *maxillary artery*, one of the terminal branches of the external carotid artery (the other being the superficial temporal artery), passes deep to the mandible and supplies blood to the mandible, the muscles of mastication, the upper part of the oral cavity, and the nasal cavity.

Veins

The veins in the neck are numerous and connect rather freely with each other. The largest, from the head and upper part of the neck, are the **internal and external jugular veins.** The internal jugular vein accompanies the common and internal carotid arteries through the neck. The external jugular vein lies largely subcutaneously and can be identified as it passes across the surface of the sternocleidomastoid muscle. On each side of the body, the external jugular vein joins the subclavian vein at the base of the neck. The internal jugular vein joins with the subclavian vein of the same side to form the *brachiocephalic vein.* The brachiocephalic veins of both sides unite to form the *superior vena cava.*

SURFACE ANATOMY

The surface anatomy of the head is largely the anatomy of the skull. The frontal, parietal, temporal, and occipital regions of the head are obviously named from the corresponding bones of the cranium. Below the **external occipital protuberance,** the prominent bump on the back of the head close to the midline, the **occipital bone** is largely covered by the muscles attaching to it. The part of the **temporal bone** on the side of the skull in front of the ear is covered by the temporalis muscle, but it can usually be palpated. The **mastoid process** of the temporal bone is easily felt posterior to the external ear. The **zygomatic process** of the temporal bone forms the back part of the **zygomatic arch,** stretching from in front of the ear to the prominence of the cheek. The **parietal and frontal bones** are largely subcutaneous.

On the face, both the **maxillary and zygomatic bones** can be palpated; the tooth-bearing **alveolar process of the maxilla** can be felt through the lips and cheek or examined by retracting the lips and cheek. Horizontal processes from the two maxillae form the anterior part of the hard palate; those of the palatine bones form the posterior part. Most of the **mandible** can be palpated. Its lower border, *body* and the posterior end of its *angle* are particularly prominent, but its *ramus* is largely covered by the masseter.

The skeletal anatomy that can be examined in the intact neck (except for parts of the vertebral column) is limited to the hyoid bone and the larynx and trachea. The **hyoid bone** is easily palpated in the anterior midline at about the level of junction of the neck and lower surface of the mandible. Its greater horns curve posteriorly on the sides of the pharynx and can be followed to their tips. Below the hyoid bone, the **thyroid cartilage** is palpable (and its projection often visible), especially close to the midline. Its two sides meet in an anterior ridge, the laryngeal prominence, and its superior border is notched above this ridge. Of the several other cartilages of the larynx, only a part of the **cricoid cartilage** can be felt. This is the rounded bar of cartilage passing across the front of the larynx immediately below the thyroid cartilage. (As noted earlier, the cricothyroid membrane spans the space between the thyroid and cricoid cartilages; this is the site where a cricothyroidotomy would be performed.) The **cartilaginous rings of the trachea** that lie inferior to the cricoid cartilage are palpable with more difficulty, but they give the trachea its rough feeling when a finger is drawn along its length (*trachea* means "rough").

Both the **masseter** and **temporalis** can be felt to contract when the teeth are clenched (the masseter where it covers the angle of the mandible and the temporalis above the zygomatic arch). Muscles of the

floor of the mouth cannot be individually identified but can be felt to contract when swallowing occurs or when the tongue is moved vigorously. The **submandibular salivary gland** can be palpated in the area just inferior to the mandible, and the **platysma** can be identified in the anterior region of the neck when the lower lip and corners of the mouth are drawn inferiorly. The **sternocleidomastoid** is best palpated and observed when the neck is flexed and the face is at the same time turned to the opposite side.

None of the nerves of the head and neck can easily be palpated, but the cutaneous innervation pattern can be reviewed by referring to Figure 21-16. Of the vessels, the **external jugular vein** may be visually evident through the skin, particularly where it crosses the sternocleidomastoid muscle. The pulse of the **common carotid artery** can be felt lateral to the larynx, and that of the **superficial temporal artery** (from the external carotid artery) can be felt just in front of the upper part of the ear. Similarly, the pulse of the **facial artery** can be felt as it crosses the inferior border of the mandible, immediately anterior to the masseter muscle.

REVIEW QUESTIONS

1 What bones form the floor of the cranial cavity? Which bone forms the anterior part of the calvaria? Which suture is located between the parietal bones?

2 The muscles of facial expression are innervated by which cranial nerve? What is the arrangement of the muscles around the oral cavity?

3 Which muscle of the neck has its origin from the manubrium of the sternum and the clavicle and its insertion on the mastoid process of the skull? What nerve provides motor innervation to this muscle? What provides sensory innervation to this muscle?

4 Name the four major muscles of mastication. Which muscles produce elevation of the mandible?

5 Which muscle is capable of depressing the tongue? How can the functional integrity of the hypoglossal nerve be tested?

6 Discuss the sequence of swallowing.

7 What are the three parts or divisions of the trigeminal nerve? Which part contains motor fibers? Which muscles do these fibers innervate?

8 At what level in the neck does the common carotid artery divide into the internal and external carotid arteries? What are the major branches of the external carotid artery?

9 Describe the anatomy of the scalene muscles. What are the relationships of the subclavian artery and vein and the brachial plexus to the scalene muscles?

10 Which cranial nerve is responsible for the cough reflex? Which is responsible for the gag reflex?

11 Which muscles have an attachment to the hyoid bone?

12 What would be the result of severing the phrenic nerve as it passes across the anterior scalene muscle?

EXERCISES

1 Identify the following by palpation:
   a external occipital protuberance
   b mastoid process
   c hyoid bone
   d thyroid cartilage
   e upper tracheal rings
   f sternocleidomastoid muscle

2 Demonstrate the effect of contraction of the left sternocleidomastoid muscle, and note the movement that occurs. Next, contract both muscles. Note the movement and palpate the full extent of the muscles as they are contracting.

22 THE THORAX

CHAPTER CONTENTS

Thoracic Wall

Pleural and Pericardial Sacs

Thoracic Viscera

Vessels

Nerves

Surface Anatomy

THORACIC WALL

Bones

The thoracic wall consists of the *sternum* anteriorly, the *vertebral column* posteriorly, and the *ribs* (costae) with their connecting muscles (Figs. 22-1 and 22-2; see Fig. 5-1). Internally, the thorax is separated from the abdomen by the diaphragm, but there is no similar separation between the neck and thorax.

The **sternum** consists of three portions: an upper part, the *manubrium;* a large middle part, the *body;* and a small inferior part, the *xiphoid process.* The manubrium and body of the sternum meet to form the *sternal angle,* at which location the second rib attaches. The clavicle and the costal cartilages of the upper seven ribs are attached to the sternum.

The **thoracic vertebrae** form the posterior aspect of the wall of the thoracic cavity. The greater portion of the thoracic wall consists of the 12 pairs of **ribs,** their cartilages, and the muscles connecting them. The majority of the ribs articulate with both the body of the sternum and a transverse process of their corresponding vertebrae (see also Chapter 13 for the discussion of the vertebral column). Freely movable joints exist between vertebral and costal elements.

The upper seven pairs of ribs are *true ribs,* for they attach directly to the sternum anteriorly. The last five pairs of ribs are termed *false ribs.* The upper three pairs of false ribs attach by their costal cartilages to each other and to that of the seventh rib. They help form the costal arch. The costal cartilages of the last two ribs of each side end freely in the musculature to which they give attachment. The last two ribs are sometimes referred to as *floating ribs.*

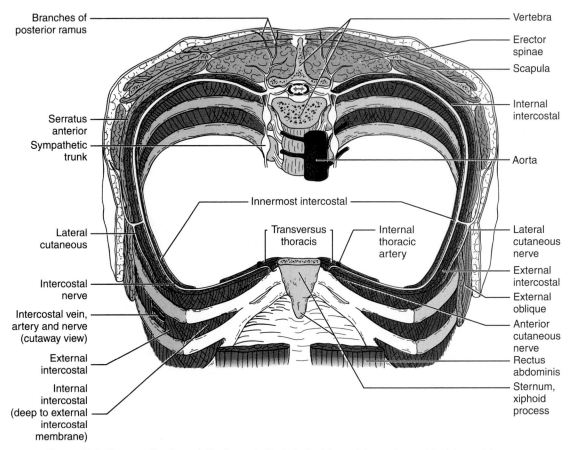

Figure 22-1 Cross-section through the thorax to illustrate the intercostal muscles and the intercostal nerves.

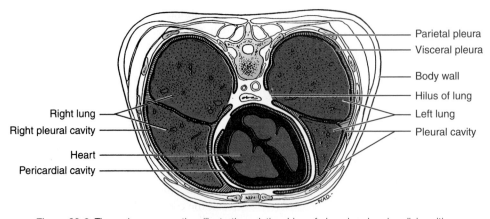

Figure 22-2 Thorax in cross-section, illustrating relationships of pleural and pericardial cavities.

Muscles

The muscles passing between two adjacent ribs are known as *intercostals*, and because they are arranged in two distinct layers, there are external and internal intercostals (Table 22-1; see Fig. 22-1; these are also shown in relation to the abdominal muscles in Fig. 23-1). Each muscle group consists of eleven pairs of muscles. Each **external intercostal** has its *origin* from the lower border of a rib, and its *insertion* on the upper border of the rib below. Their fibers slant downward and forward. Near the sternum, the external intercostal muscles are replaced by the *external intercostal membranes*. Each **internal intercostal** has its *origin* on the lower border of a rib. The muscle fibers slant downward and backward, at approximately 90 degrees to the orientation of those of the external intercostals. The internal intercostals have *insertions* on the upper border of the rib below. Internal intercostal muscles are replaced by the *internal intercostal membranes* near the vertebral column (posteriorly). Both external and internal intercostals receive *innervation* from the intercostal nerves. There is disagreement concerning the *action* of the intercostals. They can function to maintain the interspaces—that is, to keep the soft tissue of the intercostal space from bulging outward or bowing inward during respiration and to maintain the spacing between the ribs. Some accounts describe the external intercostals as inspiratory muscles and relate the function of internal intercostals to expiration; other accounts provide different interpretations. Therefore, questions still remain about their exact functional role in the elevation and depression of the ribs associated with inspiration and expiration.

In addition to the external and internal intercostals, other muscles are associated with the thoracic wall. The **innermost intercostals** have the same slant as, and lie deep to parts of, the internal intercostals; they are variable in location and may be simply deep fibers of the internal intercostals. Located only anteriorly on the inside of the thoracic wall, the **transversus thoracis** is a thin muscle that radiates upward and laterally from the posterior surface of the sternum to attach to the inner aspects of the ribs. The **subcostalis** muscles are located in the posterior region of the thoracic cavity; their shape and size vary and they are usually best developed on the lower part of the thoracic wall. These muscles all receive *innervation* from the intercostal nerves. Concerning their action, the innermost intercostals probably act with the internal intercostals; the transversus thoracis and subcostalis depress the ribs to which they attach.

Intercostal Nerves

The *intercostal nerves* (see Fig. 22-1) are the *anterior rami of the thoracic spinal nerves.* They are separated from each other by the ribs and, unlike other anterior rami, do not enter into nerve plexuses. The intercostal nerves run along the lower borders of the ribs, accompanied by intercostal arteries (for the most part, branches of the aorta) and intercostal veins. The arrangement of these structures throughout most of the intercostal space is constant and consists of (from the rib downward) the vein, artery, and nerve.

Lying deep to the internal intercostal muscles (and when the innermost intercostals are present, between them), the nerves provide motor fibers to the intercostal muscles as they course anteriorly. They provide sensory branches to the parietal pleura, the lining of the inside of the thoracic wall, and cutaneous innervation to the skin overlying the thoracic wall by giving off *lateral and anterior cutaneous branches* (see Fig. 22-1).

Table 22-1	EXTERNAL AND INTERNAL INTERCOSTAL MUSCLES			
Muscle	**Origin**	**Insertion**	**Action**	**Innervation**
External intercostals	Lower border of rib (11 pairs)	Upper border of rib below origin	Maintain intercostal space; variable reports of involvement in inspiration and expiration	Intercostal nerves
Internal intercostals	Lower border of rib (11 pairs)	Upper border of rib below origin	Maintain intercostal space; variable reports on involvement in inspiration and expiration	Intercostal nerves

Diaphragm

Between the thorax and abdomen is the **diaphragm,** a curved muscle that is convex above (Table 22-2). It completely separates the thoracic cavity from the abdominal cavity but is penetrated by structures that pass between the two cavities (see Figs. 23-2, 23-6, and 23-8). Both the inferior vena cava and the esophagus penetrate the diaphragm, but the aorta passes behind it to continue into the abdominal cavity.

FUNCTIONAL/CLINICAL NOTE 22-1

The hiatus or opening through which the esophagus passes is a potential area for the herniation of abdominal organs, particularly the stomach *(hiatal hernia).*

The diaphragm consists of skeletal muscle that has its *origin* from the inner surface of the xiphoid process and the lower ribs anterioriorly and laterally, from the bodies of the upper lumbar vertebrae, and from the fascia of the psoas major and quadratus lumborum muscles. The fibers arising from the lumbar vertebrae are called the *crura* of the diaphragm.

These muscle fibers have their *insertion* on a central tendon that completes the partition between thoracic and abdominal cavities. The diaphragm's motor *innervation* is from the phrenic nerve, which contains fibers from C3, C4, and C5. Injury to the upper cervical level of the spinal cord can eliminate fibers that contribute to the phrenic nerve and cause paralysis of the diaphragm. Because the phrenic nerve also contains sensory nerve fibers, pain from the diaphragm is sometimes felt in the neck or shoulder, where other fibers of the three cervical nerves are distributed. This is an example of referred pain. The *action* of the diaphragmatic muscle fibers is to pull down on the central tendon, which lowers its dome so that the vertical dimension (length) of the thoracic cavity is increased. This causes increased pressure within the abdominal cavity. With relaxation of the diaphragm, the elasticity of the abdominal wall pushes the viscera and the diaphragm upward in expiration.

Mechanics of Respiration

Respiration consists of inspiration and expiration. Inspiration requires an increase in the size of the thoracic cavity. Three different dimensions of the cavity can be modified to increase the capacity of the cavity: *vertical, transverse* (lateral), and *anteroposterior.* Increasing the *vertical dimension* produces the greatest change in capacity and is brought about primarily by contraction of the diaphragm. As the diaphragm contracts, it drops downward, decreasing its height and increasing the vertical dimension within the thoracic cavity. The amount of contraction and flattening of the diaphragm depends on the force of inspiration.

Movement of specific ribs produces changes in either the transverse or anteroposterior dimension of the cavity. The upper three false ribs (ribs 8 to 10) curve downward and then upward as they proceed anteriorly. When these ribs are elevated, they rotate upward and laterally, which results in an increase in the *transverse dimension* of the thoracic cavity. This movement is called the "bucket handle" movement because it is similar to that of the handle of a bucket when it is raised.

The upper ribs slope inferiorly and, when they are elevated, as a result of their articulation with the sternum, cause a hinge type of movement at the sternal angle (manubriosternal junction). In this way, the

Table 22-2	DIAPHRAGM			
Muscle	**Origin**	**Insertion**	**Action**	**Innervation**
Diaphragm	Inner surface of xiphoid process; lower ribs anteriorly and laterally; bodies of upper lumbar vertebrae as crura of diaphragm; fascia over psoas major and quadratus lumborum	Central tendon of diaphragm	Depression of central tendon to increase vertical dimension of thoracic cavity	Phrenic nerve (C3, C4, C5)

sternum is moved anteriorly and the *anteroposterior dimension* of the thoracic cavity is increased. The movement is referred to as the "pump handle" movement.

In quiet breathing, *inspiration* is brought about mainly by the action of the diaphragm. During forced inspiration, many other muscles that are attached to the ribs may assist in raising the ribs, such as the scalene and sternocleidomastoids, or in fixing the lower ribs against the pull of the diaphragm, such as the quadratus lumborum. The pectoral muscles can even be used if the arms are fixed. As stated previously, the function of the intercostals in inspiration is controversial.

Expiration can be a passive process. When the diaphragm contracts during inspiration, it compresses the abdominal organs, increasing pressure within the abdominal cavity. In expiration, this increased pressure can help to push the diaphragm upward. In forced expiration, the muscles of the abdominal wall contract to provide additional pressure on the diaphragm and to pull the lower ribs downward. The intercostals may be involved in expiration, but, again, their role is uncertain.

PLEURAL AND PERICARDIAL SACS

The thoracic cavity contains three large serous sacs lined with mesothelium. These sacs, two pleural sacs and one pericardial sac, enclose the two lungs and the heart, respectively (see Fig. 22-2). Each is a closed sac, with one wall carried inward around the organ it encloses, much as the side of a balloon may be pushed in with a fist.

The *parietal pleura* is the outer wall of each **pleural sac.** This outer layer is attached to the thoracic wall, to the diaphragm below, and to the pericardial sac medially. Where the diaphragm arises from the lower border of the rib cage, the parietal pleura is reflected off the thoracic wall and onto the surface of the diaphragm. In expiration, lung tissue is not present in this region, and the two layers of parietal pleura are in contact. The potential space created within the pleural cavity is termed the *costodiaphragmatic recess.* This recess extends around the lower border of the thoracic cavity on each side of the thorax (Figs. 22-3 and 22-4). During inspiration, as the diaphragm drops, the lung expands into the costodiaphragmatic recesses. The *visceral (pulmonary) pleura* (*pulmonary* is the adjective derived from *pulmo,* the Latin name for the lung) is the layer of the wall of the sac that has been pushed inward by the growth of the lung. It forms the smooth outer surface of the lung.

Visceral and parietal pleurae are normally in contact with themselves or each other, and the pleural cavity consists only of a potential space between the immediately adjacent surfaces of the pleurae. It is occupied by a very thin layer of fluid, which allows the two layers to slide freely on each other. Elevation of the ribs and contraction with consequent depression

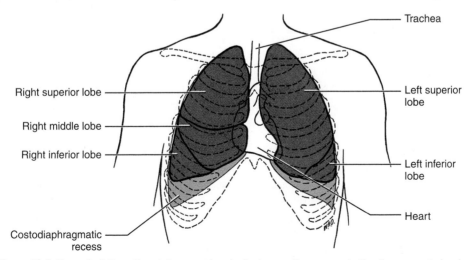

Right superior lobe

Right middle lobe

Right inferior lobe

Costodiaphragmatic recess

Trachea

Left superior lobe

Left inferior lobe

Heart

Figure 22-3 General relation of heart, lungs and costodiaphragmatic recesses to the rib cage, anterior view.

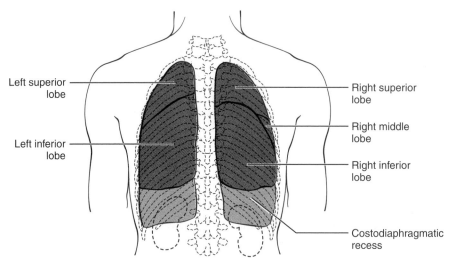

Left superior
lobe

Left inferior
lobe

Right superior
lobe

Right middle
lobe

Right inferior
lobe

Costodiaphragmatic
recess

Figure 22-4 General relation of the lungs and costodiaphragmatic recesses to the rib cage, posterior view. (*Dotted outlines* represent the kidneys.)

of the diaphragm result in an enlargement of the thoracic cavity, and the parietal pleura follows the movements of the diaphragm and thoracic wall, to both of which it is firmly attached. The outward movement of the parietal pleura naturally results in an attempt to enlarge the pleural cavity by separating parietal from visceral pleurae. The "negative" pressure within the pleural cavities causes air to move into the lungs because of atmospheric pressure, and, therefore, the lungs expand.

FUNCTIONAL/CLINICAL NOTE 22-2

Although the lungs are highly elastic, the cohesive film normally keeps them in contact with the parietal pleura. Injury to the pleura, however, either from a wound in the thoracic wall or through the lung itself, allows air to gain access to the pleural cavity, and the lung collapses. The presence of air in the pleural cavity is termed *pneumothorax*. Air may enter spontaneously through damage to the thoracic wall or the lung, or it may be introduced purposely into the pleural cavity to collapse a lung and prevent it from following the respiratory movements. Such resting of the lung may allow healing that would not progress as well if the lung was constantly being expanded and contracted. Blood can also enter the pleural cavity, which results in a *hemothorax*.

The **pericardial sac** is built upon the same fundamental plan as the pleural sacs but has an additional outer layer, the *fibrous pericardium*, which is a tough fibrous membrane. The fibrous pericardium is lined internally with mesothelium, which is termed the *parietal pericardium* (parietal lamina of the serous pericardium). Where it is attached to the great vessels as they leave the heart, the mesothelium is reflected inferiorly over these vessels and over the heart to form the *visceral pericardium* (visceral lamina of the serous pericardium or the epicardium). The pericardial cavity consists of the potential space between the parietal and visceral pericardia. Although the pericardial sac is fairly loose in order to allow for the rhythmic changes in heart volume necessary for the pump action of the heart, the pericardium is so tough that it can be expanded suddenly only very slightly. Therefore, accumulations of fluid or blood within the pericardial cavity may markedly interfere with the ability of the heart to receive incoming blood. This compression is called *cardiac tamponade,* which if severe enough, can lead to death.

THORACIC VISCERA

Lungs

The **lungs** lie laterally within the thoracic cavity and partially surround the heart (Figs. 22-5 and 22-6; see Figs. 22-2 to 22-4). They sit on the surface of the diaphragm. Their lower edges extend slightly downward into the area between the sloping diaphragm and the thoracic walls. The bronchi, vessels, nerves, and lymphatic vessels (as a group, termed the *root of the lung*) enter and leave each lung on its medial surface. The lungs are subdivided by fissures (clefts) into lobes. There are three lobes in the right lung (superior, middle, and inferior) and two in the left lung (superior and inferior). An *oblique fissure* separates the superior and inferior lobes of each lung, and a *horizontal fissure* demarcates the middle lobe from the superior lobe of the right lung. The lobes are positioned in such a way that the inferior lobe is more posteriorly placed than the superior and middle lobes.

The lungs receive air by way of the trachea and the bronchi. The *trachea* ends in the upper part of the thorax by branching into two *main bronchi,* one for each lung. The right main bronchus in turn

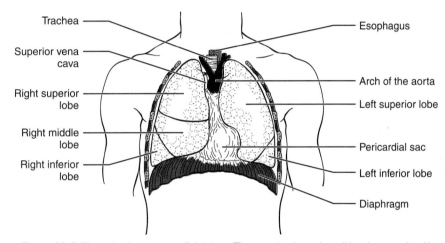

Figure 22-5 Thoracic viscera, superficial view. (The anterior thoracic wall has been omitted.)

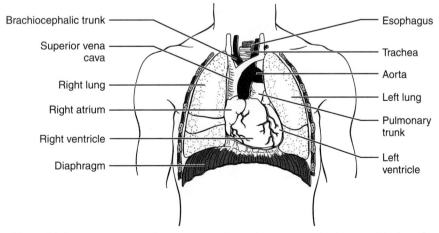

Figure 22-6 Thoracic viscera. (Anterior parts of lungs have been omitted to reveal the heart.)

branches into three *lobar bronchi*, one for each of the three lobes of the right lung, and the left main bronchus branches into two lobar bronchi. The bronchi branch repeatedly within the lungs. Their smallest subdivisions, known as *bronchioles*, finally end in connection with small, thin-walled air sacs, or *alveoli*, through the walls of which occurs the essential interchange of gases between air and the blood stream.

The lungs receive blood to be oxygenated from the *pulmonary trunk*, which arises from the right ventricle (Fig. 22-7). The pulmonary trunk divides into right and left *pulmonary arteries*, each of which tends to follow the bronchus of its own side but gives off more numerous branches into the lung than does the bronchus. The *pulmonary veins*, usually two from each lung, empty into the left atrium of the heart. Three small *bronchial arteries* provide the arterial blood supply to the lung tissue itself.

The branching of the lobar bronchi is particularly complicated, and the direction of their branching becomes important when it is necessary to drain some particular bronchus by gravity. Within a lobe, each lobar bronchus gives off from two to five smaller bronchi, each with a descriptive name but collectively known as *segmental bronchi*. These segmental bronchi usually run in different directions within a lobe.

FUNCTIONAL/CLINICAL NOTE 22-3

Only in the case of the small middle lobe of the right lung do all the segmental bronchi (there are only two here) run parallel enough with each other to allow one position to facilitate drainage of the entire lobe. For the other lobes, the patient may have to be standing in order to drain one segmental bronchus, lying on the back to drain another, or lying on one side but face down to drain another. The positions differ from lobe to lobe.

The concept of segmentation of the lungs is clinically important not only in drainage of the lung but also in such procedures as removal of diseased tissue. Each region of the lung supplied by a particular segmental bronchus is termed a *bronchopulmonary segment*. Each segment has its own arterial supply from the pulmonary and

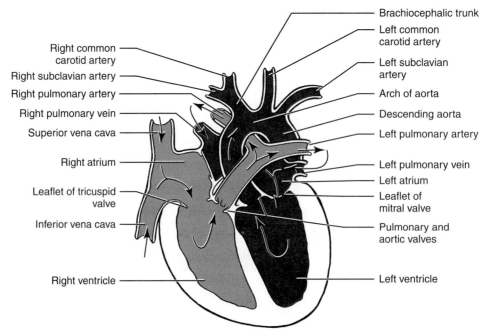

Figure 22-7 The heart and the circulation of blood through it. The *arrows* indicate the direction of flow of the blood.

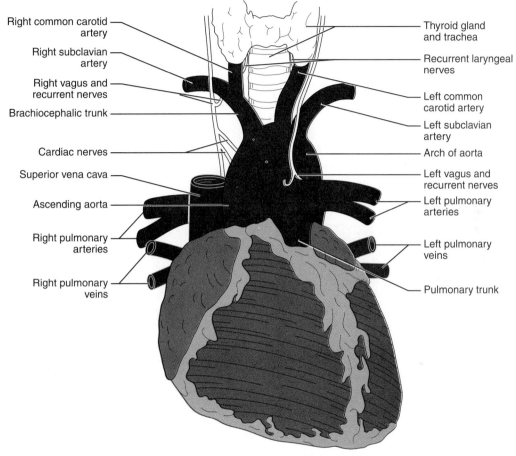

Right common carotid artery

Right subclavian artery

Right vagus and recurrent nerves

Brachiocephalic trunk

Cardiac nerves

Superior vena cava

Ascending aorta

Right pulmonary arteries

Right pulmonary veins

Thyroid gland and trachea

Recurrent laryngeal nerves

Left common carotid artery

Left subclavian artery

Arch of aorta

Left vagus and recurrent nerves

Left pulmonary arteries

Left pulmonary veins

Pulmonary trunk

Figure 22-8 The heart and great vessels. The inferior vena cava has not been included in this illustration.

bronchial arteries and its own venous drainage by the pulmonary veins. There may be, however, some limited sharing of vascular channels with adjacent segments. Such compartmentalization makes it possible to remove a diseased bronchopulmonary segment without major damage to surrounding segments.

Heart

The **heart (cor)** is a muscular pump for propelling the blood (Fig. 22-8; see Figs. 22-5 and 22-6). It contains four chambers; two, the *atria,* are thin-walled and receive incoming blood, and the

other two, the *ventricles,* are heavy-walled and propel the blood into the arterial systems (see Fig. 22-7). As is true in all pump systems, the heart contains valves to prevent backward flow of fluid and to allow a propulsive pressure to be built up within the system. By way of the superior vena cava, the right atrium receives blood returning from the head and neck, the upper extremities, and the thorax; by way of the inferior vena cava, it receives blood from the abdomen and lower extremities. This blood then passes into the right ventricle and is pumped by the right ventricle out the pulmonary trunk and arteries to the lungs, where the blood is aerated. The *tricuspid valve,* at the opening between the right atrium and ventricle, prevents backward flow from the ventricle into the atrium. The *pulmonary valve*, with three valvules somewhat resembling pockets on a vest, is located at the mouth of the pulmonary artery and prevents blood in this vessel from running back into the ventricle as the ventricle relaxes.

Blood returning from the lungs by way of the pulmonary veins enters the left atrium. It is then passed into the left ventricle, and from the left ventricle, it is pumped out into the aorta to be distributed to the body in general. The *mitral (bicuspid) valve* is located at the atrioventricular opening. An *aortic valve*, similar to the pulmonary valve, is found at the opening of the aorta.

FUNCTIONAL/CLINICAL NOTE 22-4

Any of the various valves of the heart may on occasion be thickened or otherwise defective and may fail to close properly, therefore allowing blood under high pressure to flow back into the region of less pressure. This is referred to as a leaking or "insufficient" valve and produces a sound known as a *heart murmur.*

Because the left ventricle must pump blood all over the body, whereas the right ventricle pumps blood only to the lungs, the left ventricle does considerably more work than does the right. As a result, the wall of the left ventricle is much thicker than that of the right.

VESSELS

Arteries

The **thoracic aorta** consists of three parts: the *ascending aorta*, running upward from the left ventricle; the *arch of the aorta*, curving to the left, posteriorly, and downward (see Fig. 22-8); and the *descending aorta*, which lies slightly to the left of the midline. The *thoracic aorta* as a whole descends through the thorax, passes through the diaphragm at the level of the 12th thoracic vertebra, and continues as the *abdominal aorta.*

The **right and left coronary arteries,** which supply the heart muscle, arise from the ascending aorta just above the left ventricle. The **brachiocephalic**

trunk (dividing into the right subclavian and right common carotid arteries), the **left common carotid artery,** and the **left subclavian artery** are given off in that order from the arch. Other branches of the thoracic aorta are small. The largest and most numerous are the paired **intercostal arteries,** which run beneath the lower borders of the ribs. Small branches from the aorta supply the esophagus, the walls of the bronchi, and the tissue of the lungs (bronchial arteries).

Veins

The **great veins** in the thorax consist of the *brachiocephalic veins,* the *superior and inferior venae cavae,* and the *azygos and hemiazygos venous systems.* The paired **brachiocephalic veins** are formed by the union of internal jugular and subclavian veins and therefore return blood from the head, neck, and upper limbs. The **superior vena cava** is formed by the union of the right and left brachiocephalic veins in the upper part of the thorax. The **inferior vena cava** penetrates the diaphragm to end in the immediately adjacent heart, and it therefore has a very limited thoracic course. The **azygos and hemiazygos systems of veins,** which receive blood mostly from the thoracic wall by means of the intercostal veins, empty into the superior vena cava.

The pulmonary circulation has already been briefly described in connection with the heart and lungs and need not be repeated here.

NERVES

The important nerves connected with the thoracic viscera are the paired vagus nerves and the sympathetic trunks. The **vagus nerves,** descending from the neck, pass posterior to the roots of the lungs (containing the bronchi and vessels and nerves passing to and from the lungs) to lie on the esophagus, with which they travel through the thorax and enter the abdomen. These nerves supply parasympathetic motor nerve fibers to the heart, which decrease the strength and rate of the heartbeat, and also parasympathetic motor fibers to the lungs and the esophagus.

The thoracic part of the **sympathetic trunk** consists of 11 or 12 accumulations of nerve cells called *ganglia,* connected by fibers that run up or down the trunk. This part of the trunk is continuous above with the cervical part and below with the lumbar part of the trunk. The individual ganglia are connected to spinal nerves by rami communicantes (see Chapter 13), through which they receive fibers from the spinal cord and send fibers back into the spinal nerves to be distributed with them. The heart receives its sympathetic innervation largely by branches that descend into the thorax from the cervical part of the trunk, but additional fibers also reach the heart from the thoracic part of the trunk. Vagal and sympathetic fibers unite to form plexuses in connection with the heart. Other fibers from the thoracic part of the trunk enter into plexuses supplying the lungs and the esophagus. In general, stimulation of sympathetic fibers produces effects opposite to those produced by stimulation of the vagus nerve. Therefore, sympathetic stimulation increases the rate and strength of the heartbeat. The sympathetic trunks also send large nerves, the *splanchnic nerves,* to ganglia of the prevertebral plexuses in the abdomen.

FUNCTIONAL/CLINICAL NOTE 22-5

The heart normally generates its own impulse to beat, and the sympathetic and parasympathetic fibers to it merely exert a limited control over this beat. The heart muscle also contracts in response to an appropriate electric shock. A heart that stops beating can sometimes be started again by this method, or a ventricle that is contracting irregularly can resume a steady, properly timed beat, if regularly spaced electric impulses are delivered to it through an electrode implanted in the muscle (pacemaker).

In addition to these two sets of nerve fibers, which are concerned primarily with the viscera, the thorax is traversed by the important **phrenic nerves.** These run downward, anterior to the hilus of the lungs, between pleura and pericardium, to innervate the diaphragm.

SURFACE ANATOMY

The bony framework of the thoracic wall is palpable, although anteriorly the breast and muscles of the pectoral region cover some areas. Posteriorly, the scapula and muscles attached to it prevent palpation of the upper ribs. The surface anatomy of the back and of the bones and muscles of the shoulder region has been considered in other chapters.

Anterosuperiorly, the **sternum** and **clavicle** can be palpated. The **jugular (suprasternal) notch** is evident between the medial ends of the clavicles. Immediately posterior to the notch, some of the **tracheal rings** can be felt, and superior to these, the **cricoid and thyroid cartilages** are palpable. The **cricothyroid membrane** can be felt between the cricoid and thyroid cartilages. If the **manubrium** of the sternum is followed inferiorly, the **sternal angle** can be palpated; laterally, on each side of the sternal angle, the **second rib** articulates with the sternum. This is a good landmark because the first rib is covered by the clavicle and fascia; locating the second rib in this manner enables counting of the interspaces and ribs below the second. Inferior to the manubrium, the **body of the sternum** is palpable, and the **xiphoid process** can be felt further inferiorly.

Parts of the rib cage can be palpated anteriorly, laterally, and posteriorly. The curvature of the ribs can be followed, and the **inferior costal margin** is quite apparent. The anterior ends of the **floating ribs** (ribs 11 and 12) can be located inferiorly on the lateral side of the thoracic wall. The movement of the ribs, sternum, and abdominal wall during inspiration and expiration can be observed and also felt.

The **nipple** typically lies over the fourth intercostal space in males, but its position in females varies with regard to the amount of breast tissue present. The **apex beat of the heart** (where the tip of the heart lies against the inner surface of the thoracic wall) can be palpated and sometimes observed, particularly in a thin individual, in the fifth intercostal space on the left, near the midclavicular line, an imaginary vertical line projected down from the middle of the clavicle.

The organs and structures of the thoracic cavity obviously cannot be observed, but their relative positions can be visualized by imagining their surface projections on the thoracic wall. An imaginary plane passing through the sternal angle would intersect with the disc between the fourth and fifth thoracic vertebrae. The **bifurcation of the trachea** into the two main bronchi occurs at or just below this plane, and the **arch of the aorta** passes posteriorly and to the left at this level.

The highest point of the right side of the **diaphragm** at rest is just below the right nipple and, on the left side, is approximately an inch (2.5 cm) below the left nipple. The **lungs** project into the neck approximately an inch above the first rib. They sit on top of the diaphragm, but their lower borders extend slightly into the area between the dome of the diaphragm and the thoracic wall. The **lower border of the lung** of each side (see Figs. 22-3 and 22-4) can be followed along a line that crosses the sixth rib anteriorly (at the midclavicular line), the eighth rib laterally, and the tenth rib posteriorly. The **costodiaphragmatic recesses** extend about two rib levels lower. The left lung is notched anteriorly to accommodate the heart as it projects to the left.

The position of the **heart** can be visualized by mapping its borders. The **right border** parallels the right side of the sternum, extending just past the sternum's lateral edge. Superiorly to inferiorly, it extends from the third to sixth ribs. The **superior border** on the right is at the third rib, whereas on the left it extends to the lower border of the second rib, about about three quarters of an inch (19 mm) lateral to the sternum. From that point, the **left border** extends down to the apex beat of the heart, and the **inferior border** lies on a horizontal line at the level of the junction of the xiphoid process with the body of the sternum.

REVIEW QUESTIONS

1 Describe the anatomy of the sternum. Which rib attaches to the sternum at the sternal angle?

2 How many pairs of ribs are there? How many attach directly to the sternum?

3 Describe the origin and insertion of the diaphragm.

4 What is a bronchopulmonary segment?

5 When ribs 8 to 10 are elevated, which dimension of the thoracic cavity is increased? With regard to the mechanics of respiration, to what does the "pump handle" movement refer?

6 What is the costodiaphragmatic recess?

7 Describe the course of blood flow from the superior vena cava to the arch of the aorta. Include in the description the chambers of the heart and vessels traversed, as well as the valves through which the blood passes.

8 What are the branches of the arch of the aorta?

EXERCISES

1 Demonstrate the surface projections of the lungs, costodiaphragmatic recesses, and heart.

2 By palpation, identify the following:
   a sternal angle
   b second rib
   c fifth intercostal space (apex beat of the heart on the midclavicular line)
   d jugular notch
   e cricoid cartilage

23 THE ABDOMEN AND PELVIS

CHAPTER CONTENTS

Abdominal Wall

Pelvic Floor and Perineum

Abdominal Viscera

Pelvic Viscera

Vessels

Nerves

Surface Anatomy

The abdomen is so large that it is convenient to subdivide it for purposes of description. One method of subdivision consists of the erection of imaginary lines that divide it into nine regions. The terminology employed for these regions is somewhat cumbersome, and much of it is rarely used in actual practice. The most commonly used term from this form of classification is *epigastrium* or *epigastric region*, referring to the area below the sternum and between the two costal arches.

The simplest and most convenient method of dividing the abdomen is to think of it as consisting of quadrants separated from each other by the anterior midline and a line passing horizontally through the umbilicus. In this way, the abdomen is divided into **upper right, lower right, upper left,** and **lower left quadrants.**

ABDOMINAL WALL

The abdominal wall consists functionally not only of the anterolateral abdominal muscles and the lumbar portion of the vertebral column but also of the lower ribs and the diaphragm (Fig. 23-1). Because of the domelike shape of the *diaphragm,* the abdominal viscera extend upward beneath it and are in part protected by the *lower ribs.* The diaphragm intervenes between these ribs and the abdominal viscera. Posteriorly in the midline are the bodies of the *lumbar vertebrae,* flanked on each side by the *psoas major muscle,* which acts on the lower limb (Fig. 23-2).

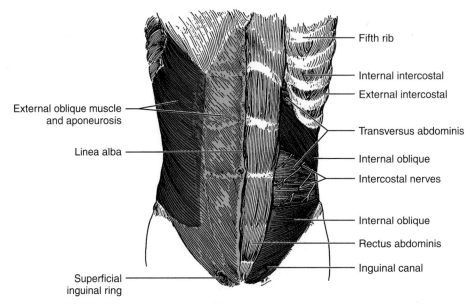

External oblique muscle and aponeurosis

Linea alba

Superficial inguinal ring

Fifth rib

Internal intercostal

External intercostal

Transversus abdominis

Internal oblique

Intercostal nerves

Internal oblique

Rectus abdominis

Inguinal canal

Figure 23-1 The musculature of the anterior and lateral aspects of the abdominal wall.

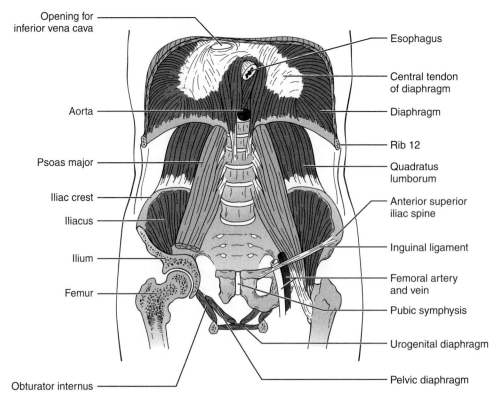

Opening for inferior vena cava

Aorta

Psoas major

Iliac crest

Iliacus

Ilium

Femur

Obturator internus

Esophagus

Central tendon of diaphragm

Diaphragm

Rib 12

Quadratus lumborum

Anterior superior iliac spine

Inguinal ligament

Femoral artery and vein

Pubic symphysis

Urogenital diaphragm

Pelvic diaphragm

Figure 23-2 The posterior abdominal wall and pelvis. Part of the pelvic region is depicted in coronal section to illustrate the pelvic and urogenital diaphragms.

Muscles of the Abdominal Wall

The anterolateral abdominal muscles serve to retain and support the abdominal viscera and also, through their attachments to the ribs and sternum, play an important part in movements of the trunk. The lateral abdominal muscles are arranged in three layers (Table 23-1; see Fig. 23-1). Two of these run obliquely and are known as the *external and internal obliques;* the third runs almost transversely and is named the *transversus abdominis.*

The **external oblique** muscle has its *origin* from about the lower six ribs and forms a broad sheet that runs downward and medially. Its *insertion* is on the anterior part of the iliac crest, the pubis, and the linea alba. The linea alba (white line) lies deep to the skin in the anterior midline. It is formed by the union of the aponeuroses of all three lateral abdominal muscles of one side with those of the other side. Most of the insertion of the external oblique is tendinous; the tendon of insertion is known as the *aponeurosis of the external oblique.* The aponeurosis extends to the anterior midline, passing anterior to the rectus abdominis muscle. The lower edge of the aponeurosis passes from the anterior superior iliac spine to the pubis and forms the **inguinal ligament.** The lateral part of the inguinal ligament is attached

to the fascia of the iliopsoas muscle, but medially it has a free edge behind which the external iliac vessels become continuous with the femoral vessels. The external oblique receives *innervation* from usually the lower six intercostal nerves.

The **internal oblique** muscle corresponds in its direction to the internal intercostal muscles, just as the external oblique muscle corresponds to the external intercostals. The internal oblique has its *origin* from the iliopsoas fascia and lateral half of the inguinal ligament, from the more anterior portion of the iliac crest, and by an aponeurotic layer that extends posteriorly to split around the muscles of the back and attach to both the spinous and transverse processes of lumbar vertebrae as the thoracolumbar fascia. The *insertion* of the internal oblique is by an aponeurosis into the linea alba. A portion of this aponeurosis passes in front of the rectus muscle to blend with the aponeurosis of the external oblique, and a second portion passes behind the rectus abdominis to blend with the aponeurosis of the transversus abdominis. The internal oblique also inserts into the lower ribs.

The **transversus abdominis** muscle, the deepest of the lateral abdominal muscles, has its *origin* from the thoracolumbar fascia, from the tips of the lower six ribs, the anterior portion of the iliac crest, and the lateral part of the inguinal ligament. This muscle also

Table 23-1	MUSCLES OF THE ABDOMINAL WALL			
Muscle	**Origin**	**Insertion**	**Action**	**Innervation**
External oblique	Lower six ribs	Anterior part of iliac crest; pubis; aponeurosis into linea alba	With internal oblique and transversus abdominis, compression of abdominal cavity; flexion and rotation of trunk	Lower intercostal nerves
Internal oblique	Iliopsoas fascia and lateral half of inguinal ligament; anterior part of iliac crest; thoracolumbar fascia	Aponeurosis into linea alba; lower ribs	Compression of abdominal cavity; flexion and rotation of trunk	Lower intercostal nerves; L1 through its iliohypogastric and ilioinguinal branches
Transversus abdominis	Thoracolumbar fascia; lateral part of inguinal ligament; tips of lower six ribs; anterior part of iliac crest	Aponeurosis into linea alba	Compression of abdominal cavity	Lower intercostal nerves; L1 through its iliohypogastric and ilioinguinal branches
Rectus abdominis	Pubic crest; ligaments of pubic symphysis	Xiphoid process; ribs 5–7	Flexion of trunk	Lower intercostal nerves

ends in an aponeurosis, the fibers of which pass, for the most part, deep to the rectus abdominis to attain an *insertion* into the linea alba. For a variable distance above the pubis, however, the aponeuroses of all three muscles pass in front of the rectus abdominis.

The internal oblique and transversus abdominis receive *innervation* from approximately the 7th to 12th intercostal nerves and from the iliohypogastric and ilioinguinal branches of the first lumbar nerve.

The external and internal oblique muscles in males are split in their lower portions to allow the structures of the spermatic cord (the ductus deferens and vessels of the testis) to make their exit from the abdominal cavity. The transversus abdominis may be involved in this, but it usually lies above the level of exit. The oblique passageway of the spermatic cord through the abdominal muscles is known as the **inguinal canal,** and it forms a weak place in the anterior abdominal wall. The abdominal end of the canal is known as the *deep inguinal ring.* Its external opening (the split in the external oblique aponeurosis) is known as the *superficial inguinal ring.*

FUNCTIONAL/CLINICAL NOTE 23-1

Approximately 97% of abdominal hernias (i.e., protrusions of abdominal viscera through the abdominal wall) in males involve all or a part of the inguinal canal. An inguinal canal is also present in females, although it is small because it transmits only a small ligament and a few tiny blood vessels. While inguinal hernias are less predominant in females, they are still the most frequent type of hernias (50%) in female patients. Other particularly weak places in the abdominal wall are the femoral canal (medial to the femoral vessels behind the inguinal ligament) and the umbilicus. Presumably because of the smallness of the inguinal canal, abdominal hernias of all types are only about one sixth as common in females as in males.

The *action* of the obliques and the transversus abdominis, working as a group, is to compress the abdomen and therefore increase the pressure on the abdominal viscera. In so doing, they may cooperate with the diaphragm to "fix" the thorax, an effect that may be brought about when especially delicate or powerful movements of the upper limb are to be carried out, at which times the breath is normally held. The external and internal obliques of both sides, acting together, aid in flexion of the trunk. The external oblique of one side is usually described as working with the internal oblique of the opposite side in flexing and rotating the trunk to the side of the internal oblique. However, this is probably carried out mostly by the internal oblique, although both external obliques become slightly active.

The **rectus abdominis** (see Fig. 23-1) is a pair of straplike muscles aligned vertically along the midline of the anterior abdominal wall. One of the pair is situated just on each side of the midline. The aponeuroses of the more lateral abdominal muscles as they pass partly in front of and partly behind the rectus abdominis muscles form sheaths for the two muscles. Each rectus abdominis has its own sheath, but the two sheaths are united at the linea alba. It takes *origin* from the pubic crest and ligaments of the pubic symphysis, and its *insertion* is onto the xiphoid process and cartilages of the fifth, sixth, and seventh ribs. The muscle is partly subdivided into segments by several fibrous bands, tendinous intersections, that cross it. In muscular individuals, the rectus abdominis muscles, even their segments, can be plainly recognized. Their curved lateral borders are called the *semilunar lines,* and they may be a prominent feature of the surface anatomy of the abdomen.

The *action* of the rectus abdominis is as an important flexor of the trunk or, at its fixed point from above, an upward rotator of the pelvis. Unlike the oblique and the transversus abdominis, the rectus abdominis does not aid in compressing the abdomen, except incidentally, as it flexes the trunk or depresses the thoracic wall. The rectus receives its *innervation* from the lower intercostal nerves that pierce the lateral wall of the muscle sheath to reach the muscle.

Posterior Muscles

A posterior muscle of the abdominal wall, situated in the lumbar region, is the **quadratus lumborum** muscle (Table 23-2; see Fig. 23-2). It is a complex muscle that has its *origin* from the medial part of the iliac crest and its *insertion* on the last rib and lower lumbar vertebrae. Some of its fibers also insert on, and some arise from, the lumbar transverse processes. Its primary *action* is to flex the vertebral column laterally; it also fixes the 12th rib to provide a stable base for contraction of the diaphragm during inspiration. Taking its fixed point from above, it tilts the side of the pelvis to which it is attached upward. Its *innervation* is provided by direct branches from T12 and L1 to L3.

The psoas major also lies on the posterior abdominal wall. Information on this muscle is presented in Chapter 16 (see Table 16-1).

Intercostal Nerves and Vessels

The lower **intercostal nerves and vessels,** continuing the downward direction of the ribs, run into the lower part of the abdominal wall. The 10th intercostal nerve ends at about the level of the umbilicus, and the 12th ends only a short distance above the pubic symphysis. *The lower intercostal nerves and the branches (iliohypogastric and ilioinguinal) from the first lumbar nerve provide innervation to the musculature and skin of the abdomen.* The main branches of the nerves run roughly parallel to each other between the internal oblique and transversus muscles. They exchange enough branches so that they form a loose plexus in this position.

Small intercostal arteries accompany the abdominal portions of the intercostal nerves and anastomose here with ascending branches from the external iliac vessels and with lateral branches of the **inferior epigastric artery,** also derived from the external iliac artery (see Fig. 23-6). In the substance of the rectus abdominis muscle, the inferior epigastric anastomoses

with the **superior epigastric artery,** a continuation of the internal thoracic artery that arises from the subclavian artery at the base of the neck. The internal thoracic artery runs downward on the inner surface of the thoracic wall a little lateral to the sternum.

An important relationship of the inferior epigastric artery close to its origin is its proximity to the deep inguinal ring, or abdominal end of the inguinal canal. The **inferior epigastric artery** lies just medial to this opening; therefore, in a hernia that traverses the entire length of the inguinal canal, an *indirect inguinal hernia,* the neck of its hernial sac is situated lateral to this vessel. The second chief type of inguinal hernia, a *direct inguinal hernia,* bulges directly toward or through the superficial inguinal ring, rather than starting at the deep ring. Therefore, it lies medial to the artery.

PELVIC FLOOR AND PERINEUM

The walls of the abdomen have already been briefly considered. The diaphragm forms the roof of the abdominal cavity, and because abdominal and pelvic cavities are continuous with each other, the floor of the pelvis is also the floor of the abdominal cavity.

The area surrounded by the coccyx, pubic symphysis, ischia, and inferior ramus of each pubic bone is known as the *pelvic outlet,* and the muscles bridging the pelvic outlet constitute the pelvic floor, or **pelvic diaphragm.** The chief muscle of the pelvic diaphragm is the **levator ani** (Fig. 23-3 and Table 23-3; see Fig. 23-2). Its *origin* on each side is from the pubis and the ischial spine and a thickening of the fascia between these two bony origins, the *tendinous arch of the levator ani.* The *insertion* of the levator ani is along the midline with the muscle of the opposite side and onto the coccyx.

Table 23-2	QUADRATUS LUMBORUM			
Muscle	**Origin**	**Insertion**	**Action**	**Innervation**
Quadratus lumborum	Medial part of iliac crest	Rib 12; lower lumbar vertebrae	Lateral flexion of vertebral column; fixation of last rib to form stable base for contraction of diaphragm	Branches from T12 and L1–L3

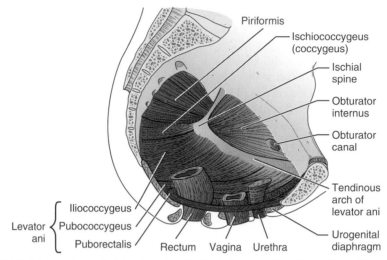

Piriformis

Ischiococcygeus
(coccygeus)

Ischial
spine

Obturator
internus

Obturator
canal

Tendinous
arch of
levator ani

Urogenital
diaphragm

Iliococcygeus

Levator
ani { Pubococcygeus

Puborectalis

Rectum   Vagina   Urethra

Figure 23-3 Medial view of a sagittally sectioned pelvis, illustrating muscles of the walls and floor of the pelvis.

Table 23-3	PELVIC DIAPHRAGM			
Muscle	**Origin**	**Insertion**	**Action**	**Innervation**
Levator ani (component parts: puborectalis, pubococcygeus, and iliococcygeus)	Pubis; ischial spine; fascia between these bony origins	Coccyx; midline around pelvic organs and with muscle of opposite side	Support of pelvic viscera, particularly during increased abdominal pressure; pulls anal canal upward	Branches from S3 and S4
Ischiococcygeus (coccygeus)	Ischial spine	Lower sacrum; upper coccyx	Pulling coccyx anteriorly; support of pelvic viscera	Branches from S4 and S5

The levator ani can be subdivided into three parts: the *puborectalis, pubococcygeus,* and *iliococcygeus* (see Fig. 23-3). The **puborectalis** is the most medial component of the levator ani muscle, arising from the medial part of the body of the pubis of each side. Its fibers are directed posteriorly, forming a muscular sling around the anorectal junction. The **pubococcygeus** lies lateral to the puborectalis, arising form the body of the pubis and anteromedial part of the tendinous arch. Its medial fibers meet with those of the opposite side along the midline, while the more lateral fibers insert on the coccyx. The most lateral component of the levator ani, the **iliococcygeus,** arises from the posterior part of the tendinous arch and the ischial spine. Its fibers insert along the midline and coccyx.

The levator ani as a whole is somewhat funnel-shaped, converging toward the rectum and anal canal at its apex. Around the anal canal, the fibers of the levator ani blend with the musculature of the canal, providing firm attachment to this terminal portion of the digestive tract as it leaves the pelvis. Anteriorly, the levator ani divides to allow the urethra to pass through. In females, it is also perforated by the vagina (see Fig. 23-7), and its attachments to the vaginal wall give support to this structure. The lower portion of the rectum and the urinary bladder or, in males, the prostate, rests on the upper surface of the levator ani. The *action* of the levator ani is to resist downward movement of the pelvic viscera caused by increased abdominal pressure and to pull the anal canal upward during defecation. The muscle receives *innervation,* usually on its pelvic surface, from branches of spinal nerves S3 and S4. The levator ani largely controls voluntary emptying of the urinary bladder and is extremely important in the support of the uterus. Weakness of this muscle (specifically of the pubococcygeus) predisposes the individual to urinary incontinence. However, exercise of this muscle and adjacent muscles may restore continence.

Posterior to the levator ani is the **ischiococcygeus (coccygeus),** the other muscle of the pelvic diaphragm. This muscle takes *origin* from the ischial spine, and its *insertion* is on the lower part of the sacrum and upper part of the coccyx. It adds little to the pelvic diaphragm, but its *action* is to pull the coccyx forward and support the pelvic viscera. Spasm of the muscle and the part of the levator ani that attaches to the coccyx has been thought to be responsible for certain cases of *painful coccyx* (coccygodynia or coccydynia). The coccygeus receives *innervation* from branches of spinal nerves S4 and S5.

External to (below) the levator ani, passing transversely from one inferior ramus of the pubis and an associated portion of the ramus of the ischium across to the corresponding bony elements on the other side, is a structure known as the **urogenital diaphragm.** This consists of muscle and fascia. Because it bridges the more anterior part of the pelvic outlet between the diverging inferior pubic rami, it affords additional support to the pelvic viscera. The urogenital diaphragm is perforated by the urethra and, in females, also by the vagina.

The external aspect of the pelvic outlet (the region between the thighs that includes both the area around the anus and the external genital organs) is known as the **perineum.** The musculature of the perineum includes the muscle in the urogenital diaphragm, special muscles in connection with the penis or the vagina and clitoris, and an external, voluntary sphincter muscle of the anus. These muscles are all innervated by the *pudendal nerve* from the lower portion (S2, S3, and S4) of the sacral plexus. The external surface of the levator ani forms the roof of the perineum. On each side between the ischial tuberosity and the levator ani, as the muscles converge on the anal canal, there is a space filled with fat and tough strands of connective tissue. This area is the **ischiorectal fossa.** The levator ani can be massaged through this tissue in the fossa.

ABDOMINAL VISCERA

The abdomen is lined by a serous membrane that is, for the most part, in intimate contact with the abdominal wall and is known as the **parietal peritoneum.** The viscera are also covered by a peritoneal layer, the **visceral peritoneum.** The peritoneal cavity lies between the visceral and parietal peritonea, and although more complicated in form, it is built upon exactly the same plan as the pericardial and pleural cavities. The walls of the peritoneal cavity can be compared to a balloon or sac, into one side of which most of the viscera have been pushed. The layer of the balloon covering the viscera (visceral peritoneum) can be followed onto the outer wall of the balloon (parietal peritoneum). As in this example, it is apparent that visceral and parietal peritonea are continuous with each other. Where the viscera have deeply invaginated the peritoneal sac, the visceral peritoneum covering them is attached to the parietal peritoneum of the body wall by a double layer of peritoneum known as a **mesentery.** The vessels and nerves to the viscera run between the two layers of mesentery.

The peritoneal cavity in males is a completely closed sac. In females, the uterine tubes open into the pelvic portion of the peritoneal cavity.

FUNCTIONAL/CLINICAL NOTE 23-2

Peritonitis, or infection of the peritoneal cavity, involves grave danger to the patient because the peritoneal surface is warm, moist, and very extensive, offering almost ideal conditions for the growth of bacteria. Infections of the peritoneal cavity in male patients usually result from rupture of an organ or penetration of the abdominal wall. Those in female patients may occur through similar causes but may also arise through infections of the genital tract with subsequent spread through the uterine tubes.

The pelvic portion of the peritoneal cavity is directly continuous with the abdominal portion, and the division between abdomen and pelvis is largely an artificial one. The portion between the flared wings of the ilia is usually described as the *greater* or *false pelvis* and is considered part of the abdominal cavity proper. The portion below a plane passing from the sacral promontory to the upper border of the pubic symphysis is described as the *lesser* or *true pelvis* (or simply as *the* pelvis).

Liver

In brief summary of the abdominal viscera, as shown in Figure 23-4, the **liver** (*hepar,* hence the adjective "hepatic") occupies the upper portion of the abdomen on the right side and extends over to the left (Fig. 23-5). It is attached to the curved dome of the diaphragm, moves with this during inspiration and expiration, and is almost completely covered by the lower ribs. The liver is by far the largest gland in the body. It secretes bile, which is stored in a blind sac, the **gallbladder,** which is attached to the posteroinferior surface of the liver. The liver

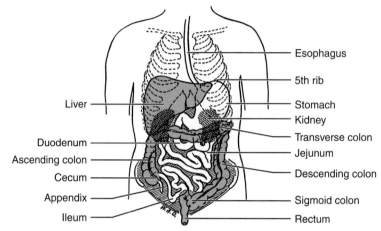

Figure 23-4 The general form and position of the chief abdominal viscera. The coils of the jejunum and ileum, which in reality largely fill the abdominal cavity, are illustrated here in a simplified, very diagrammatic manner so that the other viscera may be more clearly visible.

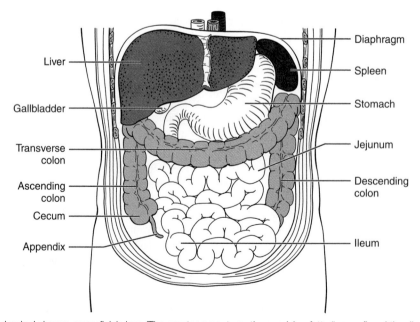

Figure 23-5 Abdominal viscera, superficial view. (The greater omentum, the overlying fatty "apron," and the ribs are omitted.)

and the gallbladder are connected to each other and to the duodenum (first part of the small intestine) by ducts. Contraction of the gallbladder discharges bile, necessary for proper digestion of fat, into the intestine. Gallstones, formed from bile, may obstruct a duct and cause painful symptoms. In addition to the secretion of bile, the liver has numerous other important functions, including metabolism of proteins, carbohydrates and lipids; breaking down metabolic waste products and other toxic substances; storage of glycogen; and storage of certain vitamins. The blood from the abdominal part of the digestive tract runs through the liver before reaching the heart.

Stomach

The **stomach** (*gaster*, hence "gastric") lies mostly to the left in the upper part of the abdomen and extends toward the right (see Fig. 23-5). Because the stomach is a hollow organ, it varies greatly in size and position according to whether it is empty or full,

according to the degree of fullness of other parts of the digestive tract, and according to the position of the individual at any particular time. The stomach not only churns the food and helps liquefy it but also breaks it down by adding hydrochloric acid and an enzyme that digests proteins. Oversecretion of acid is an important cause of *ulcers* (peptic ulcers), which usually occur in the distal end of the stomach or the adjacent first part of the small intestine.

Pancreas

The **pancreas** (Fig. 23-6) lies behind most of the abdominal viscera, across the front of the vertebral column at the level of the kidneys. The majority of its cells secrete digestive enzymes that act on all three basic foodstuffs—proteins, carbohydrates, and fats—and its main duct opens with that of the liver and gallbladder into the duodenum. In addition to its digestive function, the pancreas also has endocrine functions, the most important being the production of insulin.

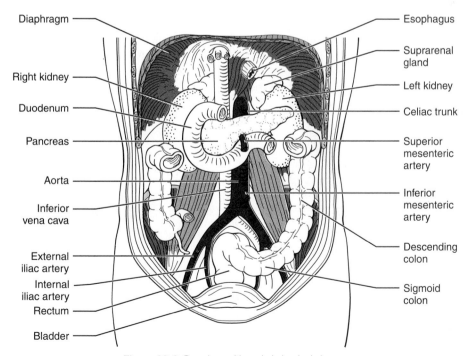

Figure 23-6 Deeply positioned abdominal viscera.

Spleen

The spleen (see Fig. 23-5) is an organ of the vascular system rather than of the digestive system, serving as a storage place for red blood cells and as a place for formation of certain types of white blood cells. It lies to the left of the stomach, against the diaphragm and ribs.

Small Intestine

The coils of the small intestine (see Fig. 23-5) occupy most of the abdominal cavity. The *duodenum* (see Fig. 23-6), or first part of the small intestine, lies against the posterior abdominal wall behind the peritoneum, but the remainder of the small intestine, the *jejunum* and *ileum,* is suspended by a fan-shaped mesentery that allows it considerable freedom of movement. Some coils of the ileum usually lie within the true pelvis, and the terminal portion of the ileum then ascends into the lower right quadrant to end in the cecum (described in next section).

Large Intestine

The small intestine joins the large intestine (see Figs. 23-5 and 23-6) not at the end of the large intestine but rather on its side. The short blind end projecting below the junction of these two parts is termed the **cecum,** to which the appendix is attached. The **appendix** was originally the end of the cecum, but in the adult, it rarely retains this position. Most commonly the appendix, originating behind the cecum, projects inferiorly, but it may lie entirely posterior to the cecum or in some other position. The **large intestine** begins with the cecum. Above the ileocecal junction the large intestine is known as the **ascending colon** and runs upward to come in contact with the lower posterior surface of the liver. Here, in the upper right quadrant, the large intestine makes a sharp bend to the left to become the **transverse colon,** which then crosses the abdominal cavity to the upper left quadrant in the region of the spleen. The transverse colon may run almost transversely or may droop markedly in its course across the abdomen. On the left side, a second bend or flexure occurs, and the **descending colon** then passes downward. Ascending and descending colons lie close against the posterior body wall and are covered with peritoneum only on their fronts and sides; they have no mesenteries. The transverse colon, however, is attached by a mesentery to the posterior abdominal wall and is also attached to a redundant mesentery of the stomach, the *greater omentum,* which hangs downward over the abdominal viscera. The descending colon is continuous with a short section of colon that has a mesentery and that is known from its shape as the **sigmoid colon.** The sigmoid colon crosses the brim of the pelvis, loses its mesentery, and becomes the **rectum** (Fig. 23-7).

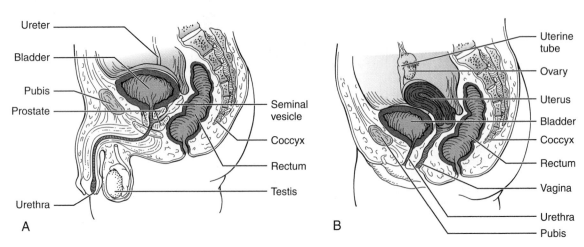

Figure 23-7 The pelvis sectioned along the median plane. **A,** Male pelvis. **B,** Female pelvis.

Kidneys and Suprarenal Glands

The **kidneys** (*renes,* hence the term *renal* related to structure of the kidney) are situated against the posterior abdominal wall on each side of the vertebral column (see Fig. 23-6). They lie behind the peritoneum. The right kidney usually lies at a slightly lower level than the left. The upper pole of the left kidney usually extends up to the level of the 11th rib as that rib attaches to the vertebral column, whereas that of the right kidney often lies at the level of the 12th rib. The ureters run downward approximately parallel to the vertebral column and pass along the lateral pelvic walls to reach the bladder.

The **suprarenal (adrenal) glands** (see Fig. 23-6) lie on the upper poles of the kidneys. They belong to the endocrine system, rather than to the digestive or urogenital system, and are discussed briefly in Chapter 3.

PELVIC VISCERA

Male Pelvis

In addition to coils of small intestine and the sigmoid colon that may be present in the pelvis, the **pelvic viscera** in the male consist of the rectum, urinary bladder, prostate, and seminal vesicles (see Fig. 23-7, *A*). The upper portion of the **rectum** is covered anteriorly and on its sides by peritoneum, and it lies against the posterior pelvic wall. The **bladder** lies against the pubis and anterior abdominal wall and is covered above and posteriorly by peritoneum. The pelvic portion of the peritoneal cavity extends downward between the bladder and rectum and ends blindly some distance above the pelvic floor, leaving the lower portions of rectum and bladder without peritoneal contact. As the bowel penetrates the levator ani, it turns posteriorly; this lower portion is the **anal canal.** The **seminal vesicles** and the **prostate,** connected with the male genital tract, lie in close connection with the base of the bladder and urethra below the level of the peritoneal cavity. Both are glands, and together they secrete most of the fluid in which the male germ cells (spermatozoa) are suspended. Because the prostate almost completely surrounds the urethra, prostatic enlargement may markedly interfere with the emptying of the bladder.

Female Pelvis

In the female pelvis, the bladder and the rectum have essentially the same peritoneal relations as in the male (see Fig. 23-7, *B*). The space between the two is occupied by the **uterus** and by the **broad ligaments** that extend from the sides of the uterus to the pelvic walls. The **uterine tubes,** in the upper border of the broad ligaments, open at their ovarian ends into the peritoneal cavity and at their uterine ends into the uterine cavity. The uterus and the broad ligaments divide the lower part of the female peritoneal cavity into two portions, one lying between the bladder and uterus, the other between the uterus and rectum. The **ovaries** lie on the lateral pelvic walls just behind the broad ligaments. The **vagina** extends downward from the uterus, lying mostly below the level to which the peritoneum reaches.

VESSELS

Arteries

The large artery of the abdomen, the **abdominal aorta** (Fig. 23-8; see Fig. 23-6), is the direct continuation of the thoracic aorta and ends below at about the level of the fourth lumbar vertebra by dividing into the two *common iliac arteries.* In its course, the abdominal aorta gives off *lumbar vessels* to the abdominal wall, *renal branches* to the kidneys, *testicular* or *ovarian branches* to the gonads, and three unpaired vessels to the digestive tract. The uppermost of the unpaired vessels, the **celiac trunk,** arises from the aorta as it lies between the crura of the diaphragm and supplies blood primarily to the stomach, liver, gallbladder, spleen, pancreas, and duodenum. The second branch, the **superior mesenteric artery,** arises from the front of the aorta directly below the celiac trunk and supplies branches to most of the small intestine and to the ascending and transverse portions of the large intestine, including the appendix and cecum. The third branch to the digestive system, the **inferior mesenteric artery,** arises somewhat lower from the front of the aorta and runs to the left, where it supplies blood to part of the transverse colon, the descending colon, sigmoid colon, and rectum.

The paired **common iliac arteries,** the large terminal branches of the aorta, proceed toward

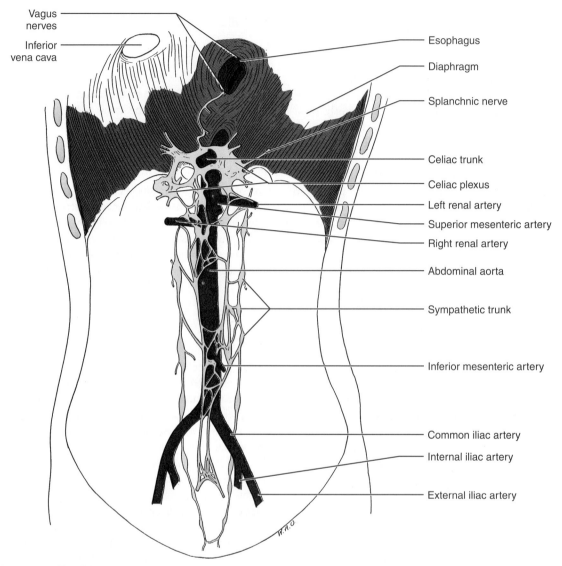

Vagus nerves

Inferior vena cava

Esophagus

Diaphragm

Splanchnic nerve

Celiac trunk

Celiac plexus

Left renal artery

Superior mesenteric artery

Right renal artery

Abdominal aorta

Sympathetic trunk

Inferior mesenteric artery

Common iliac artery

Internal iliac artery

External iliac artery

Figure 23-8 The abdominal aorta and the larger ganglia and plexuses (sympathetic and parasympathetic fibers) of the abdomen.

the pelvic brim but soon divide into the *internal* and *external iliac vessels*. The **external iliac artery** continues the course of the common iliac arteries along the pelvic brim and leaves the abdomen posterior to the inguinal ligament to continue into the thigh as the *femoral artery*. The **internal iliac artery** passes into the pelvis, and through its branches, it supplies blood to all the pelvic viscera. Some branches of this vessel also leave the pelvis to

supply the musculature of the gluteal and perineal regions.

Veins

There are two great venous systems within the abdomen, the *inferior vena cava* and the *portal vein* with its tributaries. The **inferior vena cava** parallels the abdominal aorta, lying to its right, and receives vessels corresponding to the branches of the abdominal aorta, except for veins from the digestive tract. The veins from the digestive tract parallel the branches of the celiac trunk and the superior mesenteric and inferior mesenteric arteries. However, instead of joining the inferior vena cava, they join each other to form the **portal vein.** This vein runs upward into the liver, through which all blood of the portal vein must pass in intimate contact with the hepatic cells. Blood from the liver, whether brought there by the celiac trunk or by the portal vein, is carried into the inferior vena cava by the hepatic veins just before the inferior vena cava penetrates the diaphragm.

NERVES

The **sympathetic trunks** in the abdomen (see Fig. 23-8), the continuation of the trunks within the thorax, contribute fibers to the lumbar nerves and also help form a plexus, the **abdominal aortic plexus,** across the anterior surface of the abdominal aorta The upper portion of this plexus, in the region of the celiac trunk and superior mesenteric arteries, is especially well developed and contains several ganglia, the celiac ganglia being the largest of these. The fibers to this upper portion of the plexus (celiac or solar plexus) are derived only in small part from the lumbar portions of the sympathetic trunks. The **splanchnic nerves** come into it from the thoracic part of the sympathetic trunks, carrying preganglionic sympathetic fibers synapse in the ganglia of the plexus.

From the celiac and aortic plexuses, numerous nerve fibers pass along the various arteries to supply both the blood vessels to the viscera and the smooth muscle of the visceral walls. The abdominal aortic plexus is also continued into the pelvis, where it aids in the innervation of the organs there.

The **vagus nerves** are also distributed to the digestive tract, or at least to the major portion of it. They give off branches to the stomach while they lie on the lower end of the esophagus. Parts of the vagus nerves then leave the stomach to reach the abdominal aortic plexus. Branches of this plexus are distributed to most of the abdominal viscera and to at least as far down the digestive tract as the transverse colon.

The pelvic viscera are innervated in part through the sympathetic fibers that are a continuation downward from the abdominal aortic plexus. In addition, they receive fibers from the second, third, and fourth sacral nerves. These latter fibers form the **parasympathetic roots** (pelvic splanchnic nerves), which are the chief nerves concerned with the emptying of the bladder and the rectum and supply the most important innervation of the pelvis.

In general, stimulation of the sympathetic nerves of the abdomen and pelvis produces constriction of blood vessels and cessation of movement in the gut. Parasympathetic stimulation, whether of the vagus nerves or sacral parasympathetic nerves, increases the peristaltic activity of the digestive tract.

SURFACE ANATOMY

The palpable bony landmarks of the abdominal wall are those of the rib cage and bony pelvis. Superiorly, the **inferior costal margin** can be followed on each side from the **xiphoid process** (at the midline). The **floating ribs** can be palpated posteroinferiorly. Posteriorly, the **iliac crest** can be followed on each side from the **posterior superior iliac spine** to its termination at the **anterior superior iliac spine** which is the lateral attachment for the inguinal ligament. This ligament extends medially to the **pubic tubercle,** which can be palpated on the pubic bone.

It is difficult to identify any individual muscles of the anterior abdominal wall except for the **rectus abdominis.** This muscle can be made to contract by tensing the abdominal wall and in this way can be palpated. Depending on the amount of overlying subcutaneous tissue, its outline may be visible. As a guide to the **cutaneous innervation,** skin at the level of the umbilicus is innervated by fibers from spinal nerve T10 through the 10th intercostal nerve.

Although it is possible to palpate parts of some of the abdominal viscera, it is more valuable to provide information on the surface projections of some of the organs. The positions of the other organs can then be determined by using these projections as landmarks. Most of the **liver** is deep to the rib cage and is covered by the diaphragm. It extends upward on the right side to a level just below the right nipple, and its left upper border is about an inch below the nipple.

It moves inferiorly when the diaphragm contracts. The **gallbladder** lies on the right, at the intersection of the tip of the 9th rib with the lateral edge of the rectus abdominis. The **spleen** lies laterally in the upper left quadrant; its long axis lies along the 10th rib.

The **junction of the stomach and duodenum** lies to the right of the midline on a horizontal plane that extends through the midpoint between the umbilicus and the junction of the xiphoid process with the body of the sternum. This plane projects posteriorly to the disc between the first and second lumbar vertebrae. The **pancreas** lies just inferior to this plane.

The surface projections of the kidneys are best visualized in relation to posterior structures. The upper border of the **right kidney** lies deep to the 12th rib. It extends inferiorly to the spine of the third lumbar vertebra. (For reference, the highest point of the iliac crest is at the level of the fourth lumbar vertebra.) The **left kidney** is slightly higher, with its upper part covered by both the 11th and 12th ribs.

REVIEW QUESTIONS

1 Describe the muscular arrangement, including origin and insertion, of the rectus abdominis muscles. What role do these muscles play in movement of the trunk?

2 What is the inguinal canal? Is it more prominent in females or in males? Why?

3 What role does the quadratus lumborum play in respiration?

4 Provide a brief account of the anatomy of the muscles of the pelvic diaphragm.

5 Describe the course and distribution of the vagus nerve within the abdominal cavity.

6 Which nerves provide sensory innervation to the skin around the umbilicus?

7 Where is the spleen located? Which kidney is positioned higher in the abdomen?

8 What are the three unpaired arterial branches of the abdominal aorta? Which organs does each supply with blood?

EXERCISES

1 Draw a midsagittal view of the female pelvis, illustrating the relationship of the organs.

2 By palpation identify the following:
   a inferior costal margin
   b 11th and 12th ribs
   c anterior superior iliac spine
   d iliac crest
   e rectus abdominis

SUGGESTED READINGS/REFERENCES

Agur A, Dalley A: *Grant's atlas of anatomy*, ed 12, Philadelphia, 2009, Lippincott Williams & Wilkins.

Clemente C: *Anatomy: A regional atlas of the human body*, ed 5, Philadelphia, 2007, Lippincott Williams & Wilkins.

Clemente C: *Gray's anatomy*, ed 30, American edition, Philadelphia, 1985, Lea & Febiger.

Drake R, Vogl W, Mitchell A: *Gray's anatomy for students*, Philadelphia, 2005, Churchill Livingstone.

Drake R, Vogl A, Mitchell A, Tibbitts R, Richardson P: *Gray's atlas of anatomy*, Philadelphia, 2008, Churchill Livingstone.

Federative Committee on Anatomical Terminology: *Terminologia anatomica: International anatomical terminology*, Stuttgart, Germany, 1998, Thieme.

Field D, Hutchinson J: *Field's anatomy palpation and surface markings*, ed 4, Edinburgh, 2006, Butterworth-Heinemann.

Greene D, Roberts S: *Kinesiology: Movement in the context of activity*, ed 2, St Louis, 2005, Mosby.

Kendall F, McCreary E, Provance P, Rodgers M, Romani W: *Muscles: Testing and function with posture and pain*, ed 5, Baltimore, 2005, Lippincott Williams & Wilkins.

Levangie P, Norkin C: *Joint structure and function: A comprehensive analysis*, ed 4, Philadelphia, 2005, FA Davis.

Magee D: *Orthopedic physical assessment*, ed 4, St Louis, 2006, Saunders.

Moore K, Dalley A: *Clinically oriented anatomy*, ed 5, Philadelphia, 2006, Lippincott Williams & Wilkins.

Netter F: *Atlas of human anatomy*, ed 4, Philadelphia, 2006, Saunders.

Nordin M, Frankel V: *Basic biomechanics of the musculoskeletal system*, ed 3, Philadelphia, 2001, Lippincott Williams & Wilkins.

Palastanga N, Field D, Soames R: *Anatomy and human movements: Structure and function*, ed 5, Edinburgh, 2006, Butterworth-Heinemann.

Standring S: *Gray's anatomy*, ed 39, Edinburgh, 2005, Churchill Livingstone.

GLOSSARY

Abduction Movement away from the midline.

Abduction (radial deviation) of the hand Movement at the wrist (with the hand extended) in which the hand is deviated toward the thumb (radial) side.

Abduction/adduction (of the digits) Movement of the thumb away from/toward the palm in a plane perpendicular to the plane of the palm; movement of the fingers away from/toward the long axis through the third digit; movement of the toes away from/toward the long axis through the second digit.

Adduction Movement toward the midline.

Adduction (ulnar deviation) of the hand Movement at the wrist (with the hand extended) in which the hand is deviated toward the little finger (ulnar) side.

Afferent (sensory) nerve fiber A nerve fiber that transmits impulses to the central nervous system.

Anatomical position Erect position with heels together, feet pointing somewhat laterally, arms by the sides with the palms facing anteriorly.

Antagonist A muscle that works in opposition to the prime mover.

Antebrachium (forearm) Segment of the upper limb between the elbow and wrist joints.

Anterior (ventral) Toward the front of the body.

Ape hand Lesion of the median nerve that results in rotation of the thumb into the same plane as the fingers and palm.

Aponeurosis A flat, broad tendon.

Appendicular skeleton Skeleton of the limbs, including the pectoral and pelvic girdles.

Arm (brachium) Segment of the upper limb between the glenohumeral and elbow joints.

Autonomic nervous system The sympathetic and parasympathetic systems.

Axial skeleton Skull, ribs, sternum, and vertebral column.

Bell's (facial) palsy Lesion of the facial nerve (cranial nerve VII) that results in paralysis of the muscles of facial expression.

Bilateral On both sides, or having two sides.

Brachiocephalic trunk First branch off the arch of the aorta. It divides into the right subclavian and right common carotid arteries.

Brachiocephalic vein The vein formed on both the right and left sides by union of the internal jugular and subclavian veins of those sides.

Brachium (arm) Segment of the upper limb between the glenohumeral and elbow joints.

Bursa A connective tissue sac containing a small amount of fluid.

Carpal tunnel syndrome Compression or entrapment of the median nerve at the wrist that results in possible sensory changes and/or muscle atrophy of the thenar eminence.

Cartilaginous joint A joint at which bones are united by cartilage.

Center of gravity Imaginary point around which the weight of all parts of the body is in balance. In the human body the point lies on the midline, just anterior to the level of the second sacral vertebra.

Central nervous system (CNS) The brain and spinal cord.

Circumduction Circular movement of a body part, such as the upper or lower limb, which combines flexion, abduction, extension, and adduction.

Claw hand Lesion of the ulnar nerve that results in loss of function of the interossei muscles of the hand. The interphalangeal joints are flexed, and the metacarpophalangeal joints are extended, this being most apparent in the ring and little fingers.

Concentric contraction Contraction of a muscle in which force (tension) is produced and the muscle shortens.

Cranial nerves Twelve pairs of nerves that pass through openings in the skull. All but part of cranial nerve XI are connected to parts of the brain.

Cricothyroidotomy (cricothyrotomy) An emergency procedure to create an artificial opening into the airway through the cricothyroid membrane.

Deep Farther from the surface.

Dens A vertical projection from the body of the axis (second cervical vertebra).

Dermatome Area of skin supplied by the sensory fibers of one spinal cord segment (pair of spinal nerves).

Digits of the foot The five toes (the big toe and four lateral toes), numbered as digits 1 through 5 from medial to lateral.

Digits of the hand The thumb and four fingers (index, middle, ring, and little), numbered as digits 1 through 5 from lateral to medial, with the thumb being digit 1.

Distal Farther from the trunk or point of origin.

Dorsal (posterior) Toward the back of the body.

Dorsiflexion Movement at the ankle joint in which the toes are brought closer to the anterior surface of the leg, as in standing on the heels.

Eccentric contraction Contraction of a muscle in which force (tension) is produced and the muscle increases in length.

Efferent (motor) nerve fiber A nerve fiber that transmits impulses away from the central nervous system.

Eversion Movement of turning the sole of the foot outward.

Extension Straightening out of a bent part.

Fascia Connective tissue sheet or membrane that envelops or binds together other structures.

Fibrous joint A joint at which bones are united by fibrous material.

Fingers The medial four digits (digits 2 through 5): index, middle, ring, and little fingers.

Flexion Bending at a joint that decreases the angle between two parts. In flexion of the forearm at the elbow, the forearm moves initially anteriorly in a sagittal plane; in flexion of the leg at the knee, the leg moves posteriorly.

Flexion/extension of the thumb Bending/straightening of the thumb in a plane parallel to the plane of the palm.

Forearm (antebrachium) Segment of the upper limb between the elbow and wrist joints.

Gait The manner of walking.

Gait cycle The activity that occurs from heel-strike of one limb to the next heel-strike of the same limb.

Ganglion Accumulation of nerve cell bodies outside of the central nervous system.

Gluteal region (buttock) Region posterior to the hip joint, inferior to the iliac crest, and extending to the inferior border of the gluteus maximus muscle.

Hip (coxal) bone Bone of the pelvic girdle. Each hip bone consists of the ilium, ischium, and pubis.

Inferior Toward the feet.

Insertion Attachment of the muscle that is more movable (relative to the origin).

Inversion Movement of turning the sole of the foot inward.

Isometric contraction Contraction of a muscle in which force is produced with no change in the length of the muscle.

Isotonic contraction Contraction of a muscle in which a constant force (tension) is produced and the muscle either shortens or lengthens.

Joint (articulation) Union between two or more bones.

Kyphosis Increased curvature of the thoracic region of the vertebral column (humpback).

Lateral Farther from the median plane of the body or midline of a structure.

Lateral (external) rotation Rotation about the long axis, as in the arm and thigh, so that the anterior surface is turned outward from the body.

Leg Segment of the lower limb between the knee and ankle joints.

Ligament In the skeletal system, an organized connective tissue band that binds bones together.

Line of gravity With the body in the anatomical position, a vertical line that passes through the center of gravity. The line of gravity normally passes through the junctions of the various regions of the vertebral column: the skull with the cervical vertebrae; the cervical vertebrae with the thoracic vertebrae; the thoracic vertebrae with the lumbar vertebrae; and the lumbar vertebrae with the sacrum. At the hip, the line passes posterior to the joint but lies anterior to the knee and ankle joints.

Lordosis Increased curvature of the lumbar region of the vertebral column.

Lymph node A component of the lymphatic system; commonly but incorrectly termed a lymph "gland."

Medial Closer to the median plane of the body or midline of a structure.

Medial (internal) rotation Rotation about the long axis, as in the arm and thigh, so that the anterior surface is turned inward toward the body.

Motor unit A group of muscle fibers innervated by a single nerve fiber.

Nerve plexus A mixing of sensory and motor fibers from several spinal cord segments to form branches supplying the periphery. Examples are the cervical, brachial, lumbar, and sacral plexuses.

Origin Attachment of the muscle that is more fixed (relative to the insertion).

Peripheral nervous system (PNS) The cranial and spinal nerves and the autonomic nervous system.

Plantar flexion Movement opposite of dorsiflexion, as in rising up on the toes.

Pneumothorax Presence of air into the pleural cavity.

Posterior (dorsal) Toward the back of the body.

Prime mover A muscle that carries out a movement. Also termed an *agonist*.

Pronation of the forearm/hand With the flexed forearm in a horizontal position, movement of turning the palm downward.

Protraction Moving a part of the body (such as the mandible or shoulder) anteriorly.

Proximal Closer to the trunk or point of origin.

Radicular pain Pain radiating along a peripheral nerve and its distribution.

Referred pain Pain, usually from visceral structures, that is perceived to be from another area supplied by the same spinal cord segment (or segments) that provides nerve fibers to the structure.

Retraction Moving a part of the body (such as the mandible or shoulder) posteriorly.

Rotator cuff Tendons of the supraspinatus, infraspinatus, teres minor, and subscapularis muscles that help stabilize the glenohumeral joint.

Scoliosis Lateral curvature of the vertebral column.

Segmental nerve distribution Innervation (both motor and sensory) provided by the pair of spinal nerves from one spinal cord segment.

Spina bifida Incomplete fusion of the vertebral arches in the lower region of the vertebral column.

Spinal nerves The 31 pairs of nerves that are connected to the spinal cord by the posterior and anterior roots.

Stance phase Phase in the gait cycle that begins with heel-strike and ends with toe-off of the same limb.

Sternal angle Junction of the manubrium and body of the sternum that indicates the position of attachment of the second rib to the sternum.

Superficial Closer to the surface.

Superior Toward the head.

Supination of the forearm/hand With the flexed forearm in a horizontal position, movement of turning the palm upward.

Swing phase Phase in the gait cycle that begins with toe-off and ends with heel-strike of the same limb.

Sympathetic trunks (chain) A paired series of ganglia interconnected by nerve fibers. The trunks lie on the anterolateral aspects (both right and left) of the vertebral column and extend from the second cervical vertebra to the coccyx (where they join across the midline).

Synergist Muscle that contracts at the same time as the prime mover.

Synovial joint A joint characterized by a synovial cavity; the most movable type of joint.

Synovial sheath Similar to a bursa; completely surrounds a tendon.

Tendon Connective tissue cord or band that attaches muscle to bone (or possibly to some other structure).

Thigh Segment of the lower limb between the hip and knee joints.

Unilateral On one side only or having one side.

Ventral (anterior) Toward the front of the body.

Wristdrop Lesion of the radial nerve that results in paralysis of the muscles that extend the fingers and wrist. In pronation with this condition, the hand hangs limply downward.

INDEX

A

Abdomen, 401–405. *See also*
  Abdominal wall
  nerves of, 413
  surface anatomy of, 413–414
  vessels of, 411–413
Abdominal, definition of, 2
Abdominal aorta, 398, 411
Abdominal aortic plexus, 413
Abdominal viscera, 407–411,
  408f, 409f
Abdominal wall, 401–405, 402f
  muscles of, 403–404, 403t
Abducens nerve (CN VI), 382
Abduction, 4, 66, 160, 307–308
  of arm, 96
  of fingers, 197
  of hand, 161
  of thigh, 295–296
  of thumb, 5f, 198–199
  of wrist, 163f
Abductor digiti minimi, 179–180,
  182, 342, 346, 351
Abductor hallucis, 341, 346–347,
  351
Abductor pollicis brevis, 177–178,
  182, 188, 198–199
Abductor pollicis longus,
  151–152, 182, 188, 198–199
Abductor tubercle, 249–250
Acceleration, 354
Accessory nerve (CN XI), 384
Accessory obturator nerve,
  262–263

Acetabulum, 245–247
Acetylcholine, 16
Achilles tendon. *See* Calcaneal
  tendon
Achondroplasia, 21
Achondroplastic dwarf, 21
Acromioclavicular joint, 69–70
Acromion, 66
Adduction, 4, 66, 160, 307–308
  of arm, 96–97, 98f
  of fingers, 197
  of hand, 161
  of thigh, 298
  of thumb, 5f, 198–199
  of wrist, 163f
Adductor brevis, 270, 298
Adductor canal, 270
Adductor group, 269–272, 269t
Adductor hallucis, 345, 347–348,
  351
Adductor hiatus, 270
Adductor longus, 269–270,
  297–298
Adductor magnus, 270, 294, 297
Adductor pollicis, 174–175,
  198–199
Adenosine triphosphate
  (ATP), 16
Adipose tissue, 10
Afferent fibers, 41
Alpha fibers, 34
Alveolar process, 386
Alveoli, 53
Anal canal, 53, 411

Anatomical position, 2–3
  defined, 2–3
  terms of, 3f
Anatomical snuffbox, 152
Anconeus, 110f, 115–116, 123
Anesthesia, epidural, 229
Angles, 66
Ankle joint, 307, 334–336
Ankle (tarsus), 238
  bones of, 308–310
  in weight support, 351–353
Annular ligament, 111
Annulospiral endings, 33–34
Annulus fibrosus, 213
Ansa cervicalis, 374, 384
Antagonists, 32
Antebrachial fascia, 130–131
Antebrachium. *See* Forearm
Anterior, definition of, 2
Anterior arch, 207
Anterior bands, 111
Anterior branch, 275
Anterior cerebral arteries, 364
Anterior cutaneous branch, 391
Anterior division, 73–74
Anterior fontanelle, 359–360
Anterior horns, 40
Anterior inferior iliac spine, 245
Anterior intermuscular septum,
  311
Anterior interosseous branch,
  144–145, 182, 191
Anterior longitudinal ligament,
  212

Note: Page numbers followed by *f* indicate figures; *t*, tables; *b*, boxes.

Anterior ramus, 45, 60, 73–74, 234, 384
Anterior root, 44–45, 233
Anterior sacroiliac ligament, 249
Anterior scalene, 375
Anterior superior iliac spine, 245, 255, 260, 288, 413
Anterior talofibular ligament, 335
Anterior tibial artery, 241–242, 321, 350
Anterior tibial recurrent artery, 274
Anterior tibial recurrent branch, 321
Anterior triangle, 373
Anterior wall, 73
Anterolateral fontanelle, 359–360
Anteromedial nerves, 272–277
Anteromedial vessels, 272–276
Aorta, 275f
    abdominal, 398, 411
    ascending, 398
    descending, 398
    thoracic, 398
Ape hand, 191, 192f
Apex, 73
Apex beat of heart, 399
Aponeurosis, 11
    bicipital, 114, 139
    of external oblique, 403
    palmar, 131, 173–174, 184f
    plantar, 340
Appendicular, definition of, 2
Appendicular skeleton, 58
Appendix, 410
Arachnoid mater, 229–230, 361
Arcuate arteries, 350
Arcuate popliteal ligament, 257
Arm (brachium), 57. See also
        Elbow joint; Elbow region
    abduction of, 96
    adduction of, 96–97, 98f
    arteries of, 108
    effort, 30
    extension of, 67f, 95–96, 96f
    fascia of, 112
    flexion of, 67f, 95, 95f

Arm (brachium) (Continued)
    movement of, 65–66, 107
    muscles of, 107, 114–117, 115f
    nerves of, 112, 117–121, 122t
    osteological diagram of, 110f
    posterior view of, 119f
    resistance, 30
    rotation of, 99f, 100f
    surface anatomy of, 112, 116–117
    vessels of, 112–114, 117–121
Arterioles, 50
Artery (arteries), 50. See also
        specific arteries
    anterior cerebral, 364
    anterior tibial, 241–242, 321, 350
    anterior tibial recurrent, 274
    arcuate, 350
    of arm, 108
    of axilla, 77f
    axillary, 60, 65, 78f, 79, 156f
    brachial, 60, 120, 120f
    bronchial, 396
    circumflex fibular, 274
    common carotid, 385, 387
    common iliac, 411–412
    common interosseous, 144–145
    common palmar digital, 186
    common plantar digital, 348
    coronary, 398
    deep plantar, 350
    descending genicular, 273–274
    descending scapular, 83–84
    dorsal digital, 186–189
    dorsal metacarpal, 186–187
    dorsal metatarsal, 350
    dorsalis pedis, 321, 323, 350, 350–351
    external carotid, 385, 385–386
    external iliac, 411–412
    facial, 387
    femoral, 256, 272, 274, 275f, 276, 272–274, 411–412
    fibular, 321
    of forearm, 108
    of gluteal region, 284f

Artery (arteries) (Continued)
    of hand, 128
    of head, 385–386
    iliac, 275f
    inferior epigastric, 405
    inferior mesenteric, 411
    inferior thyroid, 385
    inferior ulnar collateral, 120
    intercostal, 398
    internal carotid, 385
    internal iliac, 411–412
    lateral circumflex femoral, 272–273
    lateral plantar, 348
    lateral thoracic, 76–77
    of lower limb, 241–242
    medial circumflex femoral, 272–273
    medial plantar, 348
    metacarpal, 188–189
    middle cerebral, 364
    middle collateral, 120
    middle genicular, 274, 321
    nutrient, 120, 321
    obturator, 276
    of palm, 183f, 185f
    perforating, 272–273
    plantar, 349f
    plantar metatarsal, 348
    popliteal, 241–242, 274–275, 292, 321
    posterior cerebral, 363
    posterior communicating, 364
    posterior interosseous, 153, 155
    posterior tibial, 241–242, 321, 323
    posterior tibial recurrent, 274
    profunda brachii, 120
    proper palmar digital, 186, 188–189
    proper plantar digital, 348
    pulmonary, 396
    radial, 60, 128, 144, 145–146, 145f, 152, 155, 156f, 186–188
    radial collateral, 120
    of shoulder, 79f

Artery (arteries) *(Continued)*
   subclavian, 60, 65, 78f, 79,
      385, 398
   subscapular, 76–77
   superficial brachial, 120
   superficial cervical, 83–84
   superficial temporal, 387
   superior epigastric, 405
   superior lateral genicular, 274
   superior medial genicular, 274
   superior mesenteric, 411
   superior thyroid, 385
   supreme thoracic, 76–77
   sural, 321
   of thigh, 271f
   thoracodorsal, 76–77
   transverse cervical, 84f
   ulnar, 60, 128, 144–146, 145f,
      186, 188
   upper limb, 60
Articular disc, 68–69, 369–370
Articular processes, 211–212
Articularis genus muscle, 258, 260
Articulating surfaces, 24–25
Ascending aorta, 398
Ascending colon, 53, 410
Ascending tracts, 231
Atlanto-axial joint, 215
Atlas, 207
ATP. *See* Adenosine triphosphate
Atria, 397–398
Attachments
   distal, 26
   proximal, 26
Auricular surface, 245
Autonomic nervous system, 38,
   46–50
   functions of, 49–50
Axial skeleton, 58
Axilla, 74f
   nerves and arteries of, 77f
   upper limb, 73–79
Axillary arch muscle, 89
Axillary artery, 60, 65, 78f, 79
Axillary nerve, 60, 73, 156f
Axillary sheath, 77
Axillary vein, 61, 77

Axis, 207
Azygos system, 398

B
Back. *See also* Vertebrae; Vertebral
   column
   muscles of, 219–229, 220f
   surface anatomy of, 228–229
Ball-and-socket joints, 24,
   250–251
Base of support, 5
Basilic vein, 61, 114, 131, 145, 189
Bell palsy, 366, 383
Biceps brachii, 95, 114, 116–117,
   116t, 121–123, 160, 300
   tendon of, 139
Biceps femoris, 286, 289, 294,
   296–297, 301, 302f
Bicipital aponeurosis, 114, 139
Bifurcation of trachea, 399–400
Bipennate muscles, 28–29, 29f
Bladder, 411
Blood, 51–53
   circulation of, 396f
Blood pressure, 50
Blood vascular system, 50
Body. *See* Trunk
Bolus, 378
Bone(s), 12–14, 20–21.
   See also specific bones
   of ankle, 308–310
   of arm, 108–112
   of bony pelvis, 245–249
   carpal, 167–168
   compact, 13
   of elbow region, 148f
   ethmoid, 356–357
   features of, 20f
   flat, 20
   of foot, 308–310, 332–340,
      333f
   of forearm, 133–134, 148f
   formation, 19–20, 21–22
   frontal, 356–357, 386
   growth, 21–22
   hamate, 134, 167–168,
      172–173

Bone(s) *(Continued)*
   of hand, 128–130, 148f, 169f,
      167–173, 179f
   hip, 239–240, 247–248
   hyoid, 386
   irregular, 20
   of knee, 256–260, 282f, 312f
   lacrimal, 357–358
   of leg, 308–310
   long, 20
   maxillary, 386
   nasal, 357–358
   navicular, 339–340
   occipital, 356–357, 386
   palatine, 357–358
   parietal, 356–357, 386
   of pelvis, 282f
   pisiform, 134, 167–168, 172–173
   sesamoid, 20, 168
   short, 20
   sphenoid, 356–357
   spongy, 13
   strength, 22
   structure of, 13f
   temporal, 356–357, 386
   of thigh, 282f
   upper limb, 66–68
   of wrist, 169f
   zygomatic, 357–358, 386
Bony pelvis, 239–240
   bones of, 245–249, 282f
   joints of, 245–249, 249
   movements of, 253, 292
Borders, 66
Brachial artery, 60, 120
   branches of, 120f
Brachial fascia, 112
Brachial plexus, 60, 65, 73–76,
   75f, 79, 234
   nerve injuries to, 98–102
Brachial vein, 61, 77, 121
Brachialis, 110f, 114–117,
   121–123
Brachiocephalic trunk, 385, 398
Brachiocephalic veins, 398
Brachioradialis, 121–123,
   148–149, 152, 159

Brachium. *See* Arm
Brain, 360–364
    meninges of, 360–364
    structures of, 361f
Brainstem, 361
Branches. *See also* Nerves
    anterior, 275
    anterior cutaneous, 391
    anterior interosseous, 144–145,
        182, 191
    anterior tibial recurrent, 321
    circumflex scapular, 76–77
    deep, 141, 153–154, 347–348
    dorsal, 183
    dorsal carpal, 186–187
    dorsal digital, 141, 172
    inferior genicular, 321
    lateral cutaneous, 391
    muscular, 182
    palmar, 141
    palmar cutaneous, 182
    palmar digital, 141
    palmar metacarpal, 186–187
    perforating, 144–145, 292, 321
    posterior, 275
    posterior interosseous, 144–145
    proper palmar digital,
        183–184, 186
    radial recurrent, 144
    superficial, 141, 153, 183–184,
        347–348
    superficial palmar, 186–187
    superior genicular, 321
Broad ligaments, 411
Bronchi, 53, 395–396
    main, 377
Bronchial arteries, 396
Bronchioles, 395–396
Bronchopulmonary segment,
    396–397
Buccinator, 365
Bursae, 11, 27, 28f
    shoulder, 97–98
    subacromial, 97–98
    subdeltoid, 97–98
    upper limbs, 62
Bursitis, 27b, 98b

C

Calcaneal tendon (Achilles
    tendon), 320
Calcaneal tuberosity, 332
Calcaneofibular ligament, 335
Calcaneus, 308–310, 332,
    339–340
Calf. *See also* Leg
    muscles of, 313–314, 313t,
        315f, 315t, 316f
    nerves of, 320–321
    vessels of, 320–321
Callus, 22
Capillaries, 50
Capitate, 167–168
Capitis, 228
Capitulum, 109
Carbon dioxide, 16
Cardiac muscle, 14, 46–47
Carpal tunnel, 173–174
Carpal tunnel syndrome, 191b
Carpals, 58, 130
    bones, 167–168
Carpometacarpal joint, 23f, 130,
    172
Carpus. *See* Wrist
Carrying angle, 110b
Cartilage, 12
    cricoid, 377, 386, 399
    fibrocartilage, 12
    hyaline, 12
    thyroid, 377, 386, 399
Cartilaginous joints, 22–24, 210,
    212–215
Cartilaginous rings, 377
Cauda equina, 231, 234
Caudal, 2
Caudal analgesia, 229
Caudate nucleus, 362
Cavernous sinus, 360
Cecum, 410
Celiac trunk, 411
Center of gravity, 4–5
Centers, 363
Central nervous system, 38.
    See also Brain; Spinal cord
Central palmar compartment, 174

Cephalic vein, 61, 77, 79, 114,
    121, 131, 145, 189
Cephalon, 2
Cerebellomedullary cistern, 361
Cerebellum, 361–363
Cerebral arterial circle, 364
Cerebral cortex, 361
Cerebral hemispheres, 361–362
Cerebral hemorrhage, 364
Cerebrospinal fluid, 230
Cervical curvature, 205–206
Cervical nerves, 44
Cervical plexus, 234, 380f, 384
Cervical region, 216
Cervical rib syndrome, 76b
Cervical vertebrae, 204–205,
    207, 210
Cervicis, 228
Cervicothoracic ganglion, 384
Choroid plexus, 362
Ciliary ganglion, 49, 381
Circle of Willis, 364
Circulatory system, 50–53, 396f
Circumduction, 4, 128
Circumflex fibular artery, 274
Circumflex scapular branch,
    76–77
Cisterna magna, 361
Clavicle, 58, 64, 66–68
Clavipectoral fascia, 72–73,
    81–82
Clavipectoral triangle, 72
Claw hand, 192, 192f
Clotting, 52
Clubfoot, 327
Coccygeal nerves, 44
Coccygeus, 407
Coccyx, 204–205, 210, 245
Cold, 55
Collagen fiber, 10
Collateral ligaments, 172,
    257–258, 338–339
Colon
    ascending, 53, 410
    descending, 53, 410
    sigmoid, 53, 410
    transverse, 53, 410

Columnar cells, 8, 9f
Common carotid artery, 385, 387
Common fibular nerve, 1–2, 241, 321
distribution of, 328f
Common flexor sheath, 174–175
Common iliac arteries, 411–412
Common interosseous artery, 144–145
Common palmar digital arteries, 186
Common peroneal nerve, 1–2
Common plantar digital arteries, 348
Compact bone, 13
Concentric contraction, 31
Condylar process, 358
Condyles, 249–250, 260, 310
Condyloid joints, 23f
Coniotomy, 378
Connective tissue, 10f, 9–14
fibrous, 10–11, 369–370
Conoid ligament, 69–70
Contraction, 31
concentric, 31
consequences of, 36
eccentric, 31
isometric, 31
isotonic, 31
of muscles, 16
tetanic, 37
Conus medullaris, 231
Coracobrachialis, 95, 110f, 114–117
Coracoclavicular ligament, 69–70
Coracohumeral ligament, 71
Coracoid process, 66, 72
Cordotomy, 232
Coronal suture, 358–359
Coronary arteries, 398
Coronoid process, 109, 358
Corpus callosum, 362
Corpus striatum, 362
Corrugator supercilii, 366
Corticospinal tracts, 232
Costal facets, 207–208
Costoclavicular ligament, 69

Costoclavicular syndrome, 76b
Costodiaphragmatic recesses, 400
Coxa vara, 240
Cranial nerves, 38, 44, 49, 378–384, 380f
abducens nerve (CN VI), 382
accessory nerve (CN XI), 384
facial nerve (CN VII), 49, 366, 382–383
functions of, 380t
gastrocnemius, 299–300, 313–314, 323
glossopharyngeal nerve (CN IX), 49
hypoglossal nerve (CN XIII), 384
oculomotor nerve (CN III), 49, 381
olfactory nerve (CN I), 378–379
trigeminal nerve (CN V), 381
trochlear nerve (CN IV), 381
vagus nerve (CN X), 49, 383, 398–399, 413
vestibulocochlear nerve (CN VIII), 383
Cranial outflow, 47
Cranial venous sinuses, 360
Cranium, 2, 356, 356–357
Cricoid cartilage, 377, 386, 399
Cricothyroid membrane, 399
Cricothyroidotomy, 378
Cricothyrotomy, 378
Cruciate ligaments, 260
Crura, 392
Cubital fossa, 139
Cuboid bone, 310, 334, 339–340
Cuboidal cells, 8, 9f
Cuneate fasciculus, 231
Cuneiforms, 310, 334
Cuneocerebellar tract, 231
Cuneometatarsal interosseous ligaments, 337
Cuneonavicular joint, 335

Cutaneous innervation, 46f, 184–185, 382f, 413
of hand, 188
of head, 382f
of neck, 382f
Cylindrical grip, 200

D

Deceleration, 354
Deep arch, 188, 348
Deep branch, 141, 153–154, 347–348
Deep extensor muscles, 147
Deep fascia, 11, 72–73
Deep fibular nerve, 321, 340, 350, 352t
Deep inguinal ring, 404
Deep neck muscles, 226–227, 227t
Deep palmar arch, 186–187
Deep plantar artery, 350
Deep transverse crural fascia, 311
Deep transverse metatarsal ligaments, 338–339
Deep trochlear notch, 109
Deltoid, 86–87, 90, 95–97
posterior fibers of, 95–97
Deltoid tuberosity, 70–71, 109
Dendrites, 16–17
Denticulate ligaments, 230
Depression, 4, 367
of scapula, 91, 92f
Depressor anguli oris, 365
Depressor labii inferioris, 365
Dermatome, 45, 46f
Dermis, 10, 54–55
Descending aorta, 398
Descending colon, 53, 410
Descending genicular artery, 273–274
Descending scapular artery, 83–84
Descending tracts, 232
Development
of lower limbs, 238
of upper limbs, 57–58
Diabetes, 54

Diaphragm, 392, 392t, 400–401
pelvic, 405, 406t
urogenital, 407
Diaphysis, 20
Diencephalon, 361, 363
Digastric, 372
Digestive system, 53
Digits, 57. *See also* Finger(s); Toes
movements of, 5f
Digitus minimus, 332
Dislocation, 25b
Distal attachments, 26
Distal radioulnar joint, 169
Dorsal branch, 183
Dorsal carpal arch, 188–189
Dorsal carpal branch, 186–187
Dorsal digital artery, 186–189
Dorsal digital branches, 141, 172
Dorsal interossei, 181–182, 346
Dorsal metacarpal artery, 186–187
Dorsal metatarsal artery, 350
Dorsal metatarsal ligaments,
337
Dorsal muscles, 350t
Dorsal radiocarpal ligament,
169–170
Dorsal scapular nerve, 75–76,
84f
Dorsal surface, 332
Dorsal tarsal ligaments, 336
Dorsal tarsometatarsal ligament,
337
Dorsal venous plexus, 189,
350–351
Dorsalis pedis artery, 321, 323,
350–351
Dorsiflexion, 4–5, 128, 307
of foot, 324
Dorsum
of foot, 349–351
of hand, 188–189
surface anatomy of, 350–351
Double support, 353
Downward rotation, 65
Duodenum, 53, 414
Dura mater, 229, 360
Dwarfism, 21

E
Eccentric contraction, 31
Effort arm, 30
Effort point, 29
Elastic fibers, 10
Elbow joint, 109
anterior view of, 111f
ligaments of, 112f
movements of, 5f, 121–123
Elbow region, 190–191
bones of, 148f
osteological diagram of, 110f
views of, 136f
Electromyography, 31–32
Elevation, 4, 367
of scapula, 67f, 91, 92f
Endochondral bone formation,
19–20
Endocrine system, 53–54
Endomysium, 15
Endosteum, 22
Endothelium, 9
Entrapment syndromes, 76b
Epicondyles, 249–250, 256, 260
lateral, 109
medial, 109
Epidermis, 54–55
Epidural anesthesia, 229
Epidural space, 229
Epigastrium, 401
Epiglottis, 377
Epimysium, 15
Epinephrine, 54
Epiphyseal line, 20–21
Epiphyseal plate, 20–21
Epiphyses, 20
Epithelial tissue, 8–9
representative types of, 9f
Eponyms, 2
Erb-Duchenne paralysis, 101b,
164b
Erector spinae, 221–224, 223t, 228
Esophagus, 53, 364, 377–378
Ethmoid bone, 356–357
Ethmoidal cells, 357
Eversion, 240, 307–308
of foot, 319

Exercise, muscle and, 37–38
Expiration, 393
Extension, 4, 160
of arm, 67f, 95–96, 96f
of fingers, 196–197, 197f
of forearm, 123, 150t
of hand, 161
of leg, 299–300
of thigh, 294–295
of wrist, 162f
Extensor carpi radialis brevis,
149–150, 152, 161
Extensor carpi radialis longus,
121–123, 127, 149–150,
152, 161, 188
Extensor carpi ulnaris, 151–152,
161
Extensor digiti minimi, 150–151,
161, 182
Extensor digitorum, 150, 152,
161, 182, 188
Extensor digitorum brevis,
349–351
Extensor digitorum longus,
324–325, 351
tendon of, 320, 350
Extensor digitorum tendons,
196–197
Extensor hallucis brevis, 349–351
Extensor hallucis longus, 319,
324, 350–351
tendon of, 320
Extensor indicis, 152, 161,
182, 188
Extensor muscle masses, 60
Extensor pollicis brevis, 151–152,
182, 188, 199
Extensor pollicis longus, 151–152,
161, 182, 198–199
Extensor retinaculum, 130–131,
147–155, 311
External carotid arteries, 385–386
External iliac artery, 411–412
External intercostals, 391
External jugular vein, 387
External oblique, 403
aponeurosis of, 403

External occipital protuberance, 72, 210, 386
Extrapyramidal fibers, 232
Extrinsic muscles, 64–65

F

Facial artery, 387
Facial muscles, 364–366, 365f
Facial nerve (CN VII), 49, 366, 382–383
Facial skeleton, 356–358
False ribs, 389
Falx cerebri, 360
Fascia, 11
    antebrachial, 130–131
    of arm, 112
    brachial, 112
    clavipectoral, 72–73, 81–82
    deep, 11, 72–73
    deep transverse crural, 311
    of foot, 340–341
    of gluteal region, 281
    of hand, 130–131
    lata, 261, 281
    of leg, 310–312
    palmar, 173–174, 177
    superficial, 10–11, 72, 112
    of thigh, 261
    thoracolumbar, 210, 219
    upper limb, 72–73
Fasciculi, 40–41
Fat, 10
Female pelvis, 411
Femoral artery, 256, 272–274, 275f, 276, 411–412
Femoral canal, 272
Femoral hernia, 272
Femoral nerve, 241, 261, 263, 272, 273f
Femoral sheath, 272
Femoral triangle, 263–264, 267f
Femoral vein, 256, 272
Femur, 240, 250f, 249–253, 256
Fibers
    afferent, 41
    alpha, 34
    collagen, 10

Fibers *(Continued)*
    elastic, 10
    gamma, 34
    motor nerve, 34
    muscle, 15
    pain, 33
    parasympathetic nerve, 49, 235
    posterior, 95–97
    proprioceptive, 33
    sternocostal, 95–96
    sympathetic, 48f, 49, 234–235
Fibroblasts, 10
Fibrocartilage, 12
Fibrous connective tissue, 10–11, 369–370
Fibrous joints, 22
Fibrous sheath, 176
Fibula, 240, 256, 260, 308, 309f, 310
Fibular, 3
Fibular artery, 321
Fibular retinacula, 311
Fibularis brevis muscle, 320, 323, 346
    tendon of, 320
Fibularis longus muscle, 1–2, 320, 323, 346
Fibularis muscles, 325
Fibularis tertius, 319, 324, 346
    tendon of, 320
Filum terminale-dural part, 229
Filum terminale-pial part, 231
Final common path, 41
Finger(s), 57. *See also* Hand
    abduction of, 197
    adduction of, 197
    extension of, 196–197, 197f
    flexion of, 195–196
    joints of, 130
    movement of, 128, 197
    muscles of, 179–180, 180t
    synovial sheath of, 174–175
    tendons of, 176f
First dorsal interosseous, 182
First thoracic nerve, 73–74
Flat bones, 20
Flat muscles, 28

Flatfoot, 25b
Flavum, 212
Flexion, 4, 43b, 66, 160
    of arm, 67f, 95, 95f
    of fingers, 195–196
    of forearm, 121f
    of hand, 161
    of leg, 300
    of thigh, 297
    of thumb, 198
    of wrist, 162f
Flexor carpi radialis, 134–136, 159, 161
    tendon of, 139
Flexor carpi ulnaris, 134, 136–137, 139, 161
    tendon of, 139
Flexor digiti minimi brevis, 179–180, 345, 351
Flexor digitorum brevis, 341–342, 347, 351
Flexor digitorum longus, 314, 316, 323–324, 351
    tendon of, 343–344
Flexor digitorum profundus, 127, 134, 139, 195
Flexor digitorum superficialis, 134, 137–138, 196
    tendon of, 139
Flexor hallucis brevis, 344, 347, 351
Flexor hallucis longus, 314, 316, 323–324, 351
    tendon of, 343
Flexor muscle masses, 60
Flexor pollicis brevis, 178, 182, 198
Flexor pollicis longus, 134, 139, 198
    synovial sheath of, 174–175
Flexor retinaculum, 130–131, 134, 173–174, 311
Flexors
    of interphalangeal joints, 196f
    of metacarpophalangeal joints, 196f

Floating ribs, 389, 399, 413
Flower spray, 33–34
Fontanelles, 359–360
    anterior, 359–360
    anterolateral, 359–360
    posterior, 359–360
    posterolateral, 359–360
Foot, 238. *See also* Ankle; Toes
    arches, 334
    bones of, 308–310, 332–340, 333f
    dorsiflexion of, 324
    dorsum of, 349–351
    eversion of, 319
    fascia of, 340–341
    inversion of, 319
    joints of, 332–340
    ligaments of, 336
    movement of, 323–330
    muscles of, 241
    nerves of, 340, 352t
    surface anatomy of, 339–340, 348
    weight on, 334
    in weight support, 351–353
Foot-flat, 353–354
Footdrop, 325–327
Foramen
    greater sciatic, 248
    intervertebral, 207
    lesser sciatic, 248
    magnum, 356–357
    obturator, 246–247
    transverse, 207
    vertebral, 206–207
Forearm (antebrachium), 57
    arteries of, 108
    bones of, 133–134, 148f
    extension of, 123, 150t
    flexion of, 121f
    movement of, 107
    muscles of, 107, 126, 134–139, 134f, 135f, 137t, 138t, 147–152, 149f, 151t
    nerves of, 139–146, 140f, 144t, 152–157, 157t

Forearm (antebrachium) *(Continued)*
    posterior aspect of, 153f
    supination of, 161f
    surface anatomy of, 133–134, 139, 145–146, 152, 155
    vessels of, 139–146, 152–157
Fossa
    cubital, 139
    infraspinous, 66, 72
    intercondylar, 249–250, 256
    ischiorectal, 407
    popliteal, 255, 289
    subscapular, 66
    supraspinous, 66, 72
Fracture, greenstick, 12b
Frontal bone, 356–357, 386
Frontal plane, 3
Frontalis, 366
Funiculi, 40–41
    anterior, 40–41
    lateral, 40–41
    posterior, 40–41
Fusiform muscles, 28, 29f

G
Gait, 353–355
    cycle, 353
    running, 355
    stance phase, 353–354
    stance phase of, 353
    swing phase of, 353
Gallbladder, 408–409, 413–414
Gamma fibers, 34
Ganglia, 17
Gastrocnemius, 299–300, 313–314, 323
Genioglossus, 371
Geniohyoid, 372
Genitofemoral nerve, 262–263
Genu valgum, 240
Glenohumeral joint, 70–71, 89f
    ligaments of, 70f
    movements of, 5f
Glenohumeral ligaments, 71
Glenoid cavity, 66
Glenoid labrum, 66

Gliding movement, 370
Globus pallidus, 362
Glossopharyngeal nerve (CN IX), 49
Glossopharyngeal nerves, 383
Glucose, 16
Gluteal region, 238
    arteries of, 284f
    fascia of, 281
    muscles of, 281–286, 281f, 283t
    nerves of, 281, 284f, 289–292
    surface anatomy of, 292
    vessels of, 281, 289–292
Gluteus, 299–300
Gluteus maximus, 281–284, 288–289, 295–298
Gluteus medius, 284–285, 288–289, 295–297
Gluteus minimus, 284–285, 295–297
Golgi tendon organs, 33–34
Gomphosis, 22
Gracile fasciculus, 231
Gracilis, 270, 289, 300
Grasping, 199–201
Gravity
    center of, 4–7
    line of, 6f, 4–7
Gray matter, 39–40, 361
    anterior horns, 40
    posterior horns, 40
Great saphenous vein, 261, 276, 311–312, 323, 340, 350–351
Great veins, 398
Great vessels, 397f
Greater pelvis, 407–408
Greater sciatic foramen, 248
Greater sciatic notch, 245–246
Greater trochanter, 249–250, 255, 260, 288
Greater tubercle, 70–72
Greenstick fracture, 12b
Grips
    cylindrical, 200
    in grasping, 199–201
    hook, 200–201

Grips *(Continued)*
  pad-to-pad, 201
  pad-to-side, 201
  power, 200–201, 200f
  precision, 201
  spherical (ball), 201
  tip-to-tip (pincer) grip, 201
Grooves
  intertubercular, 70–71
  radial nerve, 109
  ulnar nerve, 109

H

Hamate bone, 134, 167–168,
    172–173
Hamstring muscles, 286–288, 298
Hand. *See also* Finger(s); Palm;
    Thumb; Wrist
  abduction of, 161
  adduction of, 161
  arteries of, 128
  bones of, 128–130, 148f, 169f,
    167–173, 179f
  cutaneous innervation of,
    187f, 188
  dorsum of, 188–190
  extension of, 161
  fascia of, 130–131
  flexion of, 161
  joints of, 128–130, 167–173
  muscles in, 126, 177–182
  nerves of, 128, 130–131, 186t,
    190–193
  surface anatomy of, 187–188
  synovial sheath, 188
  tendons of, 188
  vessels of, 130–131, 185–189
Hard palate, 357–358
Haversian canal, 13
Head, 2
  arteries of, 385–386
  cutaneous innervation of, 382f
  surface anatomy of, 386–387
Heart, 396f, 397–398, 397f, 400
  apex beat of, 399
  borders of, 400
  murmur, 398

Heat, 55
Heel-off, 353–354
Heel-strike, 353–354
Hemiazygos, 398
Hemothorax, 394
Hernia
  femoral, 272
  hiatal, 392b
Herniated disc, 214
Hiatal hernia, 392b
Hinge joint, 24
Hip, 238
  joint, 249–253, 251f
  stability of, 302–303
Hip bones, 72, 239–240, 247–248
Hook grip, 200–201
Humeroradial joint, 109–111
Humeroulnar joint, 109–111
Humerus, 58, 64, 70–72, 109, 112
  anterior view of, 108f
  head of, 70–71
  movement of, 95–97
  posterior view of, 108f
  rotation of, 99f
  shaft of, 70–71
Hyaline cartilage, 12
Hyoglossus, 370
Hyoid bone, 386
Hyperextension, 4, 127
Hypertrophy, 37b
Hypoglossal nerve
    (CN XIII), 384
Hypothalamus, 360
Hypothenar, 60
Hypothenar eminence, 126, 167

I

Ileum, 53
Iliac arteries, 275f
Iliac crest, 245, 260, 288, 413
Iliacus, 268
Iliococcygeus, 406
Iliocostalis, 222
Iliocostalis cervicis, 222
Iliocostalis lumborum, 222
Iliocostalis thoracis, 222
Iliofemoral ligament, 251–252

Iliohypogastric nerve, 262–263
Ilioinguinal nerve, 262–263
Iliolumbar ligaments, 249
Iliopsoas, 268–269, 297–298
Iliotibial tract, 261, 281
Ilium, 72, 245–247
Impingement syndrome, 98b
Inferior articular facets, 207–208
Inferior articular processes,
    207–208
Inferior border, 400
Inferior cervical ganglion, 384
Inferior costal margin, 399
Inferior epigastric artery, 405
Inferior extensor retinaculum, 311
Inferior fibular retinaculum, 311
Inferior gemellus, 285
Inferior genicular branch, 321
Inferior gluteal nerve, 289
Inferior lateral cutaneous nerves,
    112–113
Inferior mesenteric artery, 411
Inferior nasal conchae, 357–358
Inferior oblique, 366
Inferior phalangeal constrictor,
    377
Inferior recti, 366
Inferior sagittal sinus, 360
Inferior thyroid arteries, 385
Inferior ulnar collateral artery, 120
Inferior vena cava, 398, 412–413
Inferior vertebral notch, 207
Infrahyoid muscles, 373–374
Infrapatellar fat pad, 258
Infrapatellar synovial fold, 258
Infraspinatus, 87–88, 88t, 90, 97
Infraspinous fossa, 66, 72
Inguinal canal, 404
Inguinal ligament, 255, 403
Injury
  to ligaments, 335–336
  to median nerve, 190–191, 193
  to radial nerve, 193
  to ulnar nerve, 192–193
Inner ear, 357
Inner wall, 27
Innermost intercostals, 391

Innervation, 81
  cutaneous, 46f, 184–185, 188, 382f, 413
  of joints, 172, 339
  of knee, 302
  peripheral, 45, 100–101
  segmental, 45, 98–100, 141, 155
  of sternocleidomastoid, 82
  of thigh, 298–299
  of thumb, 179
Insertion, 26, 80–81
  definition of, 26
Inspiration, 393
Intercarpal joint, 130, 170–172
Intercarpal ligaments, 170–171
Interclavicular ligament, 69
Intercondylar fossa, 249–250, 256
Intercostal arteries, 398
Intercostal muscles, 391, 391t
Intercostal nerves, 234, 391, 405
Intercostal vessels, 405
Intercostobrachial nerve, 73, 112–113
Interior costal margin, 413
Intermetatarsal joint, 337
Intermuscular septa
  lateral, 112
  medial, 112
Internal capsule, 362
Internal carotid arteries, 385
Internal carotid artery, 385
Internal iliac artery, 411–412
Internal intercostals, 391
Internal oblique, 403
Interossei, 180–182, 181t, 196–197
  dorsal, 181–182, 346
  palmar, 181
  plantar, 346
Interosseous intercarpal ligaments, 170–171
Interosseous membrane, 111–112, 128–129
Interosseous muscles, 180–182
Interosseous sacroiliac ligament, 249
Interosseous tarsal ligaments, 336

Interphalangeal joints, 130, 172, 173, 173f, 339
  flexors of, 196f
Interspinales, 226
Interstitial lamellae, 13
Intertarsal joints, 336–337
Intertransversarii, 226
Intertransverse ligaments, 211
Intertrochanteric crest, 249–250
Intertubercular groove, 70–71
Intertubercular synovial sheath, 71
Intervertebral discs, 205, 213–215
Intervertebral foramen, 207
Intestine
  large, 410
  small, 410
Intramembranous bone formation, 19–21
Intrinsic muscles, 64
Inversion, 240, 307–308
  of foot, 319
Irregular bones, 20
Ischial spine, 246
Ischial tuberosity, 255, 288
Ischiococcygeus, 407
Ischiofemoral ligament, 252
Ischiorectal fossa, 407
Ischium, 246–247
Isometric contraction, 31
Isotonic contraction, 31

J

Jaw. See Mandible; Maxilla
Jejunum, 53
Joint(s), 109–111
  acromioclavicular, 69–70
  of arm, 108–112
  atlanto-axial, 215
  ball-and-socket, 24, 250–251
  of bony pelvis, 245, 249
  capsule, 25
  carpometacarpal, 23f, 130, 172
  cartilaginous, 22–24, 210, 212–215
  cavity, 258
  condyloid, 23f, 24
  cuneonavicular, 335

Joint(s) (Continued)
  distal radioulnar, 169
  examples of, 23f
  fibrous, 22
  of foot, 332–340
  of hand, 128–130, 167–173
  hinge, 24
  hip, 249–253, 251f
  innervation of, 172, 339
  intercarpal, 130, 170–172
  intermetatarsal, 337
  interphalangeal, 130, 172, 173, 173f, 196f, 339
  intertarsal, 336–337
  knee, 257–260, 276f
  of knee, 256–260, 259f, 276f
  metacarpophalangeal, 130, 172, 173, 173f, 196f
  metatarsophalangeal, 338–339
  midcarpal, 170–172
  pivot, 24
  plane, 24
  proximal radioulnar, 111–112
  radiocarpal, 169–170
  radioulnar, 159–160
  sacroiliac, 249
  saddle, 24
  of shoulder, 66–71
  sternoclavicular, 68–69
  subtalar, 308–310, 336–337
  synovial, 24–26, 210–212
  talocalcaneonavicular, 336–337
  tarsometatarsal, 337
  temporomandibular, 358, 367–370, 369f
  tibiofibular, 260, 308
  transverse tarsal, 308–310, 335
  trochoid, 111–112
  of vertebral column, 210–216
  of wrist and fingers, 130
Jugular notch, 399

K

Keratinized layer, 9
Kidneys, 53, 411, 414
Klumpke-Dejerine paralysis, 101–102b, 164b

Knee, 238. *See also* Leg
  bones of, 256–260, 282f, 312f
  innervation of, 302
  joints of, 256–260, 259f, 276f
  movements of, 255, 299–302
  stability of, 302–303
  surface anatomy, 260, 276
Kyphosis, 216–217

L

Lacrimal bones, 357–358
Lambdoid suture, 358–359
Laminae, 206–207
Large intestine, 410
Larynx, 53, 377–378
Lateral, definition of, 3
Lateral circumflex femoral arteries, 272–273
Lateral cord, 73–74
Lateral cutaneous branch, 391
Lateral cutaneous nerve, 131, 261, 263
Lateral epicondyle, 109
Lateral excursion, 367
Lateral intermuscular septa, 112, 261
Lateral ligament, 335–336
Lateral lips, 249–250
Lateral malleolus, 310, 339–340
Lateral mass, 139
Lateral patellar retinacula, 257
Lateral pectoral nerve, 74
Lateral plantar artery, 348
Lateral plantar nerve, 320–321, 340, 347–348
Lateral process, 332
Lateral pterygoid, 367
Lateral recti, 366
Lateral rotation, 4, 66
Lateral thoracic artery, 76–77
Lateral ventricles, 362
Lateral wall, 73
Latissimus dorsi, 84–85, 85t, 95–97, 210
Left border, 400

Leg, 238. *See also* Calf; Knee; Thigh
  bones of, 308–310
  extension of, 299–300
  fascia of, 310–312
  flexion of, 300
  muscles of, 241, 312–320, 318f, 318t, 319f,
  nerves of, 310–312, 320–323, 322f
  rotation of, 301–302, 301f
  surface anatomy, 310, 320–323
  vessels of, 310–312, 320–323
Lentiform nucleus, 362
Lesser pelvis, 407–408
Lesser sciatic foramen, 248
Lesser trochanter, 249–250
Lesser tubercle, 72
Levator anguli oris, 365
Levator ani, 405
Levator labii oris, 365
Levator palpebrae superioris, 367
Levator scapulae, 85–86, 86t
Levator veli palatini, 377
Levers, 29–31
  first class, 30
  second class, 30
  third class, 30, 30f
Ligamenta flava, 211
Ligament(s), 11–12, 25
  annular, 111
  anterior longitudinal, 212
  anterior sacroiliac, 249
  anterior talofibular, 335
  arcuate popliteal, 257
  broad, 411
  calcaneofibular, 335
  collateral, 172, 257–258, 338–339
  conoid, 69–70
  coracoclavicular, 69–70
  coracohumeral, 71
  costoclavicular, 69
  cruciate, 260
  cuneometatarsal interosseous, 337

Ligament(s) *(Continued)*
  deep transverse metatarsal, 338–339
  dorsal metatarsal, 337
  dorsal radiocarpal, 169–170
  dorsal tarsal, 336
  dorsal tarsometatarsal, 337
  of elbow joint, 112f
  of foot, 336
  glenohumeral, 71
  of glenohumeral joint, 70f
  iliofemoral, 251–252
  iliolumbar, 249
  inguinal, 255, 403
  injury, 335–336
  intercarpal, 170–171
  interclavicular, 69
  interosseous intercarpal, 170–171
  interosseous sacroiliac, 249
  interosseous tarsal, 336
  intertransverse, 211
  ischiofemoral, 252
  lateral, 335–336
  long plantar, 336
  medial, 335
  metatarsal interosseous, 337
  oblique popliteal, 257, 286
  palmar, 172
  palmar radiocarpal, 169–170
  palmar ulnocarpal, 169–170
  plantar, 338–339
  plantar calcaneonavicular, 335, 336
  plantar metatarsal, 337
  plantar tarsal, 336
  plantar tarsometatarsal, 337
  posterior longitudinal, 212–213
  posterior sacroiliac, 249
  posterior talofibular, 335
  pubofemoral, 252
  radial collateral, 111, 169–170
  sacrospinous, 248–249
  sacrotuberous, 248–249
  sphenomandibular, 370
  sternoclavicular, 69
  stylomandibular, 370

Ligament(s) *(Continued)*
  supraspinous, 211
  talocalcaneal interosseous,
      336–337
  transverse, 215
  transverse acetabular,
      250–251
  trapezoid, 69–70
  ulnar collateral, 111,
      169–170
  of vertebral column, 211f
  of wrist, 171f
Ligamentum nuchae, 211–212
Limbs, 2. *See also* Lower limb;
      Upper limb
Line of gravity, 4–7, 6f, 216
Linea aspera, 249–250
Liver, 408–409, 413–414
Lobar bronchi, 395–396
Long bones, 20
Long plantar ligament, 336
Long thoracic nerve, 75–76
Longissimus, 222
Longissimus capitis, 222
Longissimus cervicis, 222
Longissimus thoracis, 222
Longitudinal arch, 240, 334
Longitudinal band, 215
Longus capitis, 227, 376
Longus colli, 226–227, 376
Lordosis, 218
Low back pain, 218–219
Lower border of lung, 400
Lower limb, 241. *See also specific
      structures*
  arteries of, 241–242
  development of, 238–239
  movements of, 6f
  muscles, 241
  skeleton, 239–241
  veins of, 243
Lower ribs, 401
Lower trunk, 73–74
Lumbar curvature, 205–206
Lumbar nerves, 44
Lumbar plexus, 241, 261–263
Lumbar puncture, 212b, 231

Lumbar region, 216
  cross-section of, 219f
Lumbar spinous processes, 210
Lumbar vertebrae, 204–205,
      208–210, 401
Lumbosacral plexus, 234, 241,
      261–262
Lumbrical muscles, 174–175,
      196–197, 344, 347–348
  first, 347
Lunate, 167–168
Lung, 395, 400
  lower border of, 400
Lymph nodes, 51
Lymphatic drainage, 78b
Lymphatic vascular system,
      50–51, 51b
  drainage, 52f

M

Male pelvis, 411
Mandible, 357–358, 386
Mandibular nerve, 381
Manubrium, 72, 399
Masseter, 367, 386–387
Mastication muscles, 368f,
      367–370, 370t
Mastoid processes, 72, 210,
      357, 386
Maxilla, 357–358
Maxillary bone, 386
Maxillary nerve, 381
Medial, 3
Medial circumflex femoral artery,
      272–273
Medial cord, 73–75
Medial cutaneous nerve, 74–75,
      112–113
Medial epicondyle, 109
Medial intermuscular septa,
      112, 261
Medial ligament, 335
Medial lips, 249–250
Medial malleolus, 310, 339–340
Medial mass, 139
Medial patellar retinacula, 257
Medial pectoral nerve, 74–75

Medial plantar artery, 348
Medial plantar nerve, 320–321,
      340, 347–348, 352t
Medial process, 332
Medial pterygoid, 367
Medial rotation, 4, 66
Medial wall, 73
Median cubital vein, 61, 114, 145
Median nerve, 60, 117, 128,
      139–141, 142f, 146,
      182–188
  injury to, 190–191, 193
Median plane, 3
Medulla oblongata, 363
Medullary cavity, 20
Meninges, 229–237, 360–364
Meningitis, 43b
Menisci, 258–260
Mesentery, 407
Mesotendon, 27
Mesothelium, 9
Metacarpal arteries, 188
Metacarpals, 58, 130, 172–173,
      168
Metacarpophalangeal joint, 130,
      172–173, 173f
  flexors of, 196f
Metaphysis, 20
Metatarsal interosseous
      ligaments, 337
Metatarsals, 240, 310,
      339–340, 334
  fifth, 339–340
  first, 339–340
Metatarsophalangeal joints,
      338–339
Midcarpal joint, 170–172
Middle cerebral arteries, 364
Middle collateral, 120
Middle ear cavity, 357
Middle genicular artery, 274, 321
Middle phalangeal
      constrictor, 377
Middle phalangeal
      constrictor, 377
Middle scalene, 375
Middle trunk, 73–74
Midstance, 354
Midswing, 354

Mimetic muscles, 364
Mitral valve, 398
Motor centers, 41
Motor end plate, 34–35
Motor nerve fibers, 34–36
Motor neurons, 41–42
Motor nuclei, 378
Motor tracts, 41, 232
Motor units, 35
Mouth, 386–387
Movement. *See also* Gait;
    Running
  abduction, 4
  adduction, 4
  analysis of, 102–104b
  of arm, 65–66, 107
  of bony pelvis, 253, 292
  depression, 4
  of digits, 5f
  of elbow joint, 5f, 121–125
  elevation, 4
  extension, 4
  of fingers, 128, 197
  flexion, 4
  of foot, 323–328
  of forearm, 107
  of glenohumeral joint, 5f
  gliding, 370
  at hip, 294–299
  humeral, 95–97
  hyperextension, 4
  of knee, 255, 299–302
  lateral rotation, 4
  of lower limbs, 6f
  medial rotation, 4
  protraction, 4
  retraction, 4
  rotation, 4
  of scapula, 65–66, 67f,
  of shoulder, 77
  terms of, 4
  of thumb, 128
  of toes, 351
  of upper limbs, 5f
  of vertebral column, 216–219
  of wrist joint, 5f, 127f, 160–164

Multifidus, 225
Multipennate muscles, 28–29, 29f
Muscle(s). *See also specific muscles*
  of abdominal wall, 403–404,
    403t
  of arm, 107, 114–117
  articularis genus, 260
  of back, 219–229, 220f,
  bipennate, 28–29, 29f,
  of calf, 313–314, 313t, 315f,
    315t
  cardiac, 14, 46–47
  contraction of, 16, 36
  deep extensor, 147
  deep neck, 226–227, 227t
  dorsal, 350t
  exercise and, 37–38
  extrinsic, 64–65
  facial, 364–366, 365f,
  fibers, 15, 29f
  fibularis, 325, 346
  fibularis brevis, 320, 323
  fibularis longus, 320, 323
  of fingers, 179–180, 180t
  flat, 28
  of foot, 241
  of forearm, 107, 126, 134f,
    135f, 137t, 138t,
    147–152, 149f, 151t
  fusiform, 28
  of gluteal region,
    281–286, 281f, 283t
  hamstring, 286–288
  of hand, 126, 177–182
  infrahyoid, 373–374
  intercostal, 391, 391t
  interosseous, 180–182
  intrinsic, 64
  of leg, 241, 312–320, 318f,
    318t, 319f
  lower limb, 241
  lumbrical, 174–175, 196–197,
    344, 347–348
  of mastication, 367–370, 368f,
    370t
  mimetic, 364

Muscle(s) *(Continued)*
  multipennate, 28–29, 29f
  of neck, 375t, 376f
  nerve supply, 32–36
  of palm, 184f
  of pectoral region, 79–82, 82t
  pennate, 28, 29f
  plantar, 341–346, 342t, 344t
  quadrate, 28
  scalene, 374–376
  segmental, 226
  serratus posterior, 221, 222t
  of shoulder, 82–88
  skeletal, 15–16, 15f
  smooth, 14, 46–47
  spindles, 33–34
  splenius, 221, 221t
  strap, 28
  suboccipital, 226–227, 227t
  superficial extensor forearm, 147
  suprahyoid, 372, 373t
  of thigh, 241, 255–256, 263–
    272, 265f, 266t, 286–288,
    287f, 288t
  of thorax, 391
  of thumb, 175f, 177–179, 178t
  tissue, 14–16
  of tongue, 370–372
  transversospinalis, 224–226, 224t
  triangular, 28
  types of, 14f
  unipennate, 28–29
  upper limb, 58–60, 79–90
  variation, 89
  of wrist, 174–175
  zygomaticus, 365
Muscular action, 29–31
  determination of, 31–32
  integration of, 36
Muscular branches, 182
Muscular system, 26–38
Musculocutaneous nerve, 60,
  117–118, 122f
Musculotendinous cuff, 71b
Myelencephalon, 363
Mylohyoid, 372

Myofibrils, 15–16
Myofilaments, 15–16
Myosin, 16

N

Nasal bones, 357–358
Nasal cavity, 53
Navicular bone, 310, 334, 339–340
Neck, 2
    anterior view of, 374f
    cutaneous innervation of, 382f
    muscles of, 372–376, 375t, 376f
Nerve supply
    motor, 34–36
    muscle, 32–36
Nerve(s), 44–46, 327t. *See also*
    specific nerves
    of abdomen, 413
    abducens, 382
    accessory, 384
    accessory obturator, 262–263
    anteromedial, 272–277
    of arm, 107–108, 112–114,
        117–121, 122t
    of axilla, 77f
    axillary, 60, 73
    of calf, 320–321
    cervical, 44
    coccygeal, 44
    common fibular, 241, 328f
    cranial, 38, 44, 49, 378–384,
        380f, 380t
    deep fibular, 321, 340,
        350, 352t
    dorsal scapular, 75–76, 84f
    facial, 49, 366, 382–383
    femoral, 241, 261, 263,
        272, 273f
    first thoracic, 73–74
    of foot, 340
    of forearm, 107–108, 140f,
        144t, 152–157, 157t
    genitofemoral, 262–263
    glossopharyngeal, 49, 383
    of gluteal region, 281, 284f,
        289–292
    of hand, 128, 130–131, 186t

Nerve(s) *(Continued)*
    hypoglossal, 384
    iliohypogastric, 262–263
    ilioinguinal, 262–263
    inferior gluteal, 289
    inferior lateral cutaneous,
        112–113
    intercostal, 391, 405
    intercostobrachial, 112–113
    lateral cutaneous, 131, 261, 263
    lateral pectoral, 74
    lateral plantar, 320–321, 340,
        347–348, 352t
    of leg, 310–312, 320–323, 322f
    of lower limb, 241
    lumbar, 44
    mandibular, 381
    medial cutaneous, 74–75,
        112–113, 131
    medial pectoral, 74–75
    medial plantar, 320–321, 340,
        347–348, 352t
    median, 60, 117, 128, 131,
        139–141, 142f, 146,
        182–188, 190–191, 193
    musculocutaneous, 60, 122f,
        117–118
    obturator, 241, 253, 255–256,
        261–263, 274f, 275–276
    oculomotor, 49, 381
    olfactory, 378–379
    ophthalmic, 381
    optic, 379–381
    of palm, 183f, 185f
    palmar digital, 172
    pelvic splanchnic, 235
    phrenic, 384, 399
    plantar, 347–348
    plexus, 45
    posterior cutaneous, 112–113,
        131, 188, 290, 292
    posterior interosseous, 152–153
    pudendal, 280
    radial, 60, 118–120, 128, 131,
        152–155, 184–185, 193
    sacral, 44
    saphenous, 272, 311, 340

Nerve(s) *(Continued)*
    sciatic, 241, 255–256, 289,
        290–292, 291f
    of shoulder, 79f
    spinal, 44–46, 233–237
    to subclavius, 75–76
    superficial fibular, 311, 340
    superior gluteal, 253, 280, 289
    superior laryngeal, 383–384
    superior lateral cutaneous,
        112–113
    supraclavicular, 73
    suprascapular, 75–76
    sural, 311, 340
    of thigh, 261, 271f, 277t,
        290–292
    thoracodorsal, 75
    of thorax, 398–399
    tibial, 241, 292, 320–323, 326f
    trochlear, 381
    ulnar, 60, 74–75, 117, 128, 131,
        141, 143f, 146, 183–185,
        188, 192–193
    upper limb, 60, 61f, 73
    vagus, 49, 383, 413
    vestibulocochlear, 383
    of wrist, 182–188
    zygomaticofacial, 382
    zygomaticotemporal, 382
Nervous system, 38–50
    autonomic, 38, 46–50
    central, 38
    origin, 22
    parasympathetic, 47
    peripheral, 38
    sympathetic, 47
Nervous tissue, 16–18
Neural crest, 39
Neural tube, 39
Neuroglia, 17
Neuromuscular ending, 36–37
Neuromuscular junction, 37
Neuron(s), 16–17
    diagram of, 17f
    motor, 41–42
    postganglionic, 47–48
    preganglionic, 47

Neurotransmitters, 17
Neurovascular compression, 76b
Nipple, 399
Norepinephrine, 17, 54
Notch(es)
   deep trochlear, 109
   greater sciatic, 245–246
   inferior vertebral, 207
   jugular, 399
   radial, 109
Nucleus pulposus, 213
Nutrient artery, 20, 120, 321

O

Oblique fissure, 395
Oblique popliteal ligament, 257, 286
Obliquus capitis inferior, 226
Obliquus capitis superior, 226
Obturator artery, 276
Obturator externus, 270–272, 286, 298
Obturator foramen, 246, 247
Obturator internus, 280, 285, 289, 295–296
Obturator nerve, 241, 253, 255–256, 261–263, 274f, 275–276
Occipital bone, 356–357, 386
Occipitalis, 366
Oculomotor nerve (CN III), 49, 381
Olfactory nerve (CN I), 378–379
Omohyoid, 373–374
Ophthalmic nerve, 381
Opponens digiti minimi, 179–180
Opponens pollicis, 178, 198
Opposition, 128
   of thumb, 198
Optic nerve (II), 379–381
Oral cavity, 53
Orbicularis oculi, 366
Orbicularis oris, 365
Orbit, 366–367
Organ systems, 8, 19
Organs, 8, 19

Origin, 26, 80–81
   definition of, 26
   nervous system, 22
Osseofibrous tunnel, 176
Osteocytes, 13
Osteon system, 13
Otic ganglion, 49
Outer wall, 27
Outflow
   cranial, 47
   sacral, 47
   thoracolumbar, 47
Ovaries, 53, 411

P

Pad-to-pad grip, 201
Pad-to-side grip, 201
Pain, 55
   low back, 218–219
   radicular, 214
Pain fibers, 33
Palatine bones, 357–358
Palatoglossus, 371, 377
Palatopharyngeus, 377
Pallium, 361
Palm. *See also* Hand
   arteries of, 183f, 185f
   muscles of, 184f
   nerves of, 183f, 185f
Palmar aponeurosis, 131, 173–174, 184f
Palmar branch, 141
Palmar cutaneous branch, 182
Palmar digital branches, 141
Palmar digital nerves, 172
Palmar fascia, 173–174, 177
Palmar interossei, 181
Palmar ligaments, 172
Palmar metacarpal branches, 186–187
Palmar radiocarpal ligament, 169–170
Palmar ulnocarpal ligament, 169–170
Palmaris brevis, 179
Palmaris longus, 134–135, 139
Pancreas, 409, 414

Pancreatic islets, 54
Papillary layer, 10
Paranasal sinuses, 357
Parasympathetic fibers, 235
Parasympathetic nervous system, 47
   fibers of, 49
   ganglia of, 47
Parasympathetic roots, 413
Parathyroid gland, 14b, 54
Paravertebral ganglia, 47
Parietal bone, 356–357, 386
Parietal pericardium, 394–395
Parietal peritoneum, 407
Parietal pleura, 393
Parkinson disease, 362
Parts of body, 2
Patella, 249–250, 255–256
Patellar reflex, 42
Pectineus, 269, 297–298
Pectoral girdle, 58
Pectoral region, muscles of, 79–82, 82t
Pectoralis major, 90, 95–97, 80–81
Pectoralis minor, 90, 81–82
Pectoralis minor syndrome, 76b
Pedicles, 206–207
Pelvic diaphragm, 405, 406t
Pelvic girdle, 239–240
Pelvic outlet, 405
Pelvic splanchnic nerves, 235
Pelvic viscera, 411
Pelvis, 247. *See also* Bony pelvis
   bones of, 282f
   female, 411
   greater, 407–408
   lesser, 407–408
   male, 411
Pennate muscles, 28, 29f
Perforating arteries, 272–273
Perforating branch, 144–145, 292, 321
Pericardial sac, 393–395
Perimysium, 15
Perineum, 407
Periosteum, 21–22

Peripheral innervation, 45, 100–101
Peripheral nervous system, 38
Peritoneum
  parietal, 407
  visceral, 407
Peroneal longus muscle, 1–2
Pes valgus, 240
Petrous part, 357
Phalanges, 58, 130, 168, 172–173, 240, 310, 334, 339–340
Pharynx, 53, 377–378
  constrictors, 377
Phrenic nerve, 75–76, 384, 399
Pia mater, 230, 361
Piriformis, 280, 285, 289, 295–297
Pisiform bone, 134, 167–168, 172–173
Pituitary gland, 54
Pivot joints, 24
Plane joints, 24
Planes of body, 3
  frontal, 3
  median, 3
  sagittal, 3
  transverse, 3
Plantar aponeurosis, 340
Plantar arteries, 349f
Plantar calcaneonavicular ligaments, 335–336
Plantar flexion, 307, 323–324
Plantar interossei, 346
Plantar ligaments, 338–339
Plantar metatarsal arteries, 348
Plantar metatarsal ligaments, 337
Plantar muscles, 341–346, 342t
  deep layer of, 345–346
  second layer, 343–344, 344t
  superficial layer, 341–342
  third layer of, 344–345
Plantar nerves, 347–348
Plantar surface, 332
Plantar tarsal ligaments, 336
Plantar tarsometatarsal ligament, 337
Plantar vessels, 347–348

Plantaris, 314
Plasma, 51
Platysma, 366, 386–387
Pleural sac, 393–395
Pneumothorax, 394
Pons, 363
Popliteal artery, 241–242, 274–275, 292, 321
Popliteal fossa, 255, 289
Popliteal region, 238
Popliteal surface, 249–250
Popliteal vein, 321
Popliteal vessels, 256, 292
Popliteus, 300–301, 314–316
Portal vein, 412–413
Posterior, definition of, 2
Posterior bands, 111
Posterior branch, 275
Posterior cerebral arteries, 363
Posterior communicating arteries, 364
Posterior cord, 73–75
Posterior cutaneous nerve, 112–113, 131, 290, 292
Posterior division, 73–74
Posterior fibers, 95–96, 294–295
Posterior fontanelle, 359–360
Posterior horns, 40
Posterior inferior iliac spine, 245, 288
Posterior intermuscular septum, 311
Posterior interosseous artery, 153, 155
Posterior interosseous branch, 144–145
Posterior interosseous nerve, 152–153
Posterior longitudinal ligament, 212–213
Posterior ramus, 45, 234, 281
Posterior root, 44–45, 233
Posterior root ganglion, 44–45
Posterior sacral foramina, 209
Posterior sacroiliac ligament, 249
Posterior scalene, 375

Posterior superior iliac spine, 210, 245, 288, 413
Posterior talofibular ligament, 335
Posterior tibial artery, 241–242, 321, 323
Posterior tibial recurrent artery, 274
Posterior triangle, 373
Posterior wall, 73
Posterolateral fontanelle, 359–360
Postganglionic neurons, 47–48
Power grips, 200–201, 200f
Precision grips, 201
Preganglionic neurons, 47
  location and outflow of, 47
Prehension, 199
Pressure, 55
Prevertebral ganglia, 47
Prime movers, 32
Princeps pollicis artery, 186–187
Profunda brachii artery, 120
Pronation, 127, 159, 240, 307–308
Pronator quadratus, 127, 134, 139, 159
Pronator teres, 121–123, 134–137, 139, 159
Proper palmar digital arteries, 186, 188–189
Proper palmar digital branch, 183–184, 186
Proper plantar digital arteries, 348
Proprioceptive fibers, 33
Prostate, 411
Protraction, 4
  of scapula, 67f, 93, 94f
Protrusion, 367
Proximal attachments, 26
Proximal radioulnar joint, 111–112
Proximal row, 167–168
Pseudostratified epithelium, 9
Psoas major, 227–228, 268–269, 401
Pterygopalatine ganglion, 49
Pubic crest, 246
Pubic symphysis, 249
Pubic tubercle, 246, 260, 413
Pubis, 246–247, 260

Pubococcygeus, 406
Pubofemoral ligament, 252
Puborectalis, 406
Pudendal nerve, 280
Pulmonary arteries, 396
Pulmonary trunk, 396
Pulmonary veins, 396
Push-off, 353–354
Putamen, 362
Pyramid, 363
Pyramidal tracts, 363

Q

Quadrants of abdomen, 401
Quadrate muscles, 28
Quadratus femoris, 253, 280, 286,
    296–298
Quadratus lumborum, 228,
    404–405, 405t
Quadratus plantae, 344, 347–348,
    351
Quadriceps, 299–300
Quadriceps femoris, 265–268

R

Radial, 3
Radial artery, 60, 128, 144–146,
    145f, 152, 155, 156f,
    186–188
Radial collateral artery, 120
Radial collateral ligament, 111,
    169–170
Radial nerve, 60, 118–120,
    128, 131, 152–155,
    184–185
  groove, 109
  injury to, 193
Radial notch, 109
Radial recurrent branch, 144
Radial tuberosity, 109
Radial vein, 61
Radialis indicis artery, 186–187
Radicular pain, 214
Radiocarpal joint, 130, 169–170
Radioulnar joints, 159–160
Radius, 58, 109, 112, 130
  views of, 129f

Rami communicantes, 234–235
Rectum, 53, 410–411
Rectus abdominus, 404, 413
Rectus capitis anterior, 227
Rectus capitis lateralis, 227
Rectus capitis posterior major, 226
Rectus capitis posterior
    minor, 226
Rectus femoris, 265–268, 297
Red blood cells, 51
Red marrow, 20
Reflex arc, 42–43
Regions, 2
Reposition, 128
Resistance arm, 30
Respiration, 392–393
Respiratory system, 53
Reticular layer, 10
Reticulospinal tracts, 232
Retraction, 4
  of scapula, 93, 94f
Rhomboid major, 85–86, 86t
Rhomboid minor, 85–86, 86t
Ribs, 64, 72, 389
  false, 389
  floating, 389
Right lymphatic duct, 51, 52f
Rigidity, 34b, 44
Risorius, 365
Rotation, 4
  of arm, 99f, 100f
  of humerus, 99f
  lateral, 4, 66
  of leg, 301–302, 301f
  medial, 4, 66
  of scapula, 67f, 72, 91, 93f
  of thigh, 296–297
Rotator cuff, 71b, 88
Rotatores, 225–226
Rubrospinal tract, 232
Running, 348
Ruptured disc, 214

S

Sacral canal, 209
Sacral curvature, 205–206
Sacral hiatus, 209–210

Sacral nerves, 44
Sacral outflow, 47
Sacral plexus, 241, 279–280, 280f
Sacral vertebrae, 210
Sacroiliac joint, 249
Sacrospinous ligament, 248–249
Sacrotuberous ligament, 248–249
Sacrum, 72, 204–205, 210, 245
Saddle joints, 24
Sagittal plane, 3
Sagittal suture, 358–359
Salivary glands, 386–387
Saphenous hiatus, 261
Saphenous nerve, 272, 311, 340
Sartorius, 263–264, 295–297,
    300–301
Scalene muscles, 374–286
Scalenus anticus syndrome,
    76b, 376
Scaphoid, 152, 167–168, 172–173
Scapula, 58, 64, 66, 72
  depression of, 91, 92f
  elevation of, 67f, 91, 92f
  extension of, 67f
  flexion of, 67f
  movement of, 65–66, 67f
  protraction of, 67f, 93, 94f
  retraction of, 93, 94f
  rotation of, 67f, 72, 91, 93f
Scapulohumeral rhythm, 90–91
Scar tissue, 11b
Sciatic nerve, 241, 255–256, 289,
    290–292, 291f
Scoliosis, 216–217
Scrotum, 53
Second rib, 399
Secondary endings, 33–34
Segmental bronchi, 396
Segmental innervation, 45,
    98–100, 141–144, 155
Segmental muscles, 226
Semimembranosus, 286, 289, 294,
    297, 300–301
Seminal vesicles, 411
Semispinalis, 224–225
Semispinalis capitis, 225
Semispinalis cervicis, 225

Semispinalis thoracis, 225
Semitendinosus, 286, 289, 294, 297, 300–301
Serratus anterior, 86, 86t, 90
Serratus posterior muscles, 221, 222t
Sesamoid bones, 20, 168, 334
Sherrington, Charles Scott, 41
Short bones, 20
Shoulder, 57, 64–65
  bones of, 66–68
  bursae, 97–98
  impingement syndrome of, 98b
  joints of, 66–71
  movement of, 77
  muscles of, 82–88
  nerves and arteries of, 79f, 101t
  osteological illustrations of, 68f
  surface anatomy of, 89–90
Sigmoid colon, 53, 410
Sigmoid sinus, 360
Sinuses
  cavernous, 360
  cranial venous, 360
  inferior sagittal, 360
  sigmoid, 360
  straight, 360
  superior sagittal, 360
  transverse, 360
Skeletal muscle, 15–16
  cross-section of, 15f
Skeletal system, 19–26
Skeleton
  appendicular, 58
  axial, 58
  facial, 356–358
  lower limb, 239–241
  upper limb, 58, 59f, 65f
Skin, 54–55
Skull, 72, 356, 357f
Slipped disc, 214
Small intestine, 410
Small saphenous vein, 243, 311–312, 321, 323, 340, 350–351
Smooth muscle, 14, 46–47
Soleus, 299–300, 314, 320, 323

Spasticity, 34b
Spermatic cord, 53
Sphenoid bone, 356–357
Sphenomandibular ligaments, 370
Spherical (ball) grip, 201
Spina bifida, 219
Spinal anesthesia, 230
Spinal cord, 22, 229–235
  cross-section, 48f
  segment, 40f, 234
  tracts of, 40–41, 231–232, 232f
Spinal nerves, 38, 44–46, 233–235
Spinal reflex arc, 42
Spinalis, 223–224
Spinalis capitis, 224–225
Spinalis cervicis, 223–224
Spinocerebellar tracts, 231
Spinothalamic tracts, 232
Spinous processes, 72, 207–210
Splanchnic nerves, 49, 411
Spleen, 410, 413–414
Splenius capitis, 221
Splenius cervicis, 221
Splenius muscles, 221, 221t, 228
Spondylolisthesis, 219
Spondylolysis, 219
Spongy bone, 13
Sprain, 25–26b
Squamous cells, 8, 9f
Squamous suture, 358–359
Stability
  of hip, 302–303
  of knee, 302–303
  of vertebral column, 216
Stance phase, 353–354
Sternal angle, 389, 399
Sternalis, 89
Sternoclavicular joint, 68–69
Sternoclavicular ligaments, 69
Sternocleidomastoid, 82, 85t, 373, 386–387
  innervation of, 82
Sternocostal fibers, 95–96
Sternohyoid, 373–374
Sternothyroid, 373–374

Sternum, 58, 64, 72, 389, 399
  body of, 399
Stomach, 53, 409, 414
Straight sinus, 360
Strap muscles, 28
Styloglossus, 370
Stylohyoid, 372
Styloid process, 133–134, 173
Stylomandibular ligament, 370
Subacromial bursa, 97–98
Subarachnoid space, 230, 361
Subclavian artery, 60, 65, 78f, 79, 385, 398
Subclavian nerve, 75–76
Subclavian vein, 61
Subclavius, 90, 82, 85t
Subcostalis, 391
Subdeltoid bursa, 97–98
Subluxation, 25–26b
Submandibular ganglion, 49
Submandibular salivary gland, 386–387
Suboccipital muscles, 226–227, 227t
Subscapular artery, 76–77
Subscapular fossa, 66
Subscapularis, 87–88, 88t, 97
Subtalar joint, 308–310, 336–337
Superficial arch, 188
Superficial brachial artery, 120
Superficial branch, 141, 153, 183–184, 347–348
Superficial cervical artery, 83–84
Superficial extensor forearm muscles, 147
Superficial fascia, 10–11, 72, 112
Superficial fibular nerve, 311, 321, 340
Superficial inguinal ring, 404
Superficial palmar branch, 186–187
Superficial temporal artery, 387
Superior, definition of, 2–3
Superior articular facets, 207–208
Superior articular processes, 207
Superior border, 400
Superior cervical ganglion, 384

Superior epigastric artery, 405
Superior extensor retinaculum, 311
Superior fibular retinaculum, 311
Superior gemellus, 285
Superior genicular branch, 321
Superior gluteal nerve, 253, 280, 289
Superior laryngeal nerve, 383–384
Superior lateral cutaneous nerve, 112–113
Superior medial genicular artery, 274
Superior mesenteric artery, 411
Superior nuchal lines, 210
Superior oblique, 366
Superior phalangeal constrictor, 377
Superior recti, 366
Superior sagittal sinus, 360
Superior thyroid arteries, 385
Superior ulnar collateral artery, 120
Superior vena cava, 398
Supination, 127, 160, 240, 307–308
  of forearm, 161f
Supinator, 151, 160
Supporting weight, 351–353
Supraclavicular nerves, 73
Supracondylar ridges, 109
Suprahyoid muscles, 372, 373t
Suprapatellar bursa, 258
Suprarenal glands, 54, 411
Suprascapular nerve, 75–76
Supraspinal influences, 43–44
Supraspinatus, 87–88, 88t, 90, 96
Supraspinatus syndrome, 98b
Supraspinous fossa, 66, 72
Supraspinous ligament, 211
Supreme thoracic artery, 76–77
Sural arteries, 321
Sural nerve, 311, 340
Surface anatomy, 71–72, 79
  of abdomen, 413–414
  of arm, 112, 116–117
  of back, 228–229
  of dorsum of foot, 350–351

Surface anatomy *(Continued)*
  of foot, 339–340, 348
  of forearm, 133–134, 139, 145–146, 152, 155
  of gluteal region, 292
  of hand, 187–188
  of head, 386–387
  of knee, 260, 276
  of leg, 310, 320–323
  of shoulder muscles, 89–90
  of thigh, 272, 288–289
  of thorax, 399–400
  of vertebral column, 210
Sustentaculum tali, 332, 339–340
Sutures, 22, 23f, 356, 358–359
  coronal, 358–359
  lambdoid, 358–359
  sagittal, 358–359
  squamous, 358–359
Swallowing, 378
  sequence of, 379f
Swing phase, 353–354
Sympathetic fibers, 48f, 49, 234–235
Sympathetic nervous system, 47
Sympathetic trunks, 47, 384–385, 398–399, 413
Symphysis, 22–24, 23f
Synapse, 17, 22
Synchondrosis, 22–23, 23f
Syndesmosis, 22, 23f
Synergists, 32
Synovial fluid, 25
Synovial joints, 24–26, 210–212
Synovial membrane, 25
Synovial sheaths, 27
  of fingers, 174–175
  of flexor pollicis longus, 174–175
  of hand, 188
  of thumb, 174–175
  of wrist, 174–175
Synovium, 25, 28f

T

Tabes dorsalis, 33b
Talipes equinovarus, 327

Talocalcaneal interosseous ligament, 336–337
Talocalcaneonavicular joint, 336–337
Talus, 333, 352
Tarsals, 240, 308–310
Tarsometatarsal joint, 337
Tarsus. *See* Ankle
Tectorial membrane, 215
Temporal bone, 356–357, 386
Temporalis, 367, 386–387
Temporomandibular joint, 358, 367–370, 369f
Tendon(s), 11, 26–27
  of biceps brachii, 139
  calcaneal, 320
  extensor digitorum, 196–197
  of extensor digitorum longus, 320, 350
  of extensor hallucis longus, 320
  of fibularis brevis, 320
  of fibularis tertius, 320
  of fingers, 176f
  of flexor carpi radialis, 139
  of flexor carpi ulnaris, 139
  of flexor digitorum longus, 343–344
  of flexor digitorum superficialis, 139
  of flexor hallucis longus, 343
  of hand, 188
  strength of, 27b
  of tibialis anterior, 320
  of wrist, 174–175
Tensor fasciae latae, 264, 285, 295–297
Tensor veli palatini, 377
Tentorium cerebelli, 360
Teres major, 87–88, 88t
Teres minor, 87–88, 88t, 90, 96–97
Terminologia Anatomica: International Anatomical Terminology, 1–2
Terminology, 1–2
  introduction to, 1–2
Testes, 53
Tetanic contraction, 37

Thenar, 60
Thenar eminence, 126, 167, 177
Thigh, 238. *See also* Leg
  abduction of, 295–296
  adduction of, 298
  arteries of, 271f
  bones of, 282f
  deep artery of, 272–273
  extension of, 294–295
  fascia of, 261
  flexion of, 297
  innervation of, 298–299
  landmarks of, 255
  muscles of, 241, 255–256,
      263–272, 265f, 266t,
      286–288, 287f, 288t
  nerves of, 271f, 261, 277t,
      290–292
  rotation of, 296–297
  surface anatomy of, 272,
      288–289
  vessels of, 261, 290–292
Thoracic, 2
Thoracic aorta, 398
Thoracic curvature, 205–206
Thoracic duct, 51, 52f
Thoracic outlet syndrome, 76b
Thoracic region, 216
Thoracic spinal nerve, 60
Thoracic vertebrae, 204–205,
      207–208, 210, 389
Thoracic viscera, 395–398, 395f
Thoracodorsal artery, 76–77
Thoracodorsal nerve, 75
Thoracolumbar fascia, 210, 219
Thoracolumbar outflow, 47
Thorax
  cross section, 390f
  nerves of, 398–399
  surface anatomy, 399–400
  veins of, 398
  vessels of, 398
Thumb, 57
  abduction of, 5f, 198–199
  adduction of, 5f, 198–199
  flexion of, 198
  innervation of, 179

Thumb *(Continued)*
  movements of, 128, 197–199
    muscles of, 175f, 177–179, 178t
    opposition of, 198
    synovial sheath of, 174–175
Thyrohyoid, 373–374
Thyroid cartilage, 377, 386, 399
Thyroid gland, 54
Tibia, 240, 256, 308, 309f
Tibial, definition of, 3
Tibial nerve, 241, 292, 320–323
    distribution of, 326f
Tibial tuberosity, 256, 260
Tibialis anterior, 319, 324, 350
    tendon of, 320
Tibialis posterior, 314, 317,
      323–324
Tibiofibular joint, 260, 308
Tibiofibular syndesmosis, 308
Tip-to-tip (pincer) grip, 201
Tissue(s), 8
  adipose, 10
  connective, 9–14, 9f
  defined, 8
  epithelial, 8–9, 9f
  fibrous connective, 10–11,
      369–370
  muscle, 14
  nervous, 16–18
  scar, 11b
Toe-off, 353–354
Toes, movements of, 351.
      See also Foot
Tongue, muscles of, 370–372
Torticollis, 373b
Touch, 55
Trabeculae, 229–230
Trachea, 53, 377–378, 395–396
  bifurcation of, 399–400
  cartilaginous rings of, 377,
      386
Tracheostomy, 378
Tracheotomy, 378
Training, 37–38
Transverse acetabular ligament,
      250–251
Transverse arch, 334

Transverse band, 111
Transverse cervical artery, 84f
Transverse colon, 53, 410
Transverse crural septum, 311
Transverse dimension, 392
Transverse foramen, 207
Transverse ligament, 215
Transverse plane, 3
Transverse processes, 207–210
Transverse sinus, 360
Transverse tarsal joint,
      308–310, 335
Transversospinalis muscles,
      224–226
Transversospinalis system, 228
Transversus abdominus, 403–404
Transversus thoracis, 391
Trapezium, 152, 167–168,
      172–173
Trapezius, 82–84, 85t, 90,
      228–229
Trapezoid, 167–168
Trapezoid ligament, 69–70
Trendelenburg's sign, 295
Triangular muscles, 28
Triceps brachii, 95–96, 110f,
      115–117, 123
Triceps surae, 313–314
Tricuspid valve, 397–398
Trigeminal nerve (CN V), 381
Trigeminal neuralgia, 382
Triquetrum, 167–168
Trochlea, 109, 333
Trochlear nerve (CN IV), 381
Trochlear notch, deep, 109
Trochoid joints, 111–112
Trunk (body), 2. *See also*
      Abdomen; Abdominal wall;
      Pelvis
  surfaces of, 2
Tubercle, 207
Tuberosity, 310

U

Ulna, 58, 109, 112, 130
  views of, 129f
Ulnar, definition of, 3

Ulnar artery, 60, 128, 144–146, 145f, 186, 188
Ulnar collateral ligament, 111, 169–170
Ulnar nerve, 60, 74–75, 117, 128, 131, 141, 143f, 146, 183–185, 188
  groove, 109
  injury to, 192, 193
Ulnar vein, 61
Unipennate muscles, 28–29
Upper limb, 19. *See also specific structures*
  arteries, 60
  axilla, 73–79
  bones of, 66–68
  bursae, 62
  development, 57–58
  fascia, 72–73
  movements of, 5f
  muscle, 58, 79–90
  nerves, 60, 61f, 73
  skeleton, 58, 59f, 65f
  veins, 61, 62f
  vessels of, 76
Upper trunk, 73–74
Ureters, 53
Urethra, 53
Urinary bladder, 53
Urogenital diaphragm, 407
Urogenital system, 53
Uterine tubes, 411
Uterus, 411

V

Vagina, 411
Vagus nerve (CN X), 49, 383, 398–399, 413
Valgus, 240
Varus, 240
Vastus intermedius, 266–268
Vastus lateralis, 266–268
Vastus medialis, 266–268
Vein(s), 50. *See also specific veins*
  axillary, 61, 77
  basilic, 61, 114, 131, 145, 189
  brachial, 61, 77, 121

Vein(s) *(Continued)*
  brachiocephalic, 398
  cephalic, 61, 77, 79, 114, 121, 131, 145, 189
  external jugular, 387
  femoral, 256, 272
  great saphenous, 261, 276, 311–312, 323, 340, 350–351
  lower limb, 243
  median cubital, 61, 114, 145
  median forearm, 131
  popliteal, 321
  portal, 412–413
  pulmonary, 396
  radial, 61
  small saphenous, 243, 311–312, 321, 323, 340, 350–351
  subclavian, 61
  of thorax, 398
  ulnar, 61
  upper limb, 61, 62f
Venous plexus, 155
Venules, 50
Vertebra prominens, 207
Vertebrae, 72, 206–210
  cervical, 204–205, 207, 210
  lumbar, 204–205, 208–210, 401
  sacral, 210
  thoracic, 204–205, 207–208, 210
  types of, 206–207, 206f
Vertebral arch, 206–207
Vertebral canal, 206–207
Vertebral column, 204–206, 213f
  abnormal curvature of, 217f
  joints of, 210–216
  ligaments of, 211f
  movements of, 216
  stability of, 216
  surface anatomy of, 210
Vertebral foramen, 206–207
Vessels. *See also specific arteries and veins*
  of abdomen, 411–413
  anteromedial, 272–276

Vessels. *(Continued)*
  of arm, 117–121
  of calf, 320–321
  of forearm, 139–146, 152–155
  of gluteal region, 281, 289–292
  great, 397f
  of hand, 130–131, 185–189
  of leg, 310–312, 320–323
  plantar, 347–348
  popliteal, 292
  of thigh, 261, 290–292
  of thorax, 398
  of upper limb, 76–78
  of wrist, 182–188
Vestibulocochlear nerve (CN VIII), 383
Vestibulospinal tract, 232
Vincula, 176
Viscera. *See* Abdominal viscera; Pelvic viscera
Visceral pericardium, 394–395
Visceral peritoneum, 407
Visceral pleura, 393
Vocal folds (cords), 377
Vomer, 357–358

W

Walls
  inner, 27
  outer, 27
Weight support, 351–353
White blood cells, 51, 51–52b
White columns, 40–41
White matter, 39–40, 361
Wrist (carpus), 57. *See also* Hand
  abduction of, 163f
  adduction of, 163f
  bones of, 169f
  extension of, 162f
  flexors at, 162f
  ligaments of, 171f
  movements of, 127f, 160–163
  muscle of, 174–175
  nerves of, 182–188
  surface anatomy of, 172–173, 182
  synovial sheaths of, 174–175

Wrist (carpus) *(Continued)*
    tendons of, 174–175
    vessels of, 182–188
Wrist joint, 130
    movements of, 5f
Wristdrop, 154–155b, 192f, 193
Wryneck, 373b

X
Xiphoid process, 389, 399, 413

Z
Zona orbicularis, 251–252
Zygapophyses, 207

Zygomatic arch, 386
Zygomatic bones, 357–358, 386
Zygomatic processes, 386
Zygomaticofacial nerves, 382
Zygomaticotemporal nerve, 382
Zygomaticus muscles, 365